CW00797841

MATERIA MEDICA PURA

MATERIA MEDICA PURA

By

Samuel Hahnemann

TRANSLATED FROM THE LATEST GERMAN EDITIONS BY

R. E. DUDGEON, M.D.

WITH ANNOTATIONS BY

RICHARD HUGHES, L.R.C.P.E.

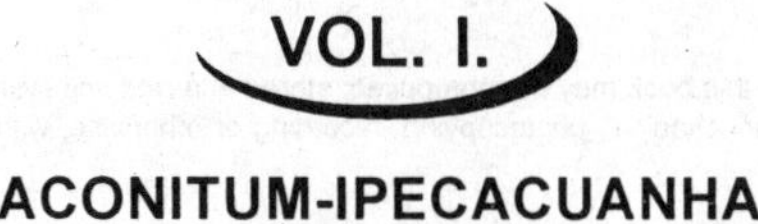

ACONITUM-IPECACUANHA

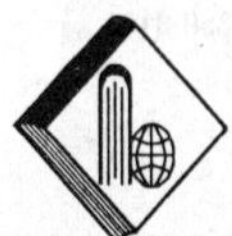

B. Jain Publishers (P) Ltd. (India)

An ISO 9001 : 2000 Certified Company

USA — EUROPE — INDIA

MATERIA MEDICA PURA

16th Impression: 2010

Published by Kuldeep Jain for

B. JAIN PUBLISHERS (P) LTD.

An ISO 9001 : 2000 Certified Company

1921/10, Chuna Mandi, Paharganj, New Delhi 110 055 (INDIA)

Tel.: 91-11-2358 0800, 2358 1100, 2358 1300, 2358 3100

Fax: 91-11-2358 0471 • *Email:* info@bjain.com

Website: **www.bjainbooks.com**

Printed in India by

J.J. Offset Printers

ISBN: 978-81-319-0215-8 (Complete set)

ISBN: 978-81-319-0216-5 (Volume I)

CONTENTS OF VOL I.

Publishers' Note to the First Indian Edition.

It would be a mere vain pretention to say anything by way of introduction to *Materia Medica Pura* by Hahnemann which occupies a magnificent place among the literary luminaries of the world.

For the first time this book happens to be published in India and we take pride in obtaining this laudable undertaking. In presenting this work of Hahnemann to the public a word or two about it may not be amiss here.

Materia Medica Pura was the maiden work of Hahnemann the Master of homœopathic philosophy and practice. The merit of this monumental work lies not so much in the prodigy of its illuminating contents as in its heralding a new epoch in the domain of treatment. The word *Pura* annexed to the title is significant and speaks a volume. It offers a challenge of purity to its counterpart of the traditional school. This challenge has remained unassailable for a century and it will remain so for all centuries to come.

Our best thanks are due to Messrs Homœopathic Publishing Co. of London for their kindly granting us the permission to publish this book.

A homœopathic teacher or, a student or, a practitioner—whatever he may be—can ill-afford to do without a copy of this book. It is indispensable to all of them as also to others who are the least interested about Homœopathy.

Publishers' Note to the First Indian Edition

It would be a mere vain pretention to say anything by way of introduction to *Materia Medica Pura* by Hahnemann which occupies a significant place among the literary luminaries of the world.

For the first time this book happens to be published in India and we take pride in executing this notable undertaking. In presenting this work of Hahnemann to the public, a word or two about it may not be amiss here.

Materia Medica Pura was the maiden work of Hahnemann in Materia Medica, [illegible] philosophy and practice. The merit of this monumental work lies not so much in the prolixity of its illuminating contents as in its heralding a new epoch in the domain of Medicine. The word *Pura* annexed to the title is significant and speaks volumes. It offers a challenge of purity to its counterpart of the traditional school. This challenge has remained unassailable for a century and will remain so for all centuries to come.

Our best thanks are due to Messrs Homoeopathic Publishing Co. of London for their kindly granting us the permission to publish this book.

A homoeopathic teacher or a student or a practitioner—whatever he may be—can ill afford to do without a copy of this book. It is indispensable to all of them as also to others who are the least interested about Homoeopathy.

TRANSLATOR'S PREFACE

THE *Materia Medica Pura* as left to us by HAHNEMANN consists of six volumes, two of which, viz. Vols. I and II, had reached a third edition, while the remainder did not get beyond the second.

The dates of the publication of these volumes are as follows :— Vol. I, 1830 ; Vol. II, 1833 ; Vols. III and IV, 1825 ; Vol. V, 1826 ; Vol. VI, 1827. In the earlier editions the pathogeneses of the various medicines are not arranged in the same way as they are in the latest. Thus, in the former, HAHNEMANN's own observations are put first and by themselves and separately numbered ; the symptoms observed by his disciples under his superintendence, and those derived from the work of other observers, being arranged together in a different list, and specially numbered.

In the third edition, to which only the first two volumes attained, the arrangement is different. Here all the symptoms of each medicine, whether observed by HAHNEMANN himself or his disciples, or taken from old-school authorities are combined in one schema and numbered continuously ; HAHNEMANN'S own observations being distinguished by having no name or sign attached, while those of his pupils are indicated by an abbreviation of the name of each appended to their respective observations. The authorities of the old school are named after the symptoms for which they are responsible.

Another peculiarity in the work as it has been left to us is, that the medicines are not arranged alphabetically. Each volume contains a varying number of medicines, arranged alphabetically according to their common German names, but there is no attempt to maintain the alphabetical arrangement in respect to the whole work.

In making a translation the work might be presented to the English reader exactly as we have it, *i. e.* each separate volume given with its own peculiar arrangement of symptoms, the medicines of each being only arranged alphabetically according to their English and Latin names. This would give six volumes of various sizes and with their contents differently arranged. It would reproduce the work as it exists in the German original, but it would, like that, be difficult to use as a book of reference ; and if the minor details of the German work were also preserved it would involve a considerable additional amount of printing without any advantage therefrom.

Though some were of opinion that the work should be presented to the English reader in the above form, it appeared to the translator that it would be paying but a poor compliment to HAHNEMANN to neglect to bring the volumes of the second edition into conformity with the perfected arrangement of those he brought out in a third.

Moreover, the translator thought that instead of publishing the work in six volumes of very unequal size, with no general alphabetical arrangement of the medicines, it would be altogether better, because more convenient to the reader and practitioner, and decidedly more artistic from a literary point of view, to arrange the medicines throughout the work alphabetically, to arrange the symptoms on the plan adopted in the latest edition, and to give out the work in two handsome volumes of equal size. Such a proceeding would involve a considerable addition to the translator's labour, but this would be fully compensated by the greater utility and the literary homogeneity of the work.

The plan has consequently been adopted, and the essays distributed throughout the original volumes have been divided between the two volumes of the translation, so as to form appropriate prefaces to each.

The alteration introduced by HAHNEMANN in his latest edition with regard to the indication of the name of the prover by an abbreviation, in place of giving the whole name, has been extended to all the medicines in this translation. These abbreviations are printed in italics. HAHNEMANN's abbreviations of his provers' names are not always the same, but uniformity has been maintained in this translation. The names of old-school authorities for symptoms are printed in small capitals, so that the student and casual reader can see at a glance whether the symptom is one produced by an intentional proving, or is the result of the generally accidental poisoning or over-dose of an old-school observer. As in the original, the symptoms with no name or abbreviations appended are those observed by HAHNEMANN himself.

Subjoined is a list of HAHNEMANN's fellow provers, the abbreviations of their names employed in this work, and the medicines proved by each.

ADAM, DR.…………	*Ad.* (cb-a., cb-v.)
AHNER, G. A.…………	*Ar.* (aco., cap., cin., men.)
ANTON, C. CHR.…………	*An.* (chi.)
BÆHR, AUG.…………	*Bhr.* (ars., bel., chi., coc.)
BECHER, HULD.…………	*Bch.* (chl., chi., dig., led., ph-x., spi., squ., ver.)
CASPARI, DR.…………	*Cas.* (cb-v.)
CLAUSS, W.…………	*Css.* (chi.)
CUBITZ, C. A.…………	*Ctz.* (dul., opi., stp.)
FLAMING, JOH. GTFD.…………	*Fg.* (coc., hyo., nx-v.)
FRANZ, CARL …………	*Fz.* (ang., arg., arn., asr., aur., ca-a., cam., can., chi., con., cyc., dig., hyo., led., mt-n., mt-s., man., men., oln., ph-x., rhs., rut., sam., spi., stn., stp., str., trx., thu., ver.)
GERSDORFF, FR. VON…………	*Gff.* (amb., cb-v.)
GROSS, W. …………	*Gss.*. (aco., ang., arg., arn., ars., aur., bel., can., chl., chi., coc., dul., dig., fer., ign., man., men., msc., oln., ph-x., rhe., rut., sam., opi., stn., stp., thu., vrb.)
GUNTHER,—…………	*Gth.* (mt-n.)
GUTMANN, SALOMO …………	*Gn.* (col., dro., men., mer., mu-x., oln., opi., ph-x., spi., spo., stp., str., trx.)
HAHNEMANN, FRIED.…………	*Fr. H—n.* (aco., arn., ars., aur.. bel., bry., can., cic., col., dro., eup., fer., hep., hyo., ign, mer., msc., nx-v., ph-x., pul., rhs., spo., str., sul., thu., ver.)

HARNISCH, ERNST..........	*Hsch.* (ang., chi., mt-n., mt-s.)
HARTLAUB, C..............	*Hb.* (see Trinks and Hartlaub.)
HARTMANN, FRANZ.........	*Htn.* (bel., bis., ca-a., chl., chi., gui., hel., mt-n., men., mer., mu-x , oln., ph-x., rut., sam., sar., spi., spo., squ., stn., stp., thu., vrb.)
HARTUNG, J. C........	*Htg.* (bel., cap., chi., cyc.)
HAYNEL, ADOLPH. FR.....	*Hnl.* (arg., coc., man., men , mu-x., spo., stn., stp., thu.)
HEMPEL, GUST..............	*Hl.* (aur., can., mt-n., thu.)
HEMPEL, H....................	*Hpl.* (bel.)
HERRMANN, CHR. TH.......	*Hrr.* (arg., aur., bel., bry., bis., cam., chl., chi., cyc., led., ph-x., rut., sar., spi., stn., stp.)
HORNBURG, CHR. G.........	*Hbg.* (aco., arn., ars., asr., bel., bry., chi., cic., coc., col., dig., hel., man., men., mer., pul., rhe., rhs., rut., spi., spo., squ., stp.)
HUGO,—........................	*Ho.* (can.)
KUMMER, ERNST............	*Kr.* (arn., bel., hel., mt-s., spi., stp., trx.)
LANGHAMMER, CHR. FR..	*Lr* (ang., arg., arn., ars., aur., bel., bis., ca-a., chl., chi., cic., cin., coc., col., con., cyc., dig., dro., eup., gui., hel., hyo., ipc., led., mt-n., man., men., mer., mu-x., oln., ph-x., rut., sam., spi., spo., stn., stp., trx., thu., vrb.)
LEHMANN, CHR. F. G.......	*Lhm.* (chi., rhs.)
LEHMANN, J. G..............	*Ln.* (bel., chi., dig., ipc., spo.)
MEYER, F......................	*Myr.* (ang., arg., ars., chl., chi., dig., ph-x., spi.)
MICHLEP, C....................	*Mch.* (ang., bry., chi., mt-n., pul., rhs.)
MOCKEL, A. F................	*Mkl.* (bel., men.)
MOSSDORF, THEOD..........	*Mss.* (ang., cap., hel., squ., vrb.)
MULLER,—......................	*Mr.* (dul.)
NENNING, CAJ................	*Ng.* (dul.)
ROSAZEWSKY,—..............	*Rz.* (fer., trx.)
RUCKERT, E. FERD..........	*Rkt.* (aco., bry., dig., dul., hel., pul., rhe., rhs.)
RUCKERT, LEOP. E.... ...	*L. Rkt.* (asr., bel., cin., col., man.)
RUMMEL, F.....................	*Rl.* (mer.)
SCHONIKE,—.......	*Sche.* (opi.)
SCHRODER,—..................	*Sr.* (rhs.)
STAPF, ERNST..........	*Stf.* (aco., arn., ars., asr., bel., bry., cam., can., cha., chi., cin., col., dig., dul., hel., hep., hyo., ipc., mt-s., man., mer., msc., mu-x., opi., ph-x., pul., rhs., rut., spi.,spo.,squ.,stp.)
TEUTHORN, J. CHR. DAV.	*Trn.* (chl., chi., dig., gui., led., man., men., ph-x., rhe., sar., squ., stp., thu., ver.)
TRINKS and HARTLAUB...	*Ts. Hb.* or *Hb. Ts.* (can., coc., dul., ign., rhs.)
URBAN, F. C..................	*Ur.* (man.)
WAGNER, GUST..............	*Wr.* (chi., dul., spo., thu.)
WAHLE, WILH................	*We.* (aco., can., coc., dul., man., nx-v.)
WALTHER FR..................	*Wth.* (chl., chi., led., spi., squ., sul.)
WENZEL, JUL..................	*Wx.* (man.)
WISLICENUS, W. E........	*Ws.* (ang., arg., arn., aur., bel., ca-a., cam., cap., chi., con., dro., eup., hel., hyo., men., mu-x., ph-x., rut., sam., spi., spo., squ., stn., thu.)

Of these provers ADAM was a Russian physician, VON GERSDORFF a nobleman residing in Eisenach, NENNING a surgeon who furnished many of the symptoms for the *Materia Medica* of HARTLAUB and TRINKS, from whose work HAHNEMANN took some symptoms, indicated by the abbreviation of their names, *Hb.*, *Ts.*, either singly or conjointly.

The remainder are more properly HAHNEMANN's own disciples, who furnished him with a written statement of the symptoms they observed, on which HAHNEMANN examined them, carefully going over all the symptoms, and correcting or altering them so as to make them, as far as possible, the exact sensation or pain observed with all its conditions and concomitants. STAPF, who resided at Naumburg, transmitted to HAHNEMANN the symptoms he observed, in a letter, and accordingly in the older editions we find after STAPF's name, "in einem Briefe," in place of the expression used after the name of those whose writings HAHNEMANN could examine their authors on—"in einem Aufsatze."

Most if not all of these provers were medical men, many of them well-known as eminent practitioners of homœopathy, and some distinguished by their valuable contributions to homœopathic literature.

Many of the symptoms have the time of the occurrence after taking the medicine. This is indicated by contractions between brackets. Here "m." means minutes, "h." hours, and "d." days.

This is not the first English translation of HAHNEMANN'S *Materia Medica Pura*. In 1846 Dr. HEMPEL published a translation. But, as Dr. HUGHES* has pointed out, HEMPEL'S translation is extremely imperfect. He has employed the third edition of the first volume, but the second edition of all the other volumes. He has omitted all names of authorities for the symptoms, which are not in separate paragraphs. His arrangement of the symptoms is sometimes, but not always, the same as HAHNEMANN'S and he has not attempted uniformity of arrangement. Several of HAHNEMANN'S medicines are omitted—as many as eighteen indeed. But not only are the entire pathogeneses of all these medicines omitted, many omissions of symptoms are made from the pathogeneses given. Mis-translations, curtailments, and omissions, are also frequent in the prefaces and notes. In short, HEMPEL'S translation is altogether very imperfect and gives the reader a very inadequate idea of the original work.

Dr. QUIN commenced a translation of the Opus Magnum of HAHNEMANN. The first volume, indeed, was completed and printed, but unfortunately the whole impression was destroyed by a fire at the printer's. The only copy saved is in the library of the British Homœopathic Society. It has no preface or introduction by the translator, nor even a title page, so we cannot for certain know his intentions with regard to the whole translation. This first volume is translated from the second edition, but the medicines it contains do not altogether correspond with those in the original. Thus, *mercurius* is omitted, but *asarum*, *chamomilla*, *cyclamen*, *pulsatilla*, *squilla*, *stramonium*, and *veratrum*, which are not in the first volume of the original, are inserted. The arrangement of the symptoms is not that of HAHNEMANN in either his second or third editions. Dr. QUIN puts together all the symptoms of HAHNEMANN and his disciples and arranges in a separate list those obtained from old-school authorities. The translation is, as might be expected from Dr. QUIN'S familiarity with the German language, fairly good. But the work, even if it had been completed as Dr. QUIN designed, would not have presented the reader with the actual *Materia Medica* of HAHNEMANN; so our regret at the interruption of the work is tempered by this consideration.

* *On the Sources of the Homœopathic Materia Medica*. Turner. London, 1877.

The present is the first attempt to give a faithful and complete English translation of the latest editions of the work. The translator must here express his obligations to his collaborator, Dr. HUGHES, for the careful revision of the proof sheets and for numerous suggestions of improved versions of the original, whereby both the faithfulness and the readableness of the translation have been greatly improved. (It is, of course, impossible to render exactly into English the expressions peculiar to the German language, or to give an exact translation of every word. All the translator can do is to give the English equivalents for German phrases where such exist, or to give the English expressions that most nearly correspond with the German originals.) This he has endeavoured to do, and he trusts he has succeeded. But he is fully aware that there are certain German words and phrases used by HAHNEMANN for which we have no precise English equivalent. In some respects German is richer than English, and so one English word has to do duty for several German analogues. On the other hand, English is in some respect richer than German, for two totally different things are sometimes expressed by one word only, and the translator has to take great care that in his translation he gives the English word for the thing intended by the original. For example, the German *Hals* is used for both *throat* and *neck* ; *Brust* is either *chest* or *mamma* ; *Fuss* is sometimes used to denote the *foot*, sometimes the *leg* up to the knee, and sometimes the whole lower extremity ; *Schenkel* is sometimes *thigh*, sometimes *leg*, and occasionally the whole lower limb ; *Schooss* is sometimes the *groin*, sometimes the *iliac region*, occasionally the whole *hypogastrium* : *Gesicht* is sometimes *sight*, sometimes *face*. Great care is required to determine in what sense these different words are used by HAHNEMANN and his fellow-provers. *Druckend* must sometimes be translated *pressive* sometimes *aching*, and it is not always easy to determine which English equivalent should be used ; no hard and fast rule can be adopted, and the translator must determine from the context, or sometimes from his "inner consciousness," which translation should be employed. As a rule *druckend* followed by *auf* or *an* must mean *pressive* whereas if followed by *in* it probably means *aching* ; but to this rule there are exceptions, and the reader must credit the translator with the possession of reasons for the particular translation he has adopted.

R. E. DUDGEON.

Dr. Dudgeon has wished me to say a few words for myself on the special matter in which I have had the pleasure of assisting him in this undertaking of his. I refer to Hahnemann's quotations from authors. These are absent from few of his pathogenesis, and in many are very numerous ; so as to number in the whole *Materia Medica Pura* upwards of 4000. It is obvious that no new edition of a work so full of citations can be satisfactory, which does not examine these in their originals for purposes of verification and (if necessary) of correction. More especially this is so when a translation has to be made, and where the author himself has rendered his cited matter into his own tongue. That one should take the German symptoms by which Hahnemann has represented the Latin, French and English authors from whom he has borrowed, and simply re-translate them, would be running a great risk of missing their true meaning.

Were it only, therefore, to make this translation of the *Materia Medica Pura* as accurate as possible, it would be desirable that all the citations contained in the work should be verified from their original sources, and rendered (or, if English, reproduced) from thence. But there is something more. It often adds to the value of a symptom that we should know the subject and circumstances of its occurrence, the dose by which it was produced, and so forth. Hahnemann rarely gives such information as to the effects of drugs he gathers from authors, but confines himself to presenting them in the same unconnected way as that which he follows in respect of his own and his fellow provers' symptoms. We long for the day-books of the experiments which gave us these : in the case of the cited symptoms we have them. From the original records we can illuminate the isolated phenomena and sensations presented to us, so as to show their occasion, their order, and their terminations.

Yet again,—examination of the sources of the symptoms in question shows that they are of very unequal value. Sometimes they are records of poisonings, when they are of unquestionable value. Sometimes they are the mere statements of systematic writers on Materia Medica, which must be taken *quantum valeant.* Very often, however, they are narratives of cases of disease treated by the drug in question, and the symptoms are such as were supposed, either by the observer or by the citer, to have resulted from (so to speak) the *obiter facta* of the medicine. It is obvious that great discrimination is needed here ; and it is the unanimous judgment of those who have enquired into the matter that Hahnemann has hardly exercised it. In my *Sources of the Homœopathic Materia Medica* (p. 16—18), I have given many instances of the wholesale way in which he has adopted symptoms from these records ; and the facts are such that, without the knowledge which enables us to judge for ourselves, we could not safely accept any symptoms so derived as genuine.

For estimation, then, as well as for verification and illumination, it is necessary to trace Hahnemann's cited symptoms to their originals. The work has been done from time to time for individual medicines,—as by Frank and Wurmb for Arsenic, by Gerstel for Aconite, by Watzke for Colocynth, by Roth for Dulcamara and others, by Langheinz for Opium, Moschus, and Cannabis. As a co-labourer with Dr. Allen in his *Encyclopædia,* I made it my task to complete these investigations and extend them to every drug in the *Materia Medica Pura* and the *Chronic Diseases.* The results are embodied in that work, after the manner suitable to it ; but remain available for such a reproduction of Hahnemann's own pathogeneses as Dr. Dudgeon is giving us. Strictly speaking, it is verification only for which they should be applied here; but it has seemed a pity that their further possibilities should not also be utilised, and I have accordingly, with the translator's approbation, extended their employment in the other directions I have indicated. On the first mention of any authority in each pathogenesis I have stated the nature of his observations; and to each symptom that has required it I have appended such explanations and corrections as might be necessary to set it forth in its full meaning and value. All this matter will be found in the notes at the bottom of the pages, designated by the small figures, [1], [2], &c., and divided by a line from Hahnemann's own annotations, which have the usual *, †, &c. At first, when any corrections were required, I made these in the text, so that any deviations to be found from Hahnemann's presentation of his cited symptoms must be charged to my responsibility. Subsequently, however, I thought it better to leave Dr. Dudgeon to render the text as it stood, and to make my emendations in the footnotes.

I am very glad to have been able to contribute this mite to the important task of giving to his English-speaking disciples the *Materia Medica* of the Master of our school.

R. HUGHES.

AUTHOR'S PREFACE.[1]

I AM not going to write a criticism of the ordinary Materia Medica, else I would lay before the reader a detailed account of the futile endeavours hitherto made to determine the powers of medicines from their colour, taste, and smell. I would show how chemistry has been applied to, in order by wet and dry distillation to extract from medicinal substances phlegma, ethereal oils, empyreumatic acids and oils, volatile salts, and from the residuary *caput mortuum* fixed salts and earths *(all nearly identical with one another).* I would set forth the methods adopted by the latest chemical science of obtaining extracts to be afterwards inspissated by dissolving their soluble parts in various fluids. I would describe the mode of separating from them resin, gum, gluten, starch, wax, albumen, salts and earths, acids and alkaloids, by means of various reagents; and I would tell how to convert them into gases. It is well known that not a single one of the innumerable medicinal substances, in spite of all these technical torturings, could be brought to reveal what sort of healing power it was possessed of. Certainly the material substances extracted from them were not the spirit animating every single substance which enables it to cure certain morbid stages. This spirit cannot be laid hold of by the hands; it can only be recognised by its effects on the living body.

The day of the true knowledge of medicines and of the true healing art will dawn when men cease to act so unnaturally as to give drugs to which some purely imaginary virtues have been ascribed, or which have been merely vaguely recommended, and of whose real qualities they are *utterly* ignorant; and which they give mixed up together in all sorts of combinations. With these delectable mixtures* a hap-hazard treatment is pursued, not of cases of disease that have been carefully investigated as to their special signs and symptoms, but of purely artificial forms and names of diseases invented by pathology. By this method no experience whatever can be gained of the helpful or hurtful

* The ordinary medical world, as long as they know no better, may go on sending their multiform complex prescriptions to be made up at the chemist's. In order to do this they do not require to know anything about the sphere of action or the special properties of each ingredient. Moreover, even should we know perfectly the powers of drugs when given singly, we can have no idea what they will do when given mixed up together.

This they call *treating* [curiren], and they may well continue to call it so until a

1 From vol. i, 3rd edit., 1830.

qualities of each medicinal ingredient of the mixture, nor can any knowledge be obtained of the curative properties of each individual drug.

The day of the true knowledge of medicines and of the true healing art will dawn when physicians shall trust the cure of complete cases of disease to a single medicinal substance, and when, regardless of traditional systems, they will employ for the extinction and cure of a case of disease, whose symptoms they have investigated, one single medicinal substance whose positive effects they have ascertained, which can show among these effects a group of symptoms very similar to those presented by the case of disease.

Among the observations from extraneous sources in the following pages are some which were observed in patients ; but as these were the subjects of chronic disease whose morbid symptoms were well known and were not confounded with the new effects caused by the medicine taken—at least GREDING seems to have carefully avoided doing so—these observations are not altogether valueless ; at all events, they serve occasionally to confirm similar or identical symptoms that may appear in pure experiments on the healthy.

As regards my own experiments and those of my disciples every possible care was taken to insure their purity, in order that the true powers of each medicinal substance might be clearly expressed in the observed effects. They were performed on persons as healthy as possible, and under regulated external conditions as nearly as possible alike.

But if during the experiment some extraordinary circumstance from without happened which might even be supposed to be capable of altering the result—for example, a shock, vexation, a fright, an external injury of considerable severity, dissipation or over-indulgence in something or other, or any other circumstances of importance—from that time no symptom that occurred in the experiment was registered ; they were all rejected, so that the observation should contain nought that had a suspicion of impurity about it.

If some little circumstance happened during the experiment, which could hardly be expected to interfere with the effects of the medicinal action, the symptoms subsequently noticed were inclosed within brackets as not certainly pure.

With respect to the *duration of action* ascribed to each medicinal substance, which I endeavoured to determine by repeated experiment, I should state that it was only learned from experiments on the healthiest possible persons. In diseases, according as they are more or

spirit of improvement wakes up within them impelling them to begin *curing* [heilen], which can only be done with simple medicinal substances.

It is only of such substances that the pure effects can be ascertained whereby we may be able to say beforehand whether this one or the other may be of use in a given case.

But what conscientious man would consent to work away at hap-hazard on a sick person hovering between life and death with tools that possess powers to hurt and destroy, without an accurate knowledge of their powers ?

No carpenter would work upon his wood with tools whose uses he was ignorant of. He knows every one of them perfectly, and hence he knows when to use the one and when the other, in order to effect *with certainty* what he intends to do ; and it is only wood he works upon, and he is but a carpenter !

less acute, more or less chronic, the duration of action of the medicine is much shorter or much longer than here stated, but can never be rightly determined if the medicine be given in a large dose or in unsuitable cases. In both these instances the duration of its action will be much shortened, for the medicine goes off, as it were, in the evacuations it causes (such as epistaxis and other hæmorrhages, catarrh, diuresis, diarrhœa, vomiting, or perspiration), and thus soon exhausts its energy. The living body spits it out quickly, so to speak, just as it often does with the miasm of infectious diseases, where it weakens the noxious agent and partly rejects it also by vomiting, diarrhœa, hæmorrhages, catarrh, convulsions, salivation, perspiration, and such-like processes and evacuations. Hence it happens that, in the ordinary practice, no one knows either the peculiar effects or the duration of action of, *e. g.* tartar emetic or of jalap, because these drugs are only given in doses so large that they excite the organism to cast them quickly out. Sometimes the organism does not do this; sometimes, that is to say, the remedy given to provoke violent evacuation is not evacuated, in which case it is vulgarly said to *stick*. When this happens there occur pure symptoms often of a very important and enduring character (the peculiar medicinal action). But it is very seldom that they have been thought worth observing and recording.

The vomiting caused by two to three grains of tartar emetic, or by twenty grains of ipecacuanha, the purging produced by thirty grains of jalap, and the perspiration excited by an infusion of a handful of elder-flowers, are not so much peculiar effects of these substances as an effort of the organism to destroy with all possible speed the peculiar medicinal effects of these drugs.

Hence the very small doses prescribed by homœopathy produce the uncommon effect they do just because they are not so large as to render it necessary for the organism to get rid of them by the revolutionary processes of evacuations. And yet these very small doses excite the system to evacuations (which shorten their duration of action) in cases of disease where the remedy has been unsuitably and not accurately homœopathically chosen.

In the *Organon of Medicine* I have taught this truth, that dynamically acting medicines extinguish diseases only in accordance with the similarity of their symptoms. He who has understood this will perceive that if a work on materia medica can reveal the precise qualities of medicines, it must be one from which all mere assumption and empty speculation about the reputed qualities of drugs are excluded, and which only records what medicines express concerning their true mode of action in the symptoms they produce in the human body. Hence the practitioner will rejoice to find here a way in which he can remove the maladies of his fellow-creatures surely, rapidly, and permanently, and procure them the blessing of health with much greater certainty.

This is not the place to give instruction as to how to select for the group of symptoms of a particular case of disease a remedy which presents in its pure effects a very similar group of peculiar symptoms. The *Organon* contains full instructions on this point, together with general directions on the subject of the doses required in homœopathy.

The smallest possible quantity of medicine in potentized development is sufficient for this purpose.

I have arranged the symptoms of the more perfectly observed medicines in a certain order, whereby the search for the desired medicinal symptom will now be facilitated. In the complex symptoms, however, there occur not unfrequently some to which, if I had had time, I would have added parallel citations referring them to their proper position.

The usual order of the symptoms is as follows:

Vertigo,
Confusion,
Deficient mental power,
Loss of memory,[1]
Headache, internal, external,
Forehead, hair,
Face in general (vultus) } or { visus,
Eyes and sight (visus) } or { vultus,
Ears, hearing (maxillary joint),
Nose, smell,
Lips,
Chin,
Lower jaw (submaxillary glands),
Teeth,
Tongue (impediments to speech),
Saliva,
Internal throat,
Fauces, œsophagus,
Taste,
Eructation, heartburn, hiccup,
Nausea, vomiting,
Desire for food and drink,* hunger,
Scrobiculus cordis (pit of stomach), stomach,
Abdomen, epigastrium, hepatic region, hypochondria,
Hypogastrium,
Lumbar region,†
Groin, inguinal region,
Rectum, anus, perinæum,
Alvine evacuation,
Urine, bladder, urethra,
Genital organs,
Sexual desire,
Sexual power, emission of semen,
Menstrual flux, leucorrhœa,

* Thirst sometimes comes after hiccup, and sometimes also among the febrile symptoms.

† Sometimes placed among the symptoms of the back and lumbar vertebræ.

1 This order is not always preserved; the mental symptoms are sometimes placed at the end of the list of symptoms. The inconvenience of separating mental and emotional symptoms is tacitly acknowledged by Hahnemann, as he places them together in the *Chronic Diseases*.

Sneezing, coryza, catarrh, hoarseness,
Cough,
Breathing,
Chest,
Heart's movements,
Sacral region, lumbar vertebræ,
Back,
Scapulæ,
Nape,
External throat*
Shoulders (axillæ),
Arms, hands,
Hips, pelvis,
Buttocks,
Thighs, legs, feet,
General corporeal sufferings and cutaneous affections,
Sufferings from open air,
Exhalation, temperature of the body, disposition to catch cold, sprains, paroxysms,
Convulsions, paralysis, weakness, fainting,
Yawning, sleepiness, slumber, sleep, nocturnal ailments, dreams,
Fever, chill, heat, perspiration,
Anxiety, palpitation of heart,† restlessness, trembling,‡
Disturbances of the disposition, affections of the mind.

SAMUEL HAHNEMANN.

KOTHEN ; *January, 1830.*

* The external throat sometimes also comes after lower jaw.

† Palpitation unattended by anxiety comes under chest symptoms.

‡ Restlessness and trembling of a merely corporeal character, in which the disposition does not participate, generally comes among the symptoms of the extremities or of the body generally.

SPIRIT OF THE HOMŒOPATHIC MEDICAL DOCTRINE *

It is impossible to devine the internal essential nature of diseases and the changes they effect in the hidden parts of the body, and it is absurd to frame a system of treatment on such hypothetical surmises and assumptions : it is impossible to divine the medicinal properties of remedies from any chemical hypotheses or from their smell, colour, or taste, and it is absurd to attempt, from such hypothetical surmises and assumptions, to apply to the treatment of diseases these substances, which are so hurtful when wrongly administered. And even were such practice ever so customary and ever so generally in use, were it even the *only one in vogue* for thousands of years, it would nevertheless continue to be a senseless and pernicious practice to found on empty surmises our idea of the morbid condition of the interior, and to attempt to combat this with equally imaginary properties of medicines.

Appreciable, distinctly appreciable to our senses must that be, which is to be removed in each disease in order to transform it into health, and right clearly must each remedy express what it can positively cure, if medical art is to cease to be a wanton game of hazard with human life, and to commence to be the sure deliverer from diseases.

I shall show what there is undeniably curable in diseases, and how the curative properties of medicines are to be distinctly perceived and employed for curative purposes.

*   *   *

What life is can only be known empirically from its phenomena and manifestations, but no conception of it can be formed by any metaphysical speculations *a priori* ; what life is, in its actual essential nature, can never be ascertained or even guessed at, by mortals.

To the explanation of human life, as also its two-fold conditions, health and disease, the principles by which we explain other phenomena are quite inapplicable. With nought in the world can we compare it save with itself alone ; neither with a piece of clock-work,

* This essay appeared in a journal twenty years ago, in those momentous days (March, 1813) when the Germans had no leisure to read and still less to reflect upon scientific matters. The consequence of this was that these words were not listened to. It may now have more chance of being perused, particularly in its present less imperfect form. [From vol. ii, 3rd edition, 1833.]

nor with a hydraulic machine, nor with chemical processes, nor with decompositions and recompositions of gases, nor yet with a galvanic battery, in short with nothing destitute of life. Human life is *in no respect* regulated by purely physical laws, which only obtain among inorganic substances. The material substances of which the human organism is composed no longer follow, in this vital combination, the laws to which material substances in the inanimate condition are subject; they are regulated by the laws peculiar to vitality alone, they are themselves animated and vitalized just as the whole system is animated and vitalized. Here a nameless fundamental power reigns omnipotent, which abrogates all the tendency of the component parts of the body to obey the laws of gravitation, of momentum, of the *vis inertiæ*, of fermentation, of putrefaction, &c., and brings them under the wonderful laws of life alone,—in other words, maintains them in the condition of *sensibility* and *activity* necessary to the preservation of the living whole, a condition almost spiritually dynamic.

Now, as the condition of the organism and its health depend solely on the health of the life which animates it, in like manner it follows that the altered health, which we term disease, consists in a condition altered originally only in its vital sensibilities and functions, irrespective of all chemical or mechanical considerations; in short it must consist in a dynamically altered condition, a changed mode of being, whereby a change in the properties of the material component parts of the body is afterwards effected, which is a necessary consequence of the morbidly altered condition of the living whole in every individual case.

Moreover, the influence of morbific injurious agencies, which for the most part excite from without the various maladies in us, is generally so invisible and so immaterial,* that it is impossible that it can *immediately* either mechanically disturb or derange the component parts of our body in their form and substance, or infuse any pernicious acrid fluid into our blood-vessels whereby the mass of our humours can be chemically altered and depraved—an inadmissible, quite unprovable, gross invention of mechanical minds. The exciting causes of disease rather act by means of their essential properties on the state of our life (on our health), only in a dynamic, very similar to a spiritual manner; and inasmuch as they first derange the organs of the higher rank and of the vital force, there occurs from this state of derangement, from this dynamic alteration of the living whole, an altered sensation (uneasiness, pains) and an altered activity (abnormal functions) of each individual organ and of all of them collectively, whereby there must also of necessity secondarily occur alteration of the juices in our vessels and secretion of abnormal matters, the inevitable consequence of the altered vital character, which now differs from the healthy state.

These abnormal matters that show themselves in diseases are consequently merely products of the disease itself, which, as long as the malady retains its present character, must of necessity be secreted, and

* With the exception of a few surgical affections and the disagreeable effects produced by indigestible foreign substances, which sometimes find their way into the intestinal canal.

thus constitute a portion of the morbid signs (symptoms); they are merely effects, and therefore manifestations of the existing internal ill-health, and they do certainly not react (although they often contain the infecting principle for other, healthy individuals) upon the diseased body that produced them, as disease-exciting or maintaining substances, that is, as material morbific causes,* just as a person cannot infect other parts of his own body at the same time with the virus from his own chancre or with the gonorrhœal matter from his own urethra, or increase his disease therewith, or as a viper cannot inflict on itself a fatal bite with its own poison.

Hence it is obvious that diseases excited by the dynamic and virtual influence of morbific injurious agents can be originally only dynamical derangements (caused almost solely by a spiritual process) of the vital character of our organism.

We readily perceive that these dynamic derangements of the vital character of our organism which we term diseases, since they are nothing else than altered sensations and functions, can also express themselves by nothing but by an aggregate of symptoms, and only as such are they cognisable to our observing powers.

Now, as in a profession of such importance to human life as medicine is, nothing but the state of the diseased body plainly cognisable by our perceptive faculties can be recognised as the object to be cured, and ought to guide our steps (to choose conjectures and undemonstrable hypotheses as our guide here would be dangerous folly, nay crime and treason against humanity), it follows, that since diseases, as dynamic derangements of the vital character, express themselves *solely* by alterations of the sensations and functions of our organism, that is, *solely* by an aggregate of cognisable symptoms, this alone can be the object of treatment in every case of disease. *For on the removal of all morbid symptoms nothing remains but health.*

Now, because diseases are only dynamic derangements of our health and vital character, they cannot be removed by man otherwise than by means of agents and powers which also are capable of producing dynamical derangements of the human health, that is to say, diseases are cured virtually and dynamically by medicinss.†

These active substances and powers (medicines) which we have at

---

* Hence by clearing away and mechanically removing these abnormal matters, acridities and morbid organisations, their source, the disease itself, can just as litte be cured as a coryza can be shortened or cured by blowing the nose frequently, and as thoroughly as possible; it lasts not a day longer than its proper course, although the nose should not be cleansed by blowing it at all.

† Not by means of the pretended solvent or mechanically dispersing, clearing-out, and expulsive powers of medicinal substances; not by means of a (blood-purifying, humour-correcting) power they possess of electively excreting fancied morbific principles; not by means of any antiseptic power they have (as is effected in dead, putrifying flesh); not by any chemical or physical action of any other imaginable sort, as happens in dead material things, as has hitherto been falsely imagined and dreamt by the various medical schools.

The more modern schools have indeed begun in some degree to regard diseases as dynamic derangements, and their intention, too, is to remove them in some sort of dynamical way by medicines, but inasmuch as they fail to perceive that the sensible, irritable, and reproductive activity of life is *in modo et qualitate* susceptible of our service effect the cure of diseases by means of the same dynamic power of altering the actual state of health, by means of the same power of deranging the vital character of our organism in respect of its sensations and functions, by which they are able to affect also the healthy individual, to produce in him dynamic changes and certain morbid symptoms, the knowledge of which, as we shall see, affords us the most trustworthy information concerning the morbid states that can be most certainly cured by each particular medicine. Hence nothing in the world can accomplish a cure, no substance, no power can effect a change in the human organism of such a character as that the disease shall yield to it, except an agent capable of absolutely (dynamically) deranging the human health, consequently also of morbidly altering its healthy state.*

On the other hand, however, there is also no agent, no power in nature capable of morbidly affecting the healthy individual, which does not at the same time possess the faculty of curing certain morbid states.

Now, as the power of curing diseases, as also of morbidly affecting the healthy, is met with in inseparable combination in all medicines, and as both these properties evidently spring from one and the same source, namely, from their power of dynamically deranging human health, and as it is hence impossible that they can act according to a different inherent natural law in the sick to that according to which they act on the healthy; it follows that it must be the same power of the medicine that cures the disease in the sick as produces the morbid symptoms in the healthy.†

Hence also we shall find that the curative power of medicines, and that which each of them is able to effect in diseases, expresses itself in no other mode in the world so surely and palpably, and cannot be ascertained by us by any purer and more perfect manner than by the morbid phenomena and symptoms (the kinds of artificial diseases) which the medicines develop in healthy individuals. For if we only have before us records of the peculiar (artificial) morbid symptoms produced by the various medicines on healthy individuals, we only require a series of pure experiments to decide what medicinal symptoms will always rapidly and permanently cure and remove certain symptoms of disease, in order to know, in every case beforehand, which of all the different medicines known and thoroughly tested as to their peculiar symptoms must be the most certain remedy in every case of disease.‡

---

as infinity of changes, and as they do not regard the innumerable varieties of morbid signs (that infinity of internal alterations only cognisable by us in their reflex) for what they actually are, to wit, the only undeceptive object for treatment; but as they only hypothetically recognise an abnormal increase and decrease of their dimensions *quoad quantitatem*, and *in an equally arbitrary manner* confide to the medicines they employ the task of changing to the normal state this one-sided increase and decrease, and thereby curing them; they thus have in their mind nothing but false ideas, both of the object to be cured and of the properties of the medicine.

* Consequently no substanc, for example, that is purely nutritious.

† The different result in these two cases is owing solely to the difference of the object that has to be altered.

‡ Simple, true, and natural as this maxim is, so much so that one would have imagined it would long since have been adopted as the rule for ascertaining the curative

If then we ask experience what artificial diseases (observed to be produced by medicines) can be beneficially employed against certain natural morbid states; if we ask it whether the change to health (cure) may be expected to ensue most certainly and in the most permanent manner :

1. by the use of such medicines as are capable of producing in the healthy body a *different* (alloeopathic) affection from that exhibited by the disease to be cured.

2. or by the employment of such as are capable of exciting in the healthy individual an *opposite* (enantiopathic, antipathic) state to that of the case to be cured.

3. or by the administration of such medicines as can cause a *similar* (homœopathic) state to the natural disease before us (for these are the

---

powers of drugs, it is yet a fact that nothing the least like it has hitherto been thought of. During the several thousands of years over which history extends, no one fell upon this natural method of first ascertaining the curative powers of medicines before giving them in diseases. In all ages down to the present times it was imagined that the curative powers of medicines could be learned in no other way than from the result of their employment in diseases themselves *(ab usu in morbis)*; it was sought to learn them from those cases where a certain medicine (more frequently a combination of various medicines) had been found serviceable in a particular case of disease. But even from the efficacious result of one single medicine given in a case of disease accurately described (which but rarely happened), we never can know the case in which that medicine would again prove serviceable, because (with the exception of diseases caused by miasms of a fixed character, as smallpox, measles, syphilis, itch, &c, and those arising from various injurious agencies that always remain the same, as *rheumatic gout*, &c.), all other cases of disease are mere individualities, that is to say, all present themselves in nature with different combinations of symptsms, have never before occurred, and can never again occur in exactly the same manner; consequently, because a medicine has cured one case we cannot thence infer that it will cure another (different) case. The forced arrangement of these cases of disease (which nature in her wisdom produces in endless variety) under certain nosological heads, as is arbitrarily done by pathology, is an unreal human performance, which leads to constant fallacies and to the confounding together of very different states.

Equally misleading and untrustworthy, although in all ages universally practised, is the determination of the general (curative) actions of medicines from special effects in diseases, where in the materia medica—when, for example, in some cases of disease *during* the use of a medicine (generally mixed up with others) there sometimes occurred a more copious secretion of urine or perspiration, the catamenia came on, convulsions ceased, there occurred a kind of sleep, expectoration, &c.—the medicine (to which the honour was attributed more than to the others in the mixture) was instantly elevated to the rank of a diuretic, a diaphoretic, an emmenagogue, an antispasmodic, a soporific an expectorant, and thereby not only was a *fallacium causæ* committed by confounding the word *during* with *by*, but quite a false conclusion was drawn, *a particulari ad universale*, in opposition to all the laws of reason; indeed the conditional was made unconditional. For a substance that does not in every case of disease promote urine and perspiration, that does not in every instance bring on the catamenia and sleep, that does not subdue all convulsions, and cause every cough to come to expectoration, cannot be said by a person of sound reason to be unconditionally and absolutely diuretic, diaphoretic, emmenagogue, soporific, antispasmodic, and expectorant! And yet this is what the ordinary materia medica does. Indeed it is impossible that in the complex phenomena of our health, in the multifarious combinations of different symptoms presented by the innumerable varieties of human diseases, the employment of a remedy can exhibit its pure, original medicinal effect, and exactly what we can expect it to do for derangements of our health. These can only be shown by medicines given to persons in health.

only three possible modes of employing them), experience speaks indubitably for the last method.

But it is moreover self-evident that medicines which act *heterogeneously* and *allœopathically*, which tend to develop in the healthy subject different symptoms from those presented by the disease to be cured, from the very nature of things can never be suitable and efficacious in this case, but they must act awry, otherwise all diseases must necessarily be cured in a rapid, certain and permanent manner by all medicine, however different. Now, as every medicine possesses an action different from that of every other, and as, according to eternal natural laws, every disease causes a derangement of the human health different from that caused by all other diseases, this proposition contains an innate contradiction (*contradictionem in adjecto*), and is self demonstrative of the impossibility of a good result, since every given change can only be effected by an adequate cause, but not *per quamlibet causam.* And daily experience also proves that the ordinary practice of prescribing complex recipes containing a variety of unknown medicines in diseases, does indeed do many things, but very rarely cures.

The *second mode* of treating diseases by medicines is the employment of an agent capable of altering the existing derangement of the health (the disease, or most prominent morbid symptom) in an *enantiopathic*, *antipathic*, or *contrary* manner (the *palliative* employment of a medicine). Such an employment, as will be readily seen, cannot effect a permanent cure of the disease, because the malady must soon afterwards recur, and that in an aggravated degree. The process that takes place is as follows :— According to a wonderful provision of nature, organized living beings are not regulated by the laws of unorganized (dead) physical matter, they do not receive the influence of external agents, like the latter, in a passive manner, but strive to oppose a contrary action to them.* The living human body does indeed allow itself to be in the first instance changed by the action of physical agents ; but this change is not in it

* The expressed, green juice of plants, which is in that state no longer living, when spread upon linen cloth is soon blanched and its colour annihilated by exposure to sunlight, whereas the colourless living plant that has been kept in a dark cellar, soon recovers its full green colour when exposed to the same sunlight. A root dug up and dried (dead), if buried in a warm and damp soil, rapidly undergoes complete decomposition and destruction, whilst a living root in the same warm damp soil sends forth gay sprouts.—Foaming malt-beer in full fermentation rapidly turns to vinegar when exposed to a temperature of 96° Fahr. in a bottle, but in the healthy human stomach at the same temperature the fermentation ceases, and it soon becomes converted into a mild nutritious juice.—Half-decomposed and strong-smelling game, as also beef and other flesh meat, partaken of by a healthy individual, furnish excrement with the least amount of odour ; whereas cinchona-bark, which is calculated powerfully to check decomposition in lifeless animal substances, is acted against by the intestines in such a manner that the most fetid flatus is developed.—Mild carbonate of lime removes all acids from inorganic matter, but when taken into the healthy stomach sour perspiration usually ensues.—Whilst the dead animal-fibre is preserved by nothing more certainly and powerfully than by tannin, clean ulcers in a living individual, when they are frequently dressed with tannin, become unclean, green, and putrid.—A hand plunged into warm water becomes subsequently colder than the hand that has not been so treated, and it becomes colder in proportion as the water was hotter.

as in inorganic substances, permanent (—as it ought necessarily to be if the medicinal agent acting in a *contrary manner* to the disease should have a *permanent* effect, and be of *durable* benefit—) : on the contrary, the living human organism strives to develop by antagonism* the exact opposite of the affection first produced in it from without,—as for instance, a hand kept long enough in ice-cold water, after being withdrawn does not remain cold, nor merely assume the temperature of the surrounding atmosphere, as a stone (dead) ball would do, or even resume the temperature of the rest of the body, no ! the colder the water of the bath was, and the longer it acted on the healthy skin of the hand, the more *inflamed* and hotter does the latter afterwards become

Therefore it cannot but happen that a medicine having an action opposite to the symptoms of the disease, will reverse the morbid symptoms for but a very short time,† but must soon give place to the antagonism inherent in the living body, which produces an opposite state, that is to say, a state the direct contrary of that transient delusive state of the health effected by the palliative (and corresponding to the original malady), which constitutes an actual addition to the now recurring, uneradicated, original affection, and is consequently an increased degree of the original disease. And thus the malady is always *certainly* aggravated after the palliative—the medicine that acts in an opposite and enantiopathic manner—has exhausted its action.‡

In chronic diseases,—the true touch-stone of a genuine healing art, —the injurious character of the antagonistically-acting (palliative) remedy often displays itself in a high degree, since from its repeated exhibition in order that it should merely produce its delusive effect (a very transient semblance of health) it must be administered in larger and ever larger doses, which are often productive of serious danger to life, or even of actual death.§

---

* This is the law of nature, in obedience to which, the employment of every medicine produces at first certain dynamic changes and morbid symptoms in the living human body (*primary* or *first action of the medicines*), but on the other hand, by means of a peculiar antagonism (which may in many instances be termed the effort of self-preservation), produces a state the very opposite of the first (the *secondary* or *after action*), as for instance, in the case of narcotic substances, insensibility is produced in the primary action, sensitiveness to pain in the secondary.

† As a burnt hand remains cold and painless not much longer than whilst it remains in the cold water, but afterwards feels the pain of the burn much more severely.

‡ Thus the pain of a burnt hand is subdued by cold water quickly, it is true, but only for a few minutes, afterwards, however, the pain of the burn and the inflammation become worse than they were previously (the inflammation as the secondary action of the cold water makes an addition to the original inflammation of the burn, which is not to be eradicated by cold water). The troublesome fulness of the abdomen in cases of habitual constipation appears to be removed, as if magically, by the action of a purgative, but the very next day the painful fulness returns together with the constipation, and becomes worse afterwards than before. The stupified sleep caused by opium is succeeded by a more sleepless night than ever. But that the state that subsequently occurs is a true aggravation, is rendered evident by this, that if we design again to employ the palliative (*e.g.* opium for habitual sleeplessness or chronic looseness of the bowels), it must be given in a stronger dose, *as if for a more severe disease*, in order that it should produce its delusive amelioration for even as short a period as before.

§ As, for instance, where opium is repeated in always stronger doses for the suppression of urgent symptoms of a chronic disease.

There remains, therefore, only a *third* mode of employing medicines in order to effect a really beneficial result, to wit, by employing in every case such an one as tends to excite of itself an artificial, morbid affection in the organism *similar* (homœopathic), best if *very similar*, to the actual case of disease.

That this mode of employing medicines is and must of necessity be the only best method, can easily be proved by reasoning, as it has also already been confirmed both by innumerable experiences of physicians who practise according to my doctrines, and by daily experience.*

It will, therefore, not be difficult to perceive what are the laws of nature according to which the only appropriate cure of diseases, the homœopathic, takes place, and must necessarily take place.

The first of these unmistakable laws of nature is : *the susceptibility of the living organism for natural diseases is incomparably less than it is for medicines.*

A multitude of disease-exciting causes act daily and hourly upon us, but they are incapable of deranging the equilibrium of the health, or of making the healthy sick ; the activity of the life-sustaining power within us usually withstands the most of them, the individual remains healthy. It is only when these external inimical agencies assail us in a

---

* I may adduce merely a few examples from daily experience ; thus, the burning pain produced by the contact of boiling water with the skin, is overpowered and destroyed, as cooks are wont to do, by approaching the moderately burnt hand to the fire, or by bathing it uninterruptedly with heated alcohol (or turpentine), which causes a still more intense burning sensation. This infallible mode of treatment is practised and found to be efficacious by lacquerers and others engaged in similar occupations. The burning pain produced by these strong spirits and their elevated temperature then remains *alone* present, and that for but a few minutes, whilst the organism, homoeopathically freed by them from the inflammation occasioned by the burn, soon restores the injury of the skin and forms a new epidermis through which the spirit can no longer penetrate. And thus, *in the course of a few hours*, the injury caused by the burn is cured by a remedy that occasions a similar burning pain (heated alcohol or turpentine), whereas if treated with the ordinary cooling palliative remedies and salves, it is transformed into a bad ulcer and usually continues to suppurate for many weeks or months with great pain. Practised dancers know from old experience that those who are extremely heated by dancing are very much relieved for the first moment by stripping themselves and drinking very cold water, but thereafter infallibly incur mortal disease, and they do not allow persons excessively heated to cool themselves by exposure to the open air or by taking off their clothes, but wisely administer a liquor whose nature is to heat the blood, such as punch or hot tea mixed with rum or arrak, and in this manner walking at the same time gently up and down the room, they rapidly lose the violent febrile state induced by the dance. In like manner no old experienced reaper, after inordinate exertion in the heat of the sun, would drink anything in order to cool himself but a glass of brandy ; and before an hour has elapsed, his thirst and heat are gone and he feels quite well. No experienced person would put a frost-bitten limb into warm water, or seek to restore it by approaching it to the fire or a hot stove ; applying to it snow, or rubbing it with ice-cold water, is the well-known homoeopathic remedy for it. The illness occasioned by excessive joy (fantastic gaiety, trembling restlessness and uneasiness, palpitation of the heart, sleeplessness) is rapidly and permanently removed by coffee, which causes a similar morbid affection in persons unaccustomed to its use. And in like manner there are many daily-occurring confirmations of the great truth, that nature intends that men should be cured of their long-standing diseases by means of similar affections of short duration. Nations, for centuries sunk in listless apathy and serfdom, raised their spirit, felt their dignity as men, and again became free, after having been ignominiously trodden in the dust by the western tyrant.

very aggravated degree, and we are especially exposed to their influence, that we get ill, but even then we only become seriously ill when our organism has a particularly impressionable, weak side (predisposition), that makes it more disposed to be affected by the (simple or compound) morbific cause in question, and to be deranged in its health.

If the inimical agents in nature that are partly physical and partly psychical, which are termed morbific noxæ, possessed an unconditional power of deranging the human health, they would, as they are universally distributed, not leave any one in good health ; every one would be ill, and we should never be able to obtain an idea of health. But as, taken on the whole, diseases are only exceptional states of the human health, and it is necessary that such a number of circumstances and conditions, both as regards the morbific agents and the individual to be affected with disease, should conjoin before a disease is produced by its exciting causes, it follows, *that the individual is so little liable to be affected by such noxæ, that they can never unconditionally make him ill, and that the human organism is capable of being deranged to disease by them only by means of a particular predisposition.*

But it is far otherwise with the artificial dynamic agents which we term medicines. For every true medicine acts at *all* times, under *all* circumstances, on every living, animated body, and excites in it the symptoms peculiar to it (even in a way perceptible to the senses if the dose be large enough) so that evidently *every living human organism must always and inevitably be affected by the medicinal disease and, as it were, infected,* which, as is well known, is not the case with respect to natural diseases.*

All experience proves incontestably, that the human body is much more apt and disposed to be affected by medicinal agents and to have its health deranged by them, than by the morbific noxæ and contagious miasms, or, what is the same thing, that the medicinal agents possess an absolute power of deranging human health, whereas the morbific agents possess only a very conditional power, vastly inferior to the former.

To this circumstance it is owing that medicines are able to cure diseases at all (that is to say, we see, that the morbid affection may be eradicated from the diseased organism, if the latter be subjected to the appropriate alteration by means of medicine) ; but in order that the cure should take place, the *second* natural law should also be fulfilled, to wit, *a stronger dynamic affection permanently extinguishes the weaker in the living organism, provided the former be similar in kind to the latter* ; for the dynamic alteration of the health to be anticipated from the medicine should, as I think I have proved, neither *differ in kind* from or be *allœopathic* to the morbid derangement, in order that, as happens in the ordinary mode of practice, a still greater derangement may not ensue ; nor should it be *opposite* to it, in order that a merely palliative delusive amelioration may not ensue, to be followed by an inevitable aggravation of the original malady ; but the medicine must have been proved by

* Even the pestilential diseases do not affect every one unconditionally, and the other diseases leave many more individuals unaffected, even when all are exposed to changes of the weather, of the seasons, and to the influence of many other injurious impressions.

observations to possess the tendency to develop of itself a state of health *similar* to the disease (be able to excite similar symptoms in the healthy body), in order to be a remedy of permanent efficacy.

Now, as the dynamic affections of the organism (caused by disease or by medicine) are only cognisable by the phenomena of altered function and altered sensation, and consequently the similarity of its dynamic affections to one another can only express themselves by similarity of symptoms; but as the organism (as being much more liable to be deranged by medicine than by disease) must yield more to the medicinal affection, that is to say, must be more disposed to allow itself to be influenced and deranged by medicine than by the similar natural morbid affection, it follows undeniably, that it will be freed from the natural morbid affection if we allow a medicine to act on it, which, while differing* in its nature from the disease, resembles it very closely in the symptoms it causes, that it to say, is homœopathic; for the organism, as a living, individual unity, cannot receive two similar dynamic affections at the same time, without the weaker yielding to the stronger similar one; consequently, as it is more disposed to be more strongly affected by the one (the medicinal affection), the other, similar, weaker one (the natural morbid affection) must necessarily give way; and the organism is therefore cured of its disease.

Let it not be imagined that the living organism, if a new similar affection be communicated to it when diseased by a dose of homœopathic medicine, will be thereby more seriously deranged, that is, burdened with an addition to its sufferings, just as a leaden plate already pressed upon by an iron weight is still more severely squeezed by placing a stone in addition upon it; or as a piece of copper heated by friction must become still hotter by pouring on it water at a more elevated temperature. No, our living organism does not behave passively, it is not subject to the laws that govern dead matter; it reacts by vital antagonism, so as to surrender itself as an individual living whole to its morbid derangement, and to allow this to be extinguished within it, when a stronger affection of a similar kind, produced in it by homœopathic medicine, takes possession of it.

Such a spiritually reacting being is our living, human organism, which with automatic power expels from itself a weaker derangement (disease), whenever the stronger power of the homœopathic medicine produces in it another but very similar affection; or in other words, which, on account of the unity of its life, cannot suffer at the same time from two similar general derangements, but must discard the primary dynamic affection (disease), whenever it is acted on by a second dynamic power (medicine), more capable of deranging it, that has a great resemblance to the former in its power of affecting the health (its symptoms). Something similar takes place in the human mind.†

* Without this difference in the nature of the morbid affection from that of the medicinal affection, a cure were impossible; if the two were not merely of a similar, but of the same nature, consequently identical, then no result (or only an aggravation of the malady) would ensue; as, for example, if we were to touch a chancre with other chancrous poison, a cure would never result therefrom.

† For example: a girl plunged into grief by the death of her companion, if taken to see a family where the poor, half-naked children have just lost their father, their

But as the human organism even in health is more capable of being affected by medicine than by disease, as I have shown above, so when it is diseased, it is beyond comparison more affectable by homœopathic medicine than by any other (whether allœopathic or enantiopathic) and indeed it is *affectable in the highest degree* ; since, as it is already disposed and excited by the disease to certain symptoms, it must now be more susceptible of the altering influence of similar symptoms (by the homœopathic medicine)—just as similar mental affections render the mind much more sensitive to similar emotions—hence only the *smallest dose* of them is *necessary* and *useful* for their cure, that is, for altering the diseased organism into the similar medicinal disease ; and *a greater one is not necessary* on this account also, because the spiritual power of the medicine does not in this instance accomplish its object by means of quantity, but by potentiality and quality (dynamic fitness, homœopathy), —and *a greater dose is not useful*, but on the contrary *injurious* because whilst the larger dose, on the one hand, does not dynamically overpower the morbid affection more certainly than the smallest dose of the most appropriate medicine, on the other hand it imposes a complex medicinal disease in its place, which is always a malady, though it passes off after a certain time.

Hence the organism will be powerfully affected and taken possession of by the power of even a very small dose of a medicinal substance, which, by its tendency to excite similar symptoms, can outweigh and extinguish the totality of the symptoms of the disease ; it becomes, as I have said, free from the morbid affection at the very instant that it is taken possession of by the medicinal affection, by which it is immeasurably more liable to be altered.

Now, as medicinal agents do of themselves, even in larger doses, only keep the healthy organism for a few days under their influence, it will readily be conceived that a small dose, and in acute diseases a very small dose of them (as it ought evidently to be in homœopathic treatment), can only affect the system for a short time ; the smallest doses, indeed, in acute diseases, only for a few hours ; and then the medicinal affection substituted for the disease passes unobservedly and very rapidly into pure health.

---

sole support, does not become more sorrowful from witnessing this touching scene, but is thereby consoled for her own smaller misfortune ; she is cured of her grief for her friend, because the unity of her mind cannot be affected by two similar passions at once, and the one passion must be extinguished when a *similar* but stronger passion takes possession of her mind, and acts as a *homœopathic* remedy in extinguishing the first. But the girl would not be tranquillized and cured of her grief for the loss of her companion, if her mother were angrily to scold her (*heterogeneous, allœopathic* influence), but, on the contrary, her mind would be still more distressed by this attack of grief of another kind ; and in like manner the sorrowing girl, if we were to cause an apparent but only *palliative* alleviation of her grief, by means of a gay entertainment, would subsequently in her solitude sink into still more profound sadness, and would weep much more intensely than previously for the death of her friend (because this affection would here be only of an *opposite enantiopathic* character).

And as it is here in psychical life, so is it in the former case in organic life. The unity of our life cannot occupy itself with, and receive, two general dynamic affections of the same kind at once ; for if the second be a similar one, the first is displaced by it, if the organism be more energetically affected by the latter.

In the permanent cure of diseases by medicines in living organisms nature seems never to act otherwise than in accordance with these her manifest laws, and then indeed she acts, if we may use the expression, with mathematical certainty. *There is no case of dynamic disease in the world* (excepting the death struggle, old age, if it can be considered a disease, and the destruction or some indispensable viscus or member), *whose symptoms can be met with in great similarity among the positive effects of a medicine, which will not be rapidly and permanently cured by this medicine.* The diseased individual can be freed from his malady, in no more easy, rapid, certain, reliable and permanent manner, by any conceivable mode of treatment,* than by means of the homœopathic medicine in small doses.

* Even those striking cures which occur in rare instances in ordinary practice, take place only by means of a homoeopathically appropriate medicine, which forms the chief agent in the receipt, into which it has been *accidentally* introduced. Physicians hitherto could not have *chosen* the medicines homoeopathically for diseases, as the positive effects of the medicines (those observed from their administration to healthy persons) had not been investigated by them, and accordingly remained unknown to them ; and even those which have been known otherwise than by my writings, were not regarded by them as capable of being utilized for treatment,—and moreover, the relation of the effects of medicines to the symptoms of the disease they resemble (the homoeopathic law of cure), which is requisite in order to effect radical cures, was unknown.

PREAMBLE.[1]

MANY persons of my acquaintance but half converted to homœopathy have repeatedly begged me to publish still more exact directions as to how this doctrine may be actually applied in practice, and how we are to proceed. I am astonished that after the very particular directions contained in the *Organon of Medicine* more special instructions can be wished for.

I am also asked, "How are we to examine the disease in each particular case?" As if special enough directions were not to be found in the book just mentioned.

As in homœopathy the treatment is not directed towards imaginary or invented internal causes of the disease, nor yet towards names of diseases invented by man of which nature knows nothing, and as every case of non-miasmatic disease is a distinct individuality, independent, peculiar, a complex of symptoms always differing in nature, never hypothetically presupposable, so no particular directions can be laid down for it (no schema, no table), except that the physician in order to effect a cure, must oppose to every aggregate of morbid symptoms in a case a group of similar medicinal symptoms as complete as can be met with in any single known drug; for this system of medicine cannot admit of more than a single medicinal substance (whose effects have been accurately tested) being given at once (see *Organon of Medicine*, 4th edit., § 270, 271).[2]

Now we can neither enumerate all the possible aggregates of symptoms of all cases of disease that may occur, nor indicate *a priori* the homœopathic medicines for these (*a priori* indeterminable) possibilities. For every individual given case (and every case is an individuality, differing from all others) the homœopathic medical practitioner must himself find them, and for this end he must be acquainted with the medicines that have till now been investigated in respect of their positive action, or consult them for every case of disease; but besides this he must do his endeavour to prove thoroughly on himself or on other healthy individuals

---

1 From vol. ii, 3rd edit. 1833. [The cases here given originally appeared in 1816 in the first edition of the *R. A. M. L.*, but the notes and most of the preliminary matter are of the date we have given, and we may therefore consider the whole to represent Hahnemann's opinion and practice, with the exception of the dose in these two cases, of the latter period.]

2 The corresponding paragraphs of the 5th edit. are 272, 273.

medicines that have not yet been investigated as regards the morbid alterations they are capable of producing, in order thereby to increase our store of *known* remedial agents,* so that the choice of a remedy for every one of the infinite variety of cases of disease (for the combating of which we can never possess enough of suitable tools and weapons) may become all the more easy and accurate.

That man is far from being animated with the true spirit of the homœopathic system, is no true disciple of this beneficent doctrine, who makes the slightest objection to institute *on himself* careful experiments for the investigation of the peculiar effects of the medicines which have remained unknown for 2500 years. Without this investigation (and unless their pure pathogenetic action on the healthy individual has previously been ascertained) all treatment of disease must continue to be not only a foolish, but even a criminal action, a dangerous attack upon human life.

It is somewhat too much to expect us to work merely for the benefit of selfish individuals, who will contribute nothing to the complete and indispensable building up of the indispensable edifice, who only seek to make money by what has been discovered and investigated by the labours of others ; and to furnish them with the means of squandering the income derived from the scientific capital, to the production of which they do not evince the slightest inclination to contribute.

All who feel a true desire to assist in elucidating the peculiar effects of medicines—our sole instruments, the knowledge of which has for so many centuries remained uninvestigated, and which is yet so indispensable for enabling us to cure the sick, will find the directions how these pure experiments with medicines should be conducted in the *Organon of Medicine*, 4th edit., § 111—136.[1]

In addition to what has been there stated I shall only add, that as the experimenter cannot, any more than any other human being, be absolutely and perfectly healthy, he must, should slight ailments to which he was liable appear during these provings of the powers of medicines, place these between brackets, thereby indicating that they are not confirmed, or dubious. But this will not often happen, seeing that during the action upon a previously healthy person of a sufficiently strong dose of the medicine, he is under the influence of the medicine alone, and it is seldom that any other symptom can show itself during the first days but what must be the effect of the medicine. Further, that in order to investigate the symptoms of medicines for chronic diseases, for example, in order to develop the cutaneous diseases, abnormal growths and so forth, to be expected from the medicine, we must not be contented with taking one or two doses of it only, but we must continue its use for several days, to the amount of two adequate doses daily, that is to say, of sufficient size to cause us to experience an

* Before the discovery of homoeopathy, medicinal substances were known only in respect to their natural history, and besides their names nothing was known regarding them but their presumed qualities, which were either imaginary or altogether false.

---

1 The corresponding paragraphs of the 5th edit. are 120—145.

action from it, whilst at the same time we continue to observe the diet and regimen indicated in the work alluded to.

The mode of preparing the medicinal substances for use in homœopathic treatment will be found in the *Organon of Medicine*, § 267—269,[1] and also in the second part of *The Chronic Diseases*. I would only observe here, that for the proving of medicines on healthy individuals, dilutions and dynamizations are to be employed as high as are used for the treatment of disease, namely, globules moistened with the decillionth development of power.[2]

The request of some friends, halting half-way on the road to this method of treatment, to give some examples of this treatment, is difficult to comply with, and no great advantage can attend a compliance with it. Every cured case of disease shows only how that case has been treated. The internal process of the treatment depends always on the same rules, which are already known, and they cannot be rendered concrete and definitely fixed for each individual case, nor can they become at all more distinct by the history of a single cure than they were already by the publication of these rules. Every case of non-miasmatic disease is peculiar and special, and it is the special in it that distinguishes it from every other case, that pertains to it alone, but that cannot serve as a model for the treatment of other cases. Now, if it is wished to describe a complicated case of disease consisting of many symptoms, in such a circumstantial manner that the reasons that influence us in the choice of the remedy shall be clearly revealed, this demands a multiplicity of details fatiguing at once for the describer and for the reader.

In order, however, to comply with the desire of my friends in this also, I may here detail two cases of homœopathic cure of the most trivial character.

Sch—, a washerwoman, somewhere about 40 years old, had been more than three weeks unable to earn her bread, when she consulted me on the 1st September, 1815.

1. On any movement, especially at every step, and worst on making a false step, she has a shoot in the pit of the stomach, that comes, as she avers, every time from the left side.
2. When she lies she feels quite well, then she has no pain anywhere, neither in the side nor in the pit of the stomach.
3. She cannot sleep after three o'clock in the morning.
4. She relishes her food, but when she has eaten a little she feels sick.
5. Then the water collects in her mouth and runs out of it, like the water-brash.
6. She has frequent empty eructations after every meal.
7. Her temper is passionate, disposed to anger.—When the pain is severe she is covered with perspiration.—The catamenia were quite regular a fortnight since.

1 The corresponding paragraphs of the 5th edit. are 269—271.

2 In place of this paragraph the 2nd edition (published in 1824) has four paragraphs describing the mode of preparing the remedies then adopted, which are superseded by the instructions in the *Organon*. In the older edition there is no mention of the decillionth potency being the appropriate dose for therapeutic and pathogenetic purposes.

In other respects her health is good.

Now, as regards Symptom 1, *Belladonna, china,* and *rhus toxicodendron* cause shootings in the pit of the stomach, but none of them *only on movement*, as is the case here. *Pulsatilla* (see Symp. 387[1]) certainly causes shooting in the pit of the stomach on making a false step, but only as a rare alternating action, and has neither the same digestive derangements as occur here at 4 compared with 5 and 6, nor the same state of the disposition.

Bryonia alone has among its chief alternating actions, as the whole list of its symptoms demonstrates, pains *from movement* and especially shooting pains, as also stitches beneath the sternum (in the pit of the stomach) on raising the arm (448), and on making a false step it occasions shooting in other parts (520, 600).

The negative Symptom 2 met with here answers especially to *bryonia* (638); few medicines (with the exception, perhaps, of *nux vomica* and *rhus toxicodendron* in their alternating action—neither of whicn, however, is suitable for the other symptoms) show a complete relief to pains during rest and when lying; *bryonia* does, however, in an especial manner (638, and many other bryonia-symptoms).

Symptom 3 is met with in several medicines, and also in *bryonia* (694).

Symptom 4 is certainly, as far as regards "sickness after eating," met with in several other medicines (*ignatia, nux vomica, mercurius, ferrum, belladonna, pulsatilla, cantharis*), but neither so constantly and usually, nor with relish for food, as in *bryonia* (279).

As regards Symptom 5 several medicines certainly cause a flow of saliva like water-brash, just as well as *bryonia* (282); the others, however, do not produce symptoms similar to the remaining ones. Hence bryonia is to be preferred to them in this part of the ailment.

Empty eructation (of wind only) after eating (Symptom 6) is found in few medicines, and in none so constantly, so usually, and to such a great degree, as in *bryonia* (253, 259).

To 7.—One of the chief symptoms in diseases (see *Organon of Medicine*, § 213) is the "state of the disposition," and as *bryonia* (772) causes this symptom also in an exactly similar manner—*bryonia* is for all these reasons to be preferred in this case to all other medicines as the homœopathic remedy.

Now, as this woman was very robust, and the force of the disease must consequently have been very considerable to prevent her by its pain from doing any work, and as her vital forces, as has been observed were not impaired, I gave her one of the strongest homœopathic doses, a full drop of the undiluted juice of bryonia root,* to be taken immediately, and bade her come to me again in 48 hours. I told my friend

* According to the most recent development of our new system the ingestion of a single, minutest globule, moistened with the decillionth (X) development of power would have been quite adequate to effect an equally rapid and complete recovery; indeed, equally certain would have been the mere olfaction of a globule the size of a mustard seed moistened with the same dynamization, so that the drop of crude juice given by me in the above case to a robust person, should not be imitated.

1 The numbers are altered so as to suit the 3rd edit., which Hahnemann neglected to do, when this edition appeared.

E., who was present, that within that time the woman would assuredly be quite cured, but he, being but half converted to homœopathy, expressed his doubts about it. Two days afterwards he came again to ascertain the result, but the woman did not return then, and, in fact, never came back again. I could only allay the impatience of my friend by telling him her name and that of the village where she lived, about a mile and a half off, and advising him to seek her out and ascertain for himself how she was. This he did, and her answer was: "What was the use of my going back? The very next day I was quite well, and could again go to my washing, and the day following I was as well as I am still. I am extremely obliged to the doctor, but the like of us have no time to leave off our work; and for three weeks previously my illness prevented me earning anything."

W—e, a weakly, pale man of 42 years, who was constantly kept by his business at his desk, complained to me on the 27th December, 1815, that he had been already ill five days.

1. The first evening he became, without manifest cause, sick and giddy, with much eructation.
2. The following night (about 2 a.m.) sour vomiting.
3. The subsequent nights violent eructation.
4. To-day also sick eructation of fetid and sourish taste.
5. He felt as if the food lay crude and undigested in his stomach.
6. In his head he felt vacant, hollow, and gloomy, and as if sensitive therein.
7. The least noise was disagreeable to him.
8. He is of a mild, soft, patient disposition.

Here I may observe :—

To 1. That several medicines cause vertigo with nausea, as well as *pulsatilla* (3), which produces its vertigo in the *evening* also (7), a circumstance that has been observed from very few others.

To 2. *Stramonium* and *nux vomica* cause vomiting of sour and sour-smelling mucus, but, as far as is known, not *at night*. *Valerian* and *cocculus* cause vomiting at night, but not of sour stuff. *Iron* alone causes vomiting at night (61, 62), and can also cause sour vomiting (66), but not the other symptoms which should be attended to here.

Pulsatilla, however, causes not only sour vomiting in the evening (349, 354) and nocturnal vomiting in general (355), but also the other symptoms of this case not found among those of *iron*.

To 3. Nocturnal eructation is peculiar to *pulsatilla* (296, 297).

To 4. Fetid, putrid (259) and sour eructation (301, 302) is also peculiar to *pulsatilla.*

To 5. The sensation of indigestibility of the food in the stomach is produced by few medicines, and by none in such a perfect and striking manner as by *pulsatilla* (321, 322, 327).

To 6. Besides *ignatia* (2) which, however, cannot produce the other ailments, the same state is produced by *pulsatilla* (39 compared with 42, 94, 98).

To 7. *Pulsatilla* produces the same state (995), and it also causes over-sensitiveness of other organs of the senses, for example, of the sight (107). And although intolerance of noise is also met with in *nux vomica*, *ignatia*, and *aconite*, yet these medicines are not homœopathic to the other symptoms and still less do they possess symptom 8, the mild character of the disposition, which, as stated in the preface to *pulsatilla*, is particularly indicative of this plant.

This patient, therefore, could not be cured by anything in a more easy, certain, and permanent manner than by *pulsatilla*, which was homœopathic to the case. It was accordingly given to him immediately; but, on account of his weakly and exhausted state, only in a very minute dose, *i. e.* half a drop of the quadrillionth of a strong drop of pulsatilla.* This was done in the evening.

The next day he was free from all ailments, his digestion was restored, and a week thereafter, as I was told by him, he remained free from complaint and quite well.

The investigation in such a slight case of disease, and the choice of the homœopathic remedy for it, is *very speedily* effected by the practitioner who has had only a little experience in it, and who either has the symptoms of the medicine in his memory, or who knows where to find them readily; but to give in writing all the reasons *pro* and *con* (which would be perceived by the mind in a few seconds) gives rise, as we see, to tedious prolixity.

For the convenience of treatment, we require merely to jot down after each symptom all the medicines which can produce such a symptom with tolerable accuracy, expressing them by a few letters (*e. g.* Ferr., Chin., Rheum., Puls.), and also to bear in mind the circumstances under which they occur, that have a determining influence on our choice; and proceed in the same way with all the other symptoms, noting by what medicine each is excited; from the list so prepared we shall be able to perceive which among the medicines homœopathically covers the most of the symptoms present, especially the most peculiar and characteristic ones,—and this is the remedy sought for.

* * *

As regards the following catalogue of medicinal symptoms there are in this part also many observations by my disciples, mostly made on themselves. Their names will be found attached, with the addition, "*in an essay*."[1] On every occasion when my Leipzic disciples delivered to me their essays I questioned them respecting the symptoms they observed (and this I would advise every teacher to do under similar circumstances) in order to get as precisely as possible the verbal expressions of their sensations and sufferings, and to ascertain with exactness the conditions under which the symptoms occurred. By this means I have, as I believe, elicited the truth. I knew also that they had faithfully

* According to our present knowledge and experience the same object would have been attained by taking one of the smallest globules of pulsatilla X (decillionth potency) and with equal certainty a single olfaction of a globule the size of a mustard seed of the same potency of pulsatilla.

1 Although this statement occurs in this "Preamble" as prefixed to the 3rd edition of vol. ii, it is not correct as applied to that edition, where the names of HAHNEMANN's disciples are indicated by their abbreviations only within square brackets. The plan he mentions was adopted in the 2nd edition of all the vols.

observed the carefully regulated diet, and had led a life undisturbed by passions during their provings, in order to be able to observe the alterations in their health purely and obviously due to the medicine taken.

By conducting their trials in this manner they become careful, delicately sensitive observers, and if with this they combine pure moral conduct and the acquisition of other useful branches of knowledge, they will become proficients in the healing art.[1]

1 It was not until the 1st vol. of the 1st edition had been published that Hahnemann obtained any assistance from others in his provings. This is the reason of the appearance of these last two paragraphs in the 2nd vol., in which vol. they are still retained in the two last editions.

ACONITUM NAPELLUS.

(*Monkshood.*)

(The freshly expressed juice of the plant at the time of the commencement of flowering mixed with equal parts of spirits of wine.)

Although the following symptoms do not express the whole significance of this most valuable plant, still they reveal to the thoughtful homœopathic physician a prospect of relieving morbid conditions in which traditional medicine has hitherto employed its most dangerous methods, *e. g.* copious blood-letting and all its complex would-be antiphlogistic treatments, often ineffectually, and almost always with disastrous consequences. I allude to the so-called pure inflammatory fevers, in which the smallest dose of aconite enables us to dispense with all the traditional antipathic treatments, and relieves rapidly and without evil effects. In measles, in purpura miliaris, and in the acute pleuritic fevers, &c., its curative power is marvellous, when, the patient being kept rather cool, it is given *alone, all other medicinal substances*, even vegetable acids, *being avoided*, in the dose of a thousandth part* of a drop of the decillionth development of power. It is seldom that a second similar dose is required thirty-six or forty-eight hours after the first.

But in order to remove from our conscientious treatment all that routine practice which is only too apt to regulate its treatment in accordance with delusive names of diseases, it is indispensable that, in all morbid conditions in which aconite is given, the chief symptoms of the malady, therefore also of the acute disease, should be found accurately reproduced among the symptoms of aconite.

The effect is then astonishing.

It is precisely in the great acute inflammatory fevers in which allopathy chiefly plumes itself as alone able to save life by means of bold, frequent venesections, and imagines that here it is superior in curative efficacy to all homœopathic treatment—it is precisely here that it is most mistaken. It is precisely here that the infinite superiority of homœopathy is manifest, that it needs not to shed a single drop of blood, that precious vital fluid (which the allopath recklessly draws off in streams, to the often irremediable disadvantage of the patient), in order to transform this dangerous fever into health in as many hours as the allopathic vitality-diminishing treatment often requires months for the perfect restoration of those who are not carried off during the process

* That is, a small globule the size of a poppy-seed moistened with it, of which more than a thousand are moistened by one drop of spirits of wine, and which are so small that 300 of them weigh only one grain.

---

1 From vol. i, 3rd edit., 1830.

by death, or, at all events, in the chronic after-affections artificially caused by the means employed.

In these acute cases of disease sometimes a homœopathic intermediate remedy is required for the morbid symptoms remaining after twelve or sixteen hours' action of the first dose of aconite; but it is very rarely that a second dose of aconite is needed after this intermediate remedy.

By means of aconite carefully administered in this way in a disease of the above mentioned character all danger is removed even in four hours, and the excited circulation resumes its tranquil vital course from hour to hour.

Although aconite, on account of the short duration of its action (which in such small doses does not exceed forty-eight hours), might seem to be useful only in acute diseases, yet it is an indispensable accessory remedy in even the most obstinate chronic affections, when the system requires a diminution of the so-called *tension of the blood-vessels* (the *strictum* of the ancients). On this subject, however, I cannot enter more fully in this place. Its utility in such cases is shown by the symptoms it produces in the healthy subject, which are partially recorded in the following pages.

Aconite is also the first and main remedy, in the minute dose indicated above, in inflammation of the wind-pipe (croup, membranous laryngitis), in various kinds of inflammation of the throat and fauces, as also in the local acute inflammations of all other parts, particularly where in addition to thirst and quick pulse, there are present anxious impatience, an unappeasable mental agitation, and agonizing tossing about.

It produces all the morbid states similar to those seen in persons who have had a fright combined with vexation, and is also the surest and quickest remedy for them.

In the selection of aconite as a homœopathic remedy particular attention should be paid to the symptoms of the disposition, so that they should be very similar.

Hence it is indispensable after fright or vexation in women during the catamenia, which without this excellent soothing remedy are only too easily, often instantaneously, suppressed by such emotional disturbances. For this purpose a single momentary olfaction at a phial containing a globule the size of a mustard-seed, moistened with the decillionth potency of aconite (which may be kept for this use for years in a well-corked phial without lossing its curative power) is quite sufficient.

Most of the apparently opposite aconite symptoms recorded below are merely alternating states, and it may be curative by means of both, but it is most so in respect of those which have a tonic character.

Vegetable acids and wine antidote its effects, and so do other medicines which correspond palliatively or homœopathically to some of its troublesome symptoms (produced by too large a dose or unhomœopathic selection).

[The names of Hahnemann's disciples who assisted him in this proving are: AHNER, GROSS, FRIEDRICH HAHNEMANN, HORNBURG, RUCKERT senior, STAPF, WAHLE

The authorities of traditional medicine quoted by him for some of the recorded effects of aconite are:

ABANO, PET. DE, *De Venenis*, cap. 30, 1496.
BACON, VINC., *Philosoph. Transactions*, xxxviii.
DURR, *Hufel Journ.*, ix, 4.
GMELIN. EBERH., *Nov. Acta Nat. Cur.*, vi. GREDING. *Vermischte Schriften.*
HELMONT, J. B. VAN, *Demens Idea*, § 12. (*Orteus Medicinæ*, 1652.)
MATTHIOLUS, *Comment in Diosc.*, lib. iv, cap. 73. MORAEUS, *Konigl. Vetensk. Acad. Handl.*, 1739.
RICHARD, CLAUD., in *P. Schenck's Obs. Med.*, lib. vii, obs. 136. RODDER, in *Alberti's Jurisprud. Med.*, tom. vi.
STOERCK, ANT. VON, *Libellus de Stram.*, *Hyos. et Acon.*

In the *Frag. de Vir.* the symptoms of aconite are 213, in the first edition of the *R.A.M.L.*, they are 314, in the second 429, and in the third 541.]

ACONITE.

Vertigo ; feeling of swaying to and fro in the brain.

Vertigo, especially when stooping ; she staggered to and fro, especially towards the right side (aft. 36 h.). *Stf. Gss.*, *Archiv. f. d. Homoopath. Heilkunst*, iv. i.[1]]

She could hardly get into bed for vertigo, in which all seemed to turn round in a circle with her (aft. 37 h.). [*Stf. Gss.*]

She has a whirling in the head, so that she dare not move it, with a feeling as if the eyes would close. [*Stf. Gss.*]

5. As if intoxicated ; all goes round with her, she staggers when walking, as if she would fall, with nausea, not on sitting, worst on rising from a seat, less when walking (aft. ½ h.). [*Stf. Gss.*]

Vertigo very much increased on shaking the head, when it became quite black before her eyes. [*Stf. Gss.*]

Vertigo and dizziness.

Giddy weight of the head, especially in the forehead and on stooping, with nausea, and qualmish feeling in the scrobiculus cordis (aft. 2 h.). [*Stf. Gss.*]

Vertigo [MATTHIOLI,[2] *Comment. in Diosc.*, lib. iv, cap. 73—VINC. BACON,[3] in *Philosoph. Transact.*, xxxviii, p. 287.]

10. Vertigo, tightness of chest and dry cough, with pain in hip. [GREDING,[4] *Vermischte Schriften.* p. 90—113.]

Giddy obscuration of sight, with unaltered pulse. [CLAUD. RICHARD, in *P. Schenck*,[5] lib. vii, obs. 136.]

---

1 In the original this is erroneously printed "V. iii." The symptoms taken from the *Archiv* were observed by Drs. Gross and Stapf on themselves and others. Hahnemann refers to the Journal in which they were first published after each symptom taken therefrom, but as Drs. Gross and Stapf were essentially fellow-workers with Hahnemann, and assisted him to prove many of his medicines, we have considered it best to give the abbreviations of their names after the symptoms for which they are responsible, as well to avoid confusion as to do honour to these able pioneers of homœopathy.

2 Narrative of two cases in which aconite was administered to criminals (male adults) to test the efficacy of the bezoar-stone as an antidote.

3 Poisoning of an adult.

4 An account of the treatment of nine patients, variously afflicted, with increasing doses of the extract.—The patient in whom these symptoms occurred had suffered from them before taking the medicine.

5 As Matthiolus (one case). See note[2].

Vertigo and headache, unaffected by active exercise (aft. ¼ h.). [*Fr. H—n.*]

Vertigo and headache in sinciput and occiput, both worst when stooping (aft. 10 m.). [*Fr. H—n.*]

Distraction of the attention when reading and writing by a frequent cessation of the thoughts. [*Rkt.*]

15. Preoccupation of the mind; he is unable to complete his description of the thoughts that he had conceived and half written down, without first making an effort to recall them (3rd day). [*We.*]

Stupid feeling of the head; as if he had a board before the forehead (aft. ¼ h.). [*Stf. Gss.*]

The head in front is as if nailed up, in the warm room. [*Stf. Gss.*]

Unsteadiness of the ideas; if she wants to pursue one train of thought a second chases this away, a third again displaces this, and so on and on, until she becomes quite confused. [*Stf. Gss.*]

Want of memory; he feels as if what he had just done were a dream, and he can scarcely recall what it was. [*Stf. Gss*]

20. **Weakness of memory** (aft. 5 and 9 h.).

Lively memory.

Weakened power of thinking. [*We.*]

He can think of nothing, consider nothing, knows nothing, and can form no idea of anything in his head, as he usually could—but he feels as if all these mental operations took place in the pit of the stomach—after two hours he has two attacks of vertigo, and then his usual thinking faculty returns into his head. [J. B. v. HELMONT,[1] in *Demens Idea*, § 12.]

In the morning vacancy and emptiness of the head, as after severe intoxication. [*Rkt.*]

25. Confusion of the head, as after intoxication, with aching in the temples.

Stupid bruised pain in the head, with bruised feeling in all the limbs (aft. 14 h).

Feeling of fulness and heaviness in the forehead, as if an outpressing weight lay there, and as if all would be forced out at the forehead (aft. ¼ h.). [*Stf. Gss.*]

Stupifying drawing in-pressing in the left temple. [*Stf. Gss.*]

Feeling as if some one drew him up by the hair. [*Stf. Gss.*]

30. **Semilateral drawing in the head.** [*Stf. Gss.*]

Aching pain in the temporal region, afterwards also in jerks in the occiput, lastly confusion of the head and contractive pain. [*Rkt.*].

Contractive pain in the forehead. [*Ar.*]

Tension all over the forehead. [*Hbg.*]

---

1 Effect of putting a piece of the root on his tongue. Of the state described in this symptom and S. 502 he writes:—"I had already often had ecstasies, but I never found myself quite like this. I have, further, repeated the experiment in vain; I have felt nothing similar again."

On stooping her forehead feels very full, as if all would come out (aft. 25 h.). [*Stf. Gss.*]

35. Headache, as if the eyes would fall out of the head (aft. ½ h.).

Headache, as if the brain pressed out.

Headache, as if here and there a part of the brain were lifted up, which is increased by slight movement, even by drinking and speaking (aft. ½ h.).

Speaking increases the headache.

Shooting, throbbing headache, as if an ulcer were inside, which sometimes prevents speaking.

40. Sometimes a fine shooting, sometimes throbbing, sometimes aching headache in the forehead when walking, relieved by sitting.

A fine throbbing here and there in the head.

Headache ; a throbbing in the left side of the forehead, whilst strong beats occur in the right side by fits (aft. 3 h.).

In the left side of the head, pain as if the head were compressed. [*Ar.*]

Headache, as if the skull were externally constricted with a ligature and drawn tightly together. [HELMONT, l. c.]

45. Very painful, sharp, pressing headache above the forehead. [*We.*]

Out-pressing pain in the forehead. [*We.*]

Tearing pain in the left temple. [*Ar.*]

In the left temple shooting pain by jerks ; stitches pass through the temple into the head. [*Stf. Gss.*]

Shooting, beating headache in the temples. [*Stf. Gss.*]

50. Shooting by jerks in the head, especially in the forehead. [*Stf. Gss.*]

Tearing pain in the left temple, with roaring noise in the ears. [*Stf. Gss.*]

Feeling of contraction of the brain under the forehead (aft. 20 h.). [*Stf. Gss.*]

Squeezing, tensive headache close behind the orbits.

A pinching and squeezing in the forehead, as if it were in the bones; she feels ill, as though about to go mad (aft. 12, 24 h.).

55. A squeezing in the forehead, above the root of the nose, as if she would lose her reason (as if wrong in the head) ; aggravated by walking in the open air (aft. 4 h.).

A feeling of crepitation (like bending gold tinsel to and fro) in the temples, nose, and forehead.

Shooting and somewhat aching headache above the orbits towards the superior maxilla, which causes nausea, or as usually occurs during the vomiting caused by an emetic (aft. 2 h.).

Aching, shooting, sick headache above the orbits and down to the upper jaw.

Feeling as if something were drawn out of the head, whereby her upper eyelids are drawn upwards (aft. ½ h.). [*Stf. Gss.*]

60. Twitching, tearing pain in the occiput. [*Ar.*]

Jerking, shooting, drawing, tearing pain in the upper part of the right side of the head. [*Ar.*]

A shoot in the occipital bone. [*Hbg.*]

Creeping on the left side of the head, as from a brush. [*Hbg.*]

Feeling as if a ball rose from the umbilical region and spread a cool air in the vertex and occiput. [MATTHIOLI, l. c.]

65. Burning headache as if the brain were moved by boiling water. [MATTHIOLI, l. c.]

Heaviness of the head. [V. BACON, l. c.]

Pain in the occiput and neck. [RICHARD, l. c.]

Headache, roaring in the ears, coryza and colic, especially in the morning, as if a chill had been taken after profuse perspiration.[1] [GREDING, l. c.]

Towards evening she got very hot in the whole head, after which there occurred tenderness of the whole head, especially of the forehead, lasting all the evening (aft. 11 h.). [*Stf. Gss.*]

70. (Puffy face and forehead).

Bluish face, black lips. [MATTHIOLI, l. c.]

Distortion of the facial muscles. [MATTHIOLI, l. c.]

Very widely dilated pupils. [*We.*]

Obscuration of the sight. [BACON, l. c.]

75. Repeated blindness, with undiminished power of speech.[2] [MATTHIOLI, l. c.]

Distortion of the eyes. [MATTHIOLI,—BACON, l. c.]

Distortion of the eyes and grinding of the teeth (about midnight).[3] [GREDING, l. c.]

On opening the eyelids pain in the interior of the eye (as if it would be pressed out), which pain spread over the region of the eye-brow into the interior of the brain (aft. 21 h.). [*Stf. Gss.*]

Dilated pupils (immediately).

80. His eyes are staring (immediately).

Desire for light, longing to look into the bright light (aft. 3 h.).

Black spots hovering before the sight.

Misty before the eyes; she does not see distinctly, with giddy feeling. [*Stf. Gss.*]

Photophobia (aft. 6 and 12 h.).*

85. Acute vision.

Dryness of the upper eyelids, which causes a sort of aching in the eyes (aft. 5 h.).

Heaviness of the eyelids; they seemed to him too heavy on raising them. [*Stf. Gss.*]

(The eyes feel cold in the open air.)

Very painful inflammation of the eyes (chemosis).

90. Sensation in the eyes as if they were greatly swollen (aft. 5 h.). [*Stf. Gss.*]

The eyes are closed with a jerk, as in irresistible sleepiness. [*Stf. Gss.*]

Protruding eyes. [MATTHIOLI, l. c.]

Aching of the eyes, most observable when looking down and

* Probably an alternating symptom with 81, so that both are primary effects.

1 This was the effect of an actual chill, not "as from a chill."

2 See S. 539.

3 In a demented and epileptic patient, subject to spasms.

when moving the eyes to and fro, at the same time with heat in them. [*Rkt.*]

Aching and burning in the left eye and over the eye-brows. [*Hbg.*]

95. Hard, red swelling of the right upper eyelid, with tensive sensation, especially in the morning. [*F. H—n.*]

Ophthalmia, with discharge, which is so painful and horrible that he longs for death. [RICHARD, l. c.]

Constant, dull, humming before the ears, followed by fainting. [BACON, l. c.]

Pain in the zygomatic process, as from an internal ulcer there.

Ringing in the ears (aft. 10 m.). [*Stf. Gss.*]

100. He feels as if something lay before the left ear. [*Ar.*]

Tickling sensation in the right ear, as if a small worm crept in. [*Ar.*]

Tearing in the left ear. [*Hbg.*]

Pain behind the left ear, like a pressure with the thumb. [*Hbg.*]

Sensation as if the cheeks were swollen to double their size. [BACON, l. c.]

105. Pain in the maxillary joint behind the zygomatic process, when chewing.

During the **perspiration** a burning pain shot several times into the left ear and upper **maxilla.**

Perspiration on the cheek on which she lies in bed.

Creeping pain on the cheeks.

Sensation of stupifying compression of the root of the nose. [*Stf. Gss.*]

110. **Epistaxis.**

Perspiration on the upper lip, under the nose.

Itching pimples on the upper lip (aft. 24 h.).

Shooting jerks in the lower jaw.

Shooting pain in various teeth (aft. 36 h.). [*We.*]

115. Aching toothache in the left upper jaw. [*We.*]

Very penetrating pain in jaws as if they would fall off. [MATTHIOLI, l. c.]

In the tongue and jaws a creeping and burning, so that the teeth seem loose. [BACON, l. c.]

Smarting sensation in the tongue, chiefly towards its tip. [*Stf. Gss.*]

Penetrating fine stitches in the tip of the tongue.

120. In the tongue a burning of long continuance. [ANT. V. STOERCK,[1] *Libellus de Stram., Hyos. et Acon.*, pp. 71, 74, 80, 91, 96, 110.]

Momentary, flying stitches in the tongue, with flow of saliva. [STOERCK, l. c.]

Coolness and dryness of the mouth, without thirst. [*Hbg.*]

Dry feeling first of the lips, then of the interior of the mouth,

1 This and the following symptom were experienced by Stoerck himself after placing a small quantity of the root on his tongue. The rest of his symptoms were observed on patients to whom he gave the drug.

with heat rising up from the chest towards the head (without redness of the cheeks).*

Transient paralysis of the tongue.

125. Dryness of the interior of the mouth (immediately).

On the middle of the tongue, sensation of dryness and roughness, without thirst (aft. 1 h.).

Feeling of dryness in the fore part of the mouth.

Feeling of soreness of the orifices of the salivary glands, as if they were excoriated.

In the throat a scraping with difficult deglutition. [*Stf. Gss.*]

130. Drawing from the side of the throat to behind the ear. [*Stf. Gss.*]

On the left side of the throat, internally, on a small spot, a shooting choking, when not, but especially when, swallowing and speaking. After ¼ of an hour it passed to the right side, whilst the painful sensation in the left side disappeared, it remained there ¼ of an hour, and went off entirely. [*Stf. Gss.*]

Prickling sensation at the back of the tongue as from pepper, with flow of saliva.

Creeping in the fauces.

Fine shooting sensation at the back of the throat, as from the prickly hairs of the dog-hip (aft. 1 h.).

135. Burning and fine shooting pain in the back of the throat (fauces).

Contractive feeling in the back of the throat, as from something astringent.

Pepper-like taste in the mouth.[1] [MATTHIOLI, l. c.]

Along with deficient appetite, bitter taste in the mouth, with pains in the chest and under the short ribs. [GREDING, l. c.]

Bitter taste.

140. Nasty, fishy taste, as from stagnant putrid water.

She felt as if the whole mouth filled with air of the taste of rotten eggs. [*Stf. Gss.*]

Sourish taste in the mouth, with loss of appetite. [*Stf. Gss.*]

What formerly had a good and strong taste is now tasteless to him. [*Stf. Gss.*]

Sweetish water rose up, like water-brash ; at the same time roaring in the ears. [*Stf. Gss.*]

145. Belching up of sweetish water, with nausea. [*Stf. Gss.*]

Scraping from the scrobiculus cordis, up into the throat, with nausea and qualmishness in the scrobiculus cordis, as if water would come into her mouth. [*Stf. Gss.*]

Empty eructation. [*Stf. Gss.*]

Ineffectual effort to eructate ; he wishes to eructate but cannot.

Thirst for beer ; but when she has drunk it, it oppresses her stomach.

* This parenthesis refers to a person who, when in good health, had generally great redness of the cheeks, which was, therefore, homœopathically removed, as aconite almost always produces heat of the cheeks.

1 Immediate local effect.

150. (She will not eat anything.)

Nausea, vomiting, thirst, general heat and profuse sweat with diuresis. [GREDING, l. c.]

She vomits lumbrici. [GREDING, l. c.]

Vomiting of green bile (aft. 1 h.). [MATTHIOLI, l. c.]

Vomiting of mucus mixed with blood for three or four successive days. [GREDING, l. c.]

155. Vomiting of blood. [GREDING, l. c.]

Qualmish, sick in the scrobiculus cordis, worse when sitting, going off almost when walking (immediately after taking it). [*Stf. Gss.*]

Disgust and sinking, qualmish feeling (aft. ¼ h.).

Long-continued disgust and anorexia.

Inclination to vomit on walking in the open air.

160. Inclination to vomit at first in the scrobiculus cordis, then beneath the sternum, lastly in the throat, without flow of saliva.

Inclination to vomit, just as if he had eaten something disgustingly sweet or greasy (aft. 1 h.).

Profuse sweat after vomiting bloody mucus. [GREDING, l. c.]

Vomiting, followed by violent thirst. [MORAEUS,[1] in *Konigl. Vetensk. Acad. Handl.*, 1739, p. 41]

Vomiting, artificially excited, only temporarily restored the patient from his state of syncope. [BACON, l. c.]

165. Vomiting with anxiety. [RICHARD, l. c.]

Inclination to vomit with severe diarrhœa. [GREDING, l. c.]

Hiccup.[2] [GREDING, l. c.]

In the morning, hiccup.[2] [GREDING, l. c.]

In the morning, long-continued hiccup.[2] [GREDING, l. c.]

170. (Hiccup after eating and drinking.)

Aching pain in the scrobiculus cordis, which increased to tightness of the chest (aft. 2½ h.).

In the scrobiculus cordis pressure as from a stone lying there, which soon afterwards extended to the back, with a squeezing-together sensation, as if she had injured herself by a strain; as if stiff. [*Stf. Gss.*]

Cardialgia. [RODDER,* in *Alberti's Jurisprud. Med.*, tom. vi, p. 724.]

Aching pain in the scrobiculus cordis when sitting, walking, and standing. [*Ar.*]

175. Pain in the scrobiculus cordis, as if it were swollen internally, with loss of appetite and attacks of dyspnœa.

Pressive pain in the stomach, like a weight (aft. 1½ h.).

Pressive pain like a weight in the hypochondria (aft. 1½ h.).

Tensive pressive pain, as from fulness or a weight pressing in the stomach and hypochondria (aft. 1½ h.).

* All the symptoms observed by RODDER were caused by applying the juice to a wound.

1 Poisoning of two adults.

2 See note to S. 77.

Contractive sensation in the stomach as from an astringent.

180. Sensation of violent constriction in the hypochondria.

Aching pain in the stomach. [*Hbg.*]

Along with repeated vomiting and frequent stools he always complains that he feels as if a cold stone lay in the stomach. [RICHARD, l. c.]

Drawing-in of the navel, especially in the morning when fasting.

A burning in the umbilical region.

185. Burning sensation in the umbilical region, which ran rapidly over her, and extended the scrobiculus cordis, with a sensation of anxious beating and shooting there ; after some time a rigor ran all over the body, with cessation of the hot feeling and of the painful sensation in the umbilical region (aft. 1½ h.). [*Stf. Gss.*]

Pinching pain in the umbilical region. [*Sft. Gss.*]

Compression of the navel ; immediately afterwards intermiting aching in the navel, like jerks. [*Stf. Gss.*]

Griping and clawing in the umbilical region. [*Stf. Gss.*]

Above the navel to the left a painless sensation, as of something cold (a cold finger) forcing itself from within outwards. [*Stf. Gss.*]

190. Aching in the region of the liver, whereby the respiration is impeded, immediately thereafter (pinching ?) bellyache in the supra-umbilical region.

Jaundice.

From both sides towards the navel, drawing pains in the abdomen, which are also produced by bending the abdomen together.

The epigastrium and hypochondria are occupied by a tense, painful swelling. [RICHARD, l. c.]

Swollen, distended abdomen, like ascites. [RICHARD,—MATTHIOLI, l. c.]

195. Violent jerks (blows) in the hepatic region that take away the breath. [*Hbg.*]

Some hours earlier than usual a hard stool, for which he must strain much.

Rolling and rumbling in the abdomen, with feeling of rawness. [*Stf. Gss.*]

Rolling and rumbling in the abdomen all night.

A sort of fermenting rumbling in the abdomen.

200. In the morning, in bed, he cries out and does not know how to compose himself for intolerable (cutting) pain in the belly, and he tosses about in bed (aft. 16 h.).

Colicky, stretching, tensive, and aching pain in the belly, as from flatulence.

On laughing loud a sharp stitch in the right side below the ribs. [*Stf. Gss.*]

On inspiring dull stitches in the left side below the ribs. [*Stf. Gss.*]

Drawing from the left side of the hypochondrium towards the back ; the side of the abdomen is painful when pressed upon. [*Stf. Gss.*]

205. **Flatulent colic in the hypogastrium as if he had taken a flatus-producing purgative,**

Very hot flatus (aft. 9 h.).

With a feeling as if only flatus were passing, unexpected discharge of thin fæces (aft. 4 h.).

Hard stool, attended with **pressing.** [*Hbg.*]

Purging. [STOERCK, l. c.]

210. Sometimes before, sometimes after the diarrhœa, nausea and perspiration. [GREDING, l. c.]

Soft, small stool, accompanied with tenesmus, from three to five per diem.

White stool.

White stool and red urine.

Watery diarrhœa.

215. The hypogastrium is painfully sensitive to touch.

Weakness of the bowels such as is apt to arise from abuse of purgatives.

Pain in the rectum (aft. 1 h.).

Shooting and aching in the anus.

Transient paralysis of the anus, involuntary evacuation.

220. Fluent hæmorrhoids.

During the diarrhœa copious flow of urine and moderate perspiration. [GREDING, l. c.]

Pressure on the bladder, with retention of urine.[1] [GREDING, l. c.]

Suppression of urine, with needle-pricks in the renal region. [RICHARD, l. c.]

Diuresis. [GREDING, l. c.]

225. Diuresis, with profuse perspiration and frequent watery diarrhœa, with bellyache. [GREDING, l. c.]

Diuresis and along with it constant perspiration. [GREDING, l. c.]

Copious diuresis. [STOERCK, l. c.]

Diuresis, with distortion of the eyes and spasmodic contraction of the feet.[2] [GREDING, l. c.]

On passing urine a slight sensation (of splashing) in the vesical region. [*Stf. Gss.*]

230. Painful urging to urinate ; she must make water very frequently, because the bladder fills rapidly with a quantity of urine as clear as water. [*Stf. Gss.*]

Urging to urinate on touching the abdomen.

Urine passed with difficulty (dysuria) (aft. 12, 18 h.).

Anxious urging to urinate (aft. 4 h.).

Urging to urinate ; the urine passed in unusually small quantity, not without difficulty, as if it would not come away properly but, without pain ; at the same time slight pinching in the umbilical region (from smelling the tincture). [*Stf. Gss.*]

235. Copious discharge of urine, which, on standing, deposits blood.

Transient paralysis of the neck of the bladder, involuntary discharge of urine.

Burning in the neck of the bladder when not urinating.

Pain of the bladder when walking (aft. 4 h.).

---

1 This patient's bladder was previously unhealthy.

2 See note to S. 77.

Tenesmus of the neck of the bladder (aft. 4 h.).

240. Brown urine passed with burning, afterwards depositing brick-coloured sediment.

On walking, pains in the loins like labour-pains.

Itching on the prepuce, relieved by rubbing, but soon returning (aft. 3 d.). [*We.*]

Shooting and pinching pain in the glans penis when urinating.

Simple pain in the testicles, like that which remains after being squeezed (aft. 2 h.).

245. Slight, not disagreeable creeping in the genitals. [*Stf. Gss.*]

He has amorous fits. [*Stf. Gss.*]

(Very much increased sexual desire, rapid alternating with relaxation.). [*Stf. Gss.*]

Diminished sexual desire.

Metrorrhagia.

250. The menses that had ceased the day before taking the drug, break out again copiously immediately (aft. $\frac{1}{4}$ h.). [*Stf. Gss.*]

Copious, viscid, yellowish leucorrhœa.[1] [Stoerck, l. c.]

Fury on the occurrence of the menses.[2] [Greding, l. c.]

* * *

Anxiety with fear of suffocation. [Rodder, l. c.]

Tightness of the chest. [Richard, l. c.]

255. Frequent violent sneezing, with pain in the abdomen. [*Stf. Gss.*]

Cannot sneeze thoroughly on account of pain in the left costal region. [*Stf. Gss.*]

Extreme sensitiveness of the olfactory nerves; disagreeable smells have a great effect on her.

Attacks of catarrh and coryza (between 8 and 12 h.).

Morning hoarseness (aft. 8 h.).

260. Attack of coryza. [Greding, l. c.]

Tussiculation from a tickle at the upper part of the larynx (immediately).

Short cough.

(Cough during the heat of the body.)

Cough after drinking.

265. Severe cough, immediately, from a little tobacco-smoke (in a person accustomed to tobacco-smoking).

He (a habitual smoker) cannot smoke, without constantly clearing his throat and coughing, either because the epiglottis allows the smoke to penetrate into the wind-pipe or because the larynx has become too sensitive (aft. 6 h.).

After midnight, every half hour, a short cough (kechekeh) from a tickle in the larynx; the more he tries to suppress it, the more frequent and the worse it was.

Hæmoptysis.

Dry cough.[3] [Greding, l. c.]

---

1 In a woman treated for "a considerable swelling in the left iliac region." This discharge coincided with the diminution and disappearance of the swelling.

2 In a maniac.

3 The patient had had this cough previously.

270. Short respiration in sleep, after midnight.

Interrupted respiration through nose, especially during sleep.

Fœtid breath.

Noisy, loud respiration, with open mouth.

Tightness of the chest, with strong, loud respiration.

275. Morbid condition (attacks of paralysis ?) of the epiglottis ; food and drink are apt to get into the wind-pipe when swallowing, so that they threaten suffocation and excite coughing ; he is apt to swallow the wrong way.

He is apt to choke on swallowing the saliva. [*Stf. Gss.*]

Anxtiety in the thoracic cavity, and oppression on the right half of the chest, then in the whole chest. [*Stf. Gss.*]

Squeezing together of the chest on the right side near the sternum ; a kind of tightness of the chest. [*Stf. Gss.*]

He feels as if the chest were contracted. [*Stf. Gss.*]

280. Compression of the chest in the region of the heart. [*Stf. Gss.*]

Anxiety that impedes respiration, with warm sweat on the forehead.

Aching pain in the chest, which is somewhat relieved by bending the upper part of the body backwards, but returns immediately on resuming the erect position (aft. 12 h.). [*We.*]

Contractive pain in the chest, as if the ribs on both sides were drawn towards one another. [*Ar.*]

He feels a weight in the chest ; it is as if the whole chest were compressed from all sides. [*We.*]

285. Painful stitches in the right side of the chest, in the region of the lowest rib, which extended towards the sacrum (aft. 10 h.). [*We.*]

Shooting, aching pain on the right side of the sternum. [*We.*]

Pinching, digging pain in the right side of the chest, between the third and fourth ribs, unaltered by anything, until it disappears of itself. [*Ar.*]

In the left side of the chest near the axilla, oppressive, obtuse stitches. [*Stf. Gss.*]

Stitches in the chest (on breathing). [*Stf. Gss.*]

290. At every breath, shooting from the lowest rib on the right side extending to the apex of the scapula, through the middle of the chest, with complaining disposition.

Shooting in the right side, with complaining lachrymose disposition.

Single, large stitches in the side through to the back (aft. 24 h.).

Pain in the chest, like a shooting, interrupting the breathing.

With anxiety and peevishness, a shooting in the side of the chest, followed by throbbing in the side of the chest, then aching headache.

295. A burning, fine shooting pain in the chest.

Sensation as if the wind-pipe under the sternum had gone asleep and were numb (aft. 8 h.).

By touching very much increased pain, as from a bruise, in the lowest rib, about which the patient makes much ado and complains.

On the middle of the sternum, pain as if bruised (also increased by external touch).

Slow blows in the cardiac region directed towards the outside of the chest. [*Stf. Gss.*]

300. **Squeezing pain in the chest.**

Aching, squeezing pain in the chest, under the sternum.

Shooting, boring, digging pain in the left side of the chest between the fourth and sixth ribs, for ten minutes. [*Ar.*]

Aching, tightening pain in the side of the chest.

A creeping pain in the chest.

305. A crawling in the chest as from beetles.

(Increase of milk in the breasts.)

Lumbar pain. [Greding, l. c.]

Aching pain in the sacrum on the left side [*Hbg.*]

Burning, corrosive pains near the dorsal vertebræ in the right side. [*We.*]

310. **Violent, shooting, digging pain** all down the left side of the spine to the sacrum, which was so much increased by inspiration that tears came repeatedly into the eyes, for four hours. [*Ar.*]

On moving painful stiffness of the sacral and hip-joints ; he is as if paralysed in the sacrum (aft. 2 h.).

Pain as if bruised in the articulation of the lowest lumbar vertebra with the sacrum ; the sacrum feels hacked off.

Tensive, aching pain in the lumbar vertebræ, or as if from a bruise ; at the same time pain in abdomen as from flatulent colic.

Pain as if bruised from the sacrum through the back up to the nape (aft. 4 h.).

315. Crawling pain in the spine as from beetles.

A cutting round from the spine to the abdomen, over the left hip, in a circle.

On the left side near the sacrum a painful boring.

A digging, boring pain from the right scapula forwards to the chest, that was increased by inspiring, but not by expiring, but never ceased, for twelve minutes.

In the nape a pain as if the flesh were detached, with a feeling as if the nape had no firmness, and as if the head would fall forwards in consequence ; on moving the head shooting in the nape. [*Stf. Gss.*]

320. **Rheumatic pain in the nape only observed on moving the neck** (between the 5th and 9th h.).

Fine shooting externally on the neck.

Single shoots in the nape on both sides. [*Rkt.*]

Aching pain in the left cervical vertebra. [*We.*]

A pain in the neck pressing inwards towards the trachea, like a pressure with the point of the finger into the neck. [*Ar.*]

325. Pain in the left shoulder-joint. [*Hbg.*]

Some flying stitches in the left shoulder. [*Stf. Gss.*]

The shoulder hurts her, and tends to sink down. [*Stf. Gss.*]

A swelling in the muscles of the shoulder, with violent pains as if bruised when touched (aft. 4 h.).

Tearing pain from the shoulder down into the arm as far as the wrist, and even the fingers, almost only on every movement ; during the pain the hand is blue (aft. 1, 14 h.).

330. After sleeping, a pain on moving in the shoulder (and hip) joint as from being crushed, or as if the bed had been too hard.

Single stitches in the middle of the right upper arm on its anterior aspect, when at rest, unaffected by motion and by pressing on it. [*Ar.*]

Sudden drawing, shooting pain in the posterior part of the right upper arm. [*Ar.*]

Trembling of the arms and hands (immediately). [*Hbg.*]

Pain in the arm and fingers.[1] [RODDER, l. c.]

335. A numbness and paralysis in the left arm (and leg), so that he can scarcely move the hand.[2] [MATTHIOLI, l. c.]

His arms are as if bruised and sink powerlessly down. [*Stf. Gss.*]

Chilliness and insensibility of the arms.

Pain on the forearm, as from a severe blow. [*Stf. Gss.*]

Drawing, shooting pain in the bone of the forearm, excitable by movement.

340. Feeling of heaviness in the arms, from the elbow to the fingers; she would like to let them sink down; with feeling of being asleep in the fingers when she grasps anything. [*Stf. Gss.*]

In the elbow-joints drawing pain. [*Stf. Gss.*]

Paralytic sensation in the right forearm and hand (when writing), which went off on stronger movement, but soon returned when writing and when at rest, but slighter. [*Ar.*]

Cramp-like pain in the whole left forearm, not relieved by anything. [*Ar.*]

Drawing, tearing pain in the external side of the right forearm. [*Ar.*]

345. Undulating, tearing pain in the upper end of the left forearm. [*Ar.*]

Twitching, drawing pain in the lower end of the inner surface of the left forearm over the wrist to the palm. [*Ar.*]

Drawing, paralytic pain in the right wrist-joint. [*We.*]

Morbid contractive pain in the left palm, so that he can hardly extend the fingers. [*Ar.*]

Tearing pain in the wrist.

350. One hand becomes icy cold and insensible, as if numb (aft. 2 h.).

Cool sweat on the palms.

Cramp-pain in the right hand. [*We.*]

Swelling of the hands, with frequent cough,[3] with good appetite. [GREDING, l. c.]

On bending the hand up and down a trembling movement in the wrist-joint. [*Rkt.*]

355. Cramp-like pain with fine stitches in the right hand, going off by moving it. [*Ar.*]

Some pulsating pricks in the right palm, as with a sharp needle. [*Ar.*]

Cutting, aching pain in the side of the right index towards the middle finger, when moving and when at rest. [*Ar.*]

---

1. Local effect. See S. 387.
2. With stupor.
3. This is the cough mentioned in note to S. 269.

Painful drawing in the left thumb. [*We.*]

Twitching pains in the right thumb. [*Ar.*]

360. When she bends the fingers down to the wrist, immediately violent stitches in the elbow-joints down to the wrist, on the external aspect of the arm. [*Stf. Gss.*]

Paralytic pain in the thumbs. [*Stf. Gss.*]

Painful movement of the right thumb-joint, as if sprained.

Creeping pain in the fingers.

Creeping in the fingers, also when writing. [*Hbg.*]

365. Tensive pressure in the thighs as from a tightly-drawn bandage, with great exhaustion, when walking. [*Rkt.*]

After sleeping, a pain, on moving, in the hip (and shoulder) joint as from being crushed, or as if the bed had been too hard.

In the head of the femur of the left leg drawing pain, when standing or sitting, still more when walking. [*Stf. Gss.*]

Fine needle-pricks in the muscles of the thigh. [*Stf. Gss.*]

After sitting, an almost paralytic weakness in the thighs and legs.

370. Powerlessness in the head of the femur, or inability to walk, on account of an indescribable, intolerable pain, almost as if the head of the femur were crushed, which sometimes declines, sometimes increases, and occurs after lying and sleep (aft. 5 h.).

Tottering walk, owing to powerlessness and pain in the head of the femur.

A numbness, like paralysis. in the left leg (and arm). [MATTHIOLI, l. c.]

Tearing pain upwards on the outer ankle of the left foot (aft. 14 h.). [*Ar.*]

Want of firmness and unsteadiness in the knees ; the knees totter on standing and walking.

375. Want of firmness of the knees, especially of one of them ; it gives way when walking (immediately and aft. 1 h.).

Heaviness of the feet (immediately).

Pains in the ankle-joints, with despairing thoughts and reflections on death.

The legs in their lower parts and the feet are as if numb and gone asleep. [*Stf. Gss.*]

Deep, slow stitch over the right knee. [*Stf. Gss.*]

380. Painful drawing in the leg from the knee to the heel and back again. [*Stf. Gss.*]

Twitching tearing on the internal side of the knees. [*Stf. Gss.*]

Paralytic drawing in the right leg and the tendo Achillis to the heel. [*Stf. Gss.*]

Coldness of the feet up to the ankles, with perspiration of the toes and soles.

Sensation on the ankles as if they were constricted by a bandage, in the morning.

385. Horrible pain in the ankles, relieved by external compression (aft. 7 h.).

Coldness of the feet, especially of the toes. [*Rkt.*]

Swelling of the part (to which the juice has been applied) and acute inflammation, followed by excessive suppuration. [RODDER, l. c.]

Sensation of tingling and burning goes gradually through the whole body, especially through the arms and legs. [BACON, l. c.]

Itching all over the body, especially on the genitals[1] [STOERCK, l. c.]

390. Fine needle-pricks here and there on the body. [*Stf. Gss.*]

Single, long-continued stitches here and there, mingled with sore feeling, at length ending in pure sore pain.

Formication, itching, and desquamation of the skin, especially on the affected parts.

Flea-bite-like spots on the hands, face, &c.

Reddish pustules filled with acrid fluid.[1] [STOERCK, l. c.]

395. Broad, red, itching pimples all over the body.[1] [STOERCK, l. c.]

The whole body is painful to the touch; the child will not allow itself to be taken hold of; it whines.

Feeling as if she was just recovering from a serious disease, and had risen from a sick-bed (aft. 6, 12 h.).

Paralytic sensation and bruisedness in the arms and legs, with violent trembling all over the body, especially of the extremities, owing to which he can hardly walk or step; at the same time excessively pale face, dilated pupils, faintness, palpitation of the heart, cold sweat on the back and bursting headache in the temples—soon followed by burning heat in the face, with a feeling of tension and redness of face, sleepiness (after dinner) (aft. 46 h.) (secondary effect?). [*Stf. Gss.*]

The paralysis on the left side soon disappeared, and quickly went into the right side.[2] [MATTHIOLI, l. c.]

400. After the cessation of the madness, pain in the stomach, head, jaws, chest, and now in one now in another joint. [RICHARD, l. c.]

Shaking of the limbs.[3] [GREDING, l. c.]

In the evening sudden cry, grinding of the teeth, then through long hiccup stiff immobility like a statue (catalepsy)[3] [GREDING, l. c.]

Gradually all parts of the body become black, the whole trunk swells, the eyes protrude from the head, the tongue hangs out of the mouth. [PET. DE ABANO,[4] *de Venenis* Cap. 30.]

All the joints are painful (aft. 7 h.).[5] [RICHARD, l. c.]

405. Great weakness of the joints, especially of the knee- and ankle-joints, with twitching in the tendons, so that he can scarcely walk. [BACON, l. c.]

Painfulness all over the body, with increased weakness.[6] [GREDING, l. c.]

Weakness and laxity of the ligaments of all the joints. (aft. 46 h.).

---

1 In cases of neuralgic pain in the extremities. As these cutaneous symptoms appeared the pains subsided.

2 See S. 335 and note.

3 See note to S. 77.

4 General statement of effects of poisoning by A.

5 See S. 400.

6 Ending in death.

Painless cracking of all the joints, particularly of the knees.

Weariness in the limbs, especially in the feet, with constant sleepiness and crossness.

410. In the morning, on waking, such great weariness, that he did not like to get out of bed, which, however, went off after getting up.

He complains of weariness of the whole body, great weakness and pain in the heart (aft. 3 h.). [MATTHIOLI, l. c.]

Sinking of the strength. [BACON, l. c.]

Progressive sinking of the strength. [EBERH. GMELIN,[1] *Nov. Acta Nat. Cur.*, vi, p. 394.]

Fainting. [PET. DE ABANO, l. c.—RODDER, l. c.]

415. Pulse intermitting and irregular, two or three beats followed rapidly in succession, and then came a pause of no long duration. [BACON, l. c.]

Syncope.

In the open air the head is free and all the symptoms ameliorated. [*Stf. Gss.*]

Disinclined for movement, she prefers to sit. [*Stf. Gss.*]

Urgent desire to lie down. [BACON, l. c.]

420. She must lie down (between the 3rd and 5th h.).

Irresistible inclination to lie down (from 2 to 5 h.).

Sleepiness and laziness ; even when walking uncommon sleepiness. [*Hbg.*]

(Interrupted yawning ; she cannot yawn perfectly.)

Yawns, often without being sleepy. [*Stf. Gss.*]

425. Yawning and stretching. [*Stf. Gss.*]

Sleepiness, sleep (aft. 2 h.).

In the afternoon great sleepiness, the eyes close, but he easily wakes at a slight noise, but always fails asleep again. [*Stf. Gss.*]

After eating unusual sleepiness. [*Stf Gss.*]

Light sleep (from 1 to 5 h.).

430. Sleeplessness (in the 4th h.).

Sleep full of dreams ; confused, vivid dreams. [*Stf. Gss.*]

He cannot lie on the right side, nor on the back ; he turns about in bed with pains, from one side to the other.

In the morning he lies in sleep on his back, the left hand opened laid under his occiput.

He sleeps sitting with head bent forward.

435. Slow respiration in sleep.

(Inspiration with double jerk, like the butting of a goat, in sleep.)

Long dreams, with anxiety in the chest, that impeded breathing, so that he woke up in consequence (nightmare).

Dreams during which he talked much.

She has vexatious dreams.

440. He starts in affright, makes many movements, and speaks in his sleep.

She starts up in sleep and says some one is seizing hold of her.

---

1 Effect of A. when given to patients for a long time.

He is delirious while awake, jumps out of bed, and thinks he is driving sheep (aft. 14 h.).

In the evening after lying down, and by day when sitting he has waking dreams, and has delutions as though he were far away from home.

Towards morning he has a very vivid dream, which gives him a correct explanation of a circumstance that was an inexplicable riddle to him when awake (aft. 20 h.).

445. He dreams half the night about a single subject, and is also occupied with it alone several hours after waking, so that nothing besides this subject possesses his mind (like the fixed idea of an insane person), which is very annoying to him and bothers him.

At night anxious dreams, and frequent waking in a fright. [*Rkt.*]

Restless night. [GREDING, l. c.]

Inability to keep awake. [MORAEUS, l. c.]

Quiet sleep for 4 or 5 hours.[1] [BACON, l. c.]

450. Desire for cold water. [MATTHIOLI, l. c.]

Feverish pulse, frequently intermitting. [RICHARD, l. c.]

Sensation as if all the blood-vessels grew cold. [MATTHIOLI, l. c.]

Sensation as if the circulation in all the blood-vessels was impeded. [BACON, l. c.]

He lies quiet, but is cold and shivers, and wishes to be covered with much bed-clothes. [BACON, l c.]

455. In the morning on waking dizzy in the head.

In the morning on waking, he feels as if he had fetid breath.

In the evening on lying down, shivering.

Rigor and frequent yawning, in the morning after rising [*Stf. Gss.*]

Anxious chilliness (aft. 3 h.).

460. Chill on the slightest movement (aft. 10 h.).

Chilliness in the abdomen. [*Stf. Gss.*]

A coldness runs continually up her arms and legs; in her face also she has a chill. [*Stf. Gss.*]

A shiver runs through her from below up into the chest. [*Stf. Gss.*]

She is chilly and shivers. [*Stf. Gss.*]

465. Rigor over back and arms. [*Stf. Gss.*]

Attack of faintness with chilliness.

At first coldness, rigor and paleness of the finger-tips, then in the fingers, afterwards sensation of cramp in the soles and calves, finally chill in the forehead (aft. $\frac{1}{4}$ h.)

Coldness all over the body.

Fever : **Chill of the whole body, with hot forehead, hot ear-lobes, and internal dry heat.**

470. Fever : coldness with stiffness of the whole body, redness and heat of one cheek, coldness and paleness of the other, with open,

---

1 Symptom of convalescence.

staring eyes, and contracted pupils, which only dilate slightly and slowly in the dark.

Towards evening, chill and coldness of hands and feet, then sickness in the middle of the sternum, which continues even when taking food that tastes well, though there is neither appetite nor dislike for it; after eating the sickness goes off, followed by heat of face, accompanied by sad despairing thoughts.

Frequent attacks (about every other hour), for a quarter of an hour at time, of the most extreme weakness and insensibility, so that he can move neither hands nor feet, nor sit up in bed, nor yet feel his former pain, nor see, hear, or speak aloud; the legs at the same time are extended (aft. a few h.).

Alternate attacks (aft. 3, 4, 6 h.): either along with redness of the cheeks, silly gaiety with sensation of heat all over the body, and headache on moving the eyes upwards and sideways;

Or, along with redness of cheeks and heat of head, shuddering all over the body, with proper taste in mouth;

475. Or, along with redness of cheeks, shivering, with weeping, accompanied by aching headache;

Or, along with redness of cheeks, an obstinate, contrary disposition, burning in the umbilical region, and aching pain in head.

Extreme redness of cheeks, with a peevish, complaining, lachrymose disposition (aft 3 h.).

Towards evening burning heat in head and face, with redness of cheeks and outpressing headache; at the same time rigor all over the body with thirst (aft. 14 h.). [*Stf. Gss.*]

Towards evening, dry heat in face with anxiety.

480. Hot on the head, with forehead hot to the touch, and rigor of the rest of the body, on the slightest movement.

Feeling of heat, first in the hands, then in the whole body, even in the chest, without perceptible external heat (aft. 4 h.).

Several times heat ran over his back. [*Stf. Gss.*]

(Heat with throwing off the clothes.)

General heat with thirst.

485. During the heat moderate thirst for beer.

(She drinks little in the heat and yet has dry lips.)

(In the heat the cough is troublesome)

(Great heat from 10 p.m. until after midnight, with short breath; she wished to cough but could not, speaking also was difficult for her; at the same time extreme restlessness and crying out from pains in the hands, feet, abdomen, and sacrum; she stamped her feet and would not allow any one to touch her.)

Perspiration with febrile rigor (aft. 3 h.).

490. **Slight perspiration all over the body.**

Sour-smelling perspiration all over the body.

Perspiration of weakness.

Slight warmth with moderate perspiration.[1] [BACON, l. c.]

1 Reaction from S. 454.

Along with profuse perspiration frequent micturition. [GREDING, l. c.]

495. Along with profuse perspiration, diarrhœa and increased flow of urine. [GREDING, l c.]

Great internal heat with thirst. [RODDER, l. c.]

Transpiration and sweat all over the body. [STOERCK, l. c.]

(Towards noon) perspiration. [GREDING, l. c.]

Profuse perspiration without exhaustion. [GREDING, l. c.]

500. Along with bold speech and sparkling eyes, cold sweat stands on the forehead, and the pulse is almost imperceptible. [MATTHIOLI, l. c.]

Nocturnal furious delirium; he cannot be kept in bed; in the morning very profuse sweat. [DURR,[1] in *Hufel. Journ.*, ix, 4, p. 108.]

He does everything in a hurry, and runs about the house. [HELMONT, l. c.]

Transient insanity.[2] [MORAEUS, l. c.]

Morose, inclined for nothing, depressed spirits, even when walking. [*Hbg.*]

505. Morose, as though she had no life in her (aft. 2 h.). [*Stf. Gss.*]

Becomes gay and inclined to sing and dance (aft. ½ h.). [*Stf. Gss.*]

More gay and excited than usual (the first h.).

Alternate attacks of opposite states of humour.[3] [MATTHIOLI, l. c.]

Sometimes he is quite rational, sometimes he talks nonsense. [MATTHIOLI, l. c.]

510. Sometimes he despairs of his recovery, sometimes he is full of hope. [MATTHIOLI, l. c.]

After vomiting, immediate revival of hope.[4] [RICHARD, l. c.]

Trembling and tendency to palpitation of the heart.

Palpitation of the heart and anxiety, and increased heat of the body, especially in the face. [*Stf. Gss.*]

Palpitation of the heart with great anxiety; oppression of the breathing and great weariness in all the limbs; it rises from thence into the head, and she is as if stupified from flying redness in the face. [*Stf. Gss.*]

515. Anxiety and peevishness, with fine shooting in the side of the chest; then beating in the scrobiculus cordis and then aching pain in the head.

Inconsolable anxiety and piteous howling, with complaints and reproaches about (often trifling) **evils** (aft. 5 h.).

Piteous, anxious complaints, with cowardly fears, despair, loud whining weeping, bitter complaints and reproaches.

Fear lest he should fall.

Anthropophobia (aft. 3 h.).

520. He is in a reverie, and sits buried in thought.

---

1 Effects of a mixture of A. and antimonial wine.

2 Not found in Moraeus' narrative.

3 The two following symptoms, and S. 536, are given as instances of this.

4 Mental effect of vomiting after the antidote had been given.

Lucid vision : he says, now my beloved (70 miles away) must have sung the difficult passage* that I was just singing.

Solicitude, grief.

The slightest noise is intolerable to him (aft. ½ h.).

Music is intolerable to her ; it goes through every limb ; she becomes quite melancholy (aft. 24 h.).

525. **Excessive tendency to be startled** (aft. ¼ h.).

He takes every joke in bad part (aft. 3 h.).

She is extremely disposed to be cross (aft. ½ h.).

She becomes quarrelsome.

She makes reproaches.

530. Quarrelsomeness, alternating from hour to hour with silly insanity —he chatters childish nonsense, and is extravagantly merry.

Angry disposition.

Obstinacy.

Misanthropy.

Composed, staid, although not cheerful humour (secondary and curative action) (aft. 8 h.).

535. Lively power of imagination.

Sometimes he appears to weep, sometimes he trills. [MATTHIOLI, l. c.]

Insane tricks. [RICHARD, l. c.]

Dread of impending death. [RICHARD, l. c.]

Mortal anxiety recurring from time to time. [MATTHIOLI, l. c.]

540. **Lamentable fears of impending death** (from 2 to 12 h.).

Fear of some misfortune happening to him.

* The passage from Beethoven : "Ah ! perfido !" she, although previously dangerously ill, had this day sung at a concert, particularly well, only five hours before her betrothal, who was particularly susceptible to mesmerism.

AMBRA GRISEA.[1]

(*Ambergris*, sometimes *Ambra ambrosiaca*, L.)

This substance, often adulterated on account of its high price, we can hope to get genuine only in first-class drug stores. The true ambergris, developed in the intestines of the sperm whale, as was proved by SCHWEDJAUR, and probably a fatty excretion from its gall-bladder, is obtained of best quality from the sea, especially after stormy weather, off the coasts of Madagascar and Sumatra. It consists of small, rough, opaque masses, which are lighter than water, of spongy consistence, and can easily be broken up into rough, uneven pieces, externally of a brownish-grey colour, internally permeated by yellowish, reddish, and blackish fibres intermingled with whitish, very odorous points, somewhat greasy to the touch, and of faint but very refreshing fragrance.

By the warmth of the fingers it becomes soft as wax, by the heat of boiling water its melts into oil, at the same time exhales a strong, very agreeable fragrance, and on heated metal burns quite away. On applying a light to it it quickly takes fire, and burns with a bright flame. Alcohol dissolves it very sparingly, but sulphuric ether dissolves it almost completely, and on adding alcohol a white wax-like substance is thrown down. Its feeble odour is much increased by this solution, as also by triturating it with other substances.

A grain of such genuine ambergris is triturated for an hour with 100 grains of milk-sugar in a porcelain mortar (every 10 minutes divided between 6 minutes of trituration and 4 minutes of scraping). Of this powder a grain is again triturated with another 100 grains of milk-sugar for an equal length of time, and in the same manner; and, lastly, of this powder so obtained one grain is again triturated with a similar quantity of milk-sugar, in the same manner, and also for an hour. This furnishes a potentized millionth attenuation of ambergris, a small portion of a grain of which is not only sufficient for a dose for most homœopathic purposes, but is often found to be quite too powerful; in which case its effects may be moderated by several small doses of camphor, but in many cases, according to the symptoms developed, bv nux vomica, and in rarer cases by pulsatilla.

The duration of the action of such a dose is, in chronic cases, at least three weeks.

(The symptoms indicated by the letters *Gff.* were observed by the State-councillor Freiherr VON GERSDORFF.).

[None of the symptoms are derived from old-school sources. Ambra first appears among Hahnemann's medicines in the 2nd edition.]

1 From vol. vi, 2nd edit., 1827.

AMBRA GRISEA.

Great vertigo.

Extraordinary, even dangerous vertigo.

Vertigo while walking in the open air, in the forenoon and afternoon.

On account of vertigo and weak feeling in the stomach she must lie down (afternoon, aft. 72 h.).

5. He is always as if in a dream.

He cannot think of anything properly; he is as if stupid (the first 24 h.).

Bad memory; the thinking power is very feeble; he must read everything three or four times over, and even then cannot take it in.

Great weakness in the head, with vertigo (aft. 48 h.).

Weakness in the head, and a kind of chill in it.

10. Every morning headache, like emptiness, as if he had been drinking over night.

Confusion in the occiput. [*Gff.*]

Tension in the head, making him stupid.

Squeezing headache from both temples. [*Gff.*]

Squeezing confusion of the head. [*Gff.*]

15. Aching confusion in the head, immediately after eating, especially when moving.

Pressure in the forehead (with anxiety lest he should go mad) (aft. 48 h.).

Aching pain in the forehead. [*Gff*]

Aching pain in occiput and nape.

Every other day down-pressing pain in the forehead and top of the head, with heat in head and burning in the eyes, with pale face from the morning onwards, only worse in the afternoon.

20. Rush of blood to the head for two days.

(Painless) feeling of pressure on the top of the head and heaviness of the head, in the evening (aft. 36 h.).

Aching in the head combined with shooting.

Aching pain on a small spot at the occiput.

Aching pain on the left frontal protuberance.

25. Aching drawing from the nape upwards and through the head to the front, whilst pressure remains on the occiput. [*Gff.*]

Tearing pressure in the whole occiput, also to the crown and in the forehead. [*Gff.*]

Transient tearing through the head. [*Gff.*]

A drawing hither and thither, or tearing in the head.

On the left side of the occiput, towards the nape and behind the ear, tearing.

30. Tearing in the left temple up to the top of the head, on the right frontal protuberance and **behind the left ear.** [*Gff.*]

Tearing headache in the forehead extending into the upper part of the face. [*Gff.*]

Very painful tearing above on the crown and as if in the whole upper half of the brain, with pale face and coldness of the left hand. [*Gff.*]

(Twitching in the head.)

Above the left temple, a stitch in the head (aft. 3 h.). [*Gff.*]

35. In the evening, several very sharp stitches upwards towards the occiput.

On exertion, a shooting and cutting headache ; he feels it at every step ; better when lying.

External headache ; also, in the nape and neck, pain as from a sprain, with tenderness to touch, the whole day (aft. 12 d.).

Headache as if catarrh would come on, sometimes more, sometimes less, and persistent. [*Gff.*]

40. On the right side of the head, a part where the hair is painful as if sore when touched. [*Gff.*]

A painful spot on the occiput.

Roaring about the temples.

The hair of the head falls out (aft. 24 h.).

Aching, tearing headache, especially over and on the head. [*Gff.*]

45. Pressure on the left eyebrow. [*Gff.*]

Pressure on the eyes, as if they lay deep (with tearing headache above from the forehead downwards, or from the ear through the occiput) (aft. 3 h.). [*Gff.*]

Short, violent pressure just above the nose, in the forehead, in frequent fits, which changes into tearing, and leaves behind it confusion in the occiput. [*Gff.*]

A painful pimple on the forehead. [*Gff.*]

A red papule on the middle of the forehead, close to the hair, touching it causes a sore pain, not suppurating. [*Gff.*]

50. In the eye, pressure and smarting, as if dust had got in it. [*Gff.*]

Smarting in the eyes and lachrymation.

Pressure on the eyes, which are opened with difficulty, and **pain in them as if they had been too tightly shut,** especially in the morning. [*Gff.*]

Distended blood-vessels in the white of the eye. [*Gff.*]

Tearing or short rends in and around the right eye. [*Gff.*]

55. Burning pain in the right eye (aft. 10 h.).

Burning in the eyelids.

Itching on the eyelid, as if it would inflame to a stye.

Around the eyes, intolerable itching tickling.

Dim vision, as if through a fog (aft. some h.).

60. Very dark before the eyes (aft. 3 d.).

Spasmodic trembling in the facial muscles.

In the evening, in bed, spasmodic twitchings in the face.

Flying heat in the face.

Jaundiced face.

65. Eruption of pimples on the face, without sensation.

Gnawing formicating itching in the face.

Tearing in the upper part of face, especially near the right ala nasi. [*Gff.*]

Red spot on the cheek, without sensation.

Eruption of pimples and itching on the whiskers.

70. Tension in the cheek, as from swelling.

(Painful swelling of the cheek on the upper jaw, with throbbing in the gums) (aft. a few h.).

Tearing in the morning, and often at other times, in the right ear.

Creping in the ears (aft. 48 h.).

Itching and tickling in the ears.

75. Roaring and whistling in the ear, in the afternoon (aft. 4 d.).

(Crepitation and creaking in the left ear, as when a watch is wound up.)

Deafness of one ear.

Hearing diminished from day to day, for five days (aft. 6 d.).

Violent tearing pain in the lobe of the ear and **behind it.** [*Gff.*]

80. Spasm of the right ala nasi towards the malar bone.

(Great dryness of the interior of the nose, although the air passes well through it.)

Dry blood collects in the nose (aft. 16 h.).

Epistaxis, especially in the morning.

Hot lips.

85. Spasm in the lower lip and sensation as if it were pressed against the gums and torn away again.

(Pain in the corners of the mouth, like soreness.)

Shooting, aching pain in the jaws.

In the jaws, pain as if they were screwed together or asunder.

Drawing pain, now in one, now in another tooth, which was aggravated by warmth, was relieved for a moment by cold, was not aggravated by chewing, and went off after eating; at the same time the gums were swollen on the inside.

90. Greatly swollen and painful gums.

Pain in a hollow tooth, in the evening.

Pain in a hollow tooth, especially in the open air, as if the nerve were touched.

After dinner, pain in a hollow tooth, more shooting than tearing, for half an hour (aft. 5 h.).

Squeezing, drawing in the right upper molars. [*Gff.*]

95. In the evening in bed aching, digging pain, as if under the left lower molars. [*Gff.*]

Drawing toothache, at one time in the right, at another in the left teeth, by day and during several nights. [*Gff.*]

Drawing in an incisor tooth, as if a draught of air penetrated it and caused a stitch. [*Gff.*]

Bleeding from the teeth.

Uncommonly profuse bleeding out of the right lower teeth. [*Gff.*]

100. Pain in a submaxillary gland, which was as if swollen (aft. 3 d.).

Fœtor of the mouth.

In the morning, on awaking, tongue, mouth, and lips, as if numb and quite dry. [*Gff.*]

In the morning, on awaking, great dryness of the mouth, with complete absence of thirst, for several days. [*Gff.*]

Smarting and soreness in the interior of the mouth ; on account of the pain she could not eat anything hard.

105. Vesicles in the mouth, which pain as if burnt.

The tongue is covered with a greyish-yellow coating. [*Gff.*]

Under the tongue lumps, like small growths, which pain like excoriation.

Contractive sensation in the salivary glands, when eating, especially during the first mouthfuls.

Rheumatic pain at the back of the tongue and in the fauces, when not swallowing. [*Gff.*]

110. Tearing pain on the palate extending into the left ear. [*Gff.*]

Scraping sensation on the palate.

Scraping in the throat. [*Gff.*]

Scraping in the throat, as in catarrh, for some days.

In the morning, dryness in the throat.

115. Feeling in her throat as if something were sticking in it.

Tearing in the interior of the throat and above, quite at the back of the fauces. [*Gff.*]

Smarting at the back of the fauces when not swallowing. [*Gff.*]

Aching, smarting paint at the back of the throat from time to time. [*Gff.*]

Pain in throat like something obstructing deglutition (aft. 8 d.). [*Gff.*]

120. (Sore throat, not when swallowing food, but during empty swallowing, and on pressing on it externally, with tension in the cervical glands, as if they were swollen) (aft. 4 d.)

(Sore throat after a draught of air ; shooting from the throat into the right ear and pain especially when moving the tongue.)

Secretion of mucus in the throat, with roughness and scraping. [*Gff.*]

Hawking of mucus, in the morning. [*Gff.*]

When hawking up mucus from the throat, almost unavoidable retching and vomiting.

125. The (accustomed) tobacco smoking greatly irritates and excites him, although it tastes good ; hiccup.

Frequently in the afternoon, rather tasteless eructation.

Frequent, empty eructation (aft. $3\frac{1}{2}$ h.) [*Gff.*]

After a meal, violent eructation.

Frequent sour eructation (aft. 48, 72 h).

130. Audible eructation, of a bitter taste.

When walking in the open air **heart-burn**, with baulked eructation. [*Gff.*]

Every evening, sensation as from disordered stomach and scrapy belching up as high as the larynx, like **heart-burn.**

(In the morning, on awaking, bitter taste in the mouth.)

After drinking milk, acidity in the mouth.

135. (After breakfast, nausea) (aft. 72 h.)

(In the stomach clawing nausea) (aft. 24 h.)

Qualmishness about the stomach.

Burning in the stomach (aft. 3 h.) [*Gff.*]

Burning in the gastric region and higher up. [*Gff.*]

140. Aching and burning under the scrobiculus cordis, which goes off by eructation. [*Gff.*]

After eating, anxiety.

After eating, pressure in the pit of the throat, as if food still stuck there, and would not go down.

During dinner tearing in the left side of the palate, and at the back of the throat. [*Gff.*]

After a meal, transient tearing first about the left, then about the right eye. [*Gff.*]

145. Immediately after eating aching confusion of the head, especially when moving.

On account of weak feeling in the stomach and vertigo she must lie down, in the afternoon (aft. 72 h.).

Tension and pressure in the gastric region.

Spasm in the stomach.

Shooting and aching in the gastric region.

150. Pressure under the scrobiculus cordis and in the hypogastrium, from time to time, also at night. [*Gff.*]

Pressure in the epigastrium, with cold hands or feet. [*Gff.*]

Pressure in the abdomen, passing into squeezing. [*Gff.*]

Aching in the umbilical region, with heart-burn, that goes off by eructation. [*Gff.*]

Pressure in the side of the abdomen over the right hip. [*Gff.*]

155. Violent spasms in the abdomen.

Continual pressure in the epigastrium, allayed by walking in the open air, returning when sitting. [*Gff.*]

An aching in the hypogastrium for several hours, equally severe when walking and when sitting (aft. 6 d.).

Aching pain in a small spot on the right side of the abdomen in the hepatic region, but not felt when touched. [*Gff.*]

Aching pain in the hepatic region. [*Gff.*]

160. Tension and distension in the abdomen, after everything **he** eats, even after every mouthful of fluid.

Tense abdomen (aft. some h.).

Distended abdomen (aft. 5 d.).

Early in the morning great compression in the abdomen.

The abdomen feels compressed.

165. Weight in the abdomen, and as if sprained and pressed from the spinal column.

After pressure in the abdomen discharge of inodorous flatus. [*Gff.*]

Squeezing pain in the right hypogastrium. [*Gff.*]

First pinching belly-ache, followed by some cutting in the epigastrium, which goes off by eructation. [*Gff.*]

Discomfort from displacement of flatus, causing pain, especially in the left side of the abdomen.

170. Immediately after midnight he wakes up with great distension of the abdomen, especially of the hypogastrium, from flatulence, which cannot pass, and excites colic, or at least severe pressing downwards ; this accumulation of flatulence goes off during subsequent sleep, without discharge of flatus, and the abdomen becomes quiet.

Fermentation and rumbling, heard but not felt, in the bowels. [*Gff.*]

Pinching in the hypogastrium, with violent fermentation and gurgling, especially in the epigastrium, when lying in bed, in the morning, diminished by rising, and renewed on again lying down, especially when lying on the back. [*Gff.*]

Violent cutting in the abdomen, in the evening.

After midnight, cutting in the abdomen in bed, even during the general perspiration of the body.

175. Cutting in the abdomen, with a soft stool, in the morning, for two successive mornings (aft. 5 d.).

Severe cutting in the abdomen, with three diarrhœic stools, on three successive days (aft. 5 d.).

(Burning in the abdomen.)

Cold feeling in the abdomen.

Coldness of one side of the abdomen for two days (aft. 48 h.).

180. Twitching in the abdominal muscles, in the evening.

Shooting over the hips, for two days (aft. 5 d.).

A sharp pressure, or obtuse stitch, over the right hip. [*Gff.*]

On drawing in the abdomen violent needle-pricks in the hypogastrium, also excited by external pressure. [*Gff.*]

Shooting belly-ache about the navel, on moving the abdomen, especially on drawing it in. [*Gff.*]

185. A frequent call to stool, but no motion occurs, and this makes her very anxious, and then the propinquity of other people is intolerable to her.

After ineffectual call to stool, a pinching pain in the hypogastrium, especially in the right side (after some days). [*Gff.*]

Tenesmus in the rectum.

Stool too scanty (aft. 24 h.). [*Gff.*]

Constipation (aft. 4. d.). [*Gff.*]

190. (Drawing in the rectum.)

Itching at the anus.

Itching in the anus (aft. some h.). [*Gff.*]

Tickling in the rectum.

Itching and smarting in the anus, which goes off by rubbing. [*Gff.*]

195. Shooting in the anus.

Four stools of ordinary character within a few hours (aft. a few h.).

Copious, soft, bright brown stool (aft. 8 d.). [*Gff.*]

(Seems to effect improvement in the hitherto sluggish stool, in the secondary action) (aft. 10, 15 d.)

Along with not hard stool, great discharge of blood (aft. 7 d.).

200. **After stool, aching deep in the hypogastrium.** [*Gff.*]

(After each stool a weakness about the scrobiculus cordis)

After passage of stool there remains in the abdomen a wanting to go (he feels as if he had not finished) for more than a minute.

Pain in the rectum and at the same time in the bladder (aft. 5 d.).

Sensation as if some drops escaped from the urethra.

205. Urine lemon coloured, almost inodorous, with a small cloud. [*Gff.*]

Urine brown.

Urine like whey.

Scanty urine, with reddish cloud, with absence of thirst. [*Gff.*]

Urine dark brown and somewhat turbid, even during its passage (aft. 20 h.)

210. **Urine turbid, even when first passed,** yellowish-brown, and depositing a brown sediment, whilst the clear urine above it was yellow.

Urine with reddish cloud. [*Gff.*]

Urine after standing a short time, of penetrating odour.

Bloody urine (aft. 7 d.)

Diminished secretion of urine (the first 3 days).

215. Scanty urine, which after some hours has a reddish sediment. [*Gff.*]

Much micturition at night.

In the morning, after rising, for two hours, urging to urinate, so that he often cannot retain the urine.

He urinates three times as much as he drinks, especially in the morning; thereafter by a dull pain in the renal region.

Copious, bright coloured, unclouded urine (aft. 4 d.).

220. Burning in the orifice of the urethra and in the anus.

Burning at the mouth of the urethra (aft. 6 d.).

(Twitching in the urethra) (aft. 12 d.).

(Twitching in the testicles) (aft. 14 d.).

Tearing in the glans penis.

225. Ulcerative pain in the glans penis.

An itching pimple above the male genitals.

Burning internally in the region of the seminal vesicles.

Burning, smarting, tickling and itching on the vulva and in the urethra when urinating.

Burning in the female genital organs, with discharge of some drops of blood, especially after walking and after a hard stool.

230. **Severe itching on the pudendum** (more rarely at the anus); she must rub the parts.

Sore pain and itching on the pudendum, also when not urinating.

Swelling and soreness of the labia pudendi, and itching there.

Itching in the glans penis, continuing while sitting, lying, standing and walking.

Violent voluptuous sensation in the interior of the genital organs, lasting for an hour, without considerable erection or irritation of the external sexual parts (aft. 4 d).

235. In the morning, on awaking, violent erection, without voluptuous sensation, with external numbness and diminished sensibility; on the

cessation of the erection, a creeping tearing in the anterior part of the urethra.

It takes away the erections (in the secondary action).

Menses three days too early (aft. 4 d.).

Menses four days too early (aft. 20 d.).

Great excitement in the abdomen, as if the menses were about to come on, which had appeared only 21 days previously (aft. 2 h.).

240. Discharge of blood from the uterus (aft. 2 h.).

During the menses the left leg becomes quite blue from distended veins, with pressing pain in the leg.

(At night, much leucorrhœa.)

(Discharge of bluish-white masses of mucus from the vagina.)

(Thick slimy leucorrhœa, increased day by day, and before each discharge a stitch in the vagina.)

* * *

245. In the forehead and eyes, sensation as before the outbreak of coryza. [*Gff.*]

Headache on blowing the nose.

Nose stopped up and sore pain in the inside of it.

Long continued, great dryness of the nose, but frequent smarting in it as if he would sneeze. [*Gff.*]

Sometimes sneezing with dry nose.

250. Creeping in the nose, as if about to sneeze.

Frequent feeling as if about to sneeze.

She sneezes almost every day, which never occurred before.

Stuffed coryza.

Scraping in the throat, as in catarrh.

255. The voice is rough and hoarse; viscid mucus collects in the throat.

Hoarseness; rough, deep voice, alternating with thick mucus in the windpipe, which he easily gets rid of by hawking and voluntary tussiculation (aft. 10, 24 h.).

Fœtid breath, in the morning after awaking.

Coryza and cough, with expectoration of white mucus.

Tickling in the throat, exciting cough.

260. Cough only at night from extreme irritation in throat—not by day.

Cough excited by scraping in the throat. [*Gff.*]

Collection of greyish mucus in the throat, which is coughed out with difficulty; at the same time scraping in the throat. [*Gff.*]

Itching in the throat and thyroid gland during the cough.

Burning, itching tickle from the larynx down into the abdomen.

265. While coughing pain in the side below the scrobiculus cordis.

Every evening cough, with pain under the left ribs, as if something were torn away there.

Cough only at night, on account of horrible irritation in the throat.

Cough comes sometimes in regular great fits.

Frightful spasmodic cough, with much eructation and hoarseness.

270. A kind of whooping-cough (aft. 48 h.).

Deep, dry cough, with flow of water into the mouth, and afterwards scraping in the throat. [*Gff.*]

When coughing, sensation as from a sore place in the throat.

Very salt expectoration when coughing.

When coughing there is a pressure in the umbilical region.

275. Sensation like rawness in the chest.

Burning in the chest.

A burning in the external parts of the chest. [*Gff*.].

On one of the right ribs, an aching burning pain, aggravated by external pressure ; then on the left side of the chest a similar pain. [*Gff*.]

A stitch in the chest extending into the back (aft. some h.).

280. A violent obtuse stitch in the right side of the chest, catching the breath. [*Gff*.]

Whistling in the chest.

Oppression on the chest. [*Gff*.]

Oppression in the back through the chest.

Oppression of the chest and in the back between the scapulæ, which goes off for a short time by eating.

285. Tight chest, with much restlessness, all day (aft. 3 d.).

Tightness of the chest ; she cannot take a deep breath nor yawn properly.

Anxiety at the heart, hindering respiration, with flying heat.

Palpitation of the heart, when walking in the open air, with pale face.

Along with violent palpitation of the heart pressing in the chest, as if a lump lay there, or the chest were stuffed there.

290. Aching sensation deep in the right side of the chest on expiring forcibly, most painful on a small spot. [*Gff*.]

Aching in the upper part of the chest, in fits of five minutes.

Aching superiorly in the chest. [*Gff*.]

Aching under (in ?) the left side of the chest.

Aching in the left side of the chest in the cardiac region [*Gff*.]

295. In the chest, above the scrobiculus cordis, an aching bruised pain, relieved by eructation. [*Gff*.]

Bruised pain on the right lowest true rib, rather posteriorly. [*Gff*.]

Rheumatic pain on the right side of the chest under the arm. [*Gff*.]

Tearing pressure in the left side of the chest. [*Gff*.]

Violent pressure on the lower part of the sacrum. [*Gff*.]

300. In the sacrum stitches, when sitting (aft. 8, 9 d.)

In the sacrum single, violent, sharp stitches, increased by the least movement. [*Gff*.]

Painful tension in the lumbar muscles.

Rheumatic pain in the back, on the right side. [*Gff*.]

Backache, as if the bowels were compressed, and a weight therein, as if he could not straighten himself.

305. A burning in the left scapula.

Shooting in the left scapula (the first days).

Rheumatic pain on the right scapula. [*Gff*.]

Aching drawing pain in the nape.

Tearing in both shoulders.

310. **Tearing in the left shoulder-Joint.** [*Gff.*]

In the evening drawing, and **as if dislocated** and paralysed **in the shoulder.**

On the right shoulder a violent obtuse stitch (aft. 2 h.). [*Gff.*]

The arms are apt to go to sleep on lying on them.

At night, in the right arm, frequently numbness and gone asleep.

315. The left arm frequently goes asleep, by day, when at rest.

Tearing, in the morning, in the right arm for five minutes.

Clucking in the arm.

Twitching in the arm.

(Paralysis in the right upper arm.)

320. Tearing in the right elbow.

Tearing on the right elbow.

Tearing in the right elbow and forearm. [*Gff.*]

Aching, drawing pain in the right forearm up into the elbow. [*Gff.*]

Falling asleep of the hands at night.

325. Cramp in the hands (aft. some h.).

In the evening the fingers are drawn crookedly inwards (aft. 7 d.).

Paralysis of the hands for some minutes (aft. 6 d.).

At night weakness of the fingers so that he can only by an effort press them upon the palm, or move them quickly. [*Gff.*]

Long,continued icy coldness of the hands (aft. 1 h.). [*Gff.*]

330. Painfull, long-continued coldness of the hands. [*Gff.*]

In the evening icy coldness of the hands ; he is chilled by it. [*Gff.*]

Tearing in the inside of the right metacarpus. [*Gff.*]

Prickings in the hands and fingers as from gadflies.

Prickings now in the right index, now in the right thumb.

335. Itching in the palms.

Rheumatic pain from the proximal joint of the thumb, through its metacarpal bone to the wrist-joint. [*Gff.*]

Tearing in the muscles of the thumb. [*Gff.*]

Trembling in the thumb, in the evening, in frequent, short fits.

Tearing in the proximal joint of the left index. [*Gff.*]

340. (The proximal joints of the fingers become stiff in the evening, and the proximal joint of the thumb swollen ; it is painful when flexed—worst when she has made no movement of the fingers during the day.)

Tearing in the right index.[*Gff.*]

Tearing in the two last fingers, in the evening, before going to sleep. [*Gff.*]

Drawing in the fingers and thumb.

Tearing in the tip of the right little finger. [*Gff.*]

345. Tearing under the nail of the right middle finger. [*Gff.*]

The skin of the finger tips is wrinkled, in the morning.

The wart on the finger pains as if sore.

Itching in the finger tips.

A small tetter appears between the thumb and index, which itches.

350. In the tip of the left thumb a shooting tearing pain, and also on

gently touching it, it feels as if a splinter were stuck in under the nail; the sensation is less on pressing strongly on it. [*Gff.*]

In the tip of the thumb a formication as if it were asleep, which goes off for a short time by external pressure. [*Gff.*]

Tearing in the left and then also in the right hip. [*Gff.*]

Aching, tearing pain anteriorly, just below the left hip. [*Gff.*]

Clucking tearing posteriorly below the left buttock. [*Gff.*]

355. Tearing in the right buttock. [*Gff.*]

Tearing in the left lower limb, in the morning.

Rheumatic tearing in the right lower limb. [*Gff.*]

Heaviness of the lower limbs.

Tension in the thigh, as if the tendons were too short, especially when walking.

360. Stretching and relaxation in the lower limbs.

The lower limbs feel gone to sleep; he cannot step firmly (aft. 8 d.).

Tearing on the right knee. [*Gff.*]

Drawing in the knees and ankles.

Paralysis of the knee for some minutes (aft. 6 d.).

365. Above the knee pain as of dislocation, especially after sitting (aft. 5 d.).

Itching on the knees.

In the morning stiffness in the hough (the first days).

Soreness in the houghs, the pain is worst in the evening.

Tearing under the left knee, at the upper part of the tibia. [*Gff.*]

370. More cold feeling in the legs than externally perceptible coldness. [*Gff.*]

The right leg is very cold, especially the knee.

Cold feet.

Very cold feet. [*Gff.*]

On both tibiæ painful spots (aft. 28 d.).

375. (The legs from the knees downwards very swollen, especially the feet) (aft. 3 d.).

Swelling of the left inner ankle; it is only painful there when walking; but on walking for a considerable time it no longer hurts (aft. 7 d.).

In the evening, after lying down, itching on the legs above the ankles; after rubbing it pains as if sore and bruised.

Intermitting tearing on the left calf. [*Gff.*]

Tearing in the lower part of the left leg. [*Gff.*]

380. **Cramp in the lower limbs and cramp in the calves almost every night.**

Grumbling in the calves and feet.

Creeping in the feet, which are as if numb (a tingling in them); when he stood up he felt faint, all became dark before his eyes; he could not remain up, he must vomit (bile), and had to lie down again.

Itching on the ankles.

Tearing in the ankles.

385. Gouty pain in the ankle-joints.

Pain on walking in the left ankle-joint.
In the left foot tearing and shooting (aft. 26 d.).
In the left foot occasional shooting.
Tension in the left foot (at noon).

390. Stiffness of the feet, which are very weary (aft. 6 d.).
Gouty pain in the ball of the big toe.
Stitch in the ball of the big toe.
Itching on the toes.
Intolerable tickling on the tip of the big toe.

395. Tearing in the middle toes of the left foot. [*Gff.*]
Tearing on the external border of the left foot. [*Gff.*]
Pain in the heel when walking.
Stitches in the heel.
Itching in the interior of the soles, not allayed by scratching.

400. Great burning in the soles.
Pain of the corns, as if sore.
By gentle walking in the open air the symptoms are alleviated, but return when sitting. [*Gff.*]
When walking, profuse perspiration chiefly on the abdomen and thighs.
Perspiration all day long (aft. 24 h.).

405. Itching almost all over, even on the abdomen.
Produces the itch-eruption on the skin, with much itching.
Causes the tetters to reappear.
A burning in several parts of the skin of the body.
In the morning on awaking the skin of the body is as if numb and insensible to the knees, without being cold ; the hands have only an indistinct sensibility—a kind of gone-to-sleep condition of the skin, but without formication. [*Gff.*]

410. He feels the pulse in the body like the ticking of a watch.
Twitching in the limbs.
Uncommon twitching in all the limbs and coldness of the body at night (aft. 5 d.).
From walking in the open air, commotion in the blood and accelerated circulation, with greater weakness of the body.
Uneasiness in all the limbs, like a formication, with a kind of anxiety—only by day.

415. In the morning (in a heated room), he became suddenly so weak that he could not walk alone, with cold sweat on the forehed and hands.
Very exhausted (aft. 8, 24 h.).
Exhaustion in the morning in bed. [*Gff.*]
In the morning great weakness in the lower limbs.
Weariness, with painfulness of all the limbs.

420. Exhaustion that goes off by walking (aft. 5 d.).
Heavy in the body and very tired (aft. 7 d.).
Faintness, sinking in the knees (aft. 3 h.).
Weakness in the feet like insensibility (aft. 48 h.).

She must lie down on account of weak feeling in the stomach and vertigo (aft. 72 h.).

425. Inclination to stretch himself.

(Sleepiness by day).

Before midnight sleeplessness.

He cannot sleep at night, he knows not why.

For several nights sleeplessness, and in the morning slumber full of fantastical dreams.

430. Frequent waking at night. [*Gff.*]

Frequent waking, and at 2 a.m. long uneasiness in the whole body, especially in the occiput.

Very late of falling asleep—then very restless sleep on account of pressure in the epigastrium, particularly the right side. [*Gff.*]

For several successive nights, always after midnight until 7 or 8 a.m., pain over the eyes, with nausea.

In the evening, late, after going to sleep in bed, aching, tearing from the occiput into the forehead. [*Gff.*]

435. The first half of the night heat in the head.

Uneasiness in the occiput after midnight.

At night he wakes up with headache, which goes off on rising.

Waking with exhaustion, dryness of mouth, and great pressure in the epigastrium, diminished by lying on the abdomen, whereupon he has tearing in the sacrum instead, which goes off when he again lies on the back. [*Gff.*]

On awaking about midnight weakness, nausea, great pressure in the scrobiculus cordis and abdomen, violent erections, without voluptuous sensation, dryness in the mouth, and insensibility of the surface of the body. [*Gff.*]

440. Very early waking; followed by frequently interrupted, but very profound sleep, with eyes fast closed. [*Gff.*]

In the morning, after waking, in bed, great weariness, especially in the upper part of the body, confusion of the head and sensation as if the eyes were very fast closed, besides some nausea in the scrobiculus cordis; he has hardly resolution to get up. [*Gff.*]

In the morning, in bed, weariness, with feeling in the eyes as if they were too firmly closed. [*Gff.*]

At night when asleep he lies on his back, the occiput supported by both hands, and with bent knees, with very vivid dreams. [*Gff.*]

Starting up in fright, in the evening, on going to sleep, with illusion as if there was too much light in the room; he sprang out of bed in anxiety (aft. some h.).

445. For three successive nights restless, with many dreams (aft. 5 d.).

While in the act of going off to sleep vivid, uneasy dreams, which almost prevented any sleep (aft. 8 d.).

The child sleeps restlessly, talks in its sleep, and wants to drink.

Sleep restless, with anxious dreams (aft. 5 d.).

The night full of uneasy, anxious dreams. [*Gff.*]

450. After falling asleep late, anxious dreams, as if he was ill used, and on account of weakness could not defend himself; he then awakes with great weakness in the upper part of the body, with squeezing

pressure under the scrobiculus cordis and nausea, sensations that recur when he lies down again and falls asleep—to which is then added pressure in the left side of the abdomen ; but on waking up and sitting up and moving the symptoms go off, with discharge of flatus, fermentation in the abdomen and eructation. [*Gff.*]

Vexatious, anxious **dreams,** and talking in sleep, for eight days (immediately).

Dreams full of business.

At night restless sleep, on account of coldness of the body and twitching in all the limbs (aft. 5 d.).

Internal chilliness at night, on account of which he cannot go to sleep, or from which he wakes up at night ; he does not become warm at all.

455. Chilliness and weariness as if he wanted to sleep, for four successive forenoons, which went off by eating his dinner (aft. 72 h.).

From early morning chill, sleep-weariness, and numb headache, which only went off by walking in the open air.

After two diarrhœic stools, chill, great weariness and headache.

Before dinner chilliness (the first days).

(Coldness of the skin of the whole body—excepting only the face, neck, and genital organs.)

460. For two successive evenings heat, from 7 to 8 p.m. (aft. 12 d.).

Every quarter of an hour heat in the face and all over the body (aft. 5, 6 d.).

Nocturnal perspiration for two successive nights (aft. 6, 7 d.).

Profuse night sweat for two successive nights (aft. 5 d.).

Always after midnight general, strong-smelling sweat, for many nights.

465. Every night a strong exhalation, almost like sweat.

Moderate night sweat all over, with great warmth of the body.

Every morning sweat, most profuse on the ailing side.

Very restless by day.

Restless all day, with tightness of chest.

470. Disposition restless and excited.

Hurriedness in intellectual occupations.

Irritable humour, as if weak in nerves and impatient. [*Gff.*]

Excited ; she spoke unusually much (loquacious), was very much exhausted thereby, could not sleep at night, got a headache, as if a great weight lay on her head ; she felt much oppressed, must sit up in bed, and had anxiety, and perspired all over the body.

Unusually long excitement.

475. Is irritated by speaking, has shaking and trembling all through the body, especially in the lower extremities, and must remain for some time alone, in order to rest.

Music sends the blood to his head.

The imagination is occupied with many lascivious ideas, even in dreams, and yet the disposition and the sexual organs are but little excited by them (in the first 24 h.).

Distorted fancies, grimaces, satanic faces take possession of the mind, and he cannot get rid of them.

Anxious thoughts arise in him.

480. **Anxious in the evening.**

Anxious and trembling (aft. 8 d.).

Great dejection (aft. 6 d.).

Sad thoughts take possession of him, with sinking feeling about the heart ; he is for a long time depressed in spirits.

Very sad (aft. 72 h.).

485. **Despair** (aft. 48 h.).

Immediately lachrymose, then peevish and quarrelsome, for two hours.

His humour is easily embittered.

Constant alternation of dejection and passionate disposition, which will not allow him to get a tranquil disposition.

Indifferent to joy and sorrow, but more dejected than calm.

Very composed disposition*.

* Secondary action produced by the organism.

ANGUSTURA.[1]

(Cortex Angusturæ or *Augusturæ.)*

The best pieces of the bark of this South American tree, called *Bonplandia trifoliata*, are about one line in thickness, slightly bent, on their external convex side covered with a greyish-white, easily scraped off, fine coating; traversed by fine transverse furrows; on the inner concave surface of a bright brownish yellow, very friable, and cinnamon coloured and porous on the fractured surface; of a disagreeable spicy smell, and of a penetrating, somewhat hot, spicy bitter taste, the powder of which resembles rhubarb powder in colour; the decoction is not precipitated by a solution of sulphate of iron. Fifty grains of this powder digested in 1000 drops of alcohol without heat so as to form a tincture are employed for medicinal purposes after appropriate dilution.)

For many years complaints have been publicly made about a substitution in commerce for this true angustura bark of a false bark, which displays dangerous and poisonous properties, and for many years the tree from which this false bark was derived was unknown.

Now the *Brucea ferruginea* is said to be the tree from which this false suspicious bark is derived; chemical investigation has shown that it furnishes the same alkaloid as nux vomica, ignatia, &c.

However, the above-described genuine angustura bark likewise possesses uncommonly great medicinal power, so that, when it is procured direct from the tree Bonplandia trifoliata at St. Thomas del Angustura, in South America, as it is now, without any doubt it can, like every other very powerful medicine, do great harm if given in immoderate doses and in unsuitable cases. In F. A. G. EMMERT's *Curgeschichte (Hufeland's Fourn.*, August, 1815, p. 75) a case is related where three tablespoonfuls of a decoction of five ounces of (presumably spurious) angustura bark, evaporated to five ounces of liquid, were given to a boy five and a half years old. This unreasonable dose, which contained about an ounce and a half of angustura power, proved fatal, as we read with a shudder, in a couple of hours, with horrible sufferings. This substance would in the same dose have a like effect not only on a boy but on an adult person.

In this fatal case described by EMMERT the boy presented the following symptoms:

Trembling, soon passing into violent convulsions (aft. ½ h.).

When the medical attendant touched the arm in order to feel the pulse tetanus suddenly ensued.

The eyelids were wide open.

The eyes were staring, projecting, and immovable.

Trismus, with wide séparation of the lips, so that the front teeth were quite exposed.

[1] From vol. vi, 2nd edit., 1827.

Tension of individual facial muscles.

The limbs were stretched out to the utmost, stiff, and stark.

The spinal column and the head strongly drawn backwards.

The trunk was from time to time shaken by violent jerking along the back, as from electric shocks, and somewhat raised.

Cheeks and lips became blue.

Respiration intermitting.

After an attack that lasted six minutes the boy breathed with great effort, panting, with blueness of the cheeks and lips.

Great and frequent longing for coffee.

Even swallowing tepid water excited tetanic spasms.

Pulse 102, spasmodic, irregular.

The tetanus sometimes returned without perceptible cause, sometimes was excited by a noise, or by touching any portion of the body; he constantly called out that no one should touch him.

After the tetanus the eyes were closed, the forehead and face covered with sweat; blueness of the cheeks and lips; groaning without (acknowledged) pains.

The whole body became flaccid and relaxed; the eye dead-like; convulsive breathing came back only after long pauses.

Death after an hour.

Half an hour after death the body was stiff and stark.

After twenty-four hours there was already a strong corpse-like smell outside and inside; on opening the veins cherry-coloured fluid blood was found.

The right lung was externally pale and bloated, internally full of blood; the left lung was externally blue, when incised blackish and very heavy from blood.

Besides the above other reports of the consequences of strong doses of angustura have been recorded, such as spasmodic twitchings, vertigo, anxiety, immobility of the muscles as from stiffening, and a report has been communicated to me by the late Dr. WÜRZNER, of Eilenburg, relating to four persons, each of whom took from ten to twelve grains of the extract in the form of pills, in whom there occurred:

Stiffness of all the muscles of the body, like tetanus; one fell to the ground suddenly, retaining his consciousness.

Closure of the jaws, trismus.

Very similar though slighter symptoms will be found in the following st of the effects of carefully selected pieces of angustura bark on the ealthy body.

I have employed for homœopathic purposes the smallest portion of a op of the billionth dilution of the above-described alcoholic tincture, have found that in some cases a still higher dilution would have n more suitable.

Camphor is not an antidote for its too violent effects, but coffee is.

AHNEMANN was aided in this proving by:—FRANZ, GROSS, HARNISCH, AMMER, MEYER, MICHLER, MOSSDORF, WISLICENUS. No old-school ties are quoted.

is 2nd edition Hahnemann has added 3 to his own symptoms, and excluded e of his disciples that appeared in the 1st edition.]

ANGUSTURA.

In the open air, vertigo (aft. 20 h.).

A feeling of vertigo comes over him when he crosses flowing water or walks at the side of a canal; he fears he will sink. [*Fz.*]

Dulness and stupid feeling in the head, as from intoxication on the previous day. [*Mlr.*]

The head is confused; throbbing in the forehead.

5. Confusion and contractive feeling in the head on walking quickly. [*Fz.*]

Suddenly great confusion of the head, as from a skin stretched over the brain, for half an hour (aft. $\frac{1}{4}$ h.). [*Mss.*]

Great distraction; when he occupies himself with something serious, other things immediately come into his head (aft. 45 h.). [*Fz.*]

Sometimes he loses himself, now in a dreamy state, now in complete absence of thought, and he readily falls asleep when reading. [*Fz.*]

In the afternoon, along with repeated (occurring the first three afternoons) warmth of the body, excessive liveliness, and very active memory; but he can think of nothing attentively on account of a not disagreeable scheme that forces itself upon him, which he almost thinks is true and feasible, and owing to which he neither sees nor hears anything beside—a kind of very strong waking dream (aft. 4 d.). [*Fz.*]

10. In the afternoon great sprightliness and vivacity of the mind; he comprehends everything much more easily than on the first day, and more readily than before, but on account of a feeling of inward restlessness as if a great happiness awaited him, and on account of a concourse of scheming ideas, he is unable to stick to his subject (aft. 35 h.). [*Fz.*]

In the morning after rising great weight in the forehead without confusion (aft. 3 d.). [*Fz.*]

In the open air he had some headache and heat (towards evening).

Cramp-like headache.

Headache: aching in the forehead above both eyes, as if all would come out there, during rest and when moving.

15. Aching in the left half of the brain on bending down the head, which is relieved by raising it up (immediately). [*Mss.*]

Aching in the temples (aft. 1 h.). [*Fz.*]

Towards evening, aching pain in the forehead, with great heat in the face. [*Fz.*]

Headache only occurred when there was heat of face. [*Fz.*]

The headaches always occur in the evening when it becomes dark and last till he goes to sleep. [*Gss.*]

20. Headache as if all moved round in the brain, with aching and boring pain, especially in the temple; if he lays his head down on the table, he feels, with the exception of some tension in the forehead,

for the moment nothing, but the pains soon come back, only not so severe; on the other hand, when he raises the head up, they again increase to their former intensity (aft. 12 h.). [*Fz.*]

Aching in the forehead. [*Hsch.*]

Bruised pain in the brain in the sinciput, increased by stooping, diminished in the open air (immediately).

Boring headache in the temples.

A stitch as from electricity darting up and down from the temples.

25. Drawing, aching pain in the temporal region. [*Hsch.*]

Headache: aching in the occiput, in the afternoon.

In the evening aching, drawing pain in the right side of the head, with aching in the lower jaw (aft. 16 h.). [*Fz.*]

Rather external tearing headache from the crown forwards over the temple (aft. 24 h.). [*Ws.*]

Intermittent needle-pricks in the right temporal region, rather externally (aft. 4 h.). [*Lr.*]

30. Continued itching stitches in the forehead and temple, externally, which are not removed by rubbing (aft. 5h.). [*Ws.*]

Stiffness, numbness in the temporal muscles, as if something were forced out there.

Tensive pain in the temporal muscles on opening the jaws.

Twitching under the skin of the left parietal region, on a small spot, which when pressed pains as if bruised (aft. 1 h.). [*Mss.*]

Whilst reading a quivering between eyebrows.

35. Some stitches above the eyes.

Contraction of the pupils (aft. $3\frac{3}{4}$ h.). [*Lr.*]

Dilatation of the pupils (aft. 13 h.). [*Lr.*]

In the afternoon and evening, several times a violent burning in the inner half of the eyes themselves and in their inner canthus.

A tension first in one then in the other eye, as from behind, in the morning.

40. Pressure on the right eye and orbit in the evening (aft. 14 h.). [*Fz.*]

In both eyes an aching, as if a dazzling light struck them, and the eyes became weak.

The eyes are red and burn from heat; in the morning they are sealed up with matter.

Sore pain of the eyelids.

Feeling of dryness under the upper eyelids.

45. Itching stitches on the upper eyelid, not removable by rubbing (aft. 1 h.). [*Ws.*]

Like a thin vapour before the eyes, soon going off.

In the morning, after rising, quite dim before the eyes, as if the cornea were dim (aft. 24 h.). [*Fz.*]

Sharper and more distinct vision at a distance than usual.* [*Hsch.*]

Long sight: he could see distant objects distinctly, though he is naturally very short-sighted* (aft. $2\frac{1}{2}$ h.). [*Lr.*]

Cramp-pain on the zygomatic arch (aft. $\frac{1}{4}$ h.). [*Ws.*]

*Curative secondary action of the organism.

The hearing is much more acute than usual* (aft. $5\frac{1}{2}$ h.). [*Fz.*]

Ringing in the right ear (aft. 33 h.). [*Lr.*]

Stitches in the anterior part of the meatus auditorius externus.

A burning in the inner ear, in the region of the membrana tympani.

55. Sensation as if something came in front of the ear and something were sticking in it.

Cramp in the external ear.

Heat in the lobe of the ear.

Tearing twitching before the left ear (aft. 1 h.). [*Ws.*]

Transient drawing several times, now in the right, now in the left ear. [*Mss.*]

60. Very painful tearing twitching in the interior of the right ear, which gradually changes into drawing (aft. 1 h.). [*Mss.*]

Behind the ears, on the side of the neck, a throbbing pain, as if the great cerebral artery was beating violently.

Tearing in a boil over the right mastoid process (aft. $\frac{1}{4}$ h.). [*Mss.*]

Heat in the ears and in both cheeks.

Smarting, sore feeling deep in the nose (immediately).

65. In the evening hot feeling on the cheek, which does not feel warm to the touch (aft. 12 h.). [*Fz.*]

Feeling of heat in both cheeks, without externally perceptible warmth.

Pain in the masseter muscles of the cheek, as if he had chewed too strongly and had tired them.

In the masseter muscles near the maxillary joint a cramp-like pain, especially when at rest, which is relieved by opening and shutting the jaw.

Great dryness of the lips and mouth without thirst (aft. 3 h.). [*Fz.*]

70. (A digging in the lower jaw) (aft. 18 h.)

Slight drawing in undefined upper molars. [*Mss*]

Drawing pain in both right upper incisors. [*Mss.*]

Drawing pain apparently among the crowns of the right middle upper molars, palliatively alleviated by applying a cold finger (aft. 1 h.). [*Mss.*]

Throbbing toothache in a hollow tooth, in the evening, after lying down (aft. 14 h.). [*Ws.*]

75. In the gums of the right upper row a shooting drawing (aft. 3 h.), [*Ws.*]

Shooting, pinching on the tip of the tongue extremely painful, even when not moving it (aft. 6 h.). [*Ws.*]

Burning on the left side of the tongue, almost on its border, as from pepper (aft. 3 h.). [*Lr.*]

White tongue, with rough sensation (aft. 12 h.). [*Lr.*]

Roughness and dryness on the back of the palate and in the fauces, without thirst, worse when swallowing (aft. 25 h.). [*Lr.*]

80. The voice is louder and bolder* (aft. $5\frac{1}{2}$ h.). [*Fz.*]

* Curative secondary action of the organism.

(Taste like peach kernels in the mouth.)

(Bread tastes sour to her.)

Bitter taste in the mouth after (accustomed) tobacco-smoking. [*Mlr.*]

Putrid, flat taste in the mouth for a short time (aft. 2 h.). [*Mss.*]

85. After dinner, which tasted good, bitter taste in the mouth, and several slight eructations (aft. 30 h.) [*Fz.*]

No desire to drink and no pleasure in doing so, and yet sensation of thirst more for warm than for cold drinks ; but cold drinks did not produce chilliness.

Much thirst for cold drinks (aft. 15 h.). [*Lr.*]

Frequent hiccup (aft. 3 h.). [*Lr.*]

Nausea, especially while eating. [*Mlr.*]

90. Sensation of nausea in the stomach (aft. 1 h.). [*Ws.*]

In the evening during slumber he had very viscid, sickly tasting, and putrid mucus in the mouth, and could not drink enough. [*Fz.*]

Although he has great appetite, food is not relished ; he feels as if it were repugnant to him, at the same time an incomplete eructation causes fulness in the chest, and yet he cannot get satiated with a very plentiful meal (aft. 6 h.) [*Fz.*]

When walking, nausea, as if he would fall down in a faint ; at the same time great exhaustion all over, which is not relieved by sitting down ; he then felt as if the nausea rose into his head, and he became hungry.

On commencing to eat a cutting pain in the stomach like sore pain, which went off on continuing to eat (aft. 3 d.). [*Fz.*]

95. After eating, much eructation of wind.

Bilious eructation.

Cramp-like, pinching pain under the scrobiculus cordis, in the evening, while sitting (aft. 13 h.). [*Fz.*]

Cutting tearing in the scrobiculus cordis, increased by moving the trunk, after dinner. [*Ws.*]

Shooting in the abdomen, followed by a drawing in it.

100. Under the short ribs, in the right side of the abdomen, a cutting on moving the trunk (aft. 48 h.). [*Gss.*]

In the left side of the abdomen, flying, shaking obtuse stitches here and there. [*Gss.*]

An obtuse shooting in the hypogastrium, on the left side, near the navel (aft. 24 h.). [*Gss.*]

In the left lumbar region cutting pain from within outwards (aft. 3 h.). [*Ws.*]

Cutting in the hypogastrium over and across the os pubis, with pressing towards the rectum (aft. $\frac{1}{4}$ h.). [*Mss.*]

5. Cramp-like pain in the abdomen when walking. [*Fz.*]

Pinching in the right lumbar region when at rest. [*Ws.*]

Drawing, bruised pain in the right side of the abdomen when walking in the open air (aft. 1 h.). [*Fz.*]

Pressure in the hypogastrium from within outwards, with anxiety (aft. 16 h.). [*Fz.*]

Above the os pubis a cramp-like pressure when sitting, as if something bored outwards there (aft. 12 h.). [*Fz.*]

110. Audible rumbling in the abdomen, with eructation. [*Fz.*]

A fermentation and rumbling in the abdomen, as if diarrhœa would ensue, with displacement of flatulence (aft. 3 h.). [*Mlr.*]

Loud gurgling in the abdomen.

On drinking warm milk a cutting and gurgling in the hypogastrium above and across the os pubis (aft. $\frac{1}{4}$ h.). [Mss.]

Painless movements, almost incessant rumbling and gurgling in the bowels, for three hours. [*Mss.*]

115. In the morning after previous cutting in the abdomen and nausea, diarrhœa ensues ; the last stool was pure mucus.

Cutting in the abdomen and purging ; the last time mucous (aft. 12, 84 h.).

Diarrhœic commotion, with penetrating drawing through all the intestines (aft. 2 h.) [*Fz.*]

Repeated sensation in the bowels as if diarrhœa would ensue. [*Mss.*]

(Crawling tickling in the rectum, as from ascarides.)

120. Frequent straining in the rectum as if diarrhœa would come on immediately, with shuddering over the face. [*Mss.*]

After every stool shuddering over the face, with goose-skin. [*Mss.*]

The stool was not so thin as the diarrhœic feeling led him to anticipate. [*Mss.*]

Feeling as if the stool had not been completely evacuated, and as if there was more to come. [*Mss.*]

Sensation in the rectum as if it would come out, followed by the evacuation of a yellow, soft, very copious stool (aft. $1\frac{1}{2}$ h.). [*Fz.*]

125. Within four hours, three evacuations of a large quantity of thin fæces. [*Mss.*]

Thin copious stool, without pains (aft. 2 h.). [*Gss.*]

Discharge of stinking flatus. [*Mss.*]

Painful pressing, as from great contraction of the anus, with swelling of the hæmorrhoidal veins, accompanied by burning pain, as if the anus was corroded, with a soft stool (aft. 3 d.). [*Fz.*]

Moderate constipation. [*Fz.*]

130. Frequent, though not urgent, call to stool ; he felt as if the stool would not come, and when he endeavoured to evacuate, only some hard pieces came away, with much pressing and straining (aft. 12 h.). [*Lr.*]

Orange-coloured urine, which soon becomes very turbid (aft. 24 h.).

Frequent urging to urinate, with scanty discharge of urine (aft. 2 h.). [*Lr.*]

(A burning after urinating ; he had frequent call to urinate, but only a few dark yellow drops were passed, which always caused burning.)

Frequent discharge of copious, white urine, preceded by pressing in the bladder; and, after urinating, ineffectual straining—strangury (aft. 36 h.). [*Fz.*]

135. **A voluptuous itching at the point of the glans, which compelled him to rub it,** when walking in the open air (aft. 6½ h.). [*Lr.*]

Itching of the scrotum.

On the prepuce shooting, sometimes itching.

(Drawing, alternating with twitching, in the left spermatic cord, with sensation of shuddering in the neighbouring parts of the scrotum and thigh.) [*Mss.*]

* * *

A stitch in the epiglottis (immediately).

140. Hoarseness caused by much mucus in the larynx (aft. 10 h.). [*Fz.*]

Tickling irritation in the upper part of the larynx, which caused dry short cough, lasting a long time (aft. 2¾ h.). [*Lr.*]

Frequent short cough, followed by a single sob (aft. 15 h.).

All day long tussiculation from an irritation deep in the larynx, which, only when walking in the open air, was associated with rattling in the chest, and with much expectoration of yellow mucus. [*Lr.*]

Violent cough from deep down in the trachea, in the morning, with expectoration of yellow mucus (aft. 24 h.). [*Lr.*]

145. Often scrapy in the throat; he must hawk, without being able to bring up anything (aft. 6 h.). [*Ws.*]

In the trachea viscid mucus, which is not easily coughed up (aft. 10, 11 h.). [*Fz.*]

Cutting pressure in both sides of the chest, at first only when inspiring, afterwards increased to cutting blows, which continue even when holding the breath (aft. 1 h.). [*Ws.*]

Transient tightness of the chest (immediately).

On walking quickly, tightness of the chest and aching in its left side (aft. 12 h.). [*Fz.*]

150. Pain in the pectoral muscles in the morning, which she moves in bed, and during the day, when she lays the arms together, they pain as if bruised; on touching the parts she feels nothing, not even when breathing.

A sharp aching, as it were pinching pain in the upper part of the chest, on a small spot (aft. 15 h.).

Cutting stitches in the last rib during inspiration, and besides that shortly before going to sleep and after lying down.

Spasm of the chest, as when suddenly exposed to serve cold. [*Myr.*]

Pressure over the whole of the right side of chest and abdomen, as if it were compressed from before and behind, with sharp inward-cutting down the sternum and behind on the spine, increased by inspiration and every movement of the trunk (aft. 5 h.). [*Ws.*]

155. Towards evening, on going upstairs, great oppression and pressure on the chest, with aching on the sides of the frontal bone and violent palpitation of the heart (aft. 2 h.). [*Fz.*]

Cutting blows on the sternum and spine, towards the interior (aft. 36 h.). [*Ws.*]

When sitting and bending forwards, violent palpitation of the heart, with painful sensation of contraction of the heart. [*Gss.*]

In the evening, in bed, while lying on the left side, he feels a violent palpitation of the heart; relieved by sitting up. [*Gss.*]

A beating pain in the cardiac region. [*Hsch.*]

160. When he takes as deep a breath as he can, it seems to stop under the upper part of the sternum; he feels there a pain, almost like obtuse shooting or pressure (aft. 72 h). [*Gss.*]

On drawing in the breath, internally a trembling feeling, like hiccup, so that he has to draw his breath, as it were, in two jerks (aft. 8 h.). [*Fz.*]

Cutting pressure out from the thoracic cavity, with feeling of anxiety (aft. ½ h.). [*Ws.*]

Single stitches on the sternum when sitting (aft. 28 h.). [*Lr.*]

Painful sensibility of the chest when he presses but lightly on it (aft. 24 h.). [*Ws.*]

165. Pressure on the chest towards the axilla and on the tendon of the pectoralis major (aft. 3 d.). [*Fz.*]

Very sharp, shooting, itching in front at the last right true rib, which at first does not go off even by scratching, but afterwards disappears spontaneously (aft. 24 h.). [*Fz.*]

In the morning, in bed, pain in the sacrum as if all were broken; after rising she could not lift anything from the ground for some hours; then hunger, followed by cutting in the abdomen and purging, at last mucous evacuations.

All night a pressing in the sacrum as if bruised; she often woke up from this pain; it was worst about 4 a.m., but when she got up it was gone.

In the morning, in bed, pain of stiffness betwixt the scapulæ and in the nape, like drawing; on getting up she could not move herself with the arms for pain nor turn her neck all the forenoon—for several successive mornings, until noon, with exhaustion of the whole body.

170. Stitches below and near the sacrum when sitting. [*Fz.*]

Dull clucking in the os sacrum (aft. 1 h.). [*Ws.*]

Sacral pain more to one side, as if bruised, and drawing aching, when sitting (aft. 35 h.). [*Fz.*].

At night in bed he often feels in the right side, near the spine, betwixt the scapulæ, when moving, a stitch, that seems to penetrate deep into the chest. [*Gss.*]

In the left cervical muscles, towards the shoulder, only when moving, a bruised pain, and as if over-stretched, which is relieved in the open air.

175. Tension in the dorsal muscles at the axilla; he has a difficulty in raising up the arms (immediately). [*Ws.*]

Cutting stitches on the scapula.

In the nape a drawing stitch.

Strong quivering in the cervical muscles of the left side (aft. 2 h.). [*Mss.*]

Even when at rest tension anteriorly on the right side of the neck, together with sharp stitches (aft. 3 h.). [*Ws.*]

180. Obtuse stitches betwixt the top of the left shoulder and the neck. [*Gss.*]

On the shoulder a quivering pain.

Aching cutting in the axilla (aft. $\frac{1}{4}$ h.). [*Ws.*]

Aching pain in the humerus, like bruised pain (aft. $1\frac{3}{4}$ h.). [*Lr.*]

The left arm is heavy when walking, with aching externally on the bend of the elbow, as if it were drawn down, when he lets it hang freely (aft. 4 h.). [*Fz.*]

185. On stretching out the arm sensation as if he had held a great weight for a long time in the hand—a kind of paralysis.

Stiffness in the elbow-joints, with weakness of the forearms.

Pain on the elbow-joint, as if in the sinews, as if he had received a blow there, increased by moving the arm and by leaning upon it (after walking in the open air) (aft. 24 h.).

Fine itching on the arms which goes off by rubbing (aft. 1 h.). [*Ws.*]

Fine tearing in the arms, rather as if in the bones, worse when at rest than when moving (aft. 2 h.). [*Ws.*]

190. Drawing in the forearm and hand, like cramp.

Single, deeply penetrating stitches above the right wrist (aft. 7 h.). [*Ws.*]

Hot feeling on the back of the left hand (aft. 6 h.). [*Fz.*]

Rheumatic drawing aching on the back of the right hand, in the evening. [*Fz.*]

Obtuse stitches on the back of the right hand, in front of the wrist (aft. $\frac{1}{2}$ h.). [*Ws.*]

195. Drawing in one finger of the left hand.

Pain in the right middle finger as if it were torn out.

Pain in the proximal finger-joints as when an ulcerated part is moved.

Insensibility of the ring-finger, as if numb, stiff, and dead.

The fingers of the right hand only are cold to the touch, with feeling of cold (aft. 8 h.). [*Fz.*]

200. Aching pain internally in the flesh of the left thumb-ball (aft. $\frac{1}{4}$ h.). [*Mss.*]

Drawing round about the thumb-joint, as if it were sprained, especially when he bends the thumb. [*Fz.*]

The whole right side of the abdomen and of the thigh and leg is as if bruised, and as if it would break on account of rheumatic drawing when walking (aft. $1\frac{1}{2}$ h.). [*Fz.*]

Sudden heaviness and exhaustion in the lower limbs (aft. $\frac{1}{4}$ h.). [*Mss.*]

In the pelvis, when walking, a drawing squeezing sensation.

205. Cramp pain on the superior border of the os ilii extending to the spine (aft. 12 h.). [*Ws.*]

Frequent pain in the hip, on moving, as if stiff, or as if dislocated, almost like cramp.

On the left os innominatum, just behind the hip-joint, obtuse stitches in short fits, increased by every movement. [*Gss.*]

The hip-joint superiorly pains as if dislocated, and is almost useless for walking. [*Fz.*]

On the sciatic nerve, on the back of the thigh downwards, a boring paralytic pain. [*Fz.*]

210. In both inguinal joints, deep in the sinews, an aching drawing pain when rising from a seat (aft. 7 h.). [*Fz.*]

Fine stitches dart through the skin of the gluteal muscles, with external formication (aft. 6 h.). [*Ws.*]

Sharp stitches in the anterior muscles of the right thigh. [*Gss.*]

Twitching stitches in the left thigh and the superior border of the os ilii, extremely painful, only when sitting (aft. ¼ h.). [*Wsl.*]

In the anterior muscles of the right thigh a tensive pain when he flexes the knee. [*Gss.*]

215. After walking in the open air, excessively tired, especially in the thighs.

A fatigue and lassitude in all the limbs, without sleepiness.

The anterior muscles of the right thigh are as if paralysed ; when moving he feels a painful tension [*Gss.*]

Fine tearing in the thighs, more as if in the bones, worse when at rest than when moving (aft. 2 h.). [*Ws.*]

On the outside of the thigh a drawing aching pain when walking. [*Fz.*]

220. Cramp pain in the middle of the posterior part of the thigh, only when walking (aft. 21 h.). [*Ws.*]

Anteriorly and superiorly on the recti muscles of the thigh a tensive aching pain on extending it (aft. 2½ h.). [*Fz.*]

Fine itching on the thighs that goes off by rubbing (aft. 1 h.). [*Ws.*]

He cannot walk at all quick ; the lower limbs feel stiff. [*Fz.*]

Weakness of the lower limbs, especially felt above the knee-joint, as after a long journey on foot.

225. In the lower extremities feeling of stiffness, almost as if contact with a sickly person had bereft him of strength.

In the right knee-joint, when walking and when lifting the leg stretched forwards, a drawing squeezing sensation.

In the external tendons of the hough stitches darting upwards, when walking in the open air (aft. 13 h.). [*Lr.*]

Intermittent needle-pricks on the left patella, when walking in the open air (aft. 6 h.). [*Lr.*]

Spasmodic stretching drawing in the calf, and from the hough into the thigh. [*Fz.*]

230. Paralytic sensation, as from contraction of the ligaments, from the middle of the hough to the calf, when at rest and when moving (aft. ½ h). [*Mss.*]

On crossing the legs he feels a spasmodic tearing drawing in the heel of the left foot that is planted firmly on the ground and in its ball, and an aching drawing on the knee of the other leg that is thrown across (aft. 10 h.). [*Fz.*]

Drawing in the tibia and the neighbouring muscles.

On the tibia and about the ankle-joint, while walking, a drawing softly pressing pain and sensation as if the tibia would break, which prevents him walking. [*Fz.*]

Obtuse stitches on the left tibia (aft. 1 h.). [*Ws.*]

235. Burning on the tibiæ when walking. [*Fz.*]

Pressure and drawing on the tibia, in the evening, when sitting (aft. 12 h.). [*Fz.*]

In the morning, when walking about, a drawing aching pain in the ankle-joints, with heat in them, and sensation as if they were dislocated, towards the outer ankle (aft. 3 d.). [*Fz.*]

The legs are numb and stiff up to the knees, but without formication.

Pressing pain, as from dislocation, on the right foot, while walking in the open air (aft. 2¼ h.). [*Lr.*]

240. Cramp in the feet, for instants.

Cramp pain in the front part of the foot without actual muscular contraction, that is to say, without spasmodic cramp, more when seated and when at rest (aft. ½ h.).

Pain in the foot, when treading.

Cramp-like pain in the foot, and the following day an aching pain and as if bruised when treading.

Paralysis in the ankle-joints. [*Hsch.*]

245. Obtuse shooting drawing in the right ankle-joint, when sitting (aft. 11 h.). [*Fz.*]

Burning sensation of heat about the right external ankle, while walking and sitting (aft. 26 h.). [*Fz.*]

Almost shooting-like tearing on the dorsum of the left foot, mostly when moving. [*Fz.*]

On the border of the left foot externally on the projection of the fifth metatarsal bone a cramp-like aching drawing, as if he had sprained it (aft. 5 h.). [*Fz.*]

The outer border of the foot and the part below the outer ankle goes to sleep when walking. [*Fz.*]

250. Shooting in the heel, when sitting, in the evening.] *Fz.*]

In the sole of the foot a sudden tearing, when sitting. [*Fz.*]

Perspiration of the feet. [*Hsch.*]

When walking he feels here and there painful tension in the muscles. [*Gss.*]

In the evening, after sitting for an hour, he is quite stiff and contracted ; after rising from his seat he cannot straighten himself (aft. 13 h.). [*Fz.*]

255. Paralytic weakness in the hands and elbow-joints ; he can hardly move them, but without stiffness or other hindrance, with chilliness and loss of vital heat (aft. 1 h.). [*Fz.*]

Cracking in almost all the joints, but inaudible.

Cracking in all the joints (aft. 26 h.). [*Fz.*]

Great irritability and strained vivacity, with drawing in the limbs, as if the tendons were stretched, in the afternoon (aft. 2 d.) [*Fz.*]

In the evening, in bed, itching; after rubbing there came flat, very painful sores.

260. Sensation in the whole body as if his strength went away, and as if especially the marrow in the bones were stiffer and more coagulated (immediately).

When not engaged in any mental work he is tolerably brisk and lively; but he becomes dazed when he reads anything, and immediately falls asleep. [*Fz.*]

In the morning discomfort, frequent yawning, and disinclination to all work (aft. 4 d.). [*Fz.*]

He falls asleep when reading whilst seated, but starts up at the slightest noise, and has a shock with great rigor which goes through and through him. [*Fz.*]

Frequent attacks of yawning without sleepiness, with a cramp-like pain in the jaws.

265. Disposition to constant stretching.

Very frequent yawning, with stretching and extending the limbs (aft. 24 h.). [*Fz.*]

In the evening great weariness and irresistible desire to sleep; he sleeps for an hour while sitting, with snoring, but when he goes to bed cannot get to sleep before 1 o'clock. [*Fz.*]

In the evening great drowsiness till 9 o'clock, then great wakefulness until after midnight. [*Fz.*]

270. Sleep disturbed by dreams until 6 a.m., then he wakes up wide, and again falls asleep; in the morning he could not free himself from sleepiness, and remains drowsy until noon. [*Fz.*]

Sleep towards morning, with dreams. [*Fz.*]

Vivid dreams, sometimes disagreeable, sometimes anxious, with frequent awaking from sleep; on again falling asleep he always dreamt of quite other things. [*Lr.*]

Restless sleep; she often wakes without cause.

Restless sleep, [*Mlr.*]

At night, restless sleep, and that only towards morning, with dreams. [*Fz.*]

275. Sleep restless and full of dreams, but without waking, and on two successive nights, pollutions. [*Fz.*]

Very confused dreams, sometimes of a horrible character. [*Gss.*]

In the morning, **chilliness** in bed, not followed by heat.

Violent rigor over the back when walking about the room, in the forenoon (aft. 25 h.). [*Fz.*]

In the afternoon (about 3 o'clock), internal shivering, with great thirst, not followed by heat, for several successive days.

280. In the afternoon (about 3 o'clock), shivering with goose-skin, allayed in the open air, and without thirst, for several successive days.

After the shivering, slight heat.

In the forenoon, much thirst, and an hour afterwards rigor over the back. [*Fz.*]

Towards evening rather warm all over the body.

In the morning, in bed, heat about the head, with perspiration on the forehead.

285. Heat at night, especially in the forehead, so that he cannot sleep after 3 a.m.; then in the forenoon, about 9 a.m., there occurs rigor.

Towards evening, for three successive days, increased warmth of the cheeks and body, with aching pain and confusion of head in the temples and the sides of the forehead. [*Fz.*]

Immediately after eating supper, internal and external heat of face [*Mss.*]

In the afternoon, feeling of warmth all over the body, especially in the cheeks, not without thirst (aft. 2 d.). [*Fz.*]

Towards evening, warmth of the whole body, with aching drawing in the side of the forehead and thirst (aft. 4 d.). [*Fz.*]

290. Warmth of all the body, except the head; the cheeks were cold.* [*Hsch.*]

In the evening, on coming into the room, great heat, he does not know how to calm himself, but without thirst (aft. 2 d.). [*Fz.*]

No confidence in himself to undertake and carry through voluntary movements.

Pusillanimity.

Sadness and crossness (aft. 24. h.). [*Ws.*]

295. Sadness, discontent with his position, disagreeable sensitiveness to jokes; slight offences fill him with bitterness (aft. 12 h.). [*Ws.*]

He is easily frightened and starts. [*Fz.*]

When walking in the open air his disposition is good and cheerful (immediately).†

Cheerfulness and self-confidence that he can undertake anything with power‡ (aft. 48 h.). [*Ws.*]

Briskness and activity of mind.§ [*Hsch.*]

* The last part of this symptom was antagonistic reaction of the vital power (secondary action), as the person had for several days heat only in the cheeks before he took angustura.

† Seems to be merely curative action.

‡ Reaction of the vital power, curative action.

§ Reaction of the vital power, secondary action, curative action.

ARGENTUM.[1]

(Silver.)

This metal in its pure state, as *leaf-silver* (argentum foliatum), from the supposed impossibility of its being dissolved in our juices—an impossibility that has no better basis than theoretical speculation—is said by the teachers of materia medica to be just as powerless as gold (which see).

At first I allowed myself to be deterred by these confident assertions from using it medicinally, and therefore employed only the solution of nitrate of silver (in the dose of a drop of the quintillionth dilution), when I had the opportunity of observing the few subjoined symptoms caused by it.

But, in spite of all the denials of theorists without experience, who always persist in regarding the stomach as a cooking or digesting machine, containing gastric juice which, judging by their trials in the vessels of their laboratory, they found to be incapable of dissolving either metallic gold or metallic silver, and therefore considered these medicines to be incapable of exciting any action upon us such as they do when chemically dissolved *lege artis* in the stomach, when they are *methodice* absorbed and introduced into the circulation of the blood ; influenced by the reasons I have adduced respecting gold, I could not refrain from employing pure silver in the metallic state. I therefore made experiments on the healthy body with leaf-silver, after triturating it for an hour to the finest powder, with a hundred parts of milk-sugar.

The few symptoms observed from it and set forth in the following pages furnish the homœopathic physician, in silver under this form, with a curative instrument in many similar morbid states, which cannot be cured by any other medicinal agent, and for which the ordinary physician fails to find a remedy in all his therapeutics, clinical experience and voluminous prescription-books.

But I subsequently found that for homœopathic use another hundred-fold attenuation, that is to say, a grain of powder containing $\frac{1}{10000}$th of silver, may be a still too large dose.

The empirical reputation of nitrate of silver in the ordinary forms of epilepsy is not well founded, and seems to have arisen from the circumstance that in some varieties of convulsions, where copper is indicated, a salt of silver containing copper has been used. But that pure silver, such as leaf-silver is, should be efficacious in the worst and commonest form of epilepsy, is not borne out by the primary symptoms as yet revealed from its administration.

[1] From vol. iv, 2nd edit., 1825.

R. BOYLE's so-called *diuretic pills*, which contain nitrate of silver, and which are so much praised by BOERHAVE, are quite unsuitable for their purpose, not only on account of the perilous size of the doses, but also because silver, as the subjoined symptoms produced by it show, only increases the urinary secretion in its primary action (consequently the opposite of the diminished urinary secretion in dropsical diseases), whereupon, by means of the ensuing reaction of the vital force, the opposite of the end aimed at must take place, which is its permanent secondary action, to wit, *a still greater diminution of the urinary secretion* ; a true antipathic and, for this case, injurious procedure.

Such hurtful mistakes must have hitherto been committed by the ordinary physicians, because they were unacquainted with the primary effects of the medicines, and knew of no way whereby they could learn them, and took no pains to discover the right way. Indeed, for five-and-twenty centuries they have had no notion of primary and secondary action of medicines, as a permanent condition, the exact opposite of their primary action, and that, consequently, in order to effect any permanent cure, medicines to be really curative must be able to produce in their primary action the *simile* of the morbid state actually present, to allow us to expect from the reaction of the organism the opposite of the medicinal primary action (and of the disease similar to it), that is to say, the destruction and alteration into health of the deranged sensations and functions.

On the other hand, silver can cure permanently some kinds of diabetes when the other symptoms of the disease correspond in similarity to the other primary symptoms of the disease.

[HAHNEMANN was assisted in this proving by—FRANZ, GROSS, HAYNEL, HARTMANN, HERRMANN, LANGHAMMER, MEYER, WISLICENUS.

The following old-school authorities were consulted for the effects of nitrate of silver :

HALL, THOM., *Phys. Med. Journal.* 1800, July, also in *Duncan's Annals of Med.* v, 1801.

KINGLAKE, *London Medical and Physical Journal*, 1801.

MOODIE, *Med. and Phys. Journal*, 1804.

No old-school writers are quoted for effects of metallic silver.

The 1st edit. gave 200 symptoms to silver, to this 2nd edit. 23 have been added.]

ARGENTUM NITRICUM.

Vertigo, with complete but transient blindness. [THOMAS HALL, in the *Phys. Med Journal*, 1800, p. 518, also in *Duncan's Annals of Med.*, 1799.[1]]

(It affected the head, as if the fit of epilepsy would come on.)

(Premonitory feeling of the impending fit.)

---

1 Effects of A. n. given to a woman, æt. 35, for convulsive attacks. This occurred twice, three hours after taking the drug. The name of this author is wrongly given by Hahnemann as "HULL."

Dimness of vision with anxiety, heat of face, and weeping eyes.

5. Spongy, easily bleeding gums, which, however, were not painful nor swollen. [MOODIE, in *Med. and Phys. Journal*, 1804.[1]]

Sensation as if the velum palati were swollen, not *per se*, but on moving the tongue and when swallowing.

Sickness, weight, and pressure in the stomach.[2] [HALL, l. c.]

Burning heat in the stomach. [KINGLAKE, in *London Medical and Physical Journal*, 1801.[3]]

Burning in the stomach and on the chest. [MOODIE, l. c.]

10. The urinary organs are at first greatly irritated.[4] [l. c.]

Disagreeable stoppage in the upper part of the nose for three days. [HALL, l. c.]

Discharge from the nose like white pus mixed with blood-clots.[5] [HALL, l. c.]

Feeling in all the limbs as if they would go to sleep and stiffen.

Exhaustion in the afternoon.

15. Profuse night sweat.

Anxiety that compels him to walk quickly.

ARGENTUM FOLIATUM.

He became suddenly dizzy, and as if a mist were before the eyes.

Vertiginous, sleepy intoxication ; his eyes closed.

Attacks of vertigo ; he cannot think properly ; also when sitting and reflecting (aft. ½ h.). [*Gss.*]

Stupid in the head. [*Gss.*]

5. His head began to creep and crawl, as from intoxication.

He is always in a kind of intoxication ; he knows not what is the matter with him. [*Fz.*]

Feeling of gloominess in the head, as if smoke were in the brain. [*Myr.*]

As if stupid and hollow in the head, the whole brain is painful, with chilliness.

Shooting burning pain in the head.

10. Severe shooting and tearing pain in the head.

(In the morning shooting headache, with redness of one eye.)

When standing and reading he had a sudden burning sensation in the scrobiculus cordis, a sensation of dull contraction of the brain from all sides, and like a threatening of vertigo, with sick nausea in the region of the sternum, such as is apt to occur after rapid violent turning round in a circle ; at the same time a sudden heat all over

---

1. General statement. Literally, "after a time, tenderness of the gums, with a disposition to bleed ; they were, however, neither painful nor swollen."
2. On three occasions, three hours after ingestion.
3. Effects of A. n. given to a man, æt 30, for epilepsy.
4. Not found ; the name of the authority being omitted, it is doubtful to which it rightly belongs.
5. After the three days of S. II. The pus is said to have been like brain-substance.

the body, but more in the face, and momentary perspiration on the chest and face.

A sensation compounded of pressure and drawing in the head, above the right ear towards the back (aft. 4 h.). [*Gss.*]

In the left temple horrible pain compounded of aching and tearing (aft. 5 h.). [*Gss.*]

15. Tearing in the left temple. [*Gss.*]

Tearing as if in the bone of the left temple and above the left mastoid process. [*Hnl.*]

Drawing pain from the occipital bone to the middle of the frontal bone, in a curved direction over the right temporal bone, externally. [*Hrr.*]

Aching tearing pain on the left and right temporal bones, increased by touch. [*Hrr.*]

Squeezing pressure on the right temple, with intermittent sharp stitches inwards (aft. 5. d.). [*Ws.*]

20. Cutting stitches, as if in the bone or on the surface of the brain, just in front of the left ear, going forwards. [*Hnl.*]

Aching pain on the temporal bones, externally. [*Hrr.*]

Aching pain on both parietal bones, externally. [*Hrr.*]

Aching pain on the left parietal bone, externally. [*Hrr.*]

A slight pressure on the head causes sore pain. [*Fz.*]

25. Slight rippling shudder over the right side of the hairy scalp. [*Hnl.*]

Aching pain with stupefaction in the sinciput, and drawing aching in the occiput.

Aching headache in the forehead above the eyebrows (aft. 2 h.). [*Ws.*]

Aching tearing headache in the left frontal protuberance (aft. 6 h.). [*Gss.*]

Aching tearing headache under the left frontal protuberance, during which the eyeball also seems to be compressed. [*Gss.*]

30. Intermittent boring pains, anteriorly on the left side of the forehead all day, aggravated after lying down in the evening (aft. 7 h.). [*Lr.*]

The nape feels stiff, and there is a strange feeling in the occiput; a kind of drawing and aching therein.

In the right temporal muscles, the right frontal muscles, the lateral cervical muscles near the thyroid cartilage, and posteriorly towards the nape, a spasmodic twitching and jumping of the muscles that pushed away the hand, with twitching pain.

A pimple on the left temple, that when touched pains like a boil.

(The borders of the upper and lower eyelids are very red and swelled, but the eyes do not suppurate.)

35. Great itching in the canthi of the eyes.

Painful gnawing aching in the facial bones of the right side, worst on the malar bone (aft. 1 h.). [*Ws.*]

Tearing on the left zygoma. [*Hrr.*]

1 [*Hartmann* in orig. evidently a misprint for *Herrmann.*]

Fine drawing pain in the facial muscles, especially on the malar bones. [*Ws.*]

Fine painful stitches on the malar bone. [*Ws.*]

40. Cutting stitches from the interior of the left ear, extending into the brain.

Sensation in the right ear as if it was stopped up.[1]

Above the left ear, on a small spot, aching tearing (aft. 12 h.). [*Gss.*]

Great itching on the external ear, causing scratching till blood comes.

Gnawing itching on the lobes of both ears, in the morning, after rising (aft. 24 h.), [*Gss.*]

45. From the depression under the lobe of the right ear to the skin of the cheek, a drawing pain, that extends to the lower jaw, as if it were in the periosteum. [*Fz.*]

On chewing, cutting sensation, as if he had taken some acrid acid, in the Eustachian tube towards the parotid gland. [*Fz.*]

Profuse epistaxis from blowing the nose (immediately after dinner), and again three hours afterwards.

Epistaxis came on after creeping and tickling in the nose.

Swelling of the upper lip, close below the nose.

50. The gums are painful *per se*, but more when touched.

(An incisor tooth pained when it was pressed forwards) (aft. 5 h.). [*Ws.*]

On the outside of the neck, left side, aching while walking in the open air. [*Fz.*]

Cutting stitches inwards under the right lower jaw, as if in a gland. [*Hnl.*]

The neck in the neighbourhood of the sub-maxillary glands is swollen, and in consequence the neck is stiff and tense when moving; at the same time swallowing is rendered difficult by internal swelling of the throat, and he must force every mouthful with an effort through the gullet (aft. 48 h.). [*Ws.*]

55. Dry feeling of the tongue, which, however, is moist. [*Fz.*]

A small vesical on the tongue with burning sore pain.

In the throat he has a raw and sore pain.

Boring and digging pain in the throat.

Soreness and rawness in the throat when expiring and swallowing. [*Fz.*]

60. Rough and scraping in the throat, lasting all day. [*Hnl.*]

On the velum palati a scraping sensation, as if a rough body were adherent there, not exactly painful but disagreeable, more felt during empty deglutition than when swallowing a morsel, but constantly felt and compelling him to swallow his saliva; after several hours this secretion goes deeper down in the fauces. [*Fz.*]

---

1 [SS. 40 and 41, though they have no name attached, are among the symptoms observed by others, therefore not by Hahnemann.]

When yawning, a painful tension in the fauces, as from a swelling. [*Gss.*]

The collection of viscid saliva in the mouth renders speaking difficult. [*Fz.*]

Collection of saliva in the mouth, with shivering shaking. [*Fz.*]

65. **Viscid, grey, gelatinous mucus in the fauces, which can be easily expectorated by hawking, in the morning.** [*Gss.*]

(Great longing for wine.)

Appetite quite gone ; he feels a loathing at food, when he merely thinks about it.

Indifference to all food, and he is easily satiated. [*Fz.*]

The morning hunger disappears. [*Fz.*]

70. Very great appetite (aft. 40 h.). [*Gss.*]

Though the stomach is full, the appetite still continues great. [*Gss.*]

Excessive gnawing hunger all day, not extinguished by eating. Afterwards, for several days, it could only be allayed for a short time by eating. [*Hnl.*]

In the morning, in the abdomen, stomach, and chest, a burning sensation as from heartburn.

Sensation similar to heartburn (aft. $1\frac{1}{2}$ h.). [***Myr.***]

75. Hiccup during (accustomed) tobacco smoking (aft. $1\frac{1}{4}$ h.). [*Lr.*]

Almost uninterrupted qualmishness and nausea. [*Fz.*]

Sick feeling in the throat, and immediately afterwards heat all over, but chiefly on the head, with redness of face, without thirst (aft. $\frac{1}{2}$ h.). [*Myr.*]

Retching, whereby a bitter, pungent, ill-tasting fluid is brought up from the stomach into the mouth, after which a scraping, scratching, very burning sensation remains permanently in the fauces (heartburn) (aft. 8 h.). [*Gss.*]

Aching in the scrobiculus cordis. [*Fz.*]

80. Pinching over the stomach and in the left hypochondrium. [*Fz.*]

After he has commenced to eat, there occurs a severe aching from the abdomen towards the pubic region, which is aggravated by inspiration, and is relieved by rising from his seat. [*Gss.*]

At night an aching painful distension in the abdomen, which went off without discharge of flatulence.

Rumbling in the abdomen at night and discharge of flatus.

Loud noises in the abdomen, on the left side, like the croaking of young frogs (aft. $\frac{3}{4}$ h.). [***Lr.***]

85. After the morning stool, contractive belly-ache, as from a chill, when sitting.

Belly-ache, as in diarrhœa. [*Fz.*]

Cutting internally, transversely through the abdomen.

Contraction of the abdominal muscles when walking, with tension in them, so that he must walk bent forwards. [*Fz.*]

In the abdominal muscles, near the last two ribs, sharp stitches from within outwards, which end in a fine pinching, and are somewhat allayed by rubbing (aft. 60 h.). [*Ws.*]

90. A boring pain in the right hypogastrium, just above the groin (aft. 34 h.). [*Lr.*]

Shooting cutting on both sides in the region of the inguinal ring (aft. 3½ h.). [*Hnl.*]

In the bend of the left groin, sensation of straining of the tendon (of the lumbar muscle) which pains as if bruised when pressed on. [*Fz.*]

Pressing in the hypogastrium during the stool, which is moderately soft, and also thereafter (aft. 72 h.). [*Ws.*]

Frequent (never ineffectual) urging to stool in the lower part of the rectum, and evacuation of a scanty soft stool (aft. 2½ h.), lasting several days.[1]

95. During the evacuation of a soft stool, a painful urging in the hypogastrium.

During the evacuation, in the afternoon, he vomited twice.

After dinner, a stool which is very dry and sandy, but is passed without difficulty (aft. 8 h.). [*Fz.*]

Very frequent micturition (aft. 6 h.). [*Gss.*]

Frequent urging to urinate and copious flow of urine for several hours (aft. 2 h.). [*Lr.*]

100. Almost every night an emission of semen.

At night pollutions, without lascivious dreams. [*Lr.*]

A pain in the left testicle, as after a contusion (aft. 49 h.). [*Lr.*]

* * *

Irritation in the nose, as if coryza were about to come (aft. 1 h.). [*Myr.*]

The nose is as if stopped up anteriorly in both nostrils, and there is smarting in the left nostril. [*Fz.*]

105. Fluent coryza ; the nose is always full of mucus. [*Gss.*]

Excessive fluent coryza, with frequent sneezing, for two days. [*Hnl.*]

Severe fluent coryza, without sneezing (aft. 10 h.). [*Lr.*]

Raw and sore pain superiorly in the larynx, when coughing, not when swallowing.

By day (not at night and not in the open air), several attacks of short rattling cough, with white, thick, easily detached expectoration, like boiled starch, but opaque, without taste or smell.

110. (In the morning, cough.)

By laughing mucus is produced in the trachea, and cough excited. [*Fz.*]

Mucus in the chest and cough with expectoration (aft. 26 h.). [*Lr.*]

On going upstairs and stooping mucus comes in the wind-pipe, which is expectorated by a single impulse of cough. [*Fz.*]

On stooping mucus comes into the wind-pipe, which is expectorated by a single impulse of cough. [*Fz.*]

115. In the morning after rising from bed, an irritating tussiculation without expectoration (aft. 48 h.). [*Lr.*]

---

1 This symptom has no name attached but being among the "observat others" must not be attributed to Hahnemann.

Obtuse cutting, passing into shooting, rises up into the wind-pipe, and compels him to cough two or three times, and thereafter continues for some time ; the cough brings watery expectoration, which does not remove the irritation to cough (aft. 24 h.). [Fz]

In the right side of the chest, from within outwards, such a violent stitch, lasting about a minute, that he can neither inspire nor expire (when sitting) (aft. 28 h.). [Lr.]

Fine stitches in the interior of the upper part of the sternum, from within outwards (aft. 48 h.). [Ws.]

Sharp stitches on the right side, near the nipple. [Hrr.]

120. Under the right nipple, a shooting, not connected with inspiration or expiration. [Gss.]

Tearing under the right nipple. [Gss.]

Gnawing scraping on the left side of the chest when at rest. [Ws.]

Cramp pain on the left side of the chest, and when it is gone the part still pains when touched (aft. 9 h.). [Ws.]

(Oppressive burning in the region of the heart. [Hnl.]

125. Feeling of pressure and oppression in the left side of the chest above the heart (aft. 78 h.). [Ws.]

A shooting, squeezing pain on the left side of the sternum, most severe when sitting bent forwards, unconnected with expiration or inspiration (aft. 8 h.). [Ws.]

Aching shooting on the right side of the chest and sternum, only slightly increased by inspiring deeply (aft. some m.). [Ws.]

On inspiring deeply an out-pressing pain on a spot the size of a florin under the second and third right ribs. [Hnl.]

On the right side of the chest, a spot with aching pain, as if something hard was pressed against the ribs. [Fz.]

130. Violent aching in the middle of the sternum, internally, very much increased by every movement, especially by stooping forwards and then rising up. [Hnl.]

Aching pain on the sternum, externally. [Hrr.]

Needle-pricks under the ensiform cartilage of the sternum. [Hrr.]

Sharp stitches on the right near the manubrium sterni (aft. 3 h.). [Hrr.]

On some ribs, a spasmodic aching tensive pain.

135. Sharp stitches between the sixth and seventh true ribs of the right side, which are aggravated by inspiring deeply. [Hrr.]

Under the last left rib a cutting stitch transversely across, on leaning over to the side and on supporting himself with his arm.

Obtuse stitches on the left side, under the last false ribs. [Hrr.]

Obtuse stitches under the third true rib of the left side, equally felt when inspiring and expiring. [Hrr.]

Slowly intermittent obtuse stitches under the cartilages of the last true ribs, on the left above the scrobiculus cordis (in the evening in bed) (aft. 31 h.). [Gss.]

140. Severe cutting from within outwards, in both sides at the lowest ribs, when inspiring deeply, only slight at other times ; if he

moves the trunk without inspiring he experiences no increase, but he does so immediately on drawing in the breath (aft. 10 h.). [*Ws.*]

Cutting stitches at the end of the ribs on the right side near the spine, especially on bending the back. [*Hnl.*]

In the side of the back, opposite the abdomen, first an aching, afterwards when standing, on the slightest movement and when breathing, a frightfully severe aching shooting, almost as if he should die; he must walk in a bent posture; it felt like the grasping pain of a malignant ulcer when he lay still; in the chest itself there was oppression, so that he could not get his breath, as if a great weight lay on the chest.

Burning shooting in the right side of the sacrum when sitting; when he rises up and when he presses on it the spot has only a burning pain, and does not shoot any more. [*Fz.*]

Drawing on the right side of the posterior portion of the pelvis and in the sacrum (aft. ¼ h.). [*Gss.*]

145. Sensation as if the sacrum were beaten (aft. 24 h.). [*Gss.*]

His sacrum is very painful, as if bruised (aft. 36 h.). [*Gss.*]

Obtuse stitches in the second lumbar vertebra. [*Hrr.*]

A tickling, itching shooting betwixt the scapulæ, as from a severe flea- or gnat-bite; he cannot scratch enough.

Sharp aching inside the scapulæ (aft. 1 h.). [*Ws.*]

150. On the upper part of the left scapula excessive tearing, when sitting, which went off on rising from the seat. [*Gss.*]

Formication, as if asleep, in the left scapula. [*Fz.*]

Tearing on the top of the shoulder and on the head of the humerus. [*Hrr.*]

Tearing in the glenoid cavity of the shoulder-joint, extending into the clavicle. [*Hrr*]

Boring stitches in the right axilla, which did not go off by touching (aft. 30 h.). [*Lr.*]

155. Aching tearing beneath the shoulder-joint. [*Gss.*]

Continued pinching on the right upper arm (aft. 1 h.). [*Ws.*]

Tearing in the left upper arm. [*Hrr.*]

A burning, very transient stitch anteriorly in the middle of the left upper arm. [*Hnl.*]

Aching pain in the flesh of the upper arm, which is increased by touching. [*Hrr.*]

160. Cramp in the middle of the upper arm on raising it; otherwise little felt (aft. 10 h.). [*Ws.*]

Tensive drawing, resembling shooting, in various parts of the arms.

In the bend of the right elbow a spasmodic, aching, drawing pain, as if the arm had been strained by violent exertion, only when moving it, but more when extending than when flexing it.

In the bend of the right and left elbow and in both knees an aching, drawing, tensive pain (under all circumstances), which only goes off for a moment by pressing strongly on it, but then returns immediately.

Paralytic sensation in the arms on moving them, especially at the elbow-joint (aft. 32 h.). [*Ws.*]

165. A kind of paralysis of the right arm and hand; it sinks down, and he can hardly write even with much effort (aft. 3 h.). [*Hrr.*]

On flexing the arm a tension externally on the point of the elbow (aft. 1 h.). [*Ws.*]

Burning in the point of the right elbow (aft. 6 h.). [*Gss.*]

On the inside of the left forearm a spasmodic, aching, drawing pain.

In the muscles betwixt the ulna and the radius of the left forearm, on the back thereof, not far from the wrist bone, a very severe, aching tearing (aft. 31 h.). [*Gss.*]

170. A not long continued jerking tearing, as if in the middle of the radius, first of the right then of the left forearm, and lastly in the proximal phalanx of the right middle finger, recurring from time to time. [*Hnl.*]

Sharp, intermittent stitches on the right radius, rather in the muscles. [*Hrr.*]

Sharp, continued stitch behind the wrist-joint, at the commencement of the radius (aft. 6 h.). [*Ws.*]

Shooting, itching burning under the skin on the inside of the left wrist-joint (aft. 32 h.). [*Ws.*]

A tickling in the right palm that compels scratching (aft. 33 h.). [*Lr.*]

175. Cramp-like drawing in the dorsum of the right hand and foot. [*Fz.*]

Aching tearing in the wrist-bones of both hands. [*Gss.*]

Tearing aching pain in the metacarpal bone of the thumb and in the metatarsal bone and proximal phalanx of the big toe of the right and left foot, increased by touching. [*Hrr.*]

Tearing in the proximal phalanx of the fourth finger of the left hand and in its metacarpal bone, with spasmodic drawing inwards of the finger, particularly when grasping anything. [*Hnl.*]

Drawing in the joints of the three middle fingers of the left hand, when moving and when at rest. [*Hrr.*]

180. Tension and drawing in the groin below the inguinal ring, in the left thigh. [*Fz.*]

In the hip and thigh a paralytic weakness.

On a spot behind the left hip, a violent pain, as if he had fallen hard upon it, only when moving; standing did not cause it (aft. 32 h.). [*Lr.*]

When running, when he treads upon the projected left foot, a painful, sharp aching in the right hip-joint. [*Gss.*]

When walking, paralytic weakness in the right hip-joint, especially when drawing forward the foot, and stitches in it when treading, which makes him limp in his gait, soon going off. [*Hnl.*]

185. Formicating humming in the left thigh, and drawing in its anterior muscles. [*Fz.*]

Twitching and palpitation in several muscular parts, especially on the right thigh. [*Gss.*]

Slight twitching on the outside of the left knee, together with a sensation like gurgling, when sitting (immediately). [*Ws.*]

Above the left knee cramp-like cutting-inwards on both sides when he is not moving (aft. 8 h.). [*Ws.*]

Tearing, obtuse stitches above the left patella, in all positions. [*Hnl.*]

190. In the left knee-joint a tearing when sitting (aft. 72 h.). [*Gss.*]

The knee pains as if bruised, more severe when sitting than when walking (aft. 1½ h.). [*Ws.*]

The knees often bend below him when walking. [*Hnl.*]

Pressing pain in the knee-joint and pressing outwards in the muscles of the left lower extremity when sitting. [*Hrr.*]

(Several papules on the tibia causing burning pain).

195. In the evening, in bed, burning, corroding stitches in the left tibia, not far from the knee, so that his foot twitched involuntarily (aft. 17 h.). [*Hnl.*]

Cramp in the left calf, worst when at rest (aft. 4 h.). [*Ws.*]

On going drown stairs the muscles of the calves pain as if they were too short. [*Hnl.*]

Bruised pain in the ankle-joints and throbbing in them, worst when sitting (aft. 3 d.). [*Ws.*]

In the ankle-joints and in the lower parts of the legs a strong beating and dull throbbing, as from being over-tired, with crawling and stitches on the skin of the leg, worst when at rest, less when moving (aft. 14 h.). [*Ws.*]

200. In the left ankle-joint a sensation as if the foot were detached there, and as if the cartilages of the joint did not touch one another, when walking. [*Fz.*]

Shooting cutting in the outer ankles, from within outwards, when sitting, scarcely at all when walking ; it is most severe when the foot is resting on a narrow ledge (aft. some h.). [*Ws.*]

Tearing in the feet, at one time on the sole, at another on the dorsum of the foot, then in the heel, then in the toes (especially in their proximal joints), then in the bones of the feet, then in the metatarsal bones, which pains do not extend beyond the ankles ; only occasionally a flying, tearing pain extends farther up. [*Hrr.*]

Pain in the heel when treading, as if numb (continued).

In the right heel and tendo Achillis a (somewhat burning) sensation of gone-to-sleep. [*Fz.*]

205. Intermittent violent burning in a corn, also when not pressed from without, for 24 hours. [*Ws.*]

On the ends of the hollow bones, near, above, or beneath their joints, on several parts of the body, an aching tearing (aft. 48 h.). [*Gss.*]

Great exhaustion of the body, especially of the thighs, when sitting and walking, with drowsiness (aft. 4 h.). [*Myr.*]

Discomfort, lassitude in all the limbs. [*Gss.*]

Chill in the back and from below to above the ankles, where it continued for two hours, and was very sensitive ; walking did not allay it (aft. 6½ h.). [*Hnl.*]

210. In the afternoon chilliness, until he went to sleep ; he could not get warm even in bed ; after midnight, perspiration.

At night, in bed, on the least raising of the bed-clothes, or letting in the air under them, febrile rigor on the upper part of the body; but when he was properly covered he had only normal warmth (aft. 4 h.).

Shivering through the whole body (aft. 1½ h.). [*Lr.*]

When walking in the open air exhaustion and heat all over, without perspiration, and anxiety as if his clothes were too tight.

In the forenoon heat and hot feeling all over the body, but less in the head, without thirst, with perspiration only on the abdomen and slightly on the chest.

215. In the evening, in bed, quick pulse, with thirst (aft. 11 h.). [***Myr.***]

The attacks recur every day at noon.

Intolerable itching, like a flea or a louse running over the head and all the body.

A burning itching here and there on the skin, *e. g.* of the face, the hands, &c., which, however, does not compel him to scratch.

Dreams of what occurred during the day.

220. Anxious dreams; after waking he was still so anxious that he imagined it had really happened as he had dreamt (aft. 65 h.).

(In her contentment she is extravagantly merry, but a trifle immediately sets her off weeping for a long time).

Greater cheerfulness of disposition and inclination to speak all day (aft. 3 h.*). [*Lr.*]

Ill-humoured.

* Curative secondary action.

ARNICA MONTANA.[1]

The root of this plant, whose favourite habitat is in shrub-grown upland plains, very soon loses in the air a considerable portion of its odour and of its medicinal power, but it loses most by boiling. Still the freshly prepared powder dried rapidly and thoroughly in the water-bath may be kept with almost unimpaired power for several years in well-corked phials.

All the artificial dogmas enunciated by the ordinary medical art, which is in its way a learned science, all its scholastic definitions, distinctions, and hair-splitting explanations were in all past centuries unable to discover the specific curative power of this plant or to find out the real remedy for the often dangerous general derangement of the health which is caused by a severe fall, by blows, knocks, contusions, sprains, or by over-stretching or laceration of the solid parts* of our body. Common people had to do this for them, and after the fruitless employment of innumerable things they found at last by accident the true remedy in this vegetable, and hence they called it *Fallkraut* (*fall plant*). Some 200 years ago a physician (FEHR) first mentioned this discovery of domestic practice to the learned medical art (this plant was then named by her "Panacea lapsorum"), which has likewise borrowed all the other still extant specific remedies she possesses without exception from the accidental discoveries of domestic practice, but was unable to find them for herself, because she never attempted to ascertain the pure effects of natural substances on the healthy human body.

The symptoms of all injuries caused by severe contusions and lacerations of the fibres are tolerably uniform in character, and, as the following record shows, these symptoms are contained in striking homœopathic similarity in the alterations of the health which arnica develops in the healthy human subject.

In severe and extensive contusion-injuries the cure is very much promoted when, in addition to a small dose of arnica taken internally (when necessary a dose every three days), the parts are also for the first twenty-four hours externally moistened with wine or equal parts of brandy and water, with one pound of either of which five to ten drops of the hundred-fold potentized dilution of arnica are mixed and strongly succussed about ten times.

But the following list of its pure powers points to several other morbid conditions in the human system for which arnica offers sure

* Hence it is very beneficial in the most severe wounds by bullets and blunt weapons, as also in the pains and other ailments consequent on extracting the teeth, and in other surgical operations whereby sensitive parts have been violently stretched, as also after dislocations of the joints, after setting fractures of the bones, &c.

1 From vol. i, 3rd edit., 1830.

homœopathic relief. It is a medicine of much utility, and although its action even in large doses does not last beyond six days, yet I have found it an indispensable auxiliary and intermediate remedy even in the most chronic diseases.

But we must never employ it in purely inflammatory acute diseases, with general heat, chiefly external, nor in diarrhœas. In such cases it will always be found to be very hurtful, the reason of which is obvious from its peculiar mode of action.

In some kinds of false pleurisy, however, it is very efficacious, in such, namely, whose symptoms correspond to those of this root.

The best preparation of this medicine for internal use is the decillionth[1] development of power. When we can obtain the plant in the green state we mix the freshly expressed juice obtained from the whole plant when near its flowering time with equal parts of spirits of wine. Two drops of the clear fluid, obtained by allowing the mixture to stand, are first diluted with ninety-eight drops of spirits of wine and potentized by two succussions. The dilution is carried on through twenty-nine other phials, always one drop of the weaker dilution added to 100 drops of spirit in the next phial, and shaken twice. In the last phial it is brought to the decillionth development of power.

But if we cannot get the plant in the green state we must be satisfied with a tincture made by adding ten grains of the finely powdered root, as fresh as it can be had, to 1000 drops of alcohol, and allowing it to digest for a week, giving it one shake per diem. Of this one drop is mixed with 100 drops of alcohol, and potentized with two succussions, and so on until the decillionth potency is reached. Two or three of the smallest globules moistened with the highest potency are the most ordinary dose for internal use.

Camphor is the antidote for large doses in unhomœopathic cases, but wine aggravates its injurious effects.

[The names of HAHNEMANN'S fellow-observers are :—AUG. BAEHR, FRANZ, GROSS, FR. HAHNEMANN, HORNBURG, KUMMER, LANGHAMMER, STAPF, WISLICENUS.

The old-school authorities quoted are :

AASKOW, *Act. Soc. Med. Hafn.*, ii.
COLLIN, *Obs. circa Morbos*, iv and v.
CRICHTON, A., *Samml. br. Abh. f. pr. Aerzte*, xiii, 3.
DE LA MARCHE, *Diss. de Arnica vera*, Halæ, 1719.
DE MEZA, *Samml. br. Abh. f. pr. Aerzte*, xiii.
Edinb. Med. Comment., Dec. ii, vol. ii.
MURRAY, *Appar. Medicam.*, i.
PELARGUS, *Obs.*, i.
STOLL, *Rat. Med.*, iii.
THOMAS A THUESSINK, *Waarnehm.*, Groning. 1805.
Veckoskrift for Lakare, viii.
VICAT, *Mat. Med.*, i.

In the *Frag. de Vir.* Arnica has 150 symptoms, in the 1st edit. 230, in the 2nd edit. 592, and in this the 3rd edit. 638.]

1 In this as in many other places Hahnemann calls the potency by the degree of its dilution, and not as on other occasions by the number of times it has been diluted by the addition of 99 or 100 parts to 1 of the stronger preparation. Thus "the hundredfold potentized dilution" is the first dilution, "the decillionth development of power" is the thirtieth dilution.

ARNICA.

During dinner sudden vertigo, as if he would fall forwards. [*Gss.*]

Giddy whilst walking. [*Stf. Gss., Archiv f. d. homoop. Heilk.*, v, iii.[1]]

Vertigo in the forehead, especially when walking, when it seems to her as if all went round with her in a circle and would tumble with her. [*Stf. Gss.*]

Vertigo ; when she sits and leans the head forward, almost unnoticed ; but when she raises or moves the head, immediately a feeling as if all went round with her. [*Stf. Gss.*]

5. Vertigo.

Confusion of head.

Confusion of head, vertigo, and anxiety, increased by artificial vomiting.

Stupefying headache in the morning.

Heaviness in the forehead (aft. 1 h.). [*Stf. Gss.*]

10. He sits buried in thought, but does not actually think of anything. [*Kr.*]

Want of memory ; he forgets the word on his lips. [*Fr. H—n.*]

Distraction of the mind ; he cannot fiix his thoughts long on one subject. [*Ws.*]

Along with cloudiness of the head and confusion of the lateral parts of the skull, contracted pupils [*Fz.*]

Dulness in the head, without any particular headache (aft. 2 h.), [*Kr.*]

15. He readily falls into a waking dream. [*Kr.*]

Internal heat, especially in the head, with heaviness of it, without thirst. *Ws.*]

Burning in the head, with aching, out-stretching pain.

Burning in the brain, the rest of the body being cool, at least not hot.

Heat in the head ; the rest of the body being cool, at least not hot.

20. Headache. [De Meza,[2] in *Samml. br. Abh. f. pr. Aerzte*, xiii.—*Edinb. Med. Comment.*, Dec. ii, v. ii, p. 350.]

In the temples an aching pain (aft. ½ h.). [*Kr.*]

After aching headache, there occurs also in the temples throbbing, aching headache.

---

1 In the original the symptoms contributed by Stapf and Gross, which first appeared in the *Archiv*, are indicated by a reference of each to that periodical. For the reason stated in regard to aconite we have substituted the names of the provers for the reference to the periodical. No explanation of these symptoms is given in the *Archiv*, save that they were observed on healthy persons.

2 A case of paraplegia induced by suppressed menstruation (from fatigue and fright) in a young girl, cured (after lasting three years) by arnica, which brought on the menses immediately, motion returning in two days. (The symptoms have been translated direct from the Latin original). See S. 339 and note.

Aching pain in the forehead.

Aching pain in the forehead, which increases when near the warm stove, as if the brain were rolled into a lump. [*Fz.*]

25. Aching and out-stretching pain, as from something soft in the crown, with drawing in the occiput and tearing towards the temples. [*Fz.*]

Aching pain over the eyes, going towards the temples, with sensation as if the integuments of the forehead were spasmodically contracted (aft. 1 h.). [*Ws.*]

First aching pain in the forehead, then shooting and jerking-shooting pain in the forehead ; with chilliness (aft. 8 h.).

Aching, pressing pain in the forehead, especially severe when walking, going up stairs, thinking and reading. [*Hbg.*]

Aching in the right frontal bone, followed by sneezing, whereupon it extended first into the left then into the right ear (aft. 2 d.). [*Hbg.*]

30. Aching, painful drawing in the left half of the skull from the ear upwards (aft. 3 h.). [*Hbg.*]

Aching, stupefying pain in the forehead, rather externally (aft. 5½ h.). [*Lr.*]

Aching pain externally, on the crown. [*Ws.*]

After sneezing twice, a pain in the left side of the forehead, as after a violent blow. [*Hbg.*]

When coughing violent shooting in the sinciput (aft. 7 h.). [***Lr.***]

35. Great shoots in the head on coughing (aft. 10 h.).

Headache ; shootings outwards, which recur when coughing and even when moving the head, and which are only allayed when he lies on the painful side of the head.

Fine shooting pain in the forehead which is aggravated by raising the eyes, with heat of face and thirst.

Shooting in the forehead.

In the forehead jerking shooting.[*Stf. Gss.*]

40. On the left temple jerking shooting. [*Stf. Gss.*]

Headache as if a nail were driven into the temple, with general perspiration, about midnight, followed by exhaustion (aft. a few h.).

From time to time recurring, fine shooting tearing headache in the left temple (aft. 4 h.).

Stitches rapidly following one another in the temporal region towards the forehead (aft. 4 h.). [*Kr.*]

In the left frontal protuberance a rapid shooting, with the sensation as if blood were extravasated in the forehead. [*Gss.*]

45. Shooting pain in the forehead. [*Hbg.*]

Obtuse stitches into the temples (aft. 1 h.). [*Ws.*]

Jerking, shooting headache on stooping, as if all would come out at the forehead ; at the same time nausea, qualmish about the heart. [*Stf. Gss.*]

Twitching, tearing headache, increased by stooping and coughing.

Twitching headache, in the sinciput (aft. 1 h.). [*Ws.*]

50. Tearing in the left temple, and, when walking in the open

air, recurrence of the aching out-stretching headache (aft. 10 h.). [*Fz.*]

Repeated tearing headache in the left temple. [*Hbg.*]

Great internal and external heat of the head. [*Bhr.*]

Transient burning on the crown and neck externally. [*Fr. H—n.*]

Formication in the forehead.

55. Formication above the orbits.

(Headache only tolerable when lying, but on rising up and sitting in bed intolerable.)

Formication on the crown, externally.

Sensation of coldness on a small spot on the forehead, as if he were touched there by a cold thumb.

A pain as if a knife were thrust through from the left side of the head across to the other side ; at the same time internal coldness in the head, so that the hair stood on end. [*Stf. Gss.*]

60. On some parts of the occiput pain as if the hair were pulled out, or like sharp electric shocks. [*Stf. Gss.*]

Shooting itching on the hairy scalp, not removed by scratching. [*Ws.*]

The scalp down to the eyebrows lies closely attached to the skull, and is almost immovable (aft. 1½ h.). [*Ws.*]

On the side of the forehead pimples, partly filled with pus (aft. 3 d.). [*Kr.*]

The face is very much fallen in. [THOMAS A THUESSINK, *Waarnehm.*, Groning., 1805.]

65. **Dry heat in the face towards evening to behind the ears, without thirst, with very cold nose** (aft. 24 h.). [*Hbg.*]

Cramp-like tearing on the left eyebrow. [*Gss.*]

Contracted pupils (aft. 2 h.). [*Lr.*]

Staring eyes, betraying anxiety.

The border of the upper eyelid, where it touches the eyeball internally, is painful when the eyeball is moved, as if it were too dry and somewhat sore.

70. Contracted pupils, with cloudiness of the head. [*Stf. Gss.*]

Sharp, fine stitches in the inner canthus. [*Stf. Gss.*]

When during the noon siesta he has the eyes closed, he feels comfortable ; on opening them nausea in the pit of the stomach. [*Stf. Gss.*]

Dilated pupils (aft. 26 h.). [*Lr.*]

Stitches in the eyes. [COLLIN,[2] *Obs. circa Morbos*, iv, p. 5, and v, p. 108.]

75. Itching in the canthi (aft. 27 h.). [*Lr.*]

Burning in the eyes.[3] [COLLIN, l. c.]

---

1 Not accessible.

2 Effects of arnica when given for paralysis, amaurosis, spasms, fever, and dysentery. SS. 74 and 76 occurred in amaurotic eyes recovering sight under the influence of the medicine (comp. note to S. 403).

3 See note (2)

Burning in the eyes, without dryness. [*Bhr.*]

Sometimes hot tears flow which burn like fire. [*Bhr.*]

The right eye protrudes somewhat from the head, and looks higher and larger than the left. [*Bhr.*]

80. Drawing pain in the right eyeball (aft. 2 h.). [*Kr.*]

On the border of the left orbit very painful, intermittent, obtuse aching. [*Gss.*]

Spasmodic aching twitching underneath the left eye on the nasal bone, which spreads over the eyeball. [*Gss.*]

On the left ear cartilage internal pain as from a blow or a bruise. [*Hbg.*]

In both ears in the neighbourhood of the membrana tympani, intermittent aching (aft. 10 h.). [*Kr.*]

85. Obtuse stitches inwards through the internal ear (aft. 1 h.). [*Ws.*]

A shooting pain darts into the right ear, immediately after into the left, at last into the eyes, with the feeling in the latter as if they were forcibly turned upwards. [*Stf. Gss.*]

Heat and burning in the lobe of the ear. [*Stf. Gss.*]

Feeling as if one ear were hot, which it is not (aft. 1 h.).

Behind the ear dull long shoots.

90. First stitches, then tearing pain in the ear (aft. 1 h.).

Aching in the ear.

Perceptibly diminished hearing (aft. 30 h.).

Much increased acuteness of hearing (aft. 10 h.).

Roaring in the ears.

95. Ringing in the left ear (aft. 3 h.). [*Kr.*]

Buzzing in the ears (aft. 7 h.). [*Lr.*]

External hot feeling on the left ear and in the cheek. [*Hbg.*]

Small-pox-like eruption on the cheeks; mostly under the eyes. [*Fr. H—n.*]

Twitching throbbing in the left cheek (aft. $\frac{1}{8}$ h.). [*Ws.*]

100. In the swollen cheek throbbing and pinching, as when two hammers are knocked together bruising the flesh. [*Bhr.*]

(Pain as if bruised in the right maxillary joint, on moving the jaw backwards and forwards, in the morning) (aft. 20 h.).

Redness and burning in one cheek, the rest of the body being cool, at least not hot.

Red swelling of the right cheek, with throbbing nipping pain, swollen lips and great heat in the head and cold body; only the feet were sometimes hot.

Heat running over the head, at the same time her face becomes bathed in perspiration. [*Stf. Gss.*]

105. Heat running over the face, in the evening (aft. 36 h.). [*Stf. Gss.*]

Hot, shining red, stiff swelling of the left cheek. [*Bhr.*]

On yawning, cramp-pain in the cheek (aft. 1 h.). [*Ws.*]

Running formication, like shivering without chilliness, on the left cheek, to the side of the occiput (aft. 6 h.).

Cramp-pain in the root of the nose (aft. 2 h.). [*Ws.*].

110. **The nose pains from above downwards, as if he had had a severe fall upon it** [*Hbg.*]

Shooting tearing pain in the nose.

Swelling of the nose.

Sensation as if the nostrils were ulcerated ; the nose is sore internally.

In and under the nose, pimples which get pus in their apices, with smarting pain.

115. Hot feeling in the nose, and yet it is cold to the touch. [*Hbg.*]

Frequent epistaxis. [*Bhr.*]

The nasal bones are the seat of obtuse pressure combined with numbness. [*Gss.*]

Sensation as if an insect was crawling near the nose ; not removed by wiping. [*Gss.*]

Itching formication on the side of the nose, going off by rubbing (aft. 1 h.). [*Ws.*]

120. Itching on the upper lip, which becomes burning on rubbing. [*Ws.*]

The outer border round about the lips, especially about the upper lip, becomes rough and as if cracked, as from cold (aft. 8 h.). [*Lr.*]

On both sides of the upper lip a pimple (aft. 2 h.). [*Kr.*]

A pimple in the depression in the middle of the upper lip, with redness round about it and tensive pain. [*Fr. H—n*]

Dry lips as if parched by thirst.

125. **Chapped lips.**

Ulcerated angles of the mouth, with burning pain, especially on moving these parts.

Formication in the lips, as if they had gone to sleep (aft, 2½ h.). [*Fz.*]

Burning heat in both lips with moderate warmth of the body. [*Ws.*]

Thick swollen lips. [*Bhr.*]

130. Violent trembling of the lower lip. [A. THUESSINK, l. c.]

Commencing paralysis of the lower jaw.

Swelling of the submaxillary glands.

In the muscles on the ramus of the lower jaw, aching jerking (intermitting tearing). [*Gss.*]

The submaxillary glands are swollen and painful, especially when he raises and turns the head, but particularly when touched (aft. 4 d.). [*Kr.*]

135. The cervical glands are projecting and swollen, and are excessively painful *per se*, but more especially when moving and when speaking. [*Bhr.*]

Rough drawing in the left cervical muscles, with bruised pain. [*Hbg.*]

Tearing pain in the neck. [COLLIN, l. c.]

Aching in the cervical muscles, as if the neckcloth was tightly tied. [*Hbg.*]

Her head is so heavy that it always sinks to one side. [*Bhr.*]

140. The head is heavy and on account of weakness of the cervical muscles so movable that it easily falls to either side (aft. 4 h.). [*Kr.*]

Pain in the teeth, as if their roots were scraped with a knife. [*Bhr.*]

In the gums formication, as if they had gone to sleep. [*Gss. Stf.*]

Slimy teeth (aft. 1 h.).

Looseness and elongation of the teeth, without pain.

145. (Toothache as from bitten out—dislocated, loose—teeth, aching throbbing, as if they were pressed out by afflux of blood ; they are more painful on being touched.)

Pressure on the lower gums internally, as from a leaden ball. [*Fz.*]

While eating, tearing pain in the left upper molars, going off after a meal. [*Fz.*]

When chewing, the gums are painful as if ulcerated, particularly also the part under the tongue. [*Fz.*]

Dryness in the mouth, without thirst. [*Fr. H—n.*]

150. Dryness in the mouth, with great thirst. [*Bhr.*]

Tongue furred quite white, with good appetite and proper taste (aft. 2 d.). [*Hbg.*]

In the morning dryness of the mouth, without thirst, with foul taste in the mouth (aft. 14 h.).

Sensation of thirsty dryness on the tip of the tongue, the palate, and the lips, with rigor over the arms and thighs (aft. 2 h.).

Smarting sensation on the tongue (aft. 4 h.).

155. Sensation of soreness of the tongue (aft. 4 h.).

Corrugating sensation on the palate as from an astringent (aft. 5 h.).

Aching pain on the hard palate.

Burning posteriorly in the throat, with sensation of internal heat, or rather of that anxiety that heat occasions (without perceptible external heat.).

Shooting posteriorly in the throat when not swallowing.

160. Pain in the gullet as if something hard and rough (*e. g.* a crust of bread) were sticking in it, in the afternoon when lying down, which goes off on standing up (aft. 6 h.).

Noise when swallowing.

Swallowing prevented by a sort of nausea as if the food would not go down.

Bitter taste in the mouth in the morning after waking.

Putrid slimy taste in the mouth.

165. (All he takes tastes sour.)

(Distaste for milk.)

The (accustomed) smoking is distasteful to him, he has no relish for it.

Distaste for meat and meat-soup.

Longing for vinegar.

170. Want of appetite in the evening.

Want of appetite, with yellow and white furred tongue.

Dysphagia. [*Bhr.*]
Rotten-egg taste in the mouth when not eating. [*Fr. H—n.*]
Mucus in the throat, which tastes bitter on being hawked up (aft. 12 h.). [*Fz.*]

175. Bitter taste in the mouth (aft. 4 h.). [*Hbg.*]
Blood in the saliva ejected (aft. 2 d.). [*Hbg.*]
After eating a kind of suppressed incomplete hiccup. [*Fz.*]
Empty eructation (aft. ¼ h.). [*Hbg.*]—(aft. ½ h.). [*Kr.*]
Tendency to eructate. (DE LA MARCHE,[1] *Diss. de arnica vera*, Halæ, 1719, pp. 15—22.]

180. On eructating a bitter mucus rises up. [*Kr.*]
Empty eructation.
In the morning eructation like rotten eggs.
Eructation bitter and like rotten eggs (aft. 2 h.).
Salt water rises up and is belched up.

185. In the morning nausea and inclination to vomit (aft. 14 h.).
Heartburn. [A CRICHTON,[2] in *Samml. br, Abh. fur pr. A.* xiii, 3.]
She wants always to drink, and knows not what, because everything is repugnant to her. [*Bhr.*]
Half-suppressed eructation. [*Stf. Gss.*]
Inordinate appetite in the evening, and after eating immediately a sensation of fulness and a colicky aching in various parts of the abdomen, especially in the sides.

190. (When eating, at noon, a perceptible warmth in one cheek.)
After the (evening) meal she weeps, is peevish, will listen to nobody, and will not hear of anything.
Total want of appetite with nausea. [*Bhr.*]
Nausea. [MURRAY,[3] *Appar. Medicam.*, i, p. 234.]
Nausea in the stomach, with empty eructation. [*Ws.*]

195. Nausea without vomiting and without stool. [DE LA MARCHE, l. c.]
On reading for a long time he grows giddy and sick. [*Hbg.*]
Retching. [STOLL,[4] *Rat. Med.*, iii, p. 162.]
Violent retching to vomit. [AASKOW,[5] *Act. soc. med. Hafn.*, ii, p. 162.]
Vomiting. [MURRAY,—COLLIN, l. c.]

200. Vomiting of coagulated blood.[6] [DE LA MARCHE, l. c.]
Empty retching, ineffectual inclination to vomit (aft. ¼ h.).
She must get up at night and retch as if to vomit, but is unable to vomit; she feels a weight like a lump in the scrobiculus cordis.

---

1. Effect of arnica in cases of injury treated with it.—This symptom preceded the vomiting of S. 200 (see note there).
2. A brief statement of the observed effects and virtues of arnica. This symptom does not appear in the English original (*Lond. Med. Journ.*, 1789, p. 236).
3. Summary of observed effects of arnica.
4. As in note (3).
5. Not found at place referred to.
6. In a case of fall from a height, where the chest was bruised.

Above the scrobiculus cordis, in the sternum, violent aching. [*Stf. Gss.*]

Violent jerks under the stomach [*Stf. Gss.*]

205. In the scrobiculus cordis a digging, and sensation as if something knotted itself there together. [*Stf. Gss.*]

After eating a fulness in the scrobiculus cordis, and a painful aching on a small spot deep in the hypogastrium, just behind the os pubis (in the bladder ?), most felt when standing, which almost constantly urges to urinate (aft. 4 h.).

The stomach is as if full ; a satiety combined with loathing.

Pressure as with a hand on the scrobiculus cordis ; this pressure rose up gradually to the throat ; then she became sick, and water collected in the mouth ; after lying down this went off, and then she had only pressure in the abdomen (aft. 1 h.).

A pinching spasmodic grasping in the stomach.

210. (A smarting pain in the stomach (immediately)).

Flatulence with stomach-ache.

In the cardiac region pain as if it was compressed, or as if it got a severe blow. [*Stf. Gss.*]

Cardialgia. [CRICHTON—STOLL, l. c.]

Pressure as if a stone lay in the stomach (immediately). [*Hbg.*]

215. Rumbling in the stomach and colic. [*Hbg.*]

Painful pressure in the scrobiculus cordis transversely across, with tightness of breath. [*Hbg.*]

Spasm in the region of the lower ribs (præcordia). [COLLIN, l. c.]

Pressure under the last ribs (aft. 2 h.). [*Ws.*]

Digging in the scrobiculus cordis (aft. ½ h.), and sensation as if something knotted itself there (aft. 24 h.). [*Hbg.*]

220. Pinching in the stomach. [*Hbg.*]

In the splenic region a pressure darting upwards, with a continual stitch (what one calls a stitch in the spleen) when walking (aft. 6 h.). [*Fz.*]

Stitches under the false ribs of the left side which take away the breath when standing. [*Hbg.*]

On the left side betwixt the scrobiculus cordis and navel squeezing beating. [*Stf. Gss.*]

Cutting above the navel, especially when breathing deeply and at every step, but not immediately before or during a motion of the bowels.

225. Cutting in the abdomen, as from a chill.

Dysenteric bellyache : a digging deep in the hypogastrium inside the hips on both sides combined with nausea and drowsiness (between the 2nd and 5th h.).

A couple of hours after a (moderate) supper, tightness and distension of the abdomen, especially of the hypogastrium, with dull general pressure in it, especially in the side of the abdomen, but without any distinct amount of flatus, which lasts all night, with heat of the limbs and dreams which strain the thinking power : he wakes up every hour, and the inodorous flatus that escapes affords no relief.

Hard distension of the right side of the abdomen, paining of itself when at rest, like an internal sore; when coughing, blowing the nose, and stepping as if painfully concussed, lacerated, or cut to pieces; and even on slightly touching it externally, as if a wound were cut into; only relieved by the discharge of flatus; occurring daily from the morning till 2 p.m.

On expiring and inspiring pressive pain as from a stone in the hepatic region, when lying on the left side. [*Stf. Gss.*]

230. Although she had eaten much, she felt as empty in the abdomen as if she had eaten nothing, but had drunk much, so that it rolled about in the abdomen. [*Stf. Gss.*]

Tearing in the abdomen above the navel.

Violent cutting on the left side of the abdomen, which darted like a stitch into the crown of the head, so that he started as from an electric spark (aft. 24 h.). [*Hbg.*]

Pinching above the navel. [*Hbg.*]

A severe jerk under the stomach. [*Hbg.*]

235. Pain in the right side of the abdomen, as from a sudden contusion when walking (aft. 36 h.). [*Fz.*]

On the left side between the scrobiculus cordis and navel, squeezing beating. [*Gss.*]

Sharp stitchess in both loins (aft. 3 h.). [*Ws.*]

Cutting pain inwards in the loins, especially when stooping (aft. 60 h.). [*Ws.*]

In the right side under the ribs obtuse stitches. [*Gss.*]

240. **Sharp blows through the hypogastrium from one side to the other** (aft. 3 h.). [*Ws.*]

In the hepatic region painful pressure (aft. 2 d.). [*Hbg.*]

Burning shooting pains in the epigastrium.[1] [Collin, l. c.]

Drawing in of the navel.[1] [Collin, l. c.]

Fine tearing in the abdominal muscles (aft. 1 h.). [*Ws.*]

245. Fine stitch in the muscles of the hypogastrium, which leaves an itching, that goes off on scratching (aft. 3 h.). [*Ws.*]

Cutting in the abdomen; an hour afterwards urging to stool, and at length a stool in broken pieces mingled with flatus. [*Gss.*]

Flatulence, rumbling in the bowels. [Stoll, l. c.]

Bellyache as if flatulence pressed.

Flatulent colic.

250. Rumbling, rolling of flatulence in the abdomen.

Fermenting flatulent disturbance in the abdomen.

Loud rumbling in the abdomen, as from emptiness (aft. 10 h.). [*Lr.*]

Rumbling and fermenting flatulent movements below the umbilical region (aft. $1\frac{1}{2}$ h.). [*Kr.*]

Whilst straining at stool discharge of flatus, after previous rumbling in the bowels (aft. 1 h.). [*Fz.*]

---

1. In a case of opisthotonos.

255. Flatus smelling like rotten eggs (aft. 3 h.). [*Kr.*]

Urging to stool followed by a copious thin or pappy, sour smelling motion, with great relief (four or five times a-day). [*Gss.*]

Ineffectual urging to stool.

Very great urging to stool every half hour, but nothing came away except mucus.

Hard, difficult stool with aching in the abdomen (aft. 36 h.). [*Hbg.*]

260. Pappy diarrhœa, with distension of the abdomen, before the motion (aft. 24 h.). [*Ws.*]

Bloody, purulent stools. [PELARGUS,[1] *Obs.*, i, pp. 263, 264.]

Pappy brown stool, with rumbling in the abdomen, as if diarrhœa was coming (aft. 1¼ h.). [*Fz.*]

In the rectum, an aching pain (aft. 6 h.). [*Kr.*]

Frequent small stools consisting of mucus only (aft. 6, 7 h.).

265. Frequent stools, after every one of which he must lie down.

White diarrhœic motions.*

(Diarrhœa like brown yeast.)

Constipation.

Nocturnal diarrhœa with aching pain in the abdomen, as from flatulence.

270. Involuntary evacuation of fæces at night in sleep.

Undigested, but not liquid, motions.

A pressure in the rectum.

Tenesmus in the anus.

Squeezing and pressing in the anus when standing (aft. 7 h.). [*Fz.*]

275. Blind hæmorrhoids.[9] [COLLIN, l. c.]

More frequent inclination to urinate than usual. [*Kr.*]

Frequent urging to urinate with great discharge of urine (aft. 1 h.). [*Lr.*]

Watery urine. [*Hbg.*]

Retention of urine with aching and pressing.

280. Strangury of the neck of the bladder, ineffectual urging to urinate.

Strangury, with involuntary dribbling of urine (aft. 1 h.).

When making water he must stand long before anything comes away. [*Stf. Gss.*]

An urging to urinate with a somewhat smarting burning, still worse after urinating, but not whilst the urine is flowing.

Cutting pain in the orifice of the urethra, at the end of micturition.

* Diarrhœa with copious evacuation of fæces seems only to be a secondary action of arnica.

1. Case of fall of a child from a height in which arnica was given.—This symptom occurred on the fourth day; and was regarded by the reporter as a sign of internal contusion or extravasation.

9. In case mentioned in note to S. 242.

285. Stitches in the urethra.

Stitches in the urethra after micturition (aft. 1 h.).

Frequent discharge of watery urine (aft. 12 h.).

Discharge of a large quantity of urine, which he cannot retain long, especially at night (aft. 30 h.).

Brown, clear urine, which immediately becomes turbid of a whitish colour (aft. 48 h.).

290. Brown urine with brick-red sediment.

Scanty red urine. [*Stf. Gss.*]

Frequent discharge of a smaller quantity of white watery urine, than he had drunk, the last drops of which he could with difficulty press out (the first 4 h.). [*Fz*]

In the morning he passes much urine, which, however, flows slowly, as if the urethra were narrowed (aft. 24 h.). [*Fz.*]

He passes more dark-red urine than he had drunk.[1] [COLLIN, l. c.]

295. Frequent urging to urinate, with little yellowish-red urinary discharge (aft. 46 h.). [*Lr.*]

Itching in the front of the urethra in the region of the glans when not urinating.

Itching or itching shooting in the glans.

A fine stitch through the glans.

On the glans, an itching, red spot.

300. On the prepuce, an itching pimple.

Single stitches in the scrotum.

(A painless pimple on the scrotum.)

After waking, strong, continued erections, without inclination for coitus and without lascivious thoughts (aft. 12 h.).

Great inclination for coitus and continued erections of the penis (in a weak old man).

305. Several pollutions in one night with lascivious dreams.

(By day) when indulging in an amorous embrace the semen comes away.

In the morning in bed, feeling of weakness with lax testicles, as if he had had a pollution the previous night in sleep, which, however, had not occurred.

Promotion of the menses.[2] [DE MEZA, l. c.]

In an otherwise healthy girl of 20 years, who had not menstruated for a year previously, immediately after taking the drug, sensation of nausea in the scrobiculus cordis, whereupon a clot of thick blood came away through the vagina. [*Stf. Gss.*]

310. Sneezing.

Severe coryza.

In the evening on going to sleep, coryza (aft. 3 h.), and in the morning on awaking, catarrh on the chest.

In the morning, hoarseness.

(Creaking in the windpipe when walking and in the evening on lying down.)

---

1. In case mentioned in note to S. 242.—The reporter says "red" merely.
2. Curative effect. See note to S. 20.

315. **Fœtid smelling breath from the mouth.**

(Constant burning on the edges of the nostrils with irritation to sneeze.)

Sneezing (aft. 2½ h.). [*Kr.*]

Frequent sneezing (aft. 48 h.). [*Lr.*]

Fetid exhalation from the mouth on expiration, for two days. [*Fr. H—n.*]

320. The breath on expiration appeared to him to cause a sensible coolness in the windpipe, as if its skin were too thin. [*Fz.*]

Feeling of internal coldness in the chest. [A THUESSINK, l. c.]

Dry tussiculation as from a tickle in the lower part of the trachea, every morning after rising. [*Lr.*]

Quite dry cough from a tickle in the lower part of the trachea (aft. 4 h.).

(Cough with expectoration, which seems to come from the posterior nasal orifices.)

325. During the midday sleep, cough from an itching irritation at the upper part of the larynx (aft. 4 h.)

Cough at night during sleep.

Even yawning provokes cough.

Crying in children with crossness and tossing about excites cough (between the 7th and 8th h.).

After weeping and whining, cough in children.

330. (When coughing, pain as if raw in the chest and clawing in the larynx.)

Hæmoptysis

Cough causing vomiting.

Cough that causes bruised pain of all the ribs.

Cough with stitches in the side of the abdomen (aft. 10 h.).

335. Bloody expectoration from the chest. [A THUESSINK, l. c.]

Short kinking breath. [A THUESSINK, l. c.]

Oppression of the breathing, rapid expiration and inspiration. [*Bhr.*]

Anxiety and pains in the chest.[1] [DE LA MARCHE, l. c.]

Oppression of the chest with anxiety, pains in the hypogastrium and headache.[2] [DE MEZA, l. c.]

340. Extreme dyspnœa.[3] [FEHR, in *Eph. Nat. Cur.*, Dec. I, Ann. 9, 10, O. 2.]

Frequent, slow, deep breathing, with pressure under the chest. [*Hbg.*]

An aching pain about the lower end of the sternum, especially severe on fetching a deep breath (aft. 12 h.). [*Kr.*]

Above the scrobiculus cordis, in the lower part of the sternum, obtuse pressure. [*Gss.*]

Aching stitches in the chest. [*Gss.*]

345. Cutting pressure outwards on both sides of the chest, increased by inspiring (aft. 1 h.). [*Ws.*]

---

1. In a case of heavy fall. Very similar symptoms were noted before arnica was given.
2. Immediately preceding the restoration of the catamenia. See note to S. 20.
3. Only an aggravation of difficulty of breathing existing before arnica was taken.

Obtuse stitches through the sternum into the thoracic cavity (aft. 2 h.). [*Ws.*]

Pain in the left side of the chest like needle pricks (aft. 29 h.). [*Lr.*]

Fine shooting pain in the sides of the chest. [*Hbg.*]

(Rapid, difficult inspiration, slow expiration.)

350. Shooting pain on one side of the chest, with a short cough that increases the pain, and constant tightness of the chest.

Fine and severe shooting pain under the last ribs.

In the right side of the chest pain like needle-pricks.

In the middle of the left side of the chest severe stitches.

In the right side close to the ribs obtuse stitches. [*Stf. Gss.*]

355. On breathing deeply stitches in the left side of the chest near the sternum. [*Stf. Gss.*]

Shooting on both sides under the ribs as from flatulence (aft. 1 h.).

Anteriorly on the sternum aching shooting pain, especially when walking.

The chest is affected, as if raw, whereby he several times spat blood with the saliva; especially when walking (aft. 36 h.). [*Stf. Gss.*]

All the joints and connexions of the bones and cartilages belonging to the chest are painful on moving and breathing as if bruised.

360. Stitches in the heart from the left to the right side. [*Bhr.*]

Squeezing of the heart. [*Bhr.*]

The beating of the heart is more like a jerking. [*Bhr.*]

In the region of the heart pain as if it was compressed or as if it got a blow (aft. 36 h.). [*Hbg.*]

The movement of the heart is at first very rapid, then suddenly extremely slow. [*Bhr.*]

365. **Pain as from dislocation in the connexions of the parts of the chest with the back.**

(A drawing pain in the chest, with anxiety.)

Anxiety, across the chest, with sickness (aft. 2 h.).

In the morning, on awaking, a weight of blood seems to have accumulated in the chest; he feels better after a little exercise.

In the middle of the left side of the chest a constrictive, painless sensation, impeding respiration, with a pain in the scrobiculus cordis when touched, which interferes with breathing.

370. (Sensation of tension over the chest to the throat, which is lessened by lying on the back, is increased by walking, and is painful on standing) (aft. 2 h.).

An aching pain in (the right side of) the chest, on a small spot, which is not increased either by movement, touch, or breathing.

Red perspiration over the chest. [VICAT,[1] *Mat. Med.*, i, pp. 20 and 362.]

Shooting itching in the sides of the chest and on the back, not removed by scratching (aft. a few m.). [*Ws.*]

1 General statement of effects.

Formicating itching on the left side of the chest (aft. 1 h.). [*Ws.*]

375. In the os sacrum pain as after a severe blow or fall. [*Hbg.*]

The sacrum pains as if beaten. [*Hbg.*]

In the sacrum pain as if something was lacerated internally. *Stf.* [*Gss.*]

Pain in the sacrum ; there was shooting in it when coughing, breathing deeply, or walking.

Rheumatic pain in the back and limbs.

380. Bruised pain in the back.

Burning pain in the back when walking in the open air.

In the back, almost under the shoulders, sensation as if something like a lump lay there, with obtuse stitches on moving, not when at rest. [*Stf. Gss.*]

At every inspiration a stitch in the right side of the back from the last ribs up to the axilla (aft. 48 h.), [*Ws.*]

Sensation as if the spinal marrow were injected, with the feeling of a shock.[1] [COLLIN, l. c.]

385. Formication in the spine. [*Hbg.*]

Formication in the dorsal spine, then in the false ribs, to the stomach.[2] [COLLIN, l. c.]

In the middle of the spine painful aching (when sitting). [*Hbg.*]

The spine is painful, as if it could not support the body. [*Bhr.*]

Aching pain between the scapulæ (aft. 2 d.). [*Hbg.*]

390. Cutting blows between the scapulæ through into the thoracic cavity, when walking (aft. 6 h.). [*Ws.*]

Shooting itching on the scapula (aft. 2 h.). [*Ws*]

On the right scapula, towards the back, pain as after a severe blow or fall. [*Hbg.*]

On the lowest cervical vertebra aching and tension, when he leans the head forwards. [*Fz.*]

Cramp-pain in the muscles of the nape, with obtuse stitches inwards (aft. 2 h.). [*Ws.*]

395. In the muscles of the nape cramp-like tensive pain on sneezing and yawning.

On the side of the nape a pimple that causes shooting and ulcerative pain when touched* (aft. 48 h.).

On the left shoulder drawing, aching pain on standing erect. [*Fz.*]

Broad, sharp stitches inwards under the axilla. [*Ws.*]

Raw, sore sensation under the shoulder. [*Fz.*]

400. The arms are tired as if beaten, so that he could not flex the fingers. [*Hbg.*]

On the anterior aspect of the arms pain as if beaten.

* This kind of pimple, so painful when touched, with an inflamed red areola, which arnica produces specifically, bears the greatest resemblance to the well-known boils (furunculi), and consequently these are homœopathically cured by arnica, and in persons who are frequently troubled with them are prevented by the use of arnica, and their future occurrence warded off, as experience has taught me.

1. See note to S. 242, The sense of concussion was felt in the body generally.
2. See note to S. 242.

Backward mounting, drawing, cramp-like pain in the bone-shafts of the fingers and forearm.

Formication in the arms.[1] [COLLIN, l. c.]

Painful blows in the arms, almost like electric shocks.[1] [COLLIN, l. c]

405. Painful stitches like blows on the upper part of the upper arm [*Gss.*]

In the left upper arm twitching as if a nerve were pulled. [*Gss.*]

Twitching in the muscles of the upper arm (immediately). [*Ws.*]

Obtuse stitches in the middle of the upper arm, so that he starts. [*Gss.*]

From the lower part of the left arm to the elbow intermittent, painful aching tearing, as if in the bone. [*Gss.*]

410. Formication in the forearms. [*Hbg.*]

On flexing the arm, stretching of the flexor muscles of the forearm, so that extension of the arm causes tensive pain (aft. 2 h.). [*Fz.*]

Sharp, broad stitches below the elbow-joint (aft. 2. h.). [*Ws.*]

Slow obtuse stitches in the left forearm, with acute pains, as if it were broken at that part (in the morning in bed). [*Gss.*]

Tearing pain in the arms and hands.

415. Burning shooting in the forearm. [*Gss.*]

In the wrist-joint dislocative pain. [*Gss.*]

In the left wrist-joint pain as if sprained (aft. 2 d.). [*Kr.*]

In the wrist-joint sharp stitches, increased by movement (aft. 2 h.). [*Ws.*]

Pain as from dislocation of the wrist (chest, back, hips).

420. In the left wrist-joint, especially when writing, tearing pain, which manifests itself particularly on the back of the hand ; on letting the hands hang down the pain is diminished. [*Kr.*]

Shooting, tearing in the wrists, chiefly in the left (aft. 3. h.). [*Kr.*]

A creeping and formication in the hands.[1] [COLLIN, l. c.]

Distended veins of the hands, with full, strong pulse. [*Hbg.*]

Powerlessnesss of the hands, especially on grasping anything (aft. 2 h.). [*Kr.*]

425. On the back of the hand painful aching. [*Hbg.*]

Cramp in the fingers of the left hand. [*Hbg.*]

Pain in the balls of both thumbs, as if they had been knocked against something hard. [*Hbg.*]

Fine shooting itching on the proximal finger-joints, completely removed by scratching (aft. 36 h.). [*Ws.*]

A pimple betwixt thumb and index, which itches, but when touched causes fine shooting pain, as if a splinter were sticking in (aft. 40. h.).

430. Stitches in both middle fingers (and in the knee).

Shooting, twitching pain in the fingers.

Fine stitches in the distal joint of the middle finger (aft. $\frac{1}{4}$ h.). [*Ws.*]

Itching stitches in the tip of the middle finger (aft. 2 h.) [*Ws.*]

---

1 In paralysed limbs, to which arnica was restoring power.

Sharp stitches in the bend of the middle joint of the index (aft. 2 h.). [*Ws.*]

435. Trembling in the lower extremities. [*Hbg.*]

Tearing pain in the lower extremities. [COLLIN, l. c.]

(Abscess of the lumbar (psoas) muscles).

Pain as from dislocation in the hips (back, chest, wrist).

440. Tearing pain in the lower extremities.

At night the lower extremities are painful when they lie on one another. [*Bhr.*]

Drawing aching pain in the left hip-joint when the leg is stretched out when sitting (aft. 5 h.). [*Fz.*]

Pain in the thigh on rising up and treading.

Twitching sensation in the muscles of the thigh.

445. Continued pinching on the outside of the thigh (aft. ½ h.). [*Ws.*].

When walking, pain on the thighs as from a blow or knock. [*Fz.*]

When sitting, drawing cram-like pressing in the muscles of the left thigh (aft. 48 h.). [*Lr.*]

Pinching twitching in the upper part of the left thigh near the scrotum. [*Gss.*]

Stitches in the knee (and both middle fingers).

450. Fine stitchtes on the thigh above the knee (aft. ¼, h.). [*Ws.*]

On the inside of the thigh above the knee itching stitches, that become more severe by rubbing (aft. 2 h.). [*Ws.*]

On the inside of the thigh a fine shooting itching, like sore feeling, ameliorated by touch. [*Fz.*]

The knee-joints have no steadfastness and totter when standing (aft. 3 h.). [*Kr.*]

The knees knuckle under him when standing (aft. 1 h.). [*Kr.*]

455. Sometimes in the knee a sudden loss of power ; they knuckle under him, whilst the feet are numb and insensible.

(In the knee and leg a cramp-like pain.)

Rheumatic pain in the foot with slight fever towards evening.

Standing causes pain.

In the right knee, on going up stairs, a pain as if he had knocked himself (aft. 3 h.). [*Kr.*]

460. **On the knee when touched a prick as with a needle** (aft. 1 h.). [*Ws.*]

Aching tearing below the left knee. [*Gss.*]

Above the calf of the right leg pain, as after a violent blow, with weariness of the legs. [*Hbg.*]

Twitching shooting pain in the tibia upwards (aft. 6 h.).

(Aching pain in the paralysed foot.)

465. A creeping formicating sensation in the feet.

Sudden swelling of the (affected) foot.

Indescribable pain in the (affected) foot, as from internal

1 See note to S. 403.

uneasiness, and as if he were lying on something hard, which compels him to lay the part here and there and to move it about, in the evening (aft. 8 h.).

Tearing pain, like boring and digging downwards on the left calf; after remaining some time there it extends upwards into the thigh, and thence around behind the coccyx; it ends on the right os ilii (aft. 6 h.). [*Kr.*]

Upward tension in the muscles of the calf and drawing therein when standing (aft. 7 h.). [*Fz.*]

470. Aching on the tibia as after a blow, only when walking (aft. 30 h.). [*Fz.*]

Gurgling from below upwards in the lower part of the leg, when at rest (aft. $\frac{1}{4}$ h.). [*Ws.*]

Undulating tearing (almost obtuse shooting) pain in the ankle-joint. [*Gss.*]

In the ankle-joint dislocation pain. [*Gss.*]

Tearing in the ankle.

475. Tearing in the heel.

Stitches in the foot through the great toe.

A shooting in the right foot, above the heel in the tendo Achillis, only on extending the ankle-joint, but not when walking (aft. 2 h.). [*Kr.*]

Stitches on the soles of feet, on one and the same place, when walking, as if a corn were there (aft. 36 h.). [*Fz.*]

Formicating stitches on the sole of the foot, on one and the same place. [*Fz.*]

480. Violent burning in the feet. [*Bhr.*]

Formication in the feet. [*Hbg.*]

Cramp in the toes of the left foot (aft. 36 h.). [*Hbg.*]

In one of the toes dull throbbing pain. [*Gss.*]

In one of the toes dull (numb) trembling pain. [*Gss.*]

485. Violent shooting in the toes when walking. [*Fz.*]

A gradually coming on shooting tearing pain in the point of the big toe on lying down for his noon-day rest.

Towards evening a gouty numb pain as from dislocation in the joint of the big toe, with some redness.

Single severe stitches in the big toe (aft. 1 h.),

A dull long stitch in the right big toe.

490. Single blows in the big toe.

Perspiration of the soles and toes.

Painful cramp in the muscles of the soles.

Shooting tearing on the inferior surface of the big toe, especially on treading on it (aft. 4 h.). [*Ws.*]

Formicating sensation in the hands and feet, and shooting pains in various joints.[1] [COLLIN, l. c.]

495. Here and there in the limbs deeply penetrating, obtuse stitches. [*Gss.*]

---

1 See note to S. 403.

A sharp pricking sensation over the whole surface of the body. [CRICHTON, l. c.]

Shooting pains. [VICAT, l. c.]

Fine shooting in almost every part of the body, especially on the nose, eyebrows, eyelids, also on the hands and fingers.

A burning pain, sometimes in one, sometimes in another part of the body, in the skin.

500. A cold pain, sometimes in one, sometimes in another part of the body, in the skin.

(Here and there in the skin a shooting, burning, itching pain on lying down for the noonday rest, which rapidly goes off on scratching, and by itself.)

Burning and cutting pains here and there.[1] [COLLIN, l. c.]

Jerks and blows in the body, as from electricity.[2] [CRICHTON, l. c.]

After touching the skin with the tincture there arises an itching miliary rash.

505. Sudden twitching of single muscle in almost all parts of the body, especially in the limbs, whereby sometimes single parts, sometimes the whole body, are shaken. [*Bhr.*]

The pains are aggravated by speaking, blowing nose, movement, and almost every noise. [*Bhr.*]

The sensations resembling tearing occur from time to time in almost every part of the body, but especially in the upper and lower extremities; in the lower mostly when sitting; the pain seemed to spread chiefly upwards. [*Kr.*]

Twitching pain in the affected part (aft. 2 h.).

A twitching in all the limbs, especially in the feet and shoulders, with heat of the feet.

510. It seemed to him as if everything on his body was too tightly tied.

Restlessness of the whole body, without mental anxiety; an excessive mobility that develops into trembling of the whole body.

The limbs on the side on which he lies go to sleep. [*Stf. Gss.*]

Painful sensibility of all the joints and of the skin on the slightest movement (aft. 4 h.).

Painful over-sensitiveness of the whole body.

515. **All his limbs are affected: a kind of paralytic pain in all the joints, and as if bruised, on moving** (aft. 8 h.).

A tingling pain in all the limbs when the body is shaken (*e. g.* in a carriage), **or when treading.**

Disagreeable, formicating, aching feeling in the part injured by a contusion.

Tearing pain in the limbs.[3] [COLLIN, l. c.]

Extremely violent pains, so that many scratch with their nails on the wall or the floor, as if they were mad, these pains, however, do not last more than an hour (immediately after taking it). [DE LA MARCHE, l. c.]

520. Trembling in the limbs. [DE LA MARCHE,—COLLIN, l. c.]

---

1 See note to S. 403.
2 Evidently taken from Collin's observations. See S. 404 and note.
3 See note to S. 403.

Pain in all the limbs, as if bruised, when at rest and when moving (aft. 10 h.). [*Lr.*]

Weariness in the feet and arms when walking in the open air (aft. $2\frac{1}{2}$ h.). [*Kr.*]

Exhaustion, fatigue, bruised feeling, that compels him to lie down. [*Stf. Gss.*]

Trembling restlessness and exhaustion. [*Stf. Gss.*]

525. When walking he becomes faint, but on standing still he recovers.

After a walk in the open air, weak in the legs ; the knees bent under her ; as soon as the weakness came in her legs she immediately grew drowsy, fell asleep at once, and dreamed immediately.

The whole right side, especially the shoulders, seemed to him, when walking in the open air, too heavy, and to hang down as if paralysed, but of this he feels nothing in the room (aft. 8 h.). [*Fz.*]

Heaviness in all the limbs, as from great fatigue. [*Hbg.*]

In the muscles under the joints of the upper and lower extremities, when walking in the open air, sensation of weight and pressure (aft. 8 h.). [*Fz.*]

530. Extraordinary heaviness of the limbs. [*Bhr.*]

Heaviness of the limbs.

Relaxed state of the limbs, as if they were all over-stretched. [*Fz.*]

Lassitude and laziness of the whole body, the legs can scarcely stand [*Hbg.*]

535. **General sinking of the strength** ; he imagines he can scarcely move a limb. [*Hbg.*]

Yawning (aft. $\frac{1}{2}$ h.). [*Kr.*]

When yawning a violent shudder passes through him. [*Gss.*]

Yawning and stretching, with dilated pupils, without sleepiness (aft. 1 h.).

Frequent yawning.

540. **In the evening frequent yawning without sleepiness. Sleepiness** (aft. $\frac{1}{2}$ h.).

Too early sleepiness in the evening.

He becomes very drowsy when he has walked long in the open air, is then not disposed either for thinking or speaking, although he was previously very wide awake. [*Stf. Gss.*]

Much sleep.

545. Sleep full of dreams.

Sleep full of dreams, which does not refresh him ; he thinks he has not slept at all.

Anxious heavy dreams from the beginning of the evening all through the night, which fatigue him greatly.

Frightful dreams, immediately in the evening (after going to sleep), about large black dogs and cats.

He has frightful dreams, cries out aloud in sleep, and wakes up in consequence.

550. Starting up in affright in sleep.

Starting and jerking the head backwards in sleep.

---

1 No. S. 534—a misreckoning.

Moaning in sleep (aft. 2 h.).

Loud incomprehensible talking in sleep, without remembered dreams.

Loud blowing expiration and inspiration in sleep (aft. 24 h.).

555. **Involuntary evacuation of fæces in sleep.**

A dream that lasts all night, in which she is always scolded and shameful reproaches (about immoral conduct) are addressed to her; on awaking she hardly knows whether the dream was not true.

A dream lasting several hours in half sleep, during which the dreamer exhibits much irresolution.

She sleeps for a couple of hours in the evening, then remains wide awake until 5 a.m., but then sleeps soundly until 9 a.m.

Sleeplessness and wakefulness until 2 or 3 a.m.; at the same time shooting and smarting itching here and there.

560. Sleepiness by day (aft. 2 h.). [*Kr.*]

In the evening he becomes sleepy too early. [*Fr. H—n.*]

Drowsiness. [A THUESSINK, l. c.]

On going to sleep sudden starting as from fright. [*Lr.*]

Anxious dreams about things he had formerly dreamt of. [*Kr.*]

565. The dreams of the previous night recur. [*Bhr.*]

Vivid dream, at first cheerful, afterwards anxious. [*Lr.*]

Vivid unremembered dreams. [*Lr.*]

Dreams of frightful things, as lightning strokes, graves, &c. [*Ws.*]

Dreams about flayed persons, very frightful to him. [*Fz.*]

570. Vivid dreams towards morning, in which he talks aloud, so as to awake himself (6th d.). [*Kr.*]

Frequent waking out of sleep with emissions of semen (2nd night). [*Lr.*]

During sleep at night he wakes up from a peculiar hot feeling in the head, followed by anxiety when awake; he dreads the recurrence of new attacks of the same sensation, and thinks he is going to have a fit of apoplexy (aft. 10 h.). [*Hbg.*]

Chilly feeling in the morning in bed, beginning before getting up and lasting all the forenoon. [*Bhr.*]

He cannot sleep in the early part of the night, but sleeps all the longer in the morning.

575. Sleeplessness with anxiety as from heat until 2 to 3 a.m.

In the morning, in bed, cold sensation on the right side, on which he lay (aft. ¼ h.). [*Fz.*]

A flush of heat over the face, and sensation of agreeable warmth of the body (aft. ½ h.). [*Fz.*]

Great internal heat with cold hands and feet, and rigor all over the body. [*Bhr.*].

Dry heat in bed with great thirst for water; the heat is intolerable; he will throw off the clothes, but on doing so, indeed, by merely moving in bed, he is chilly.

580. When he lies long without moving he becomes hot, especially on the head, which he must lay first in one place then in another in bed.

An internal continued chilliness through the whole body on awaking from sleep by day and night, but without shivering.

On yawning a violent shivering goes through him. [*Stf. Gss.*]

After awaking in the morning dry heat all over.

Flushes of heat over the back.

585. Repeated, anxious, transient perspiration all over the body, at night.

Nocturnal sour perspiration.

The exhalation smells sour.

Nocturnal thirst (aft. 48 h.).

Thirst for water.

590. **Thirst without external heat, with pupils little capable of dilatation** (aft. 1 h.).

He longs for the open air.

Sensation as if cold all over, though he is warm enough (aft. 1 h.).

Chill in the back and in the front of the thighs, in the morning.

Chill, mostly in the evening.

595. Morning fever; first chill, then attack of heat.

Very disagreeable painfulness of the periosteum of all the bones of the body, almost like a drawing in all the limbs, as in a fit of ague.

Fever; rigor all over the body, on the head, at the same time heat in the head and redness and heat of the face, with cool hands and bruised feeling in the hips, the back and the front of the arms.

Fever; on yawning before the chill, much thirst, much drinking; then in the heat also thirst, with but little drinking.

Febrile rigor, without thirst.

600. Slight repeated attacks of anxiety with flying heat all over the body.

One hour after the headache, external and internal chill and constant anxiety.

In the evening, along with dizziness in the head, ebullition of the blood; he feels the pulse all over the body (he coughs for hours until he vomits, and often wakes up at night with it).

Heat of the whole body[1]. [DE MEZA, l. c.)

Perspiration. [COLLIN, l. c.]

605. On waking from sleep, slight perspiration. [*Lr.*]

Frequent perspirations. [*Veckoskrift for. Lakare,*[2] viii.]

Attacks of anxietas. [DE LA MARCHE, DE MEZA, COLLIN, l. c., *Hbg.*]

Severe attacks of anxietas. [VICAT, l. c.]

Anxious concern about the present and the future. (3rd d.) [*Lr.*]

610. Excitable, sensitive disposition. [*Bhr.*]

Fright and starting at unexpected trifles (aft. $1\frac{1}{2}$ h.). [*Kr.*]

Dejection and absence of thought (aft. $3\frac{1}{2}$ h.). [*Kr.*]

After walking in the open air he becomes disinclined for thinking and speaking, although he was previously very lively (aft. 9 h.). [*Fz.*]

Surly humour, as after a quarrel. [*Lr.*]

615. Gay, talkative.* [*Fz.*]

* Curative and secondary action in a person of the opposite humour.

---

1 See note to S. 339. 2 Not accessible.

Composed, cheerful humour.* [*Hbg.*

Hypochondriacal anxiety.

Hypochondriacal peevishness ; he is indisposed for everything.

Uncommonly peevish, everything is repugnant to her, everything annoys her. [*Stf. Gss.*]

620. Restlessness of body and mind (but without actual anxiety), as if he was prevented doing something necessary, with complete indisposition for occupation.

All work annoys him ; he is lazy for all business.

Indifference to work, everything is indifferent to him.

(Over-busy, inclination and disposition for great and continuous literary work with no power to do it without injury to the health.)

Over-sensitiveness of the disposition ; † extreme inclination for agreeable and disagreeable mental emotions, without weakness or over-sensitiveness of the body.

625. Over-excitability ; she could easily laugh when there was no occasion for it, and when one said something annoying to her, she got angry and broke out into loud howling.

Very cross and reticent, she will not speak a word.

Surly, wants to have many things and then refuses them.

Very cross, everything annoys her, all her former cheerfulness and friendliness is gone (aft. 1 h.). [*Stf. Gss.*]

Distraction of mind, her thoughts stray unobserved from the subject in hand, and diverge into phantasies and pictures of the fancy. [*Stf. Gss.*]

630. He contradicts ; is opinionative ; no one can please him (aft. 3, 12 h.).

Quarrelsome crossness.

Cross ; he wants to quarrel with every one.

Stiff-necked obstinacy (aft. 4 h.).

Surly insolence and imperiousness (aft. a few h.).

635. **Easily startled.**

Weeping.

Fears ; anxious dread of coming evil.

Hopelessness.

* Curative and secondary action in a person of the opposite humour.

† This appeared once later as over-sensitiveness of the body, but I have seen it also alternating with the latter, and even occurring at the same time.

ARSENICUM.[1]

(The semi-oxyde of metallic arsenic in diluted solution.)

As I write down the word Arsenic, considerations the most momentous throng upon my mind.

When the beneficent Creator made iron He no doubt permitted the children of men to fashion it either into the murderous dagger or the gentle ploughshare wherewith to kill or to feed their fellow-creatures. How much happier would they be did they employ His gifts only for the purpose of doing good! This should be the aim of their life; this was His desire.

It is not to Him, the All-loving, we can impute the wickedness practised by men, who have misemployed the wonderfully powerful medicinal substances in enormous doses in diseases for which they were not suitable, guided only by frivolous ideas or some paltry authority, without having subjected them to any careful trial, and without any substantial reason for their choice.

If a careful tester of the uses of medicines and of their doses arise, they inveigh against him as an enemy to their comfort, and do not refrain from aspersing him with the vilest calumnies.

The ordinary medical art has hitherto employed, *in large and frequently repeated doses*, the most powerful drugs, such as arsenic, nitrate of silver, corrosive sublimate, aconite, belladonna, digitalis, opium, hyoscyamus, &c. Homœopathy cannot employ stronger substances, for there are none stronger. When physicians of the ordinary stamp employ them, they evidently vie with one another who shall prescribe the largest possible doses of these drugs, and make a great boast of increasing these doses to such enormous extremes. This practice they laud and recommend to their fellow practitioners. But if the homœopathic medical art employ the *same drugs*, not at random, like the ordinary method, but after careful investigation, only in suitable cases and in the smallest possible doses, it is denounced as a practice of poisoning. How prejudiced, how unjust, how calumnious is such a charge made by persons who make pretensions to honesty and rectitude!

If Homœopathy now make a fuller explanation—if she condemn (as from conviction she must) the monstrous doses of those drugs employed in ordinary practice—and if she, relying on careful trials, insist that very much less of them should be given for a dose, that where ordinary practitioners give a tenth, a half, a whole grain, and even several grains, often only a quadrillionth, a sextillionth, a decillionth of a grain is required and sufficient, then see the adherents of the ordinary school who denounce the homœopathic healing art as a system of poisoning, see how they laugh aloud at what they call childishness, and declare

1 From vol. ii, 3rd edit., 1833.

themselves convinced (convinced without trial ?) that *such a small quantity* can do nothing at all, and can have no effect whatever—is, indeed *just the same as nothing*. They are not ashamed thus to blow hot and cold from the same mouth, and to pronounce the very same thing to be inert and ludicrously small which they had just accused of being a system of poisoning, whilst they justify and praise their own monstrous and murderous doses of the same medicines. Is not this the grossest and most wretched inconsistency that can be imagined, perpetrated for the purpose of being shamelessly unjust towards a doctrine which they cannot deny possesses truth and consistency, which is borne out by experience, and which enjoins the most delicate cautiousness and the most unwearied circumspection in the selection and administration of its remedies ?

Not very long ago a highly celebrated physician* spoke of pounds of opium being consumed every month in his hospital, where even the nurses were allowed to give it to the patients according to their fancy. Opium, mind ! a drug that has sent many thousands of persons to their graves in ordinary practice ! Yet this man continued to be held in honour, for he belonged to the dominant clique to which everything is lawful, even if it be of the most injurious and absurd character. And when, a few years since, in one of the most enlightened cities † of Europe, every practitioner, from the betitled physician down to the barber's apprentice, prescribed arsenic as a fashionable remedy in almost every disease, and that in such frequent and large doses, one after the other, that the detriment to the health of the people must have been quite palpable ; yet this was held to be honourable practice, though not one of them was acquainted with the peculiar effects of this metallic oxyde (and consequently knew not what cases of disease it was suited for). And yet all prescribed it in repeated doses, *a single one of which, sufficiently attenuated and potentized, would have sufficed to cure all the diseases in the whole habitable world for which this drug is the suitable remedy*. Which of these two opposite modes of employing medicines best deserves the flattering appellation of "system of poisoning" -the ordinary method just alluded to, which attacks with tenths of grains the poor patients (who often require some quite different remedy), or homœopathy, which does not give even a droplet of tincture of rhubarb, without having first ascertained whether rhubard is the most suitable, the only appropriate remedy for the case—homœopathy, which, by unwearied multiplied experiments, discovered that it is only in rare cases that more than a decillionth of a grain of arsenic should be given, and that only in cases where careful proving shows this medicine to be the only one perfectly suitable ? To which of these two modes of practice does the title of honour, "thoughtless, rash system of poisoning," best apply ?

* * *

There is yet another sect of practitioners who may be called hypocritical purists. If they are practical physicians they, indeed, prescribe

---

* Marcus, of Bamberg.

† To what a low depth of degradation as an art must not medicine have sunk in this quarter of the globe when such a state of things could exist in a city like Berlin, which yet in all other departments of human knowledge has scarcely an equal !

all sorts of substances that are injurious when misused, but before the world they wish to pose as patterns of innocence and caution. From their professorial chairs and in their writings they give the most alarming definition of poison, so that to listen to their declamations it would appear unadvisable to treat any imaginable disease with anything stronger than quick-grass, dandelion, oxymel, and raspberry juice. According to their account poisons are absolutely (*i.e.* under all circumstances, in all doses, in all cases) prejudicial to human life, and in this category they include, as suits their humour, a lot of substances which in all ages have been extensively employed by physicians for the cure of diseases. But the employment of these substances would be a criminal offence had not *every one* of them occasionally proved of use. If, however, each of them had only been of use on one single occasion—and it cannot be denied that this sometimes happened—then this definition, besides being blasphemous, is a palpable absurdity. Absolutely and under all circumstances injurious and destructive, and at the same time beneficial, is a self-evident contradiction, utter nonsense. They seek to wriggle out of this contradictory assertion by alleging that these substances have more frequently proved injurious than useful. But, let me ask, did the injury so frequently caused by these things come of itself, or did it not come from their improper employment ? in other words, was it not caused by those physicians who made an unskilful use of them in diseases for which they were unsuitable ? These medicines do not administer themselves in diseases ; they must be administered by somebody, and if ever they were beneficial that was because they happened to be given appropriately by somebody ; it was because they might always be beneficial if nobody ever employed them otherwise than appropriately. Hence it follows that whenever these substances were hurtful and destructive, they were so only on account of having been inappropriately employed. Therefore, all the injury they did is attributable to the unskilfulness of their employer.

These narrow-minded individuals further allege, "that even when we attempt to tame arsenic by means of a corrective, *e.g.* by mixing it with an alkali, it still often does harm enough."

Nay, I reply, the arsenic must not be blamed for this ; for, as I before observed, drugs do not administer themselves, somebody administers them and does harm with them. And how does the alkali act as a corrective ? Does it merely make the arsenic weaker, or does it alter its nature and convert it into something else ? In the latter case the neutral arsenical salt produced is no longer arsenic proper, but something different. If, however, it be merely made weaker, then a simple diminution of the dose of the pure solution of arsenic would be a much more sensible and effectual mode of making it weaker and milder than leaving the dose in its hurtful magnitude, and by the addition of another medicinal substance endeavouring to effect some, but nobody knows what, alteration in its nature, as takes place when a pretended corrective is used. If you think a tenth of a grain of arsenic too strong a dose, what is to prevent you diluting the solution and giving less, a great deal less of it ?

"A tenth of a grain," I hear some one say, "is the smallest

quantity the etiquette of the profession allows us to prescribe. Who could write a prescription to be made up at the apothecary's shop for a smaller quantity without rendering himself ridiculous ?"

Oh, indeed ! A tenth of a grain sometimes acts so violently as to endanger life, and the etiquette of your clique does not permit you to give less—very much less. Is it not an insult to common sense to talk in this way ? Is the etiquette of the profession a code of rules to bind a set of senseless slaves, or are you men of free will and intelligence ? If the latter, what is it that hinders you to give a *smaller* quantity when a *large* quantity might be hurtful ? Obstinacy ? the dogmatism of a school ? or what other intellectual fetters ?

"Arsenic," they protest, "would still be hurtful, though given in much smaller quantity, even if we were to descend to the ridiculous dose of a hundredth or a thousandth of a grain, a minuteness of dose unheard of in the posological maxims of our materia medica. Even a thousandth of a grain of arsenic must still be hurtful and destructive, for it always remains an incontrollable poison. So we affirm, maintain, conjecture, and assert."

What if with all this complacent asserting and conjecturing you have for once blundered upon the truth. It is evident that the virulence of the arsenic cannot increase, but must decrease as the dose is reduced, so that we must at length arrive at such a dilution of the solution and diminution of the dose as no longer possesses the dangerous character of your regulation dose of a tenth of a grain.

"Such a dose would, indeed, be a novelty ! What kind of dose would it be ?"

Novelty is, indeed, a capital crime in the eyes of the orthodox school, which, settled down upon her old lees, subjects the reason to the tyranny of antiquated routine.

But why should a pitiful rule—why, indeed, should anything—hinder the physician, who ought by rights to be a learned, thinking, independent man, a controller of nature in his own domain, from rendering a dangerous does mild by diminishing its size ?

What should hinder him, if experience should show him that the thousandth part of a grain is too strong a dose, from giving the hundred-thousandth part or the millionth of a grain ? And should he find this last act too violently in many cases, *as in medicine all depends on observation and experience* (medicine being nothing but a science of experience), what should hinder him from reducing the millionth to a billionth ? And if this prove too strong a dose in many cases who could prevent him diminishing it to the quadrillionth of a grain, or smaller still ?

Methinks I hear vulgar stolidity croak out from the quagmire of its thousand-year-old prejudices : "Ha ! ha ! ha ! A quadrillionth ! Why, that's nothing at all !"

How so ? Can the subdivision of a substance, be it carried ever so far, bring forth anything else than portions of the whole ? Must not these portions, reduced in size to the very verge of infinity, still continue to be *something*, something substantial, a part of the whole, be it ever so minute ? What man in his senses could deny this ?

And if this (quadrillionth, quintillionth, octillionth, decillionth) continue still to be really an integral portion of the divided substance, as no man in his senses can deny, why should even such a minute portion, seeing that it is really *something*, be incapable of acting, considering that the whole was so tremendously powerful? But *what* and *how much* this small quantiy can do can be determined by no speculative reasoning or unreasoning, but by *experience alone, from which there is no appeal in the domain of facts*. It belongs to experience alone to determine if this small portion has become too weak to remove the disease for which this medicine is otherwise suitable, and to restore the patient to health. This is a matter to be settled not by the dogmatic assertion of the student at his desk, but by experience *alone*, which is the only competent arbiter in such cases.

Experience has already decided the question, and is seen to do so daily by every unprejudiced person.

But when I have finished with the wiseacre, who, never consulting experience, ridicules the small dose of homœopathy as a nonentity, as utterly powerless, I hear on the other side the hypocritical stickler for caution still inveigh against the danger of the small doses used in homœopathic practice, without a shadow of proof for his reckless assertion.

A few words here for such persons.

If arsenic in the dose of a tenth of a grain be, in many cases, a dangerous medicine, must it not be milder in the dose of a thousandth of a grain? And, if so, must it not become still milder with every further diminution of the size of the dose?

Now, if arsenic (like every other very powerful medicinal substance) can, be merely diminishing the size of the doses, be but rendered so mild as to be no longer dangerous to life, then all we have to do is merely to find by experiment how far the size of the dose must be diminished, so that it shall be small enough to do no harm, and yet large enough to effect its full efficacy as a remedy of the diseases for which it is suitable.

Experience, and that alone, not the pedantry of the study, not the narrow-minded, ignorant, unpractical dogmatism of the schools, can decide what dose of such an extremely powerful substance as arsenic is, is so small as to be capable of being ingested without danger, and yet of remaining sufficiently powerful to be able to effect in diseases all that this medicine (so invaluable when sufficiently moderated in its action, and selected for suitable cases of disease) was from its nature ordained to do by the beneficent Creator. It must, by dilution of its solution and diminution of the dose, be rendered so mild that while the strongest man can be freed by such a dose from a disease for which it is the appropriate remedy, this same dose shall be incapable of effecting any perceptible alteration in the health of a healthy infant.* This is the

* A medicine homœopathically chosen, that is to say, a medicine capable of producing a morbid condition very similar to that of the disease to be cured, affects only the diseased part of the organism, therefore just the most irritated, extremely sensitive part of it. Therefore its dose must be so small as only to affect the diseased part just a little more than the disease itself did. For this the smallest dose suffices, one so small as to be incapable of altering the health of a healthy person, who has naturally

grand problem that can only be solved by oft-repeated experiments and trials, but not settled by the sophistical dogmatism of the schools with its guesses, its assertions, and its conjectures.

No rational physician can acknowledge any such limitations to his mode of treatment as the rusty routine of the schools—which is never guided by pure experiment combined with reflection—would dictate to him. His sphere of action is the restoration to health of the sick, and the countless potent forces of the world are freely given to him by the Sustainer of life as implements of healing; nought is withheld. To him whose calling it is to vanquish the disease that brings its victim to the verge of corporeal annihilation, and effect a kind of re-creation of life (a nobler work than most other, even the most vaunted performances of mankind), to him the whole broad expanse of nature, with all her curative powers and agents, must be available, in order to enable him to perform this creative act, if we may so call it. But he must be at liberty to employ these agents in the exact quantity, be it ever so small or ever so large, that experience and trials show him to be most adapted to the end he has in view; in any form whatever that reflection and experience has proved to be most serviceable. All this he must be able to do without any limitation whatsoever, as is the right of a free man, of a deliverer of his fellow creatures, and a life-restorer, equipped with all the knowledge pertaining to his art, and endowed with a god-like spirit and the tenderest conscience.

From this God-serving and noblest of all earthly occupation let all hold aloof who are deficient in mind, in the judicial spirit, in any of the branches of knowledge required for its exercise, or in tender regard for the weal of mankind, and a sense of his duty to humanity, in one word who are deficient in true virtue! Away with that unhallowed crew who merely assume the outward semblance of health-restorers, but whose heads are crammed full of vain deceit, whose hearts are stuffed with wicked frivolity, whose tongues make a mock of truth, and whose hands prepare disaster!

* * *

The following observations are the result of doses of various strengths on persons of various sensitiveness.

For curative purposes, according to the homœopathic method, doses of very high dilution have been found, by innumerable experiments, to be amply sufficient. The dose of the smallest part of a drop containing the decillionth of a grain of white arsenic usually suffices for the cure. In order to prepare this dose, one grain of white arsenic reduced to powder is rubbed up with thirty-three grains of powdered milk-sugar in a porcelain mortar (unglazed) with an unglazed pestle for six minutes, the triturated contents of the mortar scraped for four minutes with a porcelain spatula, then rubbed a second time, without any addition to it, for six minutes, and again scraped for four minutes. To this thirty-three grains of milk-sugar are now added, triturated for six minutes, and after another four minutes of scraping, six minutes of

---

no points of contact sufficiently sensitive for this medicine, or of making him ill, which only large doses of medicine can do. See *Organon of Medicine*, § 277—279, and *Spirit of the Homoeopathic Medical Doctrine*, at the beginning of this volume.

triturating, and again four minutes of scraping, the last thirty-three grains of milk-sugar are added, triturated for six minutes, scraped for four minutes, and again triturated for six minutes, whereby, after a last scraping, a power is produced which, in every grain, contains $\frac{1}{100}$th of a grain of uniformly potentised arsenic. A grain of this powder is, in a similar way, with three times thirty-three grains of fresh milk-sugar, in one hour (thirty-six minutes of triturating, twenty-four of scraping*), brought into the state of a potentised pulverulent attenuation, one hundred times more diluted. Of this one grain (containing $\frac{1}{10,000}$th of a grain of arsenic) is rubbed up for a third hour in a similar manner with ninety-nine grains of milk-sugar; this represents a pulverulent arsenic dilution of the million-fold degree of potency. One grain of this is dissolved in 100 drops of diluted alcohol (in the proportion of equal parts of water and alcohol) and shaken with two succussions of the arm (the phial being held in the hand). This gives a solution which diluted by means of twenty-six more phials (always one drop from the previous phial added to ninety-nine drops of alcohol of the next phial, and then successed twice, before taking one drop of this and dropping it into the next phial), furnishes the required potency, the decillionth ($\overline{X}$) development of power of arsenic.

In order to prepare this highly potentised medicine for administration about ten grains of the smallest globules, made of starch and cane-sugar, such as confectioners use for sprinkling (300 to the grain), are to be placed in a small round porcelain capsule, and six to eight drops of this spirituous liquid dropped on them, and stirred with a wood chip in order that the globules may be equally moistened, then all are to be turned out on a piece of paper and spread out, and when quite dry kept in a corked phial with the name of the medicine on it.

It is much better to make a quantity of globules so saturated with the tincture for dispensing purposes than to moisten one globule every time it is required, for by this process the phial must be frequently inclined on one side, which causes it to become more highly potentised, almost as much as repeated shaking would do.

Such a globule is a sufficient dose for administration in every case of disease for which arsenic is appropriate. This dose may, if necessary, be repeated at suitable intervals, in spite of the circumstance that its action lasts for several days.

In a similar manner are moistened and kept in store the globules the size of a mustard seed (twenty of which weigh a grain), each one of which, kept in a well-corked little phial, is sufficient for olfaction. This is a mode of administering medicine which more recent *very extensive* experience teaches is greatly to be preferred in most cases to any administration of small globules by the mouth for the homœopathic cure of all chronic as well as acute diseases. But this is not the place to give the reason why this is so.

*After this operation the mortar, together with the pestle and the porcelain spatula, after being wiped with a dry cloth, should be rinsed three times with boiling water, between each rinsing rubbed dry with blotting paper, then gradually heated over a charcoal-fire to a red heat, in order that these articles may be as good as new for future trituration of medicines.

A sensible homœopathic physician will not give this remedy, even in such a minute dose, unless he is convinced that its peculiar symptoms have the greatest possible resemblance to those of the disease to be cured. When this is the case it is certain to be efficacious.

But if, owing to human fallibility, the selection has not been quite appropriate, one, two, or several olfactions of ipecacuanha hepar sulphuris, or nux vomica, according to the circumstances, will remove the bad effects.

Such an employment of arsenic has shown its curative power in countless diseased states; among the rest, in several kinds of quotidian fevers and agues of a peculiar kind; in varicose veins; in stitches in the sternum; vomiting after almost every article of food: excessive loss of blood at the menstrual period, and other disorders in connexion with that function; in constipation; in acrid leucorrhœa and excoriation caused thereby; in indurations of the liver; oppression of the chest when going up hill; fetid smell from the mouth; bleeding of the gums; hæmoptysis; aching in the sternum; gastralgia; drawing shooting here and there in the face; drowsiness in the evening; shivering in the evening and stretching of the limbs, with timorous restlessness; difficulty of falling asleep and waking up at night; weariness in the feet; bruised pain in the knee-joint; itching tetters on the knee; pain in the ball of the big toe, as if excoriated, when walking; old ulcers on the legs, with (burning and) shooting pain; tearing shooting in the hip, groin, and thigh; nocturnal drawing tearing from the elbow to the shoulder; painful swelling of the inguinal glands, &c.

(The subject of poisoning with large doses of arsenic would be out of place here. It is to be relieved as much as possible by giving carbonate of potash shaken up in oil, by a solution of hepar sulphuris, and by copious draughts of rich milk; but the complete removal of the remaining nervous symptoms must be effected by other remedies appropriate to them.)

[HAHNEMANM was aided in this proving by:—BAEHR, GROSS, FR. HAHNEMANN. HORNBURG, LANGHAMMER, STAPF.

The following authorities are quoted for the effects of the drug:

ALBERTI, *Jurisprud. Med.*, tom. i, ii, iii, iv. AMATUS LUSITANUS, *Cent.* ii. APONO, PET. DE, *De Venenis*; in *Schenck*, lib. vii.

BAYLIES, in *Samml. br. Abh. f. pr. Aerzte*, vii. BERNHARDI, *Annalen der Heilkunst*, 1811. BONETUS, *Sepulcr. Anat.*, sect. x. BORELLUS, *Hist. et Observ.*, cent. iii. BORGES, *Kopp's Jahrb. d. Staatsarzn.*, ii. BUCHHOLZ, *Beitr. z. ger. Arzn.*, iv; *Hufel. Journ.*, v. BUTTNER, *Unterricht uber die Todtlichkeit der Wunde.*

CARDANUS, *De Venenis*, i, iii, 1563. CRUGER, DAN., *Misc. Nat. Cur.*, Dec. ii. D. H., in *Kopp's Jahrb. d. Staatsarzn.*, ii. DEGNER, J. K., *Act. Nat. Cur.*, vi. DEGRANGE, *Phys. Med. Journ.*, 1800, April.

EBERS, *Hufel. Journ. f. pr. Arz.*, 1813, Sept., Oct. *Eph. Nat. Cur.*, cent. x, app.

FELDMANN, in *Commerc. Lit. Nor.*, 1743. FERNELIUS, *Therapeut.*, lib. vi. FORESTUS, P., *lib.* xvii and xviii.

FOWLER, TH., *Med. Rep. of Effects of Arsenic in Cure of Agues.* London, 1787. FRIEDRICH, in *Hufel. Journ. f. pr. Arz.*, v.

GABEZIUS. GERBITZ, in *Eph. Nat. Cur.*, Dec. iii, ann. 5, 6. GORITZ, in *Bresl. Samml.*, 1728. GREISELIUS, J. G., in *Misc. Nat. Cur.*, Dec. 1, ann. 2. GRIMM, G. C., in *Misc. Nat. Cur.*, Dec. iii. GUILBERT, *Med.-Chir. Wahrnehm.*, vol. iv, Altenb. GULDENKLEE, TIMAEUS A, *Cas. Medic.*, Lips., 1662 ; *Opp.*, Lips., 1715.

HAMMER, J. D., in *common. Lit. Norimb.*, 1738. HARGENS, in *Hufel. Journ. f. pr. Arz.*, ix. *Hartlaub und Trinks' R. A. M. L.*, iii. HARTMANN, *Diss. Aethiop. Antim. et Arsenicalis.* Halle, 1759. HEIMREICH, *Arsen. als Frebermitt.* ; in *Act. Nat. Cur.*, ii. HEINZE, in *Ebers*, l. c, HENKEL, in *Act. Nat. Cur.*, ii. HENNING, in *Hufel. Journ. f. pr. Arz.*, x. HEUN, in *Allgem. Med. Annal.*, 1805, Feby. HUBER, in *N. Act. Nat. Cur.*, iii.

ISENFLAMM-STEIMMIG, *Diss. de Remed. Suspect. et venen.*, Erlangen, 1767.

JACOBI, JOH , in *Act. Nat. Cur.*, vi. JENNER, J. C., in *Simon's Samml. d. neuest. Beobacht f. d. Jahr* 1788, Erf., 179. JUSTAMOND, *On cancerous disorders*, London, 1750.

KAISER, C. L., in *Henke's Zeitsch. f. d. Staatsarz*, vii, pt. 3. KELLNER, in *Bresl. Samml.*, 1727. KNAPE, *Annalen d. Staatsarzn.*, i. KOPP, *Jahrb. d. Staatsarzn.*, ii.

LABORDE, *Jour. de Medecine*, lxx. LOW, in *Sydenham's Opera*, II.

MAJAULT, in *Samml. br. Abhandl. f. pr. Aerzte*, viii. MARCUS, A. F., *Ephem. d. Heilk.*, heft iii. *Med. Nat. Zeit.*, 1798, Sept. *Misc. Nat. Cur.*, Dec iii, ann. 9, 10. MONTANUS, J. B., in *Schenck*, lib. 7. MORGAGNI, *De Sed. et Caus. Morb.*, lix. MUELLER, J. MAT., in *Eph. Nat. Cur.*, cent. v. MYRRHEN, A., *Misc. Nat. Cur.*, Dec. iii, ann. 9, 10.

Neue Med.-Chir. Wahrnehm., vol. 1, Altenb., 1778.

PEARSON, in *Samml. br. Abh., f. pr. Aerzte*, xiii. PFANN, *Samml. merkw. Falle*, Nurnb., 1750. PREUSSIUS, *Eph. Nat. Cur.*, cent. iii. PLY, *Samml.*, i, v, vi, viii.

QUELMALZ, *Commerc. lit. Norimb.*, 1737, heb. 28.

RAU, TH., *Act. Nat. Cur.*, ix. RICHARD, A., in *Schenck*, lib. vii.

Salzburg Med.-Chir. Zeitung. SEILER, *Progr. de Venef. per Arsen.*, Viteb., 1806. SENNERT, *Prax. Med.*, lib. 6. SIEBOLD, in *Hufel. Journ. f. pr. Arz.*, iv. STAHL, G. E., *Opusc. Chym. Phys. Med.* STOERCK, *Med. Jahrg.*, i.

TACHENIUS, O., *Hipp. Chym.*, c. 24. THILENIUS, in *Richter's Chir. Bibl.*, v. THOMSON, *Edinburgh Essays*, iv.

VAN EGGERN, *Diss. de Vacill. Dentium*, Duisb., 1787. VERZASCH, BERNARD *Obs. Med., obs.* 66. VICAT, *Observ.*

WEDEL, G. W., *Diss. de Arsen.*, Jen., 1719. WOLFF, J. PH., *Act. Nat. Cur.*, v.

The 1st Edit. gave 662 symptoms, the 2nd 948, this 3rd Edit. 1068. The *Chr. Kr.* contains 163 additional symptoms.]

Vertigo, so that she must hold on by something, when she shuts her eyes, every evening.*

Vertigo when sitting.

Vertigo (aft. 12 h.). [THOMSON,[1] *Edinburgh Essays*, iv.†—SENNERT,[2] *Prax. Med.*, lib. 6, p. 6, C. 2. ‡]

Vertigo causing obscuration of vision. § [A. MYRRHEN, *Misc. N. C.*, Dec. iii, ann. 91, 10, obs. 220.[3]]

5. Giddy in the head. [ALBERTI, *Jurisprud. Medic.*, tom. ii, pp. 527—530.[4]]

He is attacked with violent vertigo and sickness when lying ; he must rise up, in order to diminish it. [*Stf.*]

Vertigo ; when he rises up, his thoughts go away. [*Stf.*]

Vertigo only when walking, as if he would fall to the right side (aft. 9½ h.). [*Lr.*]

Vertigo and unconscious stupefaction. [EBERS, in *Hufel. Journ.*, 1813, Octob., p. 8.[5]]

10. Loss of sensation and consciousness, so that he knew not what was going on. [PYL,[6] *Samml.*, viii, pp. 98, 105, 108. ||]

She lay on the bed completely devoid of sense, muttered incomprehensible sounds, the eyes staring, cold sweat on the forehead, trembling all over the body, pulse small, hard, and very quick [EBERS, l. c., p. 9.¶]

Loss of reason and of the external and internal senses ; he did not see, for many days did not speak, did not hear, and understood nothing, and when one roared very loudly into his ears he looked at those around, like a drunken person wakened out of profound sleep. [MYRRHEN, l. c.]

Delirium recurring from time to time. [GUILBERT,[7] *Med.-Chir. Wahrnehm.*, vol. iv, Altenb.**]

Diminution of memory.

*Therefore recurring after the manner of an intermittent fever. Of such ague-like recurring symptoms, arsenic has several, *v.* SS. 265, 375, 868, 918.

† From the dust of sulphuret of arsenic.

‡ *Vide* DR. C. L. KAISER, in *Hartlaub and Trinks' R. A. M. L.*, vol. i, p. 249.[8] Sympt. 8, "Vertigo ;" Sympt. 9, "Vertigo with Headache."

§ From drawing up a solution of arsenic into the nose.

|| KAISER, l. c., Sympt. 5, "The distinct self-consciousness vanishes, or is observed in a slight degree."

¶ Ibid., S. 7, "The organs of sense seem to be in abnormal activity."

** Ibid., S. 6, "Delirium."

---

1. Poisoning of woman.
2. From inhaling realgar. (This symptom not found.)
3. From drawing a solution of A. into the nostrils for coryza.
4. Cases of poisoning in healthy adults.—This giddiness occurred during vomiting.
5. Effects of arsenite of potash in ague patients.
6. Poisoning of adult.
7. Poisoning of adult.
8. Poisoning of a whole family by A. (Quoted in *H. and T.* from *Henke's Ztsch.*, vii, pt. 3. Amalgamated with pathogenesis in *Chronischen Krankheiten.*)

15. Very defective memory for a long time. [MYRRHEN, l. c.]

His memory leaves him ; he is forgetful.

Stupid and weak in the head ; towards noon (aft. 30 h.).

When walking in the open air, giddy in the head, which is increased on coming again into the room (aft. $\frac{1}{2}$ h.).

Head is confused. [PEARSON, in *Samml. br. Abh. f. p. Aerzte*, xxii, 4. [1]]

20. Empty in the head. [*Hbg.*]

Giddy in the head ; he cannot think. [*Myr.*]

Chronic weakness of mind. [2] [EBERS, l. c., Sept., p. 48.]

Weak reason[3]. [EBERS, l. c., p. 56.]

From pains she got such a weakness in her head, and became so qualmish and weak in the scrobiculus cordis, that she was very ill.

25. Obtuseness in the head, without pain.

Great confusion of the head, in the evening (3rd d.).

After sleeping he was very dazed in the head.

(From 11 a.m. until 6 p.m.) headache, is stupid, as if from insufficient sleep.

Internal uneasiness and a stupefaction of the head, such as arises from too hasty performance of an excessive amount of business (aft. 2 d.).

30. Head stupid and empty (like a lantern), as if he had a very severe cold and is very cross.

While walking in the open air very stupid and giddy in the head, chiefly in the forehead, as if intoxicated, so that he staggered first to one side and then to the other, and feard to fall every instant (aft. $9\frac{1}{2}$ h.). [*Lr.*]

Dulness in the head. [BUCHHOLZ, *Beitr. z. ger. Arzn.*, iv, p. 164.]

Uncommon heaviness in the head with roaring in the ears, which goes off in the open air, but immediately returns when coming again into the room (aft. 16 h.).*

Head heavy and empty, so that he cannot easily rise up ; he must lie down.

35. Excessive heaviness in the head, especially when standing and sitting. [BUCHHOLZ, l. c.]

Headache. [G. C. GRIMM, *Misc. N. C.*, Dec. iii, obs. 174.][5]

Pains in the head and vertigo for several days.† [G. W. WEDEL, *Diss. de Arsen.*, Jan., 1719, p. 10.][6]

Headache (for some days), which is immediately relieved by the application of cold water, on removing which it is worse than before. [VICAT, *Observ.*, p. 197.[7]]

In the morning immediately on rising from bed, a one-sided headache, as if bruised (aft. 12 h.).

*Comp. 969.

† From the vapour of arsenic.

---

1 Effects of arsenic of potash in an epileptic.

2 See note to S. 118.

3 From suppression of ague by A.

4 Case of poisoning.

5 From the black oxide, in an adult.

6 From arsenical vapours.

7 From powdering the hair with A.

40. Semilateral headache. [KNAPE, *Annalen d. Staats-Arzn.*, i, I.[1]]

Every afternoon headache for some hours, drawing under the coronal suture.

Uncommon heaviness of the head, as if the brain was pressed down by a weight, with roaring in the ears, in the morning after rising from bed (aft. 24 h.).

(Tearing in the head and at the same time in the right eye.)

Heaviness of the head, with aching pain, in the morning (aft. 72 h).

45. Aching stupefying headache, especially in the forehead, in every position (aft. 2 h.). [*Lr.*]

Aching stupefying headache, especially on the right side of the forehead, just above the right eyebrow, which pains as if sore on wrinkling his forehead (aft. $8\frac{1}{2}$ h.). [*Lr.*]

Aching drawing pain on the right side of the forehead (aft. $2\frac{3}{4}$ h.). [*Lr.*]

Aching pain on the right temporal region, in all positions (aft. 3 h.). [*Lr.*]

Aching stitch-like pain on the left temple, which does not go off by touching (aft. $2\frac{1}{2}$ h.). [*Lr.*]

50. Aching stupefying headache (chiefly on the forehead), with fine stitches on the left temporal region near the outer canthus of the eye when walking and standing, going off when sitting (aft. $2\frac{1}{2}$ h.). [*Lr.*]

Stitch-like pain on the left temple, which went off by touching (aft. $2\frac{1}{2}$ h.). [*Lr.*]

As if beaten on the front of the head.

At night (about 2 a.m.), along with an outbreak of perspiration, a hacking (sharp hard beating) in the head, as if it would burst her skull asunder.

On moving, violent throbbing headache in the forehead. [*Stf.*]

55. In the whole head, especially in the forehead, on rising up in bed, a violent throbbing headache, with sickness. [*Stf.*]

Throbbing headache in the forehead, just above the root of the nose (aft. $\frac{1}{2}$ h.).

At noon and midnight, for half an hour, a hammering, like blows of a hammer, in the temples, very painful, after which, for a couple of hours, she is as if paralysed in the body.

A dull throbbing pain in one half of the head, to above the eye.

Pain above the nose and in the forehead, as if sore or bruised, which goes off for instants by external rubbing.

60. Periodical headache. [TH. RAU, *Acta N. C.*, ix, obs. 37.[2]]

Horrible headache. [JOH. JACOBI, *Acta N. C.*, vi, obs. 62.[3]—RAU, l. c.—(aft. 6, 7 d.) KNAPE, l. c.]

Headache in the occiput.

Tearing shooting in the left temple.

Tearing pains in the occiput. [*Bhr.*]

65. A small boil on the left side of the forehead, with smarting pain, for eight days (aft. 24 h.). [*Fr. H—n.*]

---

1 Effects of powdering hair with A.

2 From application of A. to the scalp.

3 From suppression of ague by A. in a young man.

On moving he feels as if the brain moved and struck against the skull internally.

Transient, squeezing headache above the eyes.

Headache as if stretched.

A headache compounded of weight and tearing, with sleepy exhaustion by day (aft. 4 d.).

70. Clicking sensation in the head above the ears, while walking.

The scalp pains as if festering when touched.

External headache as if bruised, which is aggravated by touch (aft. 3 h.).

Touching the hair of the head causes pain.

Formication on the integuments of the occiput, as if the roots of the hairs moved (aft. 1 h.).

75. Contractive pain in the head.

(Throbbing like pulse-beats in the eyes, and at each throb a stitch, after midnight.)

Sunken eyes, yellow complexion.

Drawing pains in the eyes, and quivering in the eyelids.

Above the left eyelid and in the upper half of the left eye-ball an aching pain, increased by looking upwards (aft. $1\frac{3}{4}$ h.).

80. (The right eye was painful quite internally, she could scarcely turn it, there came such severe stitches in its interior.)

Itching around the eyes and about the temples, as from innumerable red-hot needles.

Burning in the eyes.

In the eyes a tiresome tickling, owing to which he could not see well.

Twitching in the left eye.

85. While reading by candle-light, dryness of the eye-lids, as if they rubbed the eyes.

The eyes are dazzled by snow ; they weep.

White spots or points hover before the eyes.

The eye-lids are stuck together in the morning.

Constant trembling in the upper eye-lids, with weeping of the eyes.

90. At night, under the right eye, for an hour, an aching pain, so that from anxiety she could not remain in bed.

The borders of the eye-lids are painful on moving, as if they were dry, and rubbed upon the eye-balls (while walking in the open air and in the room.)

Red inflamed eyes. [*Neue Med. Chir. Wahrnehm.*,[1] vol. i, Altenb., 1778.*]

Aching in the left eye, as if sand had got into it (aft. 2 h.). [*Lr.*]

Itching and **watering** of the eyes ; in the morning some matter in them. [*Fr. H—n.*]

**Vide* KAISER, l. c., S. 11, "Inflammation of the conjunctiva."

---

1 Not accessible.

95. Smarting eroding itching in both eyes, compelling him to rub them (aft. $3\frac{3}{4}$ h.). [*Lr.*]*

Inflammation of the eyes. [HEUN, in *Allgem. Med. Annal.*, 1805, February.[1]]

Violent inflammation of the eyes.[2] [GUILBERT, l. c.]

Swollen eyes and lips. [KNAPE, l. c.]

Swelling of the eyes. [QUELMALZ, *Commerc. lit. Norimb.*, 1737, heb. 28.[3]]

100. Swollen eye-lids. [*Neue Med.-Chir. Wahrnehm.*, l. c.]

Burning in the eyes, nose, and mouth. [*Neue Med.-Chir. Wahrnehm.*, l. c.]

Projecting eyes filled with **tears**; the acrid tears make the cheeks sore. [GUILBERT, l. c.]†

Constant severe watering of the right eye (from 2nd to 10th d.). [*Fr. H—n.*]

Painless swelling under the left eye which partially closes the eye and is very soft (aft. 5 d.). [*Fr. H—n.*]

105. **Contracted pupils** (aft. $1\frac{1}{4}$, 5 h.). [*Lr.*]

Sensitiveness to light, photophobia.[4] [EBERS, l. c., Octob., p. 14.]

Sparks before the eyes.[4] [EBERS, l. c.]

(She sees everything indistinctly, as through a white veil.)

(Yellowness in the eyes, like jaundice.)

110. Wild look. [MAJAULT, in *Samml. br. Abhandl. f. p. Aerzte*, vii, 1, 2.[5]]

Staring[6] look. [GUILBERT, l. c.‡]

Frightfully staring[7] eyes. [MYRRHEN, l. c.]

Distortion of the eyes. [J. MAT. MUELLER,[8] in *Eph. Nat. Cur.*, cent. v. obs. 51.§]

The eye-lids are drawn to; he is tired. [*Hby.*‖]

115. Distortion of the eyes and cervical muscles. [*Eph. Nat. cur.*, cent. x, app., p. 463.[9]]

He does not recognise those about him. [A. RICHARD, in *Schenck*, lib. vii, obs. 211.[10]]

Obscuration of sight. [BAYLIES,[11] in *Samml. br. Abh. f. p. Aerzte*, vii, 2.¶]

*SCHLEGEL also observed, "Sometimes tearing in the eye." *Vide* also *Hartlaub* and *Trinks R. A. M. L.*, B., iii, p. 126, S. 3.[12]

† See also KAISER, l. c., S. 12, "Projecting eyes."

‡ Ibid., S. 15, "Staring look, without dilatation of the pupils."

§ Ibid., S. 13, "Fixed eye, directed upwards."

‖ Ibid., S. 14, "Dull eye."

¶ Ibid., S. 17, "Darkness and glittering before the eyes."

---

1. From application of A. to a cancerous ulcer of the cheek.
2. Frequently recurring.
3. Poisoning of a girl by the black oxide. See note to S. 139
4. With headache and vertigo.
5. Poisoning of several subjects with different preparations of A. (Original in *Seance Publique de la Faculte de Medecine de Paris*, 1779, p. 55.)
6. Rather, "wild." 7. Rather, "distorted." 8. General statements.
9. Poisoning of a man with twelve grains of A.
10. Poisoning of adult.
11. General statement from authors.
12. From smoking tobacco mixed with A. The symptoms quoted from *H.* and *T.* are taken from various sources, and were chiefly caused by accidental poisoning.

A weak-sighted person became almost quite blind, lost hearing for some time, and fell into a long-continued state of stupidity.[1] [EBERS, l. c., Oct., p. 15.]

Obscuration of sight; it is black before his eyes (in the 1st h.), [RICHARD, l. c.]

120. During the nausea, yellowness before the eyes. [ALBERTI, l, c., ii, p. 527.]

Long-continued weakness of sight. [MYRRHEN, l. c.]

Pimples on the forehead. [*Neue Med.-Chir Wahrnehm.*, l. c.]

Eruption on the forehead. [KNAPE, l. c.]

Red, bloated face and swollen lips. [*Stf.*]

125. Bloated face. [*Fr. H—n.*]

Pale face. [MAJAULT, l. c.*]

Pale face with sunken eyes. [J. G. GREISELIUS, in *Misc. Nat. Cur.*, Dec. i, ann. 2, p. 149.[2]]

Deadly paleness. [HENNING, in *Huf. Journ. d. p. Arzn.*, x, 2.[3]]

Deathly hue of the face.[4] [ALBERTI, l. c.]

130. Death-like appearance.[5] [ALBERTI, l. c.†]

Bluish, discoloured face.[5] [MUELLER, l. c., and *Eph. Nat. C.*, l. c.]

Earthy and leaden complexion, with green and blue spots and stripes. [KNAPE, l. c.]

Twitchings in the facial muscles. [GUILBERT, l. c.]

Distorted features, as from discontent.‡

135. Face full of ulcers. [*Neue Med.-Chir. Wahrnehm.*, l. c.]

Swelling in the face§ of an elastic character, particularly in the eyelids, especially in the morning. [TH. FOWLER, *Medical Reports of the Effects of Arsenic in the Cure of Agues.* Lond. 1787.][6]

Swelling of the face and head. [SIEBOLD,[7] in *Huf. Journ.*, iv.||]

Swelling of the face, syncopes, vertigo. [SENNERT, l. c., lib. 6, p. 237.]

Swelling of the whole head.[8] [QUELMALZ, l. c.]

140. Swelling of the head. [HEIMREICH, in *Act. N. C.*, ii, obs. 10.[9]]

Swelling of the face.¶ [JENNER, in *Simon's Samml. d neuest. Beobacht. f. d. Jahr* 1788, Erf. 1791, p. 27.[10]]

* See also KAISER, S. 20, "Paleness of face and features strikingly distorted."

† See also *Hartl.* and *Trinks*, l. c., S. 4, "Pale, yellow, cachectic appearance," and S. 5, "Sunken features."

‡ See also KAISER, l. c., S. 21, "Altered features."

§ In three among 48 persons.

|| Comp. KAISER, l. c., S. 19, "Face red and swollen,"—and *Hartl.* and *Trinks*, l. c., S. 6, "Swelling of the whole face (aft. 1 h.)." (From the external application of *Cosme's* powder in a case of labial cancer.)

¶ From internal use.

---

1 Doubtful how much is ague and how much A.
2 Observations on miners in A.
3 From application of A. to a diseased breast.—With violent vomiting.
4 During vomiting.
5 Literally—"face livid and lurid."
6 Effects of arsenite of potash in ague patients.
7 Effect of dressing pustular scalp with mixture of A. and cinnabar.
8 Should read—"Swelling of the veins of the whole head, after violent vomiting."
9 Effects of A. sprinkled on the hair.
10 Not accessible.

Enormous swelling of head and face. [Knape, l. c.]

Cutaneous swelling of the head, face, eyes, neck and chest, of natural colour. [Knape, l. c.]

Eruption of pustules on the hairy scalp and face, with burning pain. [Heimreich, l. c.]

145. The hairy scalp to the middle of the forehead covered with an ulcerous scab. [Knape, l. c.]

Ulcerous scab a finger's breadth in thickness on the hairy scalp, which fell off after some weeks. [Heimreich, l. c.]

On the hairy scalp innumerable very red pimples. [Vicat, l. c.]

On the whole hairy scalp eruption of pimples, which on being rubbed and touched pain as if festering, and the whole hairy scalp was painful as if blood was effused in it (aft. $11\frac{1}{2}$ h.). [*Lr.*]

Eroding ulcers on the hairy scalp. [Knape, l. c.]

150. Gnawing itching on the hairy scalp. [Knape, l. c.]

Gnawing itching on the whole hairy scalp, inciting him to scratch (aft. 8 h.). [*Lr.*]

Burning pain on the hairy scalp. [Knape, l. c.]

Burning itching on the hairy scalp. [Knape, l. c.]

Itching, with pain like ulceration, that incites to scratching, on the whole hairy scalp, which pains in every part, as if from effused blood, but mostly on the occiput (aft. $8\frac{1}{2}$ h.). [*Lr.*]

155. On the left parietal bone, on the hairy scalp, a pimple covered with scurf, which incites to scratching, and when rubbed pains as if festering (aft. 7 h.). [*Lr.*]

Two large pimples betwixt the eyebrows, which incite to scratching and discharge bloody water, the following day they are full of pus (aft. 2 h.). [*Lr.*]

Pimples on the left temple, inciting to scratching, discharging bloody water, and after rubbing sore pain (aft. 3 h.). [*Lr.*]

Falling out of the hair. [Baylies, l. c.]

Stitches in the nasal bones.

160. Pain in the root of the nose in the bone.

(Alternately smell of pitch and sulphur in the nose.)

Aching in the left upper jaw.

Burning in the external ear, in the evening (aft. 5 h.).

External pain in the ears, like cramp.

165. Stitches in the ear (in the morning).

Tearing in the interior of the ear.

Behind the ear, down the neck to the shoulder, drawing tearing while sitting.

Drawing tearing pain in the lobe of the left ear.

Tearing shooting outwards, in the left meatus auditorius externus, more in the evening (1st. d.).

170. Shooting in the ear (in the morning).

The left meatus externus seems to be stopped from without.

Great roaring before the ears, as from a water-weir.

Hardness of hearing, as if the ears were stopped. (aft. 60 h.).

He does not understand what is said to him. [Richard, l. c.]

175. When swallowing the ears become closed internally, like deafness.
Roaring in the ears at each attack of pains.*
Ringing noise in the whole head.
Voluptuous tickling in the right meatus auditorius, that compled him to rub (aft. 3¼ h.). [*Lr.*]
Agreeable crawling deep in both ears, for ten days (aft. 15 h.). [*Fr. H—n.*]

180. Ringing in the right ear (when sitting) (aft. 1¼ h.). [*Lr.*]
Rushing noise in the ears. [THOMSON, l. c.—BAYLIES, l. c.]
Pinching in the ears. [*Bhr.*]
An ulcer eroding all round on the lip, with tearing pain and smarting as from salt, in the evening after lying down, in the daytime when moving, worst when touched and in the open air; it prevents sleep and wakes him up in the night (aft. 14 d.).
Itching as from innumerable burning needles in the upper lip to under the nose; the following day the upper lip swelled above the red.

185. (Painful lumps in the upper lip.)
Round about the mouth red tettery skin.
Eruption (breaking out) on the lips at the edge of the red, painless (aft. 14 d.†).
(Eruption on the mouth with burning pain.)
A kind of pinching quivering on one side of the upper lip, especially when going to sleep.‡

190. A brown stripe of shrivelled epidermis, almost like a burnt part, extends through the middle of the red of the lower lip.
Eruption of ulcers about the lips. [ISENFLAMM-STEIMMIG, *Diss. de Remed. Suspect. et Venen.*, Erlang., 1767, p. 27.[1]]
Black-spotted lips. [GUILBERT, l. c.]
Bluish lips and tongue. [BAYLIES, l. c.§]
After eating, bleeding of the lower lip (aft. 1¼ h.). [*Lr.*]

195. Externally about the mouth blackish. [ALBERTI, l. c.]
Constant twitching toothache up to the temple, which is relieved or removed by sitting up in bed (aft. 8 d.)
Shooting in the gums (in the morning).
Pain of several teeth (in the gums) as if they were loose and would fall out, but the pain is not increased by chewing (aft. 1 h.).
Toothache as from loose teeth; they are loose, and pain as if sore *per se*, and still more when chewing; touching the gums likewise causes similar pain; the cheek swells on that side.

* The occurrence of other symptoms during the pains is quite peculiar to arsenic. See S. 970.

† Although in this observation the eruption on the mouth appeared very late, it is yet a primary action, and rapidly cures homœopathically a similar morbid state, if the symptoms of the disease are not unsuitable for arsenic.

‡ Twitchings on going to sleep are often observed from arsenic. Comp 708, 889, 890, 891, 899.

§ See also KAISER, l. c., S. 23, "Bluish lips."

1 General statement.

200. Toothache, rather pressive than drawing.

Tearing in the teeth and at the same time in the head, at which she became so furious that she beat her head with her fists (just before the occurrence of the menses) (the 15th d.).

A tooth becomes loose and protruding (in the morning) ; its gum is painful when touched, but still more so the external part of the cheek behind which lies the loose tooth (when touched) ; the tooth is not painful on biting the teeth together.

Nocturnal (tearing) pain of the gum at the canine tooth, which is intolerable as long as he lies on the affected side, but is removed by the heat of the stove ; the following morning the nose is swollen and painful when touched* (aft. 3 d.).

Convulsive grinding of the teeth. [VAN EGGERN,[1] *Diss. de Vacillat. Dentium*, Duisb., 1787.†]

205. All the teeth fall out. [VAN EGGERN, l. c.]

Itching on the neck under the jaw.

Swollen glands under the jaw, with pressive and contusive pain.

Great dryness in the mouth and great thirst.

Her throat feels dry ; she must always drink, and if she did dot drink she felt as if she must die of thirst.

210. Wooden dry taste in the mouth.

Absence of thirst, loss of thirst.‡

Uncommon thirst, so that he must drink much cold water every ten minutes, from morning till evening, but not in the night. [*Fr. H—n.*]§

Slimy mouth, sliminess in the throat (aft. 2 h.).

The tongue eroded at the side of the tip with smarting pain (aft. 14 d.).

215. Pricking pain as from a fish-bone in the root of the tongue, when swallowing and turning the head.

Boring pain in the right border of the tongue, during half sleep.

He feels as if he had no taste, as if the tongue were burnt dead and were without feeling.

Pain on the tongue as if there were vesicles there with burning pain.

White tongue. [ALBERTI, l. c.]

220. He must spit often. [*Hbg.*]

Feeling of dryness of the tongue. [BUCHHOLZ, in *Hufel. Journ.*, v, p. 378.[2]]

* It is a peculiarity of arsenic pains, that they are relieved by external warmth. Comp. 686, 687, 37.

† See also KAISER, l. c., S. 24, "Grinding of the teeth."

‡ A rare alternating action compared with the much more frequent one where there is constant longing for drinks, and yet only little is drunk at a time, but very often (rarely much at a time). *Vide* 362, 927.

§ See also KAISER, l. c., S. 26, "Violent thirst"—and S. 27, "Violent thirst ; drinking does not afford the patient refreshment and alleviation."

---

1 Not accessible.

2 Poisoning of several adults by black oxide. (Vol. v, part ii, p. 104.)

Great dry feeling in the mouth, with frequent severe thirst, yet he drinks but little at a time. [*Stf.*]

Great dryness in the mouth. [THILENIUS, in *Richter's Chir. Bibl.*, v, p. 540.[1]]

Dryness of the tongue. [GUILBERT, l. c.—MAJAULT, l. c.]

225. Quavering voice. [GUILBERT, l. c.]*

Speechlessness and insensibility. [*Misc. N. C.*, Dec. iii, ann. 9, 10, p. 390. [2]]

Bloody saliva. [*Neue med. chir. Wahrnehm.*, l. c.]

(A feeling in the throat as if a hair were in it.)

Sensation in the throat as from a lump of mucus, with taste of blood.

230. Behind on the velum pendulum palati a scraping scratching sensation, when not swallowing (aft. 2 h.).

Tearing pain in the œsophagus and all up the throat, also when not swallowing.

A kind of paralysis of the fauces and œsophagus ; the chewed bread could not be swallowed down, it only went **down with difficulty** with an uneasy pressure, **as if the œsophagus had no power to swallow it** ; he heard it rattle down.

Burning in the throat [RICHARD, l. c.—BUCHHOLZ, l. c.]

Long-continued rough feeling on the palate (aft. 10 h.). [*Lr.*]

235. Internal inflammation of the throat. [RAU, l. c.]

Gangrenous sore throat.† [FELDMANN, in *commerc. lit. Nor.*, 1743, p. 50.]

Difficulty of swallowing. [RAU, l. c.]

Painful deglutition. [*Neue med.-chir. Wahrn.*, l. c.]

Burning in the fauces. [RICHARD, l. c.—KNAPE, l. c.—KOPP, *Jahrbuch. d. Staatsarzn.*, ii, p. 182.[4]]

240. In the fauces and stomach a sensation as if a thread was rolled into a coil. [RICHARD, l. c.]

The œsophagus is as if constricted. [*N. m.-ch. Wahrn.*, l. c.]

Constrictive sensation in the throat. [PREUSSIUS, *Eph. N. C.*, cent. iii, Obs. 15.[5]]

He complains that he feels as if the throat would be completely closed ; as if nothing more could get through the œsophagus. [ALBERTI, l. c.]

Taste in the mouth sour ; the food too tastes sour.

245. Putrid fœtid taste in the mouth.

In the morning, taste in the mouth like putrid flesh.

In the morning the expectoration‡ is green and bitter.

* See also *Hartl.* and *Trinks.*, l. c., S. 7, "Very unequal voice, sometimes strong, sometimes weak."

† From the external application of the arsenical, so-called magnetic plaster.3

‡ But only what is hawked up from the fauces.

---

1 Effects of arsenic in a patient with mammary scirrhus.
2 Same case as Myrrhen's (see S. 4).
3 Applied for a quartan ague.
4 Poisoning of a man of 56.
5 Poisoning of a boy.

He ejects grey mucus by hawking.

The saliva he spits out tastes bitter.

250. (The first morsel she swallowed in the morning scraped and scratched her afterwards in the throat, like rancid fat.)

Salt expectoration (sputum salsum). [RICHARD, l. c.]

Bitter expectoration (sputum amarum). [RICHARD, l. c.]

Bitterness in the mouth with yellow diarrhœa. [MORGAGNI, *De Sed. et Caus. Morb.*, lix, § 6, 8.[1]]

She loathes all food; can relish nothing.

255. Absence of hunger and desire to eat, for ten days. [*Fr. H—n.*]

Anorexia. [STOERCK, *Med. Jahrg.*, i, p. 107.[2]—*Jacobi*, l. c.]*

Complete anorexia. [BUCHHOLZ in *Huf. Journ.*, l. c.]

Anorexia with violent thirst. [STOERCK, l. c.]

Loathing of food. [GORITZ, in *Bresl. Samml.*, 1728.[3]—GRIMM, l. c.]

260. Insuperable loathing of all food, so that he could not think of eating without feeling sick. [4] [EBERS, l. c., Sept., p. 56.]

Loathing of all food. [ALBERTI, l. c.]

He is unable to get the food down. [RICHARD, l. c.]

The smell of cooked meat is intolerable to him (aft. 5. h.). [RICHARD, l. c.]

He has no appetite, but when he eats it tastes well.

265. Along with proper taste of food, bitterness in the throat after eating, on alternate days (like a tertian fever) (aft. 2 h.).†

After eating, bitter taste in the mouth (aft. 3, 48 h.).‡

After eating bitter eructation, and there comes into the mouth a greenish bitter mucus.

After eating and drinking repulsive bitter taste in the mouth.

Bitter in the mouth without having eaten anything.

270. Food has a salt taste.

The food tastes as if insufficiently salted.

Taste of beer flat.

Taste of unhopped beer bitter.

(Dislike to butter.)

275. Longing for acids. [*Stf.*)

Appetite for vinegar and water.

Great longing for acids and sour fruit.

Great longing for coffee.

Great appetite for milk, which she formerly loathed.

280. Qualmishness, in the forenoon about 11 a. m., and in the afternoon about 3 p.m.

Nausea. [PFANN,[5] *Samml. merkw. Falle*, Nurnb., 1750, pp. 129, 130.—*Neue Wahrn.*, l. c.]§

* See also KAISER, l. c., S. 25, "Extinct appetite."

† Comp. 1. ‡ Alternating action with 269, 270.

‡ See also KAISER, l. c., S. 28, "Nausea."—29, "Inclination to vomit."

---

1 Poisoning of several adults.

2 Effects of arsenite of potash in ague patients.

3 Not found.

4 See note to S. 118.

5 Poisoning by cobalt ("fly-powder," a mixture of metallic arsenic with arsenious acid).

Anxiety with nausea. [ALBERTI, l. c.]

Frequent nausea, and at the same time a sweetish taste in the mouth, not immediately after eating.

Nausea in œsophagus and stomach.

285. Nausea, rather in the throat; at the same time water accumulated in the mouth.

In the open air she felt sick.

Long continued nausea, like faintness; she trembled all over, at the same time she became hot all over, afterwards shivering came on (aft. some h.).

On account of nausea and sickness he must lie down in the forenoon; at the same time tearing about the ankle and on the dorsum of the foot.*

The child† vomits after eating and drinking, and then will neither eat nor drink any more, but sleeps well.

290. Waterbrash (in the afternoon about 4 p. m.).

Incomplete excitation to flow of water from fauces and mouth, what is called **waterbrash**, shortly before and after dinner, with nausea (aft. 5 d.).

Frequent empty eructation.

Constant eructations. [GORITZ, l. c.]

Frequent empty eructation (aft. ½ h.). [*Lr.*]

295. Frequent hiccup and eructation. [MORGAGNI, l. c.]

After eating frequent hiccup, each time followed by eructation (aft. 3 h.). [*Lr.*]

Frequent hiccup (aft. 3 h.). [*Lr.*]

Convulsive hiccup. [ALBERTI, l. c.]

Sickness. [MAJAULT, l. c.]

300. When sitting, nausea; much water came into the mouth, as in waterbrash; when walking in the open air the nausea went off, and there ensued a copious pappy stool (aft. 7½ h.). [*Lr.*]

Sour eructation after dinner (aft. 6 d.).

A quarter of an hour after breakfast and after dinner an aching in the stomach for three hours, with empty eructation, whereupon a relaxed condition of the body ensued, which produced nausea.

Much eructation, especially after drinking.

Flatulence rises upwards chiefly, and causes eructation.

305. Eructation after food.

Ineffectual efforts to eructate.

In the forenoon, a constant, severe, empty eructation, with confusion of the head (aft. 36 h.).

While eating, a compressive sensation in the chest.

At night on rising up, hiccup, with scraping, disgusting taste in the mouth.

310. In the hour when the fever should come on, a long-continued hiccup.

---

* That symptoms of a not very important character (comp. 302, 605, 991, 823, 861) and otherwise trivial affections induce a sudden and complete sinking of the strength is a very important and characteristic peculiarity of arsenic.

† An infant, whose mother had taken arsenic, and was thereby cured of her ailments.

Vomiting. [MAJAULT, l. c.—GRIMM, and many others.]

He vomits immediately after each meal, without nausea. [*Fr. H—n.*]

Vomiting of all food, for several weeks. [*Salzb. m. ch. Zeitung.*[1]]

Vomiting (immediately).*[FERNELIUS, *Therapeut.*, lib. vi, cap. 18, p. 451.[2]]

315. Day and night constant vomiting with horrible cries. [HEIMREICH, l. c.]

On rising up in bed immediately uncontrollable qualmishness, nausea, and frequently rapid vomiting. [*Stf.*]†

Vomiting of a thick, glassy mucus. [RICHARD, l. c.]

He vomits mucus and green bile.[3] [ALBERTI, l. c.]

During the vomiting complaints of severe (internal) heat and great thirst. [ALBERTI, l. c.]

320. Internally severe burning, thirst, and heat, with violent vomiting. [ALBERTI, l. c., iii, p. 533.]

Excessive vomiting, with the greatest effort, of drinks, yellowish-green mucus and water, with very bitter taste in the mouth, which remained long after the vomiting had ceased. [*Stf.*]

Frequent vomiting with fear of death. [ALBERTI, l. c.]

Vomiting of bloody mucus. [*Neue Wahrn.*, l. c.]‡

Vomiting of blood. [KELLNER, in *Bresl. Samml.*, 1727.[4]]

325. Passed blood upwards and downwards [GERBITZ, in *Eph. N. C.*, Dec. iii, ann. 5, 6, obs. 137.[5]]

Excessive vomiting and purging. [PREUSSIUS, l. c.]

Violent continued vomiting and diarrhœa. [MORGAGNI, l. c.]§

When the syncope goes off, diarrhœa and vomiting. [P. FORESTUS, i, xvii, obs. 13.[6]]

Spasm in the stomach ; syncope ; very violent pain in the abdomen ; diarrhœa.‖ [LOW, in *Sydenham, Opera* ii, p. 324.[7]]

330. Empty retching. [RAU, l. c.]

Pains in the stomach. [QUELMALZ, l. c.—RICHARD and several others.].

The stomach very painful. [*Neue Wahrn.*, l. c.]

* From arsenic sprinkled on an ulcer on the breast—and after six days death.

† See also *Hartl.* and *Trinks,* l. c., S. 8, "Nausea and several times violent vomiting (3rd d.)"

‡ See also KAISER, l. c., S. 30, "Nausea and violent vomiting of a brownish mass, often mixed with blood, with great straining of the body."—S. 31, "Vomiting of a thin or thick, brownish dark mass, produced by violent effort and increase of the pains in the stomach, without subsequent relief."—S. 32, "Violent vomiting of a thin, bluish, dirty yellow mass, followed by great weakness and prostration."

§ Ibid., S. 38, "The vomiting declines, whereupon a copious very watery diarrhœa ensues."

‖ From yellow arsenic.

---

1 From application of arsenic to a fungus on the head.
2 From sprinkling arsenic on a cancerous ulcer of the breast.
3 Literally, "vomiting of green matter at night, of whitish stuff next morning."
4 Poisoning of a girl of 20.
5 From orpiment.
6 From orpiment, in a woman.
7 Not found.

Stomachache causing nausea. [RICHARD, l. c.]

Præcordial ahing ; aching pain in the scrobiculus cordis. [KELLNER, l. c.—GORITZ, l. c.—BUCHHOLZ, in *Hufel. Journ.*, l. c.]

335. Pain[1] in the stomach, as if it were forcibly distended in its whole extent, and would be torn. [D. H., in *Kopp's Jahrb. d. Staatsarzn.*, ii, p. 182.]

He felt as if the heart were pressed down. [*Stf.*]

Sensation of pressing weight in the stomach, without thirst and without fever. [MORGAGNI, l. c.]

Great oppression of the stomach as if it were troubled with flatulence, that seems, indeed, to be relieved by vomiting and diarrhœa, but afterwards becomes all the worse. [MORGAGNI, l. c., § 3.]

A very violent cardialgia with thirst. [BUCHHOLZ, in the last l. c.]

340. Burning pain in the stomach. [EBERS, l. c. Octob., 5, 8.]*

Incessant burning and great oppression in the stomach and chest. BORGES,[2] in *Kopp's Jahrb.*, l. c., p. 222.]

Aching and burning pain in the scrobiculus cordis. [GORITZ, l. c.]

Pressive pain like a weight and burning in the stomach. [MORGAGNI, l. c., § 6.]

Burning in the stomach like fire. [RICHARD, l. c.]

345. Burning in the scrobiculus cordis. [BUCHHOLZ, in the last l c.]

Eroding, gnawing pain in the stomach. [RICHARD, l. c.]

Uncommon pains in the region of the scrobiculus cordis. [J. PH. WOLFF, *Act. N. C.*, v, obs. 29.[3]]

The region under the ribs (hypochondria) and the stomach are tense and distended before the bowels are moved. [RICHARD, l. c.]†

Complaints and lamentations about indescribable[4] anxiety in the region of the scrobiculus cordis, without distension or pain in the stomach. [MORGAGNI, l. c.]

350. Great anxiety in the region of the scrobiculus cordis. [MORGAGNI, l. c.—BERNARD VERZASCH, *Obs. Med.*, obs. 66[5]—JACOBI, l. c.]

After a meal an aching at the mouth of the stomach and in the œsophagus, as if the food was retained up above ; then empty eructation.

When speaking an aching in the anterior wall of the stomach (aft. ¼ h.).

A hard pressure above the scrobiculus cordis (immediately).‡

* See also KAISER, l. c., S. 39, "Burning feeling in the scrobiculus cordis."

† Ibid., S. 40, "Inconsiderable distension in the gastric region," ahd S. 41, "The stomach begins to rise, and is warmer than the rest of the body."

‡ Ibid., S. 37, "Hot feeling, pain and pressure in the scrobiculus cordis," and S. 38, "Hot aching sensation in the præcordia."

1 "Severe pain," the author says.

2 Poisoning of an adult.

3 Poisoning of two women. "Pains" should be "anxietas."

4 In the original, "inexplicabilis."

5 Not accessible.

Her heart feels pressed down.

355. In the evening, when sitting, drawing pain from the scrobiculus cordis around beneath the left ribs, as if something was forcibly torn away there.

Dull tearing transversely across the gastric region, when walking, in the afternoon.

Cutting pain in the stomach. [THILENIUS, l. c.]

Spasmodic pain in the stomach, two hours after midnight.*

When he eats anything it presses in and about the stomach, so that he cannot bear it ; the pressure occurs always some time after, not immediately upon eating.

360. Gnawing† and pecking (fine and sharp throbbing) pain in the scrobiculus cordis, with tense feeling.

Anxiety in the scrobiculus cordis, which rises up, all night.

Burning pain round about the scrobiculus cordis.

In the evening she disliked eating, she was so full ; she had pain in the stomach when she ate.

Fulness in the epigastrium, with pinching in the abdomen.

365. Pressing ache in the liver, when walking in the open air.

Before eating nausea, and after eating or drinking distension of the abdomen, also aching and cutting.

After a meal weight in the stomach, as from a stone. [*Hbg.*]

The abdominal pain is fixed in the left side of the abdomen.

After a meal great distension of the abdomen, without pain ; he must lean his back on something in order to relieve himself.

370. After eating yawning and exhaustion, which compelled him to lie down and sleep.

He cannot keep himself warm enough, he has always an internal chilliness in the epigastric region, although that part feels warm to the touch.‡

A rumbling in the abdomen as from much flatulence, but without pain (aft. 1 h.).

Drawing pain in the umbilical region (aft. 2 h.),

Frequently a spasmodic jerk, making him start, from the scrobiculus cordis into the rectum.

375. Every morning flatulent distension ; the flatus is discharged only after some hours (aft. 14 d.).

Discharge of much flatus, preceded by loud rumbling in the abdomen (aft. 9 h.). [*Lr.*]

Discharge of putrid smelling flatus (aft. 11 h.). [*Lr.*]

In the evening, after lying down, like spasms and pinching in the abdomen, with an outburst of perspiration, followed by discharge of flatus, and then quite thin stool.§

* See also KAISER, l. c., S. 34, "Disagreeable sensation in the stomach, which soon afterwards changes into an aching, tearing, also spasmodic pain, and continues ;" further, S. 35, "Periodical spasmodic pains in the stomach and bowels ;" finally, S.36, "Violent, tearing, boring pain, and spasm in the stomach and the rest of the bowels."

† Comp. 995. ‡ Comp. 525.

§ Many arsenic symptoms occur only in the evening, and after lying down to sleep, some a couple of hours after midnight, many in the morning after rising, not a few after dinner.

In the evening, after lying down in bed, and in the morning after rising, violent colic, squeezing cutting pains in the bowels, which sometimes, also, shoot through the inguinal ring (as if they would force out a hernia) as far as the spermatic cord and perinæum ; when this colic ceases there occurs a loud rumbling and grumbling in the abdomen.

380. Tearing stitches in the left side under the short ribs, in the evening soon after lying down (aft. 3 h.).

Hypogastric pains, heat of face

Cutting pain in the side of the abdomen, under the last ribs, *per se*, but most severe when touched.

Only every morning, pinching increasing to cutting colic, deep in the hypogastrium, before and during diarrhœic stools, which pains do not cease after each stool, although they do not excite the stool.

In the morning, first great rattling in the abdomen, then a cutting twisting together of the bowels, then thrice diarrhœa.

385. Uneasiness in the abdomen, but only when at rest.

Weakness of the abdominal muscles.

On stooping, shooting dislocation pain in the right iliac and inguinal regions.

Burning pain in the abdomen, at noon and in the afternoon, going off after stool.

Violent pain in the right epigastrium. [MORGAGNI, l. c.]

390. Pain in the right epigastrium and neighbouring lumbar region, whence it spreads sometimes through the hypogastrium, at other times into the right side of the scrotum and into the flank, like renal colic (at the same time, however, the urine appears healthy). [MORGAGNI, l. c.]

Jaundice. [MAJAULT, l. c.]

Cholera.[1] [WOLFF, l. c.]

Anxiety and complaints about pain, as if the upper part of the trunk were quite cut away from the abdomen. [ALBERTI, *Jurispr. Med.* t. iv, p. 259.]

Horrible pains in the stomach and abdomen. [WOLFF, l. c.—MAJAULT, l. c.]

395. Cutting (lancinantes[2]) and gnawing pains in the stomach and bowels. [QUELMALZ, l. c.]

Swollen[3] abdomen. [GUILBERT, l. c.]

Enormously swollen abdomen. [*Eph. Nat. Cur.*, l. c.]

Distension and pains of the abdomen. [MULLER, l. c.]

Very disagreeable sensation in the whole abdomen. [MORGAGNI, l. c.]

400. Violent pains in the abdomen, with such great anxiety that he can nowhere get ease, he rolled about on the ground and gave up all hope of life. [PYL, *Samml.*, viii, pp. 98, 105, 108.]

After eating, great distension of the abdomen, without pain ; he must lean with his back supported, in order to get relief. [*Myr.*]

---

1 That is, constant vomiting and diarrhoea, with sharp nose, cold limbs, cramps and death.

2 In *Chr. Kr.*, "reissende." *i. e.* tearing.

3 "And painful," the author says.

Along with anxiety in the abdomen, fever and thirst. [MORGAGNI, l. c.]

The most violent pains in the abdomen. [DAN. CRUGER, *Misc. Nat. Cur.*, Dec. ii, ann. 4.[1]]

Twisting colic.* [RICHARD, l. c.]

405. In the right side of the abdomen, a digging aching. [*Hbg.*]

Tearing in the abdomen. [PFANN, l. c.—ALBERTI, l. c.]

Tearing and cutting in the abdomen, with icy coldness of feet and hands, and cold sweat on the face. [ALBERTI, l. c.]

Cutting pain in the abdomen. [BUCHHOLZ l. c.—KELLNER, l. c.]

In the abdomen burning, shooting, and cutting. [BUCHHOLZ, *Beitrage*, l. c.]

410. Burning in the abdomen with heat and thirst. [ALBERTI, l. c.]

Burning in the flank. [*Hbg.*]

Colics recurring from time to time. [MAJAULT, l. c.]

Rumbling in the abdomen in the morning on awaking.

Noises in the abdomen. [THILENIUS, l. c.]

Here and there wandering pains in the abdomen, yellow diarrhœa and tenesmus, with burning pains in the anus and thirst. [MORGAGNI, l. c.

415. After the stool the colic is allayed. [RICHARD, l. c.]

After the palpitation of the heart, a rattling in the abdomen, and a pinching and twisting together of the bowels, before and during the fluid motions. [*Myr.*]

Dysenteric colic[2] in the umbilical region. [GRIMM, l. c.]

Constipation of the bowels.[3] [GORITZ, l. c.—RAU, l. c.] †

He has ineffectual urging to stool.

420. Burning in the anus, for an hour, which was allayed after the evacuation of a hard, knotty stool.

Burning and pains in the rectum and anus, with constant pressing; a kind of tenesmus, as in dysentery.

After the stool there was great weakness and burning in the rectum, with trembling in all the limbs.

After the stool, palpitation of the heart and trembling weakness; he must lie down.

Spasmodic urging and pressing out at his rectum, with great pains (aft. 72 h.).

425. The fæces pass away from him unnoticed, as though they were flatus.

The fæces passed are enveloped in watery blood.

Dysentery. [CRUGER, l. c.]

Almost every moment a bloody discharge by stool, with vomiting and horrible pains in the abdomen. [GRIMM, l. c.]

*See also KAISER, l. c., S. 43, "Twisting and curling up in bed."

† Comp. *Hartl.* and *Trinks*, *Arznei M. L.*, l. c., S. 9, "Pains in the abdomen, with constipation (TREVOSSO, *The New Lond. Med. Journ.*, vol. ii, 1793) (from the vapour of wax lights rendered poisonous by arsenic)."

1 Poisoning of an adult.

2 Literally, "tormina."

3 In RAU's case, for four days.

Before the diarrhœa he has a feeling as if he would burst. [ALBERTI, l. c.]

430. Diarrhœa, alternating with constipation ; there often passed a little yellow fluid, then urging came on as if more would come, with acute pains in the abdomen about the navel. [*Stf.*]

Evacuation of fæces, sometimes more, sometimes less pappy (aft. 6, 13 h.). [*Lr.*]

Diarrhœa. [MAJAULT, l. c.—KELLNER, l. c.]*

Stools pass without his knowledge. [CHR. G. BUTTNER, *Unterricht uber die Todtlichkeit der Wunden*, p. 197.[1]]

Mucous and green evacuations by stool. [THILENIUS, l. c.]

435. Frequent discharge of a viscid bilious matter by stool, for two days. [PFANN, l. c.]

After much uneasiness and colic, discharge of a black fluid by stool, burning like fire in the anus. [RICHARD, l. c.]

Black, acrid, putrid fæcal evacuations. [BAYLIES, l. c.]

Discharge by stool of a round lump, which appeared to consist of undigested fat mixed with fibrous parts (aft. 8 d.). [MORGAGNI, l. c.]

Diarrhœa, with violent burning in the anus. [THILENIUS, l. c.]

440. (Thin mucous evacuations, as if chopped up.)

Along with urging to stool, evacuation of masses of mucus, with cutting pains in the anus, as from blind piles.

After colic small evacuations with tenesmus, at first of dark green fæces, then of dark green mucus.

Constipation.

(Rumbling in the abdomen without stool.)

445. (Itching in the anus.)

Itching, scraping, or sore pain in the anus.

The anus is painful when touched, as if sore.

At the anus, hæmorrhoids with shooting pains, when sitting and walking, not connected with the stool.

Hæmorrhoidal lumps at the anus, which, especially at night, burn† like fire, and permit no sleep, but by day the pain becomes worse, and changes into violent stitches ; worse when walking than when sitting or lying.

450. Blind hæmorrhoids with pains like slow pricks with a hot needle.

During the stool painful contraction just above the anus towards the sacrum.

Burning in the anus. [MORGAGNI, l. c.]

Tenesmus with burning. [MORGAGNI, l. c.]

Eroding itching on the perinæum, compelling him to scratch (aft. ½ h.). [*Lr.*]

455. Itching on the perinæum, especially when walking, that compels him to scratch (aft.5½ h.). [*Lr.*]

* Comp. KAISER, l. c., S. 45, "Great evacuations by stool,"—S. 46, "Diarrhœa that often becomes very severe,"—S. 47, "Involuntary discharge of fæces and urine."

† Burning is a main symptom of arsenic. Comp. 163, 362, 450, 471, 769, 777, 793, 794, 816, 819, 814, 789, 790.

1 Poisonings. This S. not found.

Painful swelling of the hæmorrhoidal veins with tenesmus. [MORGAGNI, l. c., § 8.]

Retention of stool and urine in spite of all internal feeling of wanting to pass them. [ALBERTI, *Jurisprud. med.*, tom. iv, p. 260.]

Burning in passing urine. [*Neue Wahrn.*—MORGAGNI, l. c., § 6.]

Bloody urine. [O. TACHENIUS, *Hipp. Chym.*, c. 24, p. 149.[1]]

460. Suppression of urine. [*N. Wahrn.*, l. c.—GUILBERT., l. c.]

Diminished flow of urine.[2] [TH. FOWLER, l. c.]

Increased flow of urine.[3] [TH. FOWLER, l. c.]

Frequent urging to urinate, with copious flow of urine (aft. 2, 3, 4, 5½, 16, 17 h.). [*Lr.*]

After urinating great feeling of weakness in the epigastrium, so that she trembled.

465. On passing urine contractive pains in the left iliac region.

Involuntary micturition; she could not get to the utensil; the urine ran away from her, and yet there was but little of it.

He must rise at night three or four times to pass urine, and each time he passes a great deal, for several successive days.

Burning in the bladder, and urging to urinate every minute.

In the morning burning in the anterior part of the urethra at the commencement of urination (aft. 24 h.).

470. Retention of the urine as from paralysis of the bladder.

But little water passes, and it burns during the flow.

(Urine almost colourless.)

Very turbid urine (aft. 5 d.)

(In the urethra smarting pain.)

Deep in the urethra frequent pain, like tearings (in the afternoon).

475. Single, severe, slow stitches on both sides of the pudendum in the flanks (aft. 3 h.).

(In the inguinal swelling) a burning and digging; even a slight touch (with the bed-clothes, for example) excites the pain.

(Itching of the pudendum.)

Severe itching on the glans penis without erection of the penis.

Nocturnal emission of semen with voluptuous dreams. [*Lr.*]

480. Nocturnal emission of semen without voluptuous dreams, followed by long continued erection of the penis (aft. 20 h.). [*Lr.*]

Erection of the penis in the morning without pollution. [*Lr.*]

The glans penis is bluish-red, swollen, and cracked with rhagades [PFANN, l. c.]

On the penis, near the scrotum, eroding itching compelling scratching (aft. 5¼ h.). [*Lr.*]

Inflammatory swelling of the genital organs, going the length of mortification, with horrible pains. [J. H. DEGNER, *Act. Nat. Cur.*, vi.[4]]

485. Extremely painful swelling of the genitals. [*Neue Wahrn.*, l. c.]

Sudden occurrence of mortification in the male genitals. [G. E. STAHL, *Opusc. Chym. Phys. Med.* p. 454.[5]]

1 From inhaling sublimed arsenic. 2 Sometimes. 3 Often.

4 Effects of applying a solution of arsenic for itch, in two men.

5 Poisoning of two adults. "Mortification" is "sphacelatio."

Swelling of the testicles.[1]* [ALBERTI, *Jurispr. Med.*, tom. i, p. 167.]

Lasciviousness in a woman; she desires coitus twice a day, and when it is not accorded a discharge takes place of itself.

Shooting pain in the hypogastrium down into the vagina.

490. Leucorrhœa, of a yellowish and thick character, about a cupful. in the twenty-four hours, with smarting erosion where it runs, the parts on both sides of the vulva become excoriated by it, for ten days

When standing the leucorrhœa drops away during a discharge of flatus (aft. 24 h.)

Menses too soon.

Excitation of too profuse menstrual flux.

During the menses sharp shooting in the rectum into the anus and vulva.

495. After the cessation of the menses bloody mucus passes.

During the menses pinching, shooting, cutting from the scrobiculus cordis to the hypogastrium, also in the back and sides of the abdomen; she must bend herself together, standing and cowering down, on account of pain, with loud groaning, complaints, and weeping and with loud eructation.

* * *

A profuse bleeding of the nose after severe vomiting. [HEIMREICH, *Arsen. als. Fiebermittel.*]

(During vexation) profuse flow of blood from the nose (aft. 3 d.).

Dryness of the nasal cavity.

500. Severe continued sneezing.

Frequent sneezing without coryza (aft. 3, 6 d.). [*Lr.*]

Frequent sneezing with fluent coryza (aft. 11 h.). [*Lr.*]

Discharge of acrid fluid from the nose. [MYRRHEN, l. c.]

Stopped-up coryza combined with fluent coryza.

505. Every morning on waking sneezing and coryza, which each time goes off quickly.

Watery mucus flows from the nose, smarting and burning at the nostrils, as if they became sore from it.

Severe fluent coryza.

Excessive† coryza with hoarseness and sleeplessness.

In the morning his throat is rough and hoarse (aft. 24 h.).

510. Dryness of the larynx.

Rough speech and hoarseness.

* From the internal use of arsenic.

† There is scarcely any heroic remedy, which is not sometimes capable of producing this kind of crisis (a violent coryza, and, at other times, vomiting, diarrhœa, perspiration, salivation, diuresis, &c.) in healthy persons or in cases of disease in which it is improperly given, where nature endeavours to remove and, as it were, to eject what is prejudicial to the life of the body; and thus suddenly destroys a large, often the largest, portion of the remaining medicinal power of the remedy. But yet these corporeal actions which destroy the other medicinal disease are, at the same time characteristic medicinal symptoms, and the coryza of arsenic remains very different in many essential and, as yet, not sufficiently accurately observed circumstances from that produced by the magnet, belladonna, nux vomica, mezereum, &c.

1 For "testicles," read "scrotum."

Palpitation of the heart. [MAJAULT, l. c.]

At night, about 3 a.m., an irregular but so violent palpitation, that he thinks he hears it, combined with anxiety. [*Myr*]

Excessive, very troublesome palpitation of the heart. [*Stf.*]

515. When he lies on his back, the heart beats much quicker and stronger. [*Stf.*]

In the scrobiculus cordis, anxiety. [*Hbg.*]

Very viscid mucus in the chest, that can with difficulty be coughed up. (aft. 48 h.).

Streaks of blood in the mucus expectorated.

He hawks up mucus with blood streaks ; then follows nausea.

520. Sensation of rawness and soreness in the chest.

Pains in the chest. [PEARSON, l. c.]

Much pain in the chest. [*N. Wahrnehm.*, l. c.]

Internal pain in the upper part of the chest (aft. 5 h.).

Shooting tearing pain in the uppermost right rib.

(Formication in the left side of the chest).[1]

525. Towards evening, a chilliness internally in the chest, also after supper.†

Tensive pain in the chest, especially when sitting.‡

Stitches superiorly in the right side of the chest, especially felt when drawing the breath, like pressure, that ends in a stitch (aft. 1½ h.).

Violent shooting on the left side of the chest only during expiration, which is thereby rendered difficult (aft. 7½ h.). [*Lr.*]

Aching on the chest. [BUCHHOLZ, *Beitrage*, l. c.]

530. Burning in the chest. [STORCK, l. c.]

Burning in the right side of the chest extending to the flank, where it ached. [*Hbg.*]

After a meal, a sweet taste of blood, with a scraping shooting pain in the throat, as if he had swallowed a fish-bone, for a quarter of an hour, followed by short cough with hæmoptysis, at first like coagulated blood ; after the spitting of blood nausea, and after two hours anxiety. [*Myr.*]

Great heat in the chest to below the diaphragm. [*Hbg.*]

A long-continued burning in the region of the sternum. [STORCK, l. c.]

535. Violent morning cough.

Constant tickling in the whole wind-pipe, which excites him to cough, also independent of breathing.

In the morning, after the (accustomed) tea-drinking, a short cough.

Dry violent cough (aft. 2 h.).

When he drinks without thirst, it causes coughing.

540. **Cough especially after drinking.**

At night, when the cough comes on, he must sit up.

* See also KAISER, l. c., S. 50, "The heart's beat generally excited."

† Comp. 371. ‡ Comp. note to 677.

1 A mis-reckoning here.

In the evening, immediately after lying down, cough; she must sit up, thereafter a contractive pain in the scrobiculus cordis and gastric region, keeping up the cough, which exhausted her.

In the evening, in bed, a cough lasting some minutes, with nausea and having to vomit.

Cough immediately after lying down.

545. Cough woke him up at night; severe bursts of it, so that he felt like to choke, and his throat swelled.

Deep, dry, short, incessant cough after midnight.

(The chest feels like to burst from the cough.)

On walking in the open air she feels such a smothering sensation that she must cough.

Hard cough, difficult to loosen, which causes sore pain in the chest.

550. Cough when she comes into the cold open air.

Dry cough during bodily exertion.*

Twitching in the hip followed by dry cough, which seems to be excited by the former.

During the cough heat in the head.

With violent cough much water flows from the mouth, like water-brash.

555. During the cough bruised pain in the abdomen, as if crushed (aft. 2 h.).

During the cough shooting in the scrobiculus cordis.

When hawking, drawing shooting pain under the left short ribs up into the chest.

During the cough shooting, first in the side of the chest, then (two days afterwards) in the side of the abdomen.

During the cough shooting pain in the sternum upwards.

560. When drawing a deep breath stitches in the left side of the chest, which compel him to cough.

When stooping dull stitches in the chest.

Shooting in the side under the short ribs, he dare not lie on that side.†

By coughing increased stitches under the ribs and increased headache as from heat in it.

A constrictive sensation up in the wind-pipe (in the region of the pit of the throat), as from sulphur vapour, which excites cough.

565. In the evening, after getting into bed as gently as possible and lying down very carefully, his breath goes immediately, and such fine whistling in the (constricted) wind-pipe as if a fine harp-string sounded.

Excitation to short cough in the wind-pipe, without expectoration (aft. 3½ h.). [*Lr.*]

Dry tussiculation. [Storck, l. c.]

Dry fatiguing cough. [Storck, l. c.]

In the evening tightness of the chest and dry cough.

570. Great tightness of chest.[1] [Pyl, *Samml.*, viii, p. 98, &c.]

* Which often makes him very quickly breathless.

† Comp. 621.

1 For a long time.

Constrictive sensation in the chest. [PREUSSIUS, l. c.*]
Painful respiration. [*N. Wahrnehm.*, l. c.]
Oppression of the chest.[1] [RAU, l. c.]
Oppression of the chest, difficult breathing. [THILENIUS, l. c.]
575. Difficult respiration. [TACHENIUS, l. c.]
Anxious groaning respiration.[2] [GUILBERT, l. c.]

Piteous lamentation, that an intolerable anxiety and a very oppressive sensation in the abdomen hinders respiration. [MORGAGNI, l. c.] †

Frequently recurring tightness of chest. [MORGAGNI, l. c., S. 6.]

Tightness of chest for an hour, which threatens suffocation. [GREISELIUS, l. c.] ‡

580. Long-continued tightness of chest. [TIMAEUS A GULDENKLEE, *Opp.*, Lips., 1715, p. 280.[3]]

He feels like to suffocate ; sticks his tongue out. [WEDEL, l. c.]

Choking rheum.[4] [*Misc. Nat. Cur.*, Dec. iii, ann. 9, 10, p. 390.]

On moving (walking) sudden tightness of chest and want of breath, weakness, and excessive prostration.[5]‖ [MAJAULT, l. c.]

Nocturnal sudden catarrh, threatening suffocation.[4]¶ [MYRRHEN, l. c.]

585. First oppression of the chest, then pain in the chest with short cough and salt expectoration.[6] [EBERS, l. c., Oct., pp. 8 and 11.]

Great anxiety, as if all would be constricted, with anxiety in the scrobiculus cordis.

During the abdominal pains, difficult breathing, as if the chest were compressed.

Frequent short, difficult respiration, and dry short cough, with ulcerative sore pain in the scrobiculus cordis up to the middle of the chest.

Frequent oppressive, anxious, short breathing in the chest, in all positions.

590. Oppression during the cough and on walking quickly, or on going upstairs.

* See also *Hartl.* and *Trinks*, *A. M. L.*, l. c., S. 11, "The chest contracted, so that he could hardly speak a word and almost fainted (3rd d.)", and S. 12, "Constant tussiculation and contraction in the chest (3rd d.)."

† See also KAISER, l. c., S. 49, "The breathing oppressed, the anxiety increases."

‡ See also *Hartl.* and *Trinks*, l. c., S. 10, "Short breath."

§ From arsenical vapour, during the preparation of arsenicum fixum.

‖ As the symptoms mentioned are not observed in the mass from any other known medicine, it is evident how arsenic is homœopathic to inflammation of the chest, and that it can and does cure it specifically.

¶ I cured myself rapidly with arsenic of a similar suffocative catarrh that always came on more severely every evening after lying down, which brought me near to death ; the dose I used was of a minuteness that passes all belief. The other symptoms of my malady were certainly also met with among the symptoms of arsenic.

1 In the original "anxietates pectoris."

2 Literally "breathing difficult, and often interrupted by sighs."

3 From the vapour.

4 These two symptoms describe the same attack of suffocative bronchitis, brought on by drawing a solution of arsenic into the nostrils for coryza, and ending in convulsions and death.

5 The original is simply "much lassitude and oppression of breathing in walking."

6 See note to S. 118.

In the evening, great anxiety and restlessness, and the chest as if contracted.

Dyspnœa for eight days, oppression in the region of the sternum, on breathing deeply.

Always immediately after coughing the breath is so short, as if his whole chest was contracted.

Frequent, quite short, dry cough, excited by a suffocative sensation in the larynx, such as is apt to occur from sulphur fumes.

595. Pain under the scrobiculus cordis, which takes away the breath.

When he gets vexed he has tightness of chest.

When he has fatigued himself he gets a tightness of the chest, such as is apt to arise from anxiety.

Eruption of yellow spots on the chest. [WEDEL, l. c.]

Distortion of the cervical muscles.[1] [MULLER, l. c.]

600. Tensive stiffness of the neck. [*Bhr.*]

(At night and in the morning) stiffness in the nape, as if bruised or strained, and a similar pain above the hips (aft. 12 h.).

External swelling of the neck without pain. [*Stf.*]

On stooping low the artery of the left side of the neck swells out to an extraordinary degree. [*Bhr.*]

All round the neck, on the shoulders and in the sides, a kind of colourless smarting eruption. [*Fr. H—n.*]

605. Drawing pain between the scapulæ, which comples him to lie down (aft. 5 h.)*

Drawing from the sacrum up into the shoulders, and at the same time stitches in the sides, during which flatulence moves about in the abdomen, which, not being able to be discharged, presses upwards, as it were, then eructation ensues, and he gets relief.

(Stiffness in the spine, from the coccyx upward.)

The sacrum is painfully stiff all day.

Want of strength in the small of the back.

610. Drawing pain in the back (in the forenoon) (aft. 6 d.).

Drawing up and down in the back.

Along with pain in the back restlessness and attacks of anxietas. BUTTNER, l. c.]

Only when lying on the right side strong clucking movements in the muscles of the left side of the back. (aft. $3\frac{3}{4}$ h.). [*Lr.*]

Bruised pain in the back and over the scapulæ as if beaten (aft. 4 d.)

615. In the sacrum pain as if bruised (aft. 4 h.).

In the loins (renal region) stitches when breathing and sneezing.

Excoriation beneath the arms in the axillæ. [KLINGE, in *Huf. Journ. d. p. A.*, vi, p. 904.[2]]

Tearing shooting pain in the right armpit.

A painful lump on the arm. [*Neue Wahrn.*, l. c.]

620. At night, in bed. **tearing** in the elbow and wrist-joint (aft. 4 h.).

* See note to 288.

1 Not found.

2 Observation on miners in arsenic.

At night pain in the arm of the **side lain on**.*

(When he lies on the right side the right arm goes to sleep.)

Eroding itching on the left forearm near the wrist-joint, inciting to scratch (aft. $1\frac{1}{2}$ h.). [*Lr.*]

Great formication in the hands at night.

625. Painful swelling of the hands. [*N. Wahrn.*, l. c.]

Stiffness and insensibility of the hands.[1] [PYL, *Samml.*, viii, p. 98, &c.]

Fine tickling in the left palm, causing him to rub it (aft. 7 h.). [*Lr.*]

Cold hands. [*Stf.*]

Small lumps on the hands. [*N. Wahrn.*, l. c.]

630. Always towards evening in both wrists a drawing pain.

Tickling itching on the inside of the right middle finger, compelling him to scratch (aft. 5 h.). [*Lr.*]

Tearing shooting pain in the bones of the hand and of the little finger (aft. 2 h.).

Drawing pain in the middle fingers.

✓ Drawing **tearing** in the fourth and fifth metacarpal bones, in the morning.

635. Drawing and twitching (tearing) from the finger-tips up to the shoulder.

Cramp in the fingers of the right hand when he stretches them straight out.

Painful cramp in the proximal joints of the fingers of both hands.

From morning till noon a painful spasm in the finger-tips, calf, and toes (aft. 5 d.)

Inflexibility of the fingers, as if they were stiff.

640. Finger-joints painful when moved.

Discoloured nails. [BAYLIES, l. c.]

Paralysis of the lower limbs.[2] [EBERS, l. c., Octob., p. 18.]

Gout in the hip (sciatica).† [BORELLUS, *Hist. et Observ.* cent. iii, obs. 36.]‡

Excoriation betwixt the thighs, with itching. [KLINGE, l. c.]

645. **Eroding itching on the right thigh, near the groin, causing him to scratch** (aft. $4\frac{1}{2}$ h.). [*Lr.*]

Eroding itching on both thighs, causing scratching, in the evening on undressing (aft. 13 h.). [*Lr.*]

Convulsions of the knees and thighs.§ [ALBERTI, l. c., tom. i.]

Spasm (cramp) in the lower extremities (thighs). [PYL, *Samml.* i, p. 245.]

Pain and shooting in the knees (aft. 2 h.). [RICHARD, l. c.]

650. Paralysis in both knees. [J. B. MONTANUS, in *Schenck*, lib. 7, obs. 209.[3]]

* Comp. 562.

† Worn as an amulet in the pocket. [The original is simply "sciatica."]

‡ See also *Hartl.* and *Trinks*, l. c., S. 13, "In the morning after a rather sleepless night, violent, drawing tearing pain in the hips and left foot (3rd d.)."

§ Shortly before death.

1 Lasting for a long time. 2 Not found. 3 Poisoning of a woman.

In the hough tension, as if tendons were too short, when sitting and standing, but not when walking.

Paralysis of the legs, so that he can hardly walk. [PET. FORESTUS, lib. 18. Schol. ad. obs. 28.]

Emaciated legs. [MAJAULT, l. c.]

Tearing pains in the bones. [*Bhr.*]

655. Cramp in the calf when walking, and in the hand on moving it (aft. 2 h.).

Tearing pain in the right calf (when sitting) (aft. 11 h). *Lr.*]

In the ankle and knee-joints tearing, only when moving.

A weakness in the knees, so that he can only sit down with difficulty.

At night profuse sweat on the lower extremities, especially the knees.

660. In the left knee dislocated and bruised pain, especially on rising up from sitting.

(In the right knee great want of firmness, it bends under him.).

Drawing tearing in the right hough down to the heel, as from a sprain.

Drawing tearing in the anterior side of the thigh down to the knee and ankle-joint when walking.

Sharp drawing in the tibia.

665. In the tibia single, violent tearings making him cry out.

A boring pain in the right tibia.

Tearing shooting internally, at the lower part of the leg, on a small spot.

Under the knees sensation as if the legs were tightly bound there.

Formication in the lower extremities, as if they were asleep.

670. In the morning spasmodic pain in the foot, which changes into a vibration and tingling in it. (aft. 96 h.).

Tearing in the lower extremities from above downwards to the lower part; he could not tread, sit, or lie, either in bed or on a bench; day and night he must either keep the foot swinging to and fro or limp about with it, and he could not rest upon it; worst at night.*

A **tearing shooting**, as if in the periosteum, down the thigh and leg as far as the tip of the big toe. (aft. 24 h.).

At night he often cannot lie, must lay the feet first in one place then in another, or must walk about to get relief.

Drawing in the foot; he cannot keep it still; at the same time he can walk gently with care, but not quickly.

675. In the afternoon, when sitting, a twitching in the feet.

On making a false step with the affected foot there occurs a jerk in it that gives a shock to the whole limb.

On the side of the knee a point that pains as if bruised, only when touched, as if the flesh was loose there, only when seated, not when walking.†

* From fever-drops, which in Saxony the wandering pedlars lately used to sell to the country people in small four-sided bottles, and which I found to contain a very strong solution of arsenic.

† The alternating action of arsenic, in which symptoms are produced or renewed

(When the feet hang down perpendicularly when sitting they have drawing pains.).

Heaviness, fatigue, and drawing pain in the legs with knuckling (unsteadiness and weakness) of the knees, especially in the morning.

680. Weariness in the lower extremities.*

Morning sweat on the legs (the first night).

Feet so heavy, he can hardly lift them.

Continual cold feet when he sits still ; he can scarcely warm them in bed.

In the calves an aching pain.

685. The calf became hard and pressed flat with intolerable pain almost like cramp pain (but much worse), making her scream for an hour and a half ; the whole limb was stiff, she could not move it at all, and quite cold and insensible ; there remained tension in the calf and a kind of paralysis in the thigh (aft. 50 h.).

Feet swollen, the swelling extending up over the calves ; previously tearing in the calf, which was removed by applying warm cloths† (aft. 3 d.).

The ankles swell without being red, and have tearing pains, which are relieved by external warmth.

Shining hot swelling of the feet (dorsum and soles), to above the ankles, with round, red spots, which cause a burning pain (aft. 3 d.).

The swelling of the feet itches.

690. On treading, on the top of the instep, in the ankle, pain as if ricked or sprained (aft. 72 h.).

Shooting and tearing in both the ankle-joints ; when treading and walking stitches in them, as if the feet were sprained, so that she is like to fall ; the ankles are painful when touched. (aft. 12 h.).‡

A tearing, drawing, and twitching, from the ankles up to the knees.

Tearing in the ankles.

Coldness of the knees and feet, with cold sweat on them ; they cannot be warmed.

695. (Cold sensation in the soles of the feet.)

Tearing in the heels. [*Bhr.*]

Tearing in the lower extremities. [Pyl, l. c.]

Violent pains in the legs, especially in the joints. [Majault, l. c.]

When she does not set down her foot straight, or when she makes a false step, she has a pain in it as if dislocated. [*Bhr.*]

700. The pains in the foot are aggravated by movement. [*Bhr.*]

by movement, is much rarer than that in which the symptoms are produced or increased when at rest, when (lying and) sitting, or are diminished by standing or moving ; the latter alternating action is therefore much more important for homœopathic curative action by arsenic. Comp. 526, 671, 674, 675, 707, 776, 777, 779, 780, 821.

* See also *Hartl.* and *Trinks*, l. c., S. 21, "Great weariness (aft. 1 h)."—S. 22, "On going upstairs a sensation as if the legs would break down under him (7th d.).

† Comp. note to 203.

‡ See also *Hartl.* and *Trinks*, l. c., S. 18, "The ankles are painful to the touch."

After vomiting, paralysis of the feet. [CARDANUS, *De Venen.* i, iii, 1563.[1]]

Coldness of the feet with contracted pulse. [MORGAGNI, l. c., § 8.]

Swelling, stiffness, insensibility and numbness of the feet; occasionally they were full of great pains. [PYL, *Samml.*, viii, p. 97, &c.]*

On awaking the heels are painful, as if she had lain on something hard.

705. Under the left heel, on treading, single stitches up to the back of the thigh.

Several stitches in the sole (aft. ½ h.).

When lying† he has nausea and tearing about the ankles and dorsum of the feet.

(In the evening, in bed, the toes are drawn backwards, and some muscular fibres in the calves and thigh are contracted with a spasmodic pain for three hours, whereupon he became very exhausted.)

Cramp in the calves and fingers frequently, especially in bed at night.

710. The whole of the left side of the body affected with a numb pain. [*Bhr.*]

The right foot has numb pains; when seated she can only lift it with the help of the hands. [*Bhr.*]

Tickling running itching on the right big toe, something like the healing of a wound, compelling him to rub (aft. 1½ h.). [*Lr.*]

Swelling of the whole of the right side to the hips and left thigh. [THILENIUS, l. c.]

General anasarca.[2] [EBERS, l. c.]

715. Complete anasarca[3] (aft. 4 d.). [EBERS, l. c., p. 56]

Swelling of the face and feet, dry mouth and lips, distended abdomen, diarrhœa, colic, vomiting.[4] [EBERS, l. c., Sept., p. 28.]

Great swelling of the face and the rest of the body. [FERNELIUS, l. c.]

Swelling of the feet. [JACOBI, l. c.]

Swelling on various parts of the body, of an elastic kind. [TH. FOWLER, l. c.]

720. Pains in the feet. [TIM. A GULDENKLEE, *Opp.*, p. 280.]

Violent pains in the soles, which sometimes bring on convulsions. [PFANN, l. c.]

Convulsive attack: at first she struck outwards with her arms, then she lost all consciousness, lay like a dead person, pale but warm,

* See also *Hartl.* and *Trinks*, l. c, SS. 14—17, "Intolerable pains in the lower extremities, with swelling of one of them (aft. 8 weeks)."—"First on the right, then on the left foot a hard, reddish-blue, greenish-yellow, and very painful swelling (aft. 28 d.)."—"Great pains, tearing and stiffness in the limbs, as if he could not move them (14th d.)."—"Stiffness of the limbs, especially of the knees and feet, alternating with tearing pains (28th d)."

1 General statement from authors.
2 See note to S. 118.
3 From suppression of ague by arsenic.
4 As S. 714.

turned the thumbs in, twisted the hands, which were shut, drew the arms slowly up and pushed them slowly down ; after ten minutes she drew the mouth hither and thither, as if she waggled her jaw ; at the same time no respiration could be detected ; after this had lasted a quarter of an hour the fit ended with a jerk through the whole body like a single thrust forwards with arms and legs, and then immediately full consciousness returned, only great exhaustion remained.

Twitching, like something alive (felt when touched), in some muscular parts of the thighs and legs, with spasmodic pain in them by jerks.

Attacks of tetanus. [*Salzb. Med.-Ch. Zeitung.*]*

725. Spasms. [HENNING, l. c.—KELLNER, l. c.]

Convulsions. [FORESTUS, lib. 17, obs. 13.—CRUGER, l. c.—WEDEL, l. c.]

The most violent convulsions. [VAN EGGERN, l. c.]

(Before death) convulsions. [ALBERTI. l. c.—(aft. 4 d.) BONETUS, *Sepulcr. Anat.*, sect. x, obs. xiii, part 1, l. c.]†

Convulsions and miserable distortions of the limbs.‡ [MORGAGNI, l. c.]

730. Epilepsy. § [CRUGER, l. c.—BUTTNER, l. c.]

Trembling of the limbs. [*N. Wahrn.*, l. c.—BUCHHOLZ, *Beitrage*, l. c. —BONETUS, l. c.—HEIMREICH, l. c.—GREISELIUS, l. c.]||

Trembling and shaking with perspiration on the face. [ALBERTI, l. c.]

Trembling in all the limbs. [JUSTAMOND, *On Cancerous Disorders*, Lond., 1750.][1]

He trembles in every part. [*Hbg.*]

735. Trembling all over the body. [GUILBERT, l. c.]

After vomiting trembling of the limbs. [CARDANUS, l. c.]

Trembling in the arms and feet.

Paralysis of the feet. [HEIMREICH, l. c.]

Paralysis ; contraction. [PET. DE APONO, in *Schenck*, lib. vii, obs. 214.]

740. Contraction of the limbs. [J. D. HAMMER, in *Commerc. lit. Norimb.*, 1738, Hebd. 24.]

Stiffness of all the joints. [PET. DE APONO, *de Venen.*, cap. 17.] ¶

Immobility of all the joints. [PET. DE APONO, l. c.]

Paralysis of the lower extremities. [BERNHARDI. in the *Annalen der Heilkunst*, 1811, January, p. 60.[2]]

* See also KAISER, l. c., S. 56, "Tetanus."

† See also KAISER, l. c., S. 59, "Death with and without spasms."

‡ Shortly before death—just as most of the considerable convulsions from arsenic are nothing but secondary action and transition to death.

§ Only secondary action and transition to death. Probably not actual epilepsy, but convulsions similar to those observed by the other authors.

|| See also KAISER, l. c., S. 55, "Trembling." Also *Hartl.* and *Trinks*, l. c., S. 19, "Trembling in the limbs even after very moderate walking."

¶ From sulphuret of arsenic, realgar.

---

1 From arsenic given to a woman with cancer of the tongue.

2 Not accessible.

Paralysis ; inability to walk. [CRUGER, l. c.]

745. Paralysis of the lower extremities, with loss of sensation. [HUBER, *N. Act. Nat. Cur.*, iii, obs. 100.[1]]

She becomes much emaciated, with earthy complexion, blue rings round the eyes, great weakness in all the limbs, disinclination for all work, and constant desire to rest (aft. 8 d.).

Emaciation.[2] [STORCK, l. c—JACOBI, l. c.]

Complete emaciation. [GREISELIUS, l. c.]

Gradual emaciation (and death within the year). [AMATUS LUSITANUS, *Cent.* ii, cur. 4, 65.[3]]

750. (Fatal) marasmus. [*Saltzburger Med.-Ch. Zeit.*]

Wasting. [MAJAULT, l. c.]

Phthisical fever.[4] [STORCK, l. c.]

Horrible pains in the limbs. [PFANN, l. c.]

In the morning in bed sudden tearing twitching or shooting, which changes into burning, in the thumb or big toe.

755. In the evening in bed drawing pain in the middle finger of the hand, and in the foot (aft. 7 d.).

(At night in the back, sacrum and thighs a drawing, shooting and throbbing pain (aft. 3 h.).

Drawing from the abdomen to the head, where there was throbbing and still more tearing ; it then came into the left side, where one or two stitches came in jerks (aft. 8 d.)

Pain in the sacrum and back, especially after riding (in one accustomed to ride).

Gouty pains in the limbs, without inflammation.

760. During a sedentary occupation such peevish restlessness that she must rise up and walk about.

Drawing pain in the joints of the knees, ankles, and wrists.

Indescribably painful and extremely disagreeable feeling of illness in the limbs.

Severe tearing in the arms and legs, owing to which he cannot lie on the side, where it tears ; it becomes most tolerable by moving about the part where the tearing pain is.

All her limbs are painful.

765. Throbbing in all the limbs, and also in the head.

All his limbs are painful, whether he walks or lies.

Extreme painfulness of the skin of the whole body.

Fine pricks all over the body.

Here and there slow pricks, as with a red-hot needle.

770. (The pains become slighter and leave off by compressing the part.)

Tearing pains in the hollow bones.

(On the occurrence of the pains, heat of face and body.)

The nocturnal pains only become tolerable when he walks

1 Statement that the author knows a woman so affected by arsenic.
2 See note to S. 118.
3 Poisoning of a youth.
4 See note to S. 118.

about; they are unendurable when sitting, and particularly when lying still.

The pains are felt at night when asleep.

775. The pains are intolerable, they make the sufferer furious.

The pain of the affected part is even felt during (light) sleep, and wakes him up occasionally during the night, especially before midnight.

On the affected part a pain as if an abscess had passed into suppuration there and would burst; observed when sitting (aft. 4 h.).

On the affected part a pain as if the bone was swollen there; observed when sitting.

An ulcer that is particularly painful in the morning, which contains a dark, brown, bloody matter under a thin scab, with single stitches whilst sitting, which are relieved by standing, but most effectually by walking.

780. After the (midday) meal, whilst sitting, the pains increase, but they are relieved by standing and moving the body.

Conversation addressed to him by others is intolerable to him; it increases his pains enormously (aft. ½ h.).

Tearing pain in the ulcers.

On the affected part, in the ulcer, a burning as from a live coal.

(From dipping the hands in a cold solution of arsenic, a frightful burning pain in the fourth finger, as if the part were burnt with boiling fat (for 4 hours) (aft. ½ h.).

785. The ulcer gets very elevated borders.

The old ulcers, hitherto painless, became painfully sensitive.

The ulcer discharges much black coagulated blood.

Ulcers on the heels with bloody pus.[1] [GUILBERT, l. c.]

Itching in the ulcer passing into burning. [HEUN, l. c.]

790. Burning pain in the ulcer [HARGENS, in *Huf. Journ. d. pr. A.*, ix, i.][2]

Cancerous ulcer which rendered it necessary to amputate the limbs.[3] [HEINZE, in *Ebers*, l. c., Octob., p. 38.]

The ulcer becomes inflamed all around, bleeds on being bandaged, and gets a superficial dry scab. [HARGENS, l. c]

An ulcer appears on the leg, which is covered with a grey scab, has burning pain, and an inflamed border.

Burning pain in the ulcers.

795. Around the ulcer (not in the ulcer itself) burning pain, like fire; it has a very fetid smell and discharges little; at the same time exhaustion and drowsiness in the daytime.

After the burning about the border of the ulcer, an itching in the ulcer itself.

A burning itching on the body.

Much itching on the right thigh and on the arms.

Itching running sensation as from fleas on the thigh up to the abdomen, also on the loins and nates, making him scratch.

800. Burning itching, and after scratching the part is painful.

---

1 In the original, "ichorose Stoff."

2 From application of arsenic to a cancerous ulcer.

3 In a refiner of arsenic.

Intolerable burning in the skin. [HEIMREICH, l. c.]
Burning eroding pains. [PREUSSIUS, l. c.—GABEZIUS, l. c.]
Burning pains. [QUELMALZ, l. c.—HENKEL, *Act. N. C.*, ii, obs. 155.]
Needle pricks on the skin. [*N. Wahrn.*, l. c.]

805. Inflamed measle-like spots over the body, especially on the head, face and neck.[1] [THOMSON, l. c.]

Spots here and there on the skin. [BAYLIES, l. c.]

Thick eruption of little white elevations the colour of the skin, of the size of a lentil and smaller, with smarting pain, which is usually worst at night. [*Fr. H—n.*]

Cutaneous eruption.[2] [MAJAULT, l. c.]

Miliary eruption all over the body which falls off in scales (aft. 14 d.). [GUILBERT, l. c.]*

810. The whole body, even the hands and feet, full of small spots with white points, which resemble millet seeds. [DEGRANGE, in *Phys. Med. Journ.*, 1800, April, p. 299.[3]]

Eruption of a copious red scorbutic miliary rash. [HARTMANN, *Diss. Aethiop. Antim. et Arsenicalis*, Halle, 1759, p. 49.[4]]

Eruptions[5] resembling urticaria. [FOWLER, l. c.]

Very painful black pocks.† [B. VERZASCH, l. c.]

Eruption of black pocks, which cause burning pain (aft. 8d.). [PFANN, l. c.]

815. Pimples very difficult to heal.[6] [AMATUS LUSITANUS, *Cent.* ii, cur. 34.]

Eruption of small pimples on several parts, also on the forehead and under the jaw, which cause burning pain and slight itching.

(On the appearance of small pointed pimples, itching which goes off on scratching, not followed by soreness or burning.)

With burning itching, as from gnat-bites, an eruption comes out on the hands, between the fingers (at the union of the fingers), and on the abdomen, consisting of whitish, pointed pimples, which contain watery fluid in their apices ; scratching causes the fluid to escape, and the itching goes off.

In the eruption of pimples there is such burning that she can scarcely remain quiet from anxiety.

820. In the evening (from 6 to 8 o'clock) great anxiety, with violent aching and pressing in the head, transient sweat, and extreme anorexia (aft. 106 h.).

Weariness and pain in the joints, an hour before dinner, more felt when sitting than when walking.

* See also KAISER, l. c., S. 60, "Blue spots on the abdomen, genitals, and white of the eye."

† On the spot on which the suspended arsenical amulet hung.

---

1 After opium as an antidote.
2 Not found.
3 From rubbing arsenic into the head.
4 Not accessible.
5 Slight.
6 The symptoms 815, 917, and 1031 were observed on patients affected with itch, that had been suppressed by an arsenical ointment (FRANK, *Hygea*. xix.)

She becomes quite stiff, cannot move or stir, she can only stand (aft. 72 h.).

After eating great weariness.

Astonishing exhaustion, anxiety, she cannot recollect herself, she has a difficulty in giving her attention, and is at the same time very giddy.

825. During the depression, weakness; on returning cheerfulness, stronger.

Faintings. [BUCHHOLZ, *Beitrage*, l. c.—PET. FORESTUS, l. c.—HENCKEL, l. c.—[MORGAGNI, l. c.—VERZASCH, l. c.—TIM. A GULDENKLEE, *Cas. Medic.*, Lips., 1662, lib. 7. cap. ii.]

Frequent syncope, with weak pulse[1] (aft. 3 h.). [FERNELIUS, l. c.]

Severe faintings. [GUILBERT, l. c.—MORGAGNI, l. c.]

Profound syncope (from the smell of orpiment). [SENNERT, *Prax. Med.*, lib. 6, p. 6, c. 9.]

830. Commencing debility. [FRIEDRICH, in *Hufel. Journ. d. pr. A.*, v, p. 172[2]]

Exhaustion (aft. 6 h.). [BUCHHOLZ, *Beitrage*, l. c.]

For several days weakness of the whole body, weak pulse, must lie down for several days. [WEDEL, l. c.]*

Great weakness, especially in the legs. [PYL, *Samml.*, viii, p. 98, &c.]

Weakness so that he could scarcely walk across the room.[3] [EBERS, l. c.]

835. He trembled from loss of strength, and could hardly leave his bed. [EBERS, l. c., p. 56.]

Extreme weakness. [GORITZ, l. c.]

Sinking of the strength. [STORCK, l. c.—GUILBERT, l. c.—RAU, l. c.—GRIMM, l. c.—HAMMER, l. c.]

So weak he cannot walk alone (before the vomiting) (aft. 3 h.). [ALBERTI, l. c., tom. i, app., p. 34.]

On attempting to walk he falls down, though he retains his senses. [PYL, *Samml.*, vi, p. 97.]

840. He cannot step properly; he is as if paralysed in all his limbs. [*Hbg.*]

Walking is extremely difficult for him; he thinks he will fall. [*Hbg*]

Great exhaustion; he cannot walk across the room without sinking down. [*Stf.*]

Great exhaustion for several days, so that he can scarcely stand up. [*Stf.*]

Death—without vomiting, with only extreme anxiety and excessive sinking of the strength (aft. 16 h.). [SEILER, *Progr. de Venefic. per Arsen.*, Viteb., 1806.[4]]

845. Death—without vomiting or convulsions, only from sinking of the strength. [BONETUS, l. c.[5]]

* See also KAISER, l. c., S. 53, "General weakness in the body, especially in the legs, which can scarcely be moved," and S. 54, "The strength becomes more and more lost."

1 With vomitings. 2 Poisoning of a woman. 3 See note to S 118. 4 Not accessible. 5 Case of poisoning.

Death—more from rapid sinking of the strength than from the violence of the pains, or convulsions (aft. 12 h.). [MORGAGNI, l. c., § 3.]

Violent vertigo, complete exhaustion, continual vomiting, hæmaturia, and rapid extinction of life (without convulsions, fever or pain).*

Uncommon prostration and weakness of the limbs, which compels him to lie down. [GORITZ, l. c.]

He must lie down and becomes confined to bed. [*Fr. H—n.*]

850. Lying down. [ALBERTI, l. c., tom. ii.]

Sleeplessness. [BUCHHOLZ, *Beitrage*, l. c.—(aft. 14 d.) KNAPE, l. c.—DEGNER, l. c.—GRIMM, l. c.]

Yawning and stretching, as if he had not slept enough (aft. $2\frac{3}{4}$, 11 h.). [*Lr.*]

(Incomplete yawning, short yawning, he cannot yawn fully.)

Extremely frequent yawning.

855. In the day-time, frequent paroxysm of sleep, when sitting.

After dinner excessive yawning and great fatigue (aft. 100 h.).

Exhaustion, as if suffering loss of strength from want of food.

The strength of the hands and feet as if lost, and they are very trembling, in the morning (aft. 12 h.).

He keeps lying down all day.

860. **He can scarcely walk across the room without sinking down.**

When he walks but little, he feels immediately an extraordinary weakness in the knees.

He wishes to rise up, but when he rises he can hardly maintain himself.

In the morning he cannot get out of bed, he feels as if he had not had enough sleep, and is weary in his eyes.

When she gets out of bed she immediately falls in a heap on account of weakness and vertigo, the headache also is then worse.

865. In the morning faint and anxiously weak.

She emaciates much, with earthy complexion, blue rings round the eyes, great weakness in all the limbs, disinclination for all work, and constant inclination to repose (aft. 8 d.)

Emaciation of all the body, with very profuse sweats.

Paralytic weakness of the limbs, daily at a certain hour, like a fever.

Sleeplessness with restlessness and moaning.

870. He talks and scolds in his sleep.

From 3 a. m. she only sleeps interruptedly and tosses about.

At night (about 3 a. m.) pricking pain in the left meatus auditorius as from within outwards.

For two successive nights, in sleep, feeling of illness.

The whole night much heat and restlessness, on account of which she cannot fall asleep, at the same time pulsation in the head.

* GEHLEN died thus from inhalation of arseniureted hydrogen. [*Halle Allg. Lit. Zeit.*, 1815, No. 181.]

875. Only at night much thirst, on account of great dryness in the throat, which ceases in the morning.

In the evening (at night) while lying in bed, some pricking tearing in a corn.

Sleepless tossing about at night in bed, with a crawling in the abdomen.

In sleep he lies on his back, the left hand supporting the head.

In the evening in sleep loud moaning.

880. During sleep, turning about in bed, with moaning, especially about 3 a. m.

Grinding of the teeth in sleep.

She cannot get warm in bed at night.

After midnight feeling of anxious heat, with desire to throw off the clothes.

In the morning in bed, at sunrise, general heat, sweat on the face and dryness of the front of the mouth, without thirst.

885. In the morning in bed a dull headache, that goes off on getting up.

In the morning in bed qualmish, sick up into the chest, then vomiting of white mucus, but with bitter taste in the mouth.

After waking, great peevishness ; she knew not how to compose herself, owing to ill-humour, pushed and threw the pillows and bed-clothes away from her, and would look at and listen to nobody.

In the evening in bed, immediately before going to sleep, she has a choking feeling in the throat like sulphur fumes, making her cough.

In the evening after lying down, at the commencement of sleep, violent twitching in the limbs.

890. Movements of the fingers and hands in sleep.

Twitching on going to sleep.

Sleep restless ; she wakes up very early. [*Bhr.*]

Could not get to sleep, and occasionally fell into faints [TIM. A GULDENKLEE, *Opp.*, p. 280.]

Great inclination to sleep; he falls asleep again immediately after having had a conversation (from the 6th to the 10th day). [*Fr. H—n.*]*

895. Sleep full of the most violent startings and shudderings.[1] [THOMSON, l. c.] †

Vivid vexatious dreams (aft. 19 h.). [*Lr.*]‡

Rambling at night. [SIEBOLD, l. c.]

Spasmodic starting of all the body (aft. 36 h.).[2] [THOMSON, l. c.]

In the evening, on going to sleep, startling twitches, like shaking blows on the affected part, which are excited by a slight ailment on a distant part, by a tearing, an itching, &c. (aft. 4 d.).

* See also KAISER, l. c., S. 63, "Great, almost irresistible, inclination to sleep, alternating with great restlessness, without particular fear of death."

† See also KAISER, l. c., S. 64, "Sleepiness, which is interrupted by uneasy dreams and great anxiety."

‡ See also *Hartl.* and *Trinks*, l. c., No. 25, "The night full of uneasy dreams."

1 After opium had been given as an antidote.

2 As S. 895. Should be after 12, not 36 hours.

900. Immediately after lying down he dreams that he was about to knock his foot against a stone, whereupon he has a sudden jerk in the knee, and thereafter he is awakened as if by an electric shock.

When he is going to sleep an anxious dream, he would like to cry out, but can hardly bring out a word, and he suddenly wakes up by a call which he continues to hear.

He dreamed all night incessantly of storms, conflagration, black water, and darkness.

He sleeps disturbed by dreams full of care, distress, and fear.

At night anxious frightful dreams.

905. Dreams full of cares and dangers, from each of which he wakes up, sometimes with a cry, and he always dreams something new.

In the morning slumber he hears every sound and every noise, and yet he dreams all through it.

Care-beset dreams; he wakes up, and after going to sleep again dreams the same thing.

Dreams full of threatenings, and apprehensions, or remorse.

Dreams accompanied by fatiguing reflections.

910. On awaking frequently at night **she has burning in all the blood-vessels.**

Towards evening drowsiness, with chilliness, with, at the same time, a disagreeable feeling of illness through the whole body, as in ague when the fit is quite or nearly over—recurring at the same hour two days later—after midnight profuse perspiration on the thighs.

Towards evening he feels very uncomfortable in the body, like fever, and when he lies down his head becomes hot, especially the ears, but the knees are cold (aft. 36 h.).

Almost constant yawning.

Fever.[1] [HEUN, l. c.]

915. (During the febrile attack) increased tension in the hypochondria, lying on the side is almost impossible. [EBERS, l. c., p. 68.]

Violent fever. [KNAPE, l. c.—DEGNER, l. c.]

(Fatal) fever.[1] [AMATUS LUSITANUS, l. c.]

Renewal of the same arsenical disease[2] in the quartan type, at the same hour in the forenoon. [MORGAGNI, l. c., § 8.]

Thirst, fever. [MORGAGNI, l. c., § 6.]

920. Thirst. [PET. DE APONO, l. c.—RAU, l. c.—PREUSSIUS, l. c.]

Great thirst. [ALBERTI, l. c., tom. ii.]

He drinks much and often. [*Stf.*]

Incessant, great thirst. [BUTTNER, l. c.]

Sweat and excessive thirst; he is always wanting to drink. [*Hbg.*]

925. Violent thirst. [MAJAULT, l. c.]

He cries out about choking thirst. [FORESTUS, lib. 17, obs. 13.]

Burning thirst. [MAJAULT, l. c.]

He is thirsty, yet drinks but little at a time. [RICHARD, l. c.]

---

1 See 815, note.

2 More correctly in the *Chr. Kr.* "Arsenik-Beschwerden." The recurrence only took place once.

Unquenchable thirst. [BUCHHOLZ, *Beitrage*, l. c.—KELLNER, l. c. —GUILBERT, l. c.—CRUGER, l. c.]

930. Unquenchable thirst, with dryness of the tongue, fauces, and larynx. [TIM. A GULDENKLEE, *Opp.*, p. 280.]

After the occurrence of diarrhœa thirst and internal heat (aestus). [MORGAGNI, l. c.]

Violent thirst not without appetite for food. [KNAPE, l. c.]

Violent rigor. [FERNELIUS, l. c.]*

Shivering. [BUCHHOLZ, *Beitrage*, l. c.]

935. Febrile rigor. [*Med. Nat. Zeit.*, 1798, Sept.]

Febrile rigor through the whole body, with hot forehead, warm face and cold hands, without thirst and without subsequent heat (aft. 3 h.). [*Lr.*]

Rigor all over the body, with warm forehead, hot cheeks, and cold hands, not followed by heat (aft. $3\frac{3}{4}$ h.). [*Lr.*]

In the afternoon stretching and drawing in the limbs, with rigor in the integuments of the head, as in sudden shuddering from fear; thereafter chill, with goose skin. This was followed in the evening, from 8 to 9 o'clock, by heat in the body, especially in the face, without sweat, with cold hands and feet.

After drinking a shudder as from disgust. [ALBERTI, l. c., tom. iii.]

940. The limbs are cold. [RICHARD, l. c.—FERNELIUS, l. c.]

External coldness of the limbs and internal heat, with anxious unrest and weak variable pulse. [ALBERTI, l. c., tom. iii.]

Chill, febrile rigor.

After dinner shivering.

A chilliness in the external skin over the face and feet.

945. **After drinking**, chill and shivering (immediately).

An attack of fever, which recurs daily at a certain hour.

Febrile rigor, without thirst (immediately).

By day much chilliness, after the chill thirst, in the evening much heat in the face.

Chilliness, with inability to get warm, without thirst, with crossness, and when she spoke or moved, a flush of heat ran over her, she became red in the face, and yet was chilly.

950. In the chill no thirst.

(In the forenoon violent rigor without thirst; he has at the same time spasms in the chest, pains throughout the body, and cannot collect his thoughts; after the chill heat with thirst, and after the heat perspiration with roaring in the ears (aft. 20 h.).

The rigor goes off after dinner.†

Every afternoon about 3 o'clock chill attended with hunger; after eating the chill became still more severe.

(In the afternoon chill, cutting in the abdomen and diarrhœic stool, and thereafter continued cutting in the abdomen.)

* See also KAISER, l. c., S. 65, "Chilliness up to the greatest degree of cold."—S. 66, "General coldness, with copious sweat on the skin."—S. 67, "The body feels cold to the touch and dryness of the skin alternates with cold sweat."

† A (rare) alternating action compared with the more frequent one in which symptoms occur after dinner.

955. The rigor returns always about 5 p.m.
In the evening, immediately before lying down, rigor.
Towards evening chill with coldness.
Every evening a febrile rigor.
Chilliness internally, heat externally, with red cheeks, in the afternoon.
960. He was chilly, the feet were cold ; he began to perspire.
In the evening coldness and chilliness in the feet, and even the abdomen is cold to the touch.
In the evening chilliness on the legs, from the calves down to the feet.
She is either too cold in the whole body and yet is nowhere cold to touch ; or she is too warm, and yet is nowhere hot to touch, except slightly in the palms.
In the evening, after lying down, great chilliness, in bed.
965. He cannot get warm in bed ; thinks he has caught cold in bed.
During the febrile rigor tearing in the legs.
Shivering when out of bed.
When walking in the open air shivering occurs.
When he comes into the room* from the open air there occurs chilliness, followed hy long-continued hiccup, then general perspiration, and then again hiccup.
970. During the pain, rigor, after the pain, thirst.†
At one time chilliness, at another heat. [ALBERTI, l. c., tom. iii.]
Internal heat.‡ [GORITZ, l. c.]
Heat all through the body, internally and externally, as from drinking wine, with thirst for beer. [*Myr.*]
Anxious heat.[1] [PET. DE APONO, l. c.]
975. General anxious warmth. [*Hbg.*]
Sensation as if the blood ran too quickly and too hot through the blood-vessels, with small, quick pulse. [*Stf.*]
In the evening, at 10 o'clock, heat and redness all over the body ; after the heat, sweat. [*Stf.*]
Violent palpitation in the night. [*Bhr.*]
Excessive ebullition of the blood.[1] [GRIMM, l. c.]
980. After the febrile heat, sick feeling (aft. 15 h.).
Nocturnal heat without thirst and without perspiration.§
At 7 p. m. heat of face lasting an hour.
In the evening after a short sleep she wakes with toothache.
At the commencement of sleep, in the evening after lying down, perspiration, which goes off during subsequent sleep.

* Comp. 33.

† As, according to the characteristic peculiarity of the action of arsenic, another symptom occurs during the attack of pain (see note to 176), and here (970) chilliness and rigor in particular ; so, again, pains are associated with the arsenical febrile rigor, as we see in 960 and 995.

‡ See also KAISER, l. c., S. 69, "Great heat."—S. 70, "Dry heat of the skin, after preceding chill."—S. 71, "Skin dry and hot."

§ Characteristic for arsenic.

1 The original of both these symptoms is "exæstuatio," the real meaning of which is best rendered in 979.

985. At the commencement of sleep* perspiration only on the hands and thighs, which goes off during subsequent sleep, and is not perceived any more after waking (aft. 6 h.).

About 2 a. m. increased warmth, sweat on face and between the legs, and colic-like painful tension in the epigastrium and the region beneath the ribs, which causes anxiety.

The perspiration each time comes on only when the fever has come to an end.†

Morning sweat from waking until rising, all over the body.

Sweat on three successive nights.

990. Sweat only on the face, on waking in the morning.

(The perspiration exhausts him, as he lies in bed, almost to the production of syncope.)

During the perspiration his skin, and especially his eyes, acquired a yellow tinge.[1] [EBERS, l. c., p. 69.]

Perspiration.[2] [MAJAULT, l. c.]

Cold clammy sweat.[3] [HENNING, l. c.]‡

995. Along with febrile rigor and shivering and heat of the external ear, anxiety and gnawing§ pain in the scrobiculus cordis, as from fasting long, mingled with nausea.

Fever every alternate day: the first afternoon, about 6 o'clock, chilliness and fatigue, and bruised feeling in the thighs; the third afternoon, about 5 o'clock, at first inclination to lie down, then rigor all over without thirst, then heat without thirst, with aching pain in the forehead.

In the morning rigor alternating with heat.

In the forenoon perspiration, heaviness of the head, roaring in the ears, trembling.

Very slow pulse, only thirty-eight beats in the minute. [PEARSON, l. c.]

1000. Small, quick pulse. [*N. Wahrn.*, l. c.—MAJAULT, l. c.]

Quick, weak pulse.[4] [MAJAULT, l. c.]

Very rapid, small, weak pulse. [MORGAGNI, l. c.]

Tense pulse. [KNAPE, l. c.]

Extremely quick, intermittent,[5] weak pulse. [GUILBERT, l. c.]

1005. Very febrile pulse. [KNAPE, l. c.]‖

* Characteristic.

† Characteristic, and to be met with almost only with arsenic.

‡ See also KAISER, l. c., No. 72, "Cold sweat alternating with cold dryness of the skin.

§ Comp. 360.

‖ The variations of the pulse are given thus by KAISER, l. c., SS. 73—78: "Small, quick, hard pulse."—"Pulse weak and small."—"Pulse small and intermitting."—"The pulse becomes irregular, intermittent, small, and at last quite extinct."—"Pulse frequent, not full, and irritated. The heart's beat is very violent, tumultuous."—"Absence of the pulse, with quick, very irritated, frequent beat of the heart."

---

1 See note to S. 118.

2 With vomiting.

3 Stated to be the effect of aniseed given as an antidote.

4 Not found.

5 Rather, "irregular."

After dinner a sad melancholy disposition with headache (aft. 80 h.).

The child is full of restlessness, cross, and whines.

He can find rest in no place, continually changes his position in bed, will get out of one bed and into another, and lie now here, now there.*

About 1 a.m. excessive anxiety; sometimes she is hot, sometimes as though she would vomit.

1010. She cannot fall asleep before midnight on account of anxious heat, for many days.

In the evening, after lying down, and at about 3 a.m. (after waking), anxiety.†

Anxiety, anxietates. [*N. Wahrn.*, l. c.—*Med. Nat. Zeit.*, l. c.—MYRRHEN, l. c.—QUELMALZ, l. c.]

Anxiety so that he frequently fainted, besides a violent pain in the place, and black pocks on the spot.‡ [BERN. VERZASCH, *Obs. Med.*, obs. 66]

The most intolerable anxiety.[1] [FORESTUS, l. c.]

1015. Talks little, only complains of anxiety. [ALBERTI, l. c.]

Deathly anxiety.[2] [HENNING, l. c.]

Præcordial anxiety, interrupted by the occurrence of faintings.[3] [FRIEDRICH, l. c.]

Long-continued anxiety.[4] [TIM. A GULDENKLEE, l. c.]

Anxiety, trembling, and quaking, with cold sweat in the face. [ALBERTI, l. c.]

1020. Anxiety and restlessness in the whole body (aft. 1 h.). [RICHARD, l. c.]

On account of increasing pains he appeared to lie at the last gasp, with unspeakable anxiety. [MORGAGNI, l. c.]

Restlessness, with pains in the head, abdomen, and knees. [RICHARD, l. c.]

Sadness and restlessness and tossing about in bed, with unquenchable thirst § (aft. 24 h.). [BUTTNER, l. c.]

Piercing lamentations, interrupted by the occurrence of faintings.[5] [FRIEDRICH, l. c.]

1025. He wept and howled, and spoke little and but few words at a time. [*Stf.*]

Piteous lamentations, that the most intolerable anxiety, with extremely disagreeable sensation in the whole abdomen, took away

* Scarcely occurs so markedly in any other medicine.

† Characteristic.

‡ When arsenic was worn in a bag on the bare chest for four days.

§ From external application on the head in two children. Death ensued after two days, and revealed inflammation of the lungs and great inflammation in the stomach and small intestines.

---

1 Not found.

2 With vomiting.

3 See note to S. 1024.

4 In the original "præcordiorum angustia."

5 The attacks were of weakness (Schwachheiten), not faintings (Ohnmachten).

his breath and compelled him to curl himself together now here now there, then again to rise up and walk about. [MORGAGNI, l. c., § 8.]

Trembling, anxious, he is afraid that he cannot refrain from killing some one with a sharp knife, [A. F. MARCUS, *Ephem. d. Heilk.*, pt. iii][1]

Driven by great anxiety he turns and twists about in bed. [BUTTNER., l. c.—TIM. A GULDENKLEE, *Opp.*, p. 280.]

He wants to get out of one bed into another. [MYRRHEN, l. c.]

1030. Great anxiety, trembling, and shaking, with severe tearing in the abdomen. [ALBERTI, l. c., iii, p. 533.]

He became furious, must be bound, and seeks to run away.[2] [AMATUS LUSITANUS, l. c.]

Mania : first headache, horrible anxiety, noise before the ears, as from a number of large bells, and when he opened the eyes, he always saw a man who had (formerly) hung himself on the ground-floor of the house, who incessantly beckoned him to cut him down ; he ran thither with a knife, but as he could not cut him down, he became overwhelmed with despair and wished (as his friends assured him) to hang himself ; but being prevented from doing so, he became so restless that he could hardly be kept in bed, he lost the power of speech, though complete consciousness remained, and on attempting to express himself by writing, he could only put down unmeaning signs, whilst he trembled, wept, his forehead bedewed with the sweat of anxiety, and he knelt down and raised his hands in a supplicating manner. [EBERS, l. c.]

He despairs of his life.[3] [RICHARD, l. c.]

Hypochondriac anxiety, such as is wont to occur from sitting much in a room, just as if it came from the upper part of the chest ; without palpitation of the heart (aft. some minutes).

1035. He is cold, shivers and weeps, and thinks, in his despair, that nothing can help him, and he must die ; followed by general exhaustion.

In the evening, in bed, anxious sad fancies, *e. g.* that something bad must have happened to his relatives.

Easily startled.

When he is alone he is beset by thoughts about disease and other thoughts of an indifferent character, of which he cannot get rid.

Persistent anxiety, like a qualm of conscience, just as if he had failed to do his duty, but without knowing wherein.*

1040. Over-sensitiveness and excessive tenderness of disposition ; dejected, sad, lachrymose, is distressed and anxious about the slightest trifle.

Very sensitive to noise.

Irritated state of the disposition, he vexes himself

* See also KAISER, l. c., SS. 1—3, "Internal anxiety,"—"Great feeling of anxiety." —"High degree of anxiety, oppression of the chest and difficulty of breathing."

1 In a fever patient, after taking arsenite of potash.
2 See 815, note.
3 Not found.

about trifles and cannot leave off talking about the faults of others.

Discomfort, he has pleasure in nothing.

Recurring fits of irresolution; he wishes something and when one attempts to gratify his wish the merest trifle will alter his resolution, and he wishes it no longer.

1045. Her desire is greater than her need; she eats and drinks more than is good for her; she walks further than she need do or can bear.

Having not the least appetite, she allows herself to be pressed to take something, but gets furiously angry about it (aft. 7 d.).

Very cross, irritable, whimsical, takes every word in bad part, and becomes angry when she should answer.

Cross about trifles.

Discontented with everything, finds fault with everything; everything is too strong and too irritating, all conversation, all noise, and all light.

1050. **Anxiously impatient.**

Ill-humour in bed in the morning; he peevishly knocks the pillows about, throws off the bed-clothes and uncovers himself, he looks at nobody and does not want to know about anything.

Variable humour; **ill-humour** alternating with mild friendliness; in the ill-humoured state will not look at any one nor hear about anything; he weeps also.

Weak in body and mind (down-hearted), he does not speak and yet is not morose.

(Talking nonsense, with open eyes, without being conscious of having fancies either before or after.)

1055. Great indifference and want of interest.

Life appears to him naught; he attaches no value to it.*

Uncommonly tranquil disposition; quite unconcerned about their approaching death, they neither hoped nor wished to recover.†

Religious melancholy and reserve.[1] [EBERS, l. c., p. 18.]

Tranquillity of mind (in a despairing melancholic). [LABORDE, in *Journ. de Medicine*, lxx.][2]

1060. Tranquil serious mood; he remained undisturbed throughout all the events that occurred. [*Lr.*]

Good humoured; he has pleasure in entertaining himself with others. [*Lr.*]

More disposed to gaiety and inclined to be always occupied. [*Lr.*]

* See also KAISER, l. c., S. 4, "Indifference to life."

† A secondary or curative action observed in two suicides, who in the most intolerable depression of mind took one a drachm the other about two scruples of powdered arsenic, and in a few hours died with the greatest calmness of mind.

---

1 Not found.

2 LA MOTTE in Hahnemann. A woman taking arsenic for suicide. The calmness was rather mental, from her determination, than physical.

Sensitive peevish disposition ; the least thing can annoy him and almost cause him to be angry. [*Lr.*]

All day long discontented with himself and very cross with himself ; he imagines he has not done enough, and reproaches himself bitterly. [*Lr.*]

1065. The first minutes great calmness of mind and cheerfulness,* after half an hour, however, extreme anxiety, restlessness ; he had a great dread of the effects of the poison and desired to live. [*Stf.*]

Great seriousness.

After death, the lips and nails of the hands and feet quite blue, as also the glans penis and scrotum quite blue ; the whole body, and especially the limbs, quite stiff and contracted ; the large intestine very much contracted. [PYL, *Samml.* v, p. 106.]

The corpse was still fresh and undecomposed after 16 days. [PYL, *Samml.*, vi, p. 97.]†

* In a despairing suicide, in whom the preliminary calmness of mind was a curative action.

† For the sake of comparison I will here give the history of the poisoning of a horse by arsenic from the *Anzeiger der Leipziger okonomischen Societat.*

Amid frightful symptoms there gushed streams of green water from the nose, the eyes stuck out of the head and were severely inflamed, the pupils of the eyes were round and preternaturally dilated ; the nostrils widely opened, and on account of the rapid, short, difficult, and anxious respiration in constant motion ; the gums, palate, and tongue swollen, dry, and bluish-red ; the pulse excessively small and tremulous ; the restlessness indescribable ; the abdomen extremely tense ; the whole body covered with cold sweat.

If we had performed many similar (and still more careful) experiments on these useful domestic animals with several simple drugs we should then have for them a pure materia medica, and should be able to cure them also rationally (homœopathically), quickly, permanently, and surely, in place of the present impotent quackery with a multitude of unsuitable mixtures.

ORPIMENT (*Auripigmentum*).

While walking in the open air a severe giddiness in the whole head as from intoxication (aft.5½ h.) [*Lr.*]

Stupefaction of the whole head; too many irrelevant things occurred to him (aft. 8½ h.). [*Lr.*]

Throbbing stitches on the right side of the forehead (aft. 2½ h.). [*Lr.*]

Needle pricks externally on the right side of the forehead (aft. 5 h.). [*Lr.*]

5. On stroking the hair of the occiput, a tensive sensation behind the right ear, as if something was sticking behind the ear which pressed the ear forwards (aft. 1½ h.). [*Lr.*]

Eye gum in the canthi of the eyes (aft. 33 h.). [*Lr.*]

On chewing the food the teeth were painful as if they were loose (aft. 5 h.). [*Lr.*]

At noon after eating violent nausea (aft. 5¾ h.). [*Lr.*]

In the morning on waking violent cutting in the abdomen, as from a chill (aft. 25 h.). [*Lr.*]

10. Needle pricks from within outwards in the right side of the chest (aft. 6 h.) [*Lr.*]

In the evening on going to sleep a fright as if he fell out of bed. (aft. 18 h.). [*Lr.*]

ASARUM.[1]

(The spirituous tincture of the dry root of *Asarum europæum* or the juice of the whole plant mixed with alcohol.)

Even when the ordinary physicians have taken the trouble, which they but seldom did, to ascertain by their own experiments the powers of simple medicinal substances, we can see how carelessly they went to work by such an example, among others, as the labours in this direction of COSTE and WILLEMET, who, in their prize essay entitled ***Essais sur quelques plantes indigenes*** (Nancy, 1778), pretend to give us among others a complete proving of *Asarum*. And what then did they discover from the trials they themselves made of it? Nothing of all the remarkable symptoms recorded below, except that, when given in doses of from twenty-eight to forty grains, it caused vomiting five or six times. But what was the peculiar character of this vomiting, or by what dangerous symptoms it was accompanied, of this they give us no hint. Further, that forty-eight grains given to a porter caused severe colic pains and violent vomiting and purging, which had to be allayed by a clyster of milk. And hence, as they imagine, this root must be regarded as identical in its action with ipecacuanha. And did it do nothing more than this? And is this all the curative action that can be expected from it? How carelessly must they have acted in such an important matter when they observed nothing more and discovered no more medicinal uses for it!

No! asarum is as little adapted for employment as an emetic in the place of ipecacuanha (which also causes many other changes in the health of human beings) as many other substances, which when taken in excess are also rejected from the system by forcible vomiting, such as arsenic, sulphate of zinc, acetate of copper, veratrum album &c. Do all these substances, which when taken in excess cause dangerous vomiting, merely exist in nature in order that we may use them as emetics? What short-sightedness, what dangerous superficiality! And my remarks do not apply only to COSTE and WILLEMET, but the same complaint may be made of all our ordinary (non-) observers. *Mutato nomine de te fabula narratur.* They will see, and have seen, almost nothing from the administration of all medicinal substances but evacuations by the skin, kidneys, bowels, &c., for they have always sought to sweep out material morbid stuff that has seldom any existence, and have no idea of effecting cures in any other way.

If we take into consideration what these authors relate about their

---

1 From vol. iii, 2nd edit., 1825.

porter in an offhand manner, as if it were a mere nothing because he did not die on the spot, together with what may be read in the following observations, it would seem to be highly probable that this root, when given in such a large dose as that it shall excite that evacuation upwards of which the saburralists are so fond, is capable of putting a human being in imminent danger of his life, and that consequently it may actually produce a fatal result, as was, indeed, seen by WEDEL. That would, indeed, be a splendid inestimable remedy which should remove the (imaginary) foulness of the stomach with no other disadvantage than—palpable danger to life! Preserve us from acting so barbarously towards our sick fellow-creatures!

No! the beneficent Preserver of life created this root for much nobler objects. To cure natural morbid vomiting accompanied by threatening symptoms like those of asarum with the smallest dose of the excessively diluted tincture of asarum, this is the first noble employment that we have to make of it—exactly the opposite of that murderous misuse of it in which it was recommended in large doses as an emetic.

What else it can do in the way of homœopathic help may be seen from its other symptoms detailed below, which, to the thoughtful physician, require no elucidation, nor is it necessary to give any other indication of the diseases curable by it.

The homœopathic practitioner who does exactly the opposite of that which the ordinary medical school has hitherto enjoined knows how to make a better use of this mighty gift of God; he never misuses it for the production of such involuntary break-neck upsettings of the human organism; even our domestic animals should be spared those cruelties practised under the name of veterinary medicine.

No, the Creator wished that we might learn to overcome great diseases by means of powerful medicines having similar symptoms (homœopathically) in doses of the smallest size, and therefore incapable of doing harm. He did not create them in large quantities in order that we should by giving them in large doses inflict injury on the noble human race without affording relief, as is the case in the ordinary allopathic treatment. These substances are ordained by nature for very different ends and purposes, all of which we do not yet know, and for which they have been produced in great quantities; nothing has been created for one single object; on the contrary, the purposes of their useful production are manifold. And if among these their utility as medicines is included, the large supply nature affords us of them cannot warrant us to misuse them in great doses for diseases. Thus for instance, arsenic has undoubtedly other important uses in the divine economy, for we can only employ a very small portion of the many hundred tons of it which the Saxon Erzgebirge alone can furnish for a useful medicinal purpose.

According to COSTE and WILLEMET vinegar is an antidote to asarum. Camphor is apparently efficacious in alleviating the injurious effects of its employment in unsuitable cases or in large doses.

A quadrillionth of a grain (in the form of diluted solution) of the alcoholic tincture, and the quintillionth dilution of the freshly-expressed juice mixed with an equal quantity of alcohol (in the dose of a drop or a small portion of a drop), appear to be the best doses for homœopathic purposes.

[HAHNEMANN was assisted in the proving of this medicine by C. FRANZ, C. G. HORNBURG, L. RUCKERT, E. STAPF.

The following old-school authorities are cited:

COSTE and WILLEMET, in *Samml. br. Abh. f. pr. A.*, iv.

HELMONT. J. B. van, *Pharmac, mod.*

MURRAY, *Appar. Med.*, iii.

RAY, *Hist. univ. Plant.*, i.

WEDEL, G. W., *Amœnit. Mat. Med.*

The 1st edit. had 268 symptoms; only 2 new symptoms appeared in the 2nd edit.]

ASARUM.

Vertigo, as from slight intoxication, on rising from a seat and walking about (aft. 10 m.). [*Stf.*]

He does not notice things about him. [*Fz.*]

Mental condition as if just falling asleep; a gradual vanishing of the thoughts. [*Fz.*]

Thoughts so overstrained that they vanish completely. [*Fz.*]

5. He is quite stupid in his head and has no inclination for anything. [*L. Rkt.*]

Incapacity for any work, and he can do nothing; his mental powers fail him (before each attack of vomiting, afterwards somewhat better); as a rule his reason is defective all throughout the medicinal disease. [*L. Rkt.*]

Sensation of vertigo, as if he could not stand very surely, in the evening (aft. 4 d.). [*L. Rkt.*]

Confusion, like stupidity of the whole head, with tension in the region of the ears. [*L. Rkt.*]

In the morning, on rising, dizzy in the head, with headache in the left side of the forehead (aft. 22 h.). [*Stf.*]

10. When he wishes to work with his head and to reflect, the want of thinking power immediately returns and the drawing pressure in the forehead, so that he must immediately leave off. [*L. Rkt.*]

As often as he attempts to reflect a little, the head affections and the sick feeling increase perceptibly; he must quickly cease thinking, which would besides be in vain, as he is quite stupid. [*L. Rkt.*]

Aching, stupefying, dull headache in the forehead, as if he had been wakened too soon from sleep. [*Stf.*]

Dull headache (aft. ½ h.). [*Hbg.*]

Headache, like confusion in the left temple, thereafter under the parietal bones, lastly in the occiput. [*Hbg.*]

15. **Confusion of the head,** less observable when walking, more when sitting, and pressing in the eyes as with a blunt point from within outwards, especially under the right eyelid (aft. ¼ h.). [*Fz.*]

Tensive painful confusion of the head. [*Stf.*]

The head is heavy and confused, at the same time pressure above the sagittal suture, as if he were intoxicated (aft. 3 h.). [*Stf.*]

The head becomes heavy, as if there were something that shook or swayed in it, which, after bending it fowards or backwards, lets its weight be felt. [*Fz.*]

Pressure in the brain, chiefly anteriorly (aft. $\frac{3}{4}$ h.). [*L. Rkt.*]

20. Aching in the left side of the occiput extending towards the side of the head (aft. 3 m.) [*Stf.*]

Out-pressing pain on both sides of the head. [*L. Rkt.*]

Very acute headache in the left temple and behind the ears, like compression, which becomes worse when walking and shaking the head, but is alleviated by sitting (aft. 12 h.). [*Stf.*]

Pressure from without inwards over the greatest portion of the brain (aft. $2\frac{3}{4}$ h.). [*L. Rkt.*]

Pressure in the brain from above downwards as with a stone, on a spot of the forehead (af. $\frac{1}{4}$ h.). [*L. Rkt.*]

25. Violent pressure downwards in the forehead upon the eyes, which then water (aft. $2\frac{1}{4}$ h.). [*L. Rkt.*]

Pressure combined with other sensations here and there in the brain. [*L. Rkt.*]

Sensation of pressure of alternating severity from above downwards in the forehead. [*L. Rkt.*]

Aching pain in the temples, especially the left. [*Fz.*]

Sharp aching headache above the root of the nose. [*Fz.*]

30. Tearing aching pain in the left temple. [*Stf.*]

Violent, drawing pressure in the brain under the forehead (increased every time he retches). [*L. Rkt.*]

Drawing headache, as if it would draw into the temple (at noon) ; it appears to be alleviated in the open air and by lying. [*Stf.*]

A (stupefying) drawing here and there in the brain, ear, and nape. [*Stf.*]

When he has stooped and rises up again, for some seconds, lacerating pain in the forehead. [*L. Rkt.*]

35. Tearing, pulse-like throbbing pain in the forehead. [*L. Rkt.*]

In the morning on rising from bed, throbbing pain in the forehead (aft. 24 h.). [*L. Rkt.*]

By stooping forwards, throbbing headache is excited in the forehead. [*L. Rkt.*]

He feels the beat of the arteries in the occiput, afterwards throughout the body. [*L. Rkt.*]

Tension of the whole scalp so that he is (painfully) conscious of the hairs. [*L. Rkt.*]

40. Itching commencing with fine pricks under the left temple. [*Fz.*]

A cold sensation on a small spot of the left side of the head, a couple of inches above the ear. [*Stf.*]

Formication under the upper eye-lid, especially of the left eye. [*Fz.*]

The left upper eye-lid is somewhat swollen ; the eye cannot bear much reading. [*L. Rkt.*]

Twitching of the lower lid of the right eye. [*Fz.*]

45. Sensation of twitching in the left upper eyelid from within out-

wards, by fits, but only when he holds the eyelid still; but when he elevates it in order to look at anything, it goes off immediately (aft. 9 h.). [*L. Rkt.*]

In the outer canthus of the right eye a feeling of cold as form a cold breath. [*Stf.*]

When he uses the eyes for reading, there occurs in each of them a feeling as if it was forced asunder. [*L. Rkt.*]

Pressure in the left eye. [*Stf.*]

Tearing pain in the interior of the right eye synchronous with the pulse (aft. $1\frac{1}{2}$ h.). [*L. Rkt.*]

50. Sensation of dryness and drawing in the eyes. [*L. Rkt.*]

Dry burning in the eyelids and inner canthi, especially in the left eye. [*Stf.*]

Painful dry feeling in the interior of the eye. [*Stf.*]

Warm feeling and slight pressure in the eyes; they have lost much of their brightness and look duller. [*L. Rkt.*]

Obscuration of the eyes (aft. $\frac{1}{4}$ h.). [*Fz.*]

55. The whole of the right outer ear is hot to the touch, frequently recurring during the whole medicinal disease. [*L. Rkt.*]

Sensation of warmth at the orifice of the right meatus auditorius and feeling as if a thin skin were over it (aft. $\frac{1}{2}$ h.). [*L. Rkt.*]

Dull roaring in the left ear, like a distant wind; in the right clear singing. [*Fz.*]

In the ear, externally as well as internally, a pinching feeling, like earache. [*Hbg.*]

Aching behind and below the left ear. [*Hbg.*]

60. On bending the head towards the left, a pain, as if from over-exertion a fasciculus of muscular fibres was out of its place, which spreads over the left temple and behind the ear towards the left shoulder, and in unison with the pulse increases as that rises, and diminishes as it falls. [*Stf.*]

Continued pressive and tensive pain at the orifice of the meatus auditorius. [*L. Rkt.*]

In the left ear a sensation observed outwardly and inwardly, as if the cartilages of the ear contracted. [*Hbg.*]

Diminished hearing of the left ear, as if it were closed by the hand; it is as if the cartilages went closer together, or as if cotton-wool plugged the ears. [*Fz.*]

He feels as if a skin were stretched over the right meatus auditorius (immediately). [*L. Rkt.*]

65. A sensation in the external meatus as if the orifice in front of the membrana tympani were pasted up. [*Hbg.*]

In front of both ears he feels as if they were stopped. [*Fz.*]

He hears worse with the right than with the left ear (aft. 1 h.). [*L. Rkt.*]

He feels as if a membrane were before the orifice of the meatus auditorius, with sensation as if it was compressed (aft. $\frac{1}{4}$ h.). [*L. Rkt.*]

It is as if a membrane were stretched over the right meatus auditorius, with a tensive pressure therein—almost continuously for seven days, but always worse during the chill. [*L. Rkt.*]

70. The feeling of tension and pressure on the right meatus auditorius scarcely ever remits, and when it does it extends to the right lower jaw, and when it is severe a large quantity of apparently cold saliva flows from the right side of the mouth (aft. ½ h.). [*L. Rkt.*]

Burning, shooting pain on the left cheek, [*Fz.*]

Feeling of warmth in the left cheek (aft. 4 h.). [*Stf.*]

Feeling of warmth in the cheeks (aft. 10 h.). [*L. Rkt.*]

On washing the face with cold water the vertigo, headache, burning on the tongue and in the mouth, contraction of the left cervical muscles and the weakness of the knees went off, but after drying the face they returned. [*Stf.*]

75. Fine shooting on the right cheek. [*Fz.*]

On the left cheek a contractive pain accompanied by gentle, but sharp blows, with drawing pain in the third molar tooth. [*Fz.*]

Produces in the nose* a discharge of bloody mucus [MURRAY, *Appar. Med.*, iii, p. 519.[1]]

Dryness of the inside of the lower lip. [*Fz.*]

A feeling of coldness, like a cold breath, in the upper incisors. [*Stf.*]

80. Sensation in the left row of teeth as if they were hollow. [*Hbg.*]

Cutting pain, with cramp, at the maxillary joint. [*Fz.*]

Much cool saliva collects in the mouth. [*Stf.*]

Frequent sensation of contraction in the interior of the mouth, causing flow of watery saliva. [*L. Rkt.*]

The saliva in the mouth seems to be quite viscid (aft. 24 h.). [*L. Rkt.*]

85. The saliva ejected was burning hot in the mouth (aft. ½ h.). [*Stf.*]

Tongue furred white (aft. 26 h.). [*L. Rkt.*]

A smarting sensation on the tongue and gums. [*Stf.*]

Sensation of burning transversely across the middle of the tongue, then burning and dryness in the whole of the mouth (aft. 20 m.). [*Stf.*]

Mucus in the mouth, with sweetish flat taste. [*Fz.*]

90. Taste in the mouth as if the stomach were deranged. [*L. Rkt.*]

Tobacco smoking is not relished. [*L. Rkt.*]

Tobacco when smoked tastes bitter. [*Fz.*]

Bread tastes bitter. [*L. Rkt.*]

The dry bread eaten tastes bitter (in the evening). [*Fz.*]

95. Dryness of the throat, with shooting. [*Fz.*]

Scraping in the throat. [*Stf.*]

In the throat such viscid mucus that he could not bring it up nor hawk it out, for eight days. [*L. Rkt.*]

Swallowing is difficult, as from swelling of the cervical glands. [*L. Rkt.*]

Hiccup (aft. 1½ h.). [*L. Rkt.—Hbg.*]

100. Hunger in the morning. [*Fz.*]

Frequent eruption. [*L. Rkt.—Hbg.*]

* Snuffed up into the nose.

1 Statement.

Frequent empty eructation. [*Stf.*]

When walking in the open air a rising up as of air, out of the stomach, and when it came to the mouth he must yawn a couple of times, then for an hour empty eructation and copious discharge of flatus. [*Stf.*]

Incomplete eructation up to the upper part of the chest. [*Fz.*]

105. Shivering from nausea. [*L. Rkt.*]

Nausea (aft. 1 h.). [*Hbg.*]

General discomfort and nausea. [*L. Rkt.*]

Nausea and loathing with shuddering (immediately). [*Fz.*]

Constant nausea and sickness in the fauces. [*L. Rkt.*]

110. Nausea, with aching in the forehead, and great flow of water into the mouth. [*L. Rkt.*]

Empty retching, with flow of water into the mouth (aft. ½, 1½ h.). [*L. Rkt.*]

The retching is always more violent the oftener it comes; the eyes become filled with water. [*L. Rkt.*]

When retching all the symptoms are increased, except the stupidity of the head, which decreases. [*L. Rkt.*]

Vomiting (an hour after the first retching), with great straining of the stomach, in five or six paroxysms, each time as if the head would burst in the region of the ears; only a little greenish, slightly sour, gastric juice is ejected (aft. 1½ h.). [*L. Rkt.*]

115. Vomiting, with great anxiety. [J. B. v. HELMONT, *Pharmac. mod.*, § 47.[1]]

Vomiting, diarrhœa—death. [G. W. WEDEL, *Amœnit. Mat. Med.*, p. 240.[2]]

Vomiting with great effort and violent pressure in the stomach; the effort to vomit takes away his breath, so as almost to suffocate him, and yet nothing but sourish water is ejected (aft. 2¼ h.) [*L. Rkt.*]

Vomiting, with sensation of straining of the stomach and violent compression in the epigastrium, and a similar feeling in the head (aft. 2¼ h.). [*L. Rkt.*]

There always remains some nausea in the stomach, with disinclination to work, sensation of want of thinking power and laziness. [*L. Rkt.*]

120. (After the vomiting alleviation of the head symptoms.) [*L. Rkt.*]

Fulness in the stomach, with hunger. [*Fz.*]

Pinching in the stomach (aft. 1½ h.). [*Hbg.*]

Slight pinching in the stomach or just ovet it. [*Fz.*]

In the stomach a pressure as with a blunt point. [*Hbg.*]

125. Troublesome pressure on the scrobiculus cordis, which prevents him feeling whether he is hungry or not—all day. [*L. Rkt.*]

Hard pressure on the region of the stomach and scrobiculus cordis for two successive days. [*L. Rkt.*]

Pressure on the gastric region on inspiring. [*L. Rkt.*]

---

1 General statement.

2 Case of poisoning of a strong man.

Feeling of constriction in the region of the diaphragm. [*L. Rkt.*]

From time to time sharp cutting round about in the epigastrium, which is always relieved by the discharge of some flatulence. [*L. Rkt.*]

130. Cutting in the epigastrium (aft. 2 h.). [*L. Rkt.*]

Horrible colic and vomiting. [Coste and Willemet, in *Samml. br. Abh. f. pr. A.*, iv, 2.[1]]

Fulness in the abdomen, and yet at the same time appetite and hunger. [*Fz.*]

Qualmishness in the abdomen, with repeated aching pain along the coronal suture (aft. 8 h.). [*Stf.*]

A painless and gentle working about in the abdomen. [*Stf.*]

135. Explosion of flatulence in the abdomen which is not discharged. [*Fz.*]

Pressure in the abdomen. [*L. Rkt.*]

Feeling of aching and painful pressing on the left side of the abdomen, observed when moving. [*L. Rkt.*]

Single painful sensations in the left side of the abdomen, obliquely below the navel. [*Stf.*]

Before the stool cutting in the abdomen and sharp stitches in the rectum from above downwards (in the morning). [*L. Rkt.*]

140. He has hurried urging to stool (1½ hour after the first stool) with cutting in the abdomen and rectum before and during the (looser) stool. [*L. Rkt.*]

Stool in hard small pieces. [*L. Rkt.*]

The usual morning stool was delayed for some hours, and then it was scanty, yellow like an egg (slimy) and of slender form. [*Stf.*]

Diarrhœa. [Coste and Willemet, l. c.]

Diarrhœic, viscid slimy, as it were resinous stool; ascarides pass in shaggy masses of mucus, for six days. [*Stf.*]

145. Stool whitish-grey and ash coloured, with bloody mucus on the top.

Pressure on the bladder, during and after urinating. [*Fz.*]

Constant urging to urinate. [*Fz.*]

(A drawing in the urethra.)

A wild, acute pain in the left groin, which darted quickly through the urethra into the glans penis, and there a smarting, contractive, violent internal pain remained for a long time. [*Stf.*]

150. Premature birth, expulsion of the fœtus.[3] [Ray, *Hist. univ. Plant.*, i.]

* * *

(Stuffed coryza; the left nostril is stopped up). [*Stf.*]

(Violent sneezing.)

A tickling runs through the nose (as from the positive galvanic pole), which, after ineffectual urging, causes sneezing and a flow of clear fluid. [*Stf.*]

Sensation as if the breath and saliva were hot, but without dry feeling in the mouth. [*L. Rkt.*]

---

1 General statement.

2 This represents Ray's statement that A. is abortifacient.

155. Repeated coughing on account of mucus in the chest, which first rises up into the throat and causes difficulty of breath, and at length cough, with expectoration. [*Fz.*]

Inspiration causes an irritation in the throat, which excites cough. [*L. Rkt.*]

Very short breath (at night).

(Angry and cross before the cough.)

Great expectoration of mucus by hawking and coughing.

160. (At the commencement of the cough the respiration is whistling.)

Short breath ; the throat is constricted and this causes hacking cough. [*L. Rkt.*]

Obtuse stitch, impeding respiration, quite low down, as if in the left lung, at every inspiration (aft. 15 h.). [*L. Rkt.*]

He can only breathe short and by jerks on account of stitches and constriction in the larynx ; short coughing relieved the constriction for a little time. [*L. Rkt.*]

Obtuse stitch on the left near the scrobiculus cordis (aft. 9 h). [*L. Rkt.*]

165. **In the right lobe of the lung stitches when inspiring** (aft. 12 h.). [*L. Rkt.*]

Frequent, obtuse **stitches in both lungs, during inspiration,** for eight days. [*L. Rkt.*]

Stitches in the chest during respiration (aft. 24 h.). [*L. Rkt.*]

When he takes a rather deep breath immediately obtuse stitches in both lungs. [*L. Rkt.*]

Sensation of pressure on the whole of the chest. [*L. Rkt.*]

170. In the region of the last ribs a sharp pressure as if with the back of a knife. [*Hbg.*]

In the right side of the chest a severe, forcible pressing at regular intervals (aft. $1\frac{1}{2}$ h.). [*Hbg.*]

Visible twitching and palpitation in the muscles of the region of the clavicle. [*Hbg.*]

Stretching pain in the left side (aft. $\frac{3}{4}$ h.). [*Fz.*]

Sensation as if the left lung were constricted or cut into by a string or wire. [*L. Rkt.*]

175. Pain round about in both lungs, as if they were constricted by a sharp wire. [*L. Rkt.*]

In the right side of the chest a burning sensation, more externally than internally. [*Hbg.*]

Burning pain with shooting in the sacrum, while sitting. [*Fz.*]

From one crista ilii to the other over the spine, pain as if the flesh of the muscles were rent outwards, in tearing jerks, when walking. [*L. Rkt.*]

Paralytic pain, as if bruised, in the back, as long as he remains erect, stands or sits, but does not lie. [*L. Rkt.*]

180. Bruised pain in the back. [*L. Rkt.*]

Obtuse stitches under the scapulæ. [*L. Rkt.*]

At the inner border of the right scapula a pain as from a knock or blow, especially felt on touching the scapula or drawing it inwards (aft. 25 h.). [*Stf.*]

Pain in the nape on the left side as if by over-exertion a bundle of muscular fibres had got out of their place, the pain then spreads over the head and shoulders (aft. 6 h.). [*Stf.*]

Paralytic pain in one of the muscles of the nape, as if it were bruised, on moving the neck. [*L. Rkt.*]

185. On the muscles of the nape a sensation as from a too tight neck cloth, and as if a blunt knife were pressed on it. [*Fz.*]

Feeling of weight on the neck and sensation as if the muscles were compressed by bandages. [*Hbg.*]

Spasmodic contraction of the left cervical muscles, with perceptible bending of the head to that side. [*Stf.*]

Violent tearing stitches in both shoulders during motion and rest. [*L. Rkt.*]

In the axilla, as if in the axillary glands, a rapidly occurring obtuse pain. [*Stf.*]

190. A pressure in the left axilla, as with a rough piece of wood. [*Hbg.*]

Under the right axilla towards the front an itching, as from a flea-bite. [*Fz.*]

Pain in the shoulder, as if dislocated, on moving the arm. [*Fz.*]

On the deltoid muscle of the upper arm a contractive tensive pain, on lying the hand on the table, and also when it is left lying there. [*Fz.*]

Paralytic weakness in the arm. [*L. Rkt.*]

195. He cannot keep the arm lying on the table long without discomfort and feeling of exhaustion ; but when he allows the arm to hang down he feels nothing. [*L. Rkt.*]

Aching tearing in the left arm in all positions. [*L. Rkt.*]

Drawing paralytic pain in the left wrist-joint. [*Stf.*]

Quick, drawing burning pain from the wrist through the thumb and index finger (aft. 3 h.). [*Hbg.*]

A drawing in the fingers, in the evening, while lying in bed.

200. Occasional twitching tearing pains in the upper and lower extremities. [*L. Rkt.*]

Bruised feeling and sometimes transient painful tearing in the upper and lower extremities. [*L. Rkt.*]

Painful sensation on the hip. [*Fz.*]

In the right hip an obtuse aching. [*Hbg.*]

In the head of the left thigh and beyond, especially when walking, a (drawing tensive) pain. [*Stf.*]

205. In the hips a drawing aching pain (when walking). [*Hbg.*]

When walking or moving after sitting, as also when touching, a dull pain in the hip-joint and in the middle of the thigh. [*Stf.*]

Sensation from the right hip-joint to the knee, as if the limb were going to sleep. [*Stf.*]

When he treads he has a violent pain in the hip-joint and in the middle of the thigh, and the limb is as if paralysed by it ; he cannot tread properly. [*Stf.*]

Sudden, digging pain in the upper muscles of the left thigh. [*Fz.*]

210. Tearing, shooting pain in the left thigh. [*L. Rkt.*]

Spasmodic contraction of the muscles of the right thigh, near the knee, which goes off on stretching out the leg. [*Fz.*]

A drawing in the knee.

A drawing in the tendons of the hough, in the evening while lying in bed.

(Clucking in the hough.)

215. Violent tearing stitches in the knees, on moving and when at rest. [*L. Rkt.*]

Fatigue of the thighs on going upstairs, for many days. [*L. Rkt.*]

Exhausted feeling in the thighs as if he had not obtained rest by sleep. [*L. Rkt.*]

Feeling of weakness in the knees with visible staggering when walking, when he does not take great care (aft. 15 m.). [*Stf.*]

Exhaustion and bruised feeling of the thighs and knees, as in a fit of ague. [*L. Rkt.*]

220. Restlessness in the left knee-joint, which forces him to move (aft. ½ h.). [*Fz.*]

Above the right hough a pressure as with some hard blunt substance. [*Hbg.*]

The left leg is as if asleep, and the foot, as when very cold, insensible and as if dead. [*Fz.*]

Visible twitching and palpitation in the muscles of the calf. [*Hbg.*]

In the left tibia sensation as if bruised. [*Hbg.*]

225. In the sole of the foot quick shooting pains (aft. 3½ h.). [*Hbg.*]

A drawing in the toes, in the evening when lying in bed.

(On both feet the little toes are painful as if frozen.) [*Stf.*]

Over-sensitiveness of all the nerves; when he thinks (which he cannot help doing constantly) of someone scratching gently with the finger-tip or nail on linen or something similar, a very disagreeable sensation runs through him, which for an instant stops all his thoughts and actions (aft. 11 h.). [*L. Rkt.*]

After dinner great fatigue. [*Stf.*]

230. Every afternoon great exhaustion and constant yawning. [*L. Rkt.*]

Laziness, slowness, and dislike to all work. [*L. Rkt.*]

General feeling of exhaustion and sometimes bruised feeling. [*L. Rkt.*]

Agility in all the limbs; he does not know that he has a body. [*Fz.*]

When walking in the open air the headache, heat of the cheeks and sleepy crossness go off. [*Stf.*]

235. When walking in the open air he seems to be floating like a disembodied spirit. [*Fz.*]

Frequent yawning. [*L. Rkt.*]

Towards evening he becomes so weak, with sick feeling, that when he sits upright he feels as if he would every moment succumb and die, he must lie down in bed. [*L. Rkt.*]

Very great drowsiness by day (aft. 12, 13, 14 d.). [*L. Rkt.*]

Drowsiness, crossness. [*Stf.*]

240. (On alternate nights restless sleep ; he cannot readily fall asleep.)

During sleep such a violent shooting in the dorsum of the left foot, that he dreamt he got a stab during the application of a blister ; on awaking he felt nothing. [*Hbg.*]

At night vexatious and annoying dreams of being put to shame, &c. [*Fz.*]

In the evening, in bed, an ebullition in the blood that prevented him going to sleep, for two hours.

Shaking all over the body (immediately). [*Fz.*]

245. Slight shiver over the body (aft. ½, 1½ h.), [*L. Rkt.*]

Shiver (with loathing and nausea) (immediately). [*Fz.*]

A rigor in the back (which came on suddenly on biting a hard crust). [*Stf.*]

Rigor and chilliness, without thirst. [*L. Rkt.*]

Uninterrupted chilliness, goose-skin ; hands and face cold, blueness of complexion. [*L. Rkt.*]

250. The hands are icy cold, but the arms and the rest of the body warm, yet covered with goose-skin, and he is very chilly. [*L. Rkt.*]

In the evening rigor with extreme weakness, especially in the knees and sacrum, without thirst; the hands are cold, but the rest of the body as warm as usual, the forehead, however, hot. [*L. Rkt.*]

Shivering with heat in the face. [*L. Rkt.*]

All day long chilliness ; when he sits still or lies and keeps himself covered, he feels nothing (except a pain in the eyes, pressure in the forehead and on the scrobiculus cordis, and sometimes external heat) ; but when he moves about in the room ever so little, or sits out in the open air without moving, he is excessively chilly, almost entirely without thirst ; but when he walks quickly out of doors or comes from the open air into the warm room, or when he becomes heated by animated conversation in the room, or after dinner as also when lying in the warm bed, he feels well and warm enough, he has, indeed, some heat with thirst for beer. [*L. Rkt.*]

Chill when drinking. [*L. Rkt.*]

255. Cold sensation on the body, as if a cold wind blew on him ; at the same time he felt cold to the touch, almost always with goose-skin ; after a few hours warmth returned somewhat increased (in the afternoon), with slimy mouth, dryness in the throat and thirst ; hereafter a similar coldness, and in the evening (an hour before bed-time) again increased warmth, which lasted in bed, during which he must put the hands outside the bed-clothes, also with great dryness on the palate. [*Fz.*]

All day long fever : in the forenoon chilliness, which does not go off either by moving in the open air or by external warmth ; after the midday siesta external feeling of heat, with internal rigor and thirst. [*L. Rkt.*]

When seated and not well covered up, or when he moves, immediately chilliness, but when he covers himself up he instantly becomes hot, though sometimes with rigor. [*L. Rkt.*]

After the cessation of the hot feeling, while heat of the head and face remains, chilliness comes on, so that he shivers on the slightest movement. [*L. Rkt.*]

Heat of the forehead and scalp, the rest of the body of normal temperature, with shivering and chilliness without thirst, and strong and quick pulse. [*L. Rkt.*]

260. After the chilliness feeling of heat and actual heat, especially of the face and palms, whereupon the pains in the ear return. [*L. Rkt.*]

Feeling of warmth, as if sweat would break out (aft. 4 h.). [*L. Rkt.*]

Unusual warmth of the body all day (aft. 24 h.). [*Fz.*]

Slight sweat only on the upper part of the body and the upper extremities. [*Hbg.*]

In the evening in bed, immediately after lying down, perspiration.

265. Profuse night sweat. [*L. Rkt.*]

Warm perspiration, even when sitting still. [*L. Rkt.*]

He perspires very readily from a slight cause. [*L. Rkt.*]

Melancholy peevishness.

Lachrymose sadness and anxiety. [*Stf.*]

270. Great gaiety (aft. 6 to 12 h.), alternating with calmness or even sadness for some moments. [*L. Rkt.*]

AURUM.[1]

(*Gold*, the well-known metal.)

Just as superstition, impure observations, and credulous assumptions have been the source of innumerable falsely ascribed remedial virtues of medicines in the Meteria Medica ; in like manner physicians by their failure to resort to the test of experiment and by their futile theorizing, have quite as unreasonably denied the possession of any medicinal power whatever to many substances that are very powerful, and consequently of great curative virtue ; and by so doing they have deprived us of these remedies.

In this place I will only speak of *gold*, and not of this metal altered by the ordinary chemical processes, consequently not of it dissolved by the action of acids nor precipitated from its solution (fulminating gold), both of which have been declared to be, if not useless, then absolutely noxious, apparently because they cannot be taken without dangerous consequences when given in what is called a *justa dosis*, or, in other words, in excessive quantity.

No ! I speak of pure gold not altered by chemical manipulations.

Modern physicians have pronounced this to be quite inactive ; they have at length expunged it out of all their Materia Medicas, and thereby deprived us of all its mighty curative virtues.

"It is incapable of solution in our gastric juices, hence it must be quite powerless and useless." This was their theoretical conclusion, in the medical art, as is well known, such *theoretical dicta* have always availed more than *convincing proof*. Because they did not question experience, the only possible guide in the medical art which is found on experience alone ; *because it was easier to make mere assertions*, therefore they usually preferred bold dicta, theoretical empty assumptions and arbitrary maxims to solid truth.

It is no excuse for them that the older physicians have also deemed gold to be quite useless and powerless, that, for example, FABRICIUS (in *Obs. Med.*) says :—"What effect can the low temperature of our stomach have on gold-leaf, seeing that it is unaltered by the most intense heat ?" Or NICHOLAS MONARDES (*De Ferro*, pp. 32, 33) :—"Patients may take my word for it, and spare themselves the expense of employing gold as a medicine—they can never obtain any medicinal virtue from it for their maladies." Or ALSTON (*Mat. Med.*, i, p. 69) :—"Seeing that gold in its metallic state cannot be dissolved or altered by the vital power, it can consequently have no medicinal action, but what it exerts on the intestines by virtue of its weight, hardness, and mechanical form." Or, lastly, J. F. GMELIN (*Appar.*

---

1 From vol. iv, 2nd edit., 1825.

Med. Min., i, p. 445) :—"As gold is not destructible, not resolvable into vapour, and is hence incapable of union with juices of the animal body, therefore it cannot possess curative virtues."*

Nor are they excused when they adduce a number of other older physicians as deniers of the medicinal properties of gold, and refer to such names as ANT. MUSA BRASSAVOLUS, FEL. PLATERUS, HIER. CARDANUS, JO. BRAVUS PETRAFIT, FRANC. PIC. MIRANDOLA, MERINUS MERCENIUS, DURETUS, CAMERARIUS, CORDOSUS, CONRINGIUS, LEMERY, ANGELUS SALA, or JOH. SCHRODER, who in other matters is so extremely credulous.

They were all wrong, and so are all the modern physicians.
Gold has great, peculiar medicinal powers.

At first I allowed myself to be deterred by these deniers from hoping for medicinal properties in pure gold ; but as I could not persuade myself to consider any metal whatsoever as destitute of curative powers, I employed it at first in solution. Hence the few symptoms from the solution of gold recorded below. I then gave, in cases where the symptoms guided me to the homœopathic employment, the quintillionth or sextillionth of a grain of gold in solution for a dose, and observed curative effects somewhat similar to those I afterwards experienced from pure gold.

But because, as a rule, I do not like, when I can avoid it, to give the metals dissolved in acids (when I cannot avoid doing so, I prefer their solution in vegetable acids), and least of all in mineral acids, as that detracts from their noble simplicity, for they must assuredly undergo some alteration in their properties when acted on by these acids—as we must perceive on a comparison of the curative effects of corrosive sublimate with those of the black oxyde of mercury—I was delighted to find a number of Arabian physicians unanimously testifying to the medicinal powers of gold in a finely pulverized form, particularly in some serious morbid conditions, in some of which the solution of gold had already been of great use to me. This circumstance inspired me with great confidence in the assertions of the Arabians.

The first trace of this we meet with in the eighth century, when GEBER (*De Alcimia traditio*, Argent. ap. *Zetzner*, 1698, lib. ii, p. iii, cap. 32) vaunts gold as a "materia laetificans et en juventute corpus conservans."

Towards the end of the tenth century SERAPION the younger (*De Simplicibus Comment.*, Venet. fol. ap. Junt., 1550, cap. 415, p. 192), recommends it in these words :—"Powdered gold is useful in melancholy and weakness of the heart."

Then at the commencement of the eleventh century AVICENNA (*Canon.*, lib. ii, cap. 79) says :—"Powdered gold is one of the medicines against melancholy, removes fœtor of the breath, is, even when given internally, a remedy for falling out of the hair, strengthens the eyes, is

* It was very stupid to attempt to decide theoretically the question whether gold *can* possess remedial properties—the only proper thing to do was to convince oneself by trial and experience whether it had remedial powers or not. If it has curative virtues then all the theoretical denials are ridiculous.

useful in pain of the heart and palpitation, and is uncommonly serviceable in dyspnœa."*

Abulkasem (Albucasis), at the commencement of the twelfth century, is the first who describes (in *Libro Servitoris de præp. Med.*, p. 242) the preparation of this gold powder in these words :—"The gold is rubbed on a rough linen cloth in a basin filled with water, and the fine powder that falls to the bottom of the water is to be employed for administration." Johann von St. Amand (in the thirteenth century) describes the same method of its preparation (in the Appendix to Mesue, *Opera*, Venet., 1561, p. 245,4 E.).

This mode of preparation was imitated by Zacutus, the Portuguese, and he records (*Histor. Medic.*, lib. i, obs. 333) the history of the case of a nobleman who had long been troubled by melancholy ideas, whom he cured in a month by the *sole* use of a fine powder obtained by rubbing gold on a grind-stone.

I may refer here to the laudations of gold powder and of gold by Jo. Platearius (*quæst. Therap.*), Rodericus a Castro (*De Meteor. Microcosm.*, cap. 3), Abraham a Porta leonis (*Dialog. de Auro*), Zaccharias a Puteo, Joh. Dan. Mylius (*Anatomia Auri*), Horn (*Ephem. Nat. Cur.*, Dec. ii, ann. 3, obs. 159), Fr. Baco (*Historia Vitæ et Mortis*), Fr. Joseph Burrhi (*Epist. 4 ad. Thom. Barthol. de Oculis*), Jo. Jacob Waldschmiedt (*Diss. de Auro*, Marb., 1685), Chph. Helwig (*Diss. de Auro ejusque in Medic. viribus*, Gryphisv., 1703), Lemnius, Pet. Forestus, Ol. Borrichius, Rolfinck, Andr. Lagner, Ettmuller, Tackius, Helcher (*Diss. de Auro*, Jen., 1730), Poterius, J. D. Horstius, Hollerius, Hœfer, and Zwelfer (*Pharm. August*). But leaving these authorities out of the question, I thought I might attach more value to the testimony of the Arabians as to the curative powers of finely powdered gold than to the theoretical unfounded doubts of the moderns, so I triturated the finest gold-leaf (its fineness is 23 carats, 6 grains) with 100 parts of milk-sugar for a full hour, for internal medical use.

I will not attempt to determine if in this fine powder the gold is only triturated smaller, or if by this energetic trituration it has become to some degree oxydated. Enough, that in proving it on some healthy adults, 100 grains of this powder (containing one grain of gold), and on others, 200 grains (containing two grains of gold), dissolved in water, sufficed to excite very great alterations in the health and morbid symptoms, which are recorded below.

From these it will be perceived that the assertions of the Arabians are not without foundation, as even small doses of this metal given in the form mentioned caused even in healthy adults morbid states very similar to those cured (in unconscious *homœopathic* manner) by those Orientals, who deserve credit for their discovery of remedies.

Since then I have cured quickly and permanently of melancholia resembling that produced by gold many persons who had serious thoughts of committing suicide, by small doses, which for the whole

* The Arabic word for this last has two meanings ; according to the accentuation of the word it means either "taking to himself," or "dyspnœa." Experience of the curative power of gold shows the last to be the true meaning.

treatment contained altogether from the $\frac{3}{100}$th to the $\frac{9}{100}$th of a grain of gold ; and in like manner I have cured several other severe affections, resembling the symptoms caused by gold. I do not doubt that much higher attenuations of the powder and much smaller doses of gold would amply suffice for the same purpose.

* * *

Some time after writing the above I had an opportunity of convincing myself that a hundred-fold higher attenuation of the above preparation (made by triturating gold with a hundread parts of milk-sugar), consequently $\frac{1}{10000}$th part of a grain of gold for a dose, showed itself not less powerful in a curative point of view, especially in caries of the palatal and nasal bones, caused by the abuse of mercury prepared with mineral acids.* In the subjoined schema the symptoms of gold homœopathic to these affections will be readily observed.

By further triturations and dilution the power of gold is still more developed and spiritualized, so that I now employ for all curative purposes only a very small portion of a grain of the quadrillion-fold dilution for a dose.

Would our physicians, by their customary method of fabricating the virtues of medicines out of airy hypothesis, and constructing a materia medica of such fanciful materials, ever have discovered this remarkable power of a metal which their learned speculations had consigned to the category of utterly powerless substances ? And which other of the favourite methods of our materia-medica-manufacturers would have taught us these remedial properties of gold ? These have been clearly and certainly taught to the homœopathic physician by the symptoms it produces, which resemble the morbid states it is capable of curing.

Poor, fabulous materia medica of the ordinary stamp, how far dost thou lag behind the revelation which medicines in their action on the healthy human body clearly make by the production of morbid symptoms, which the homœopathic physician can employ with infallible certainty for the cure of natural disease !

The duration of the action of gold in not extremely small doses is at least twenty-one days.

[HAHNEMANN'S disciples who helped him with this proving are—FRANZ, GROSS, FR. HAHNEMANN, HEMPEL, HERRMANN, LANGHAMMER, MICHLER, WISLICENUS.

The only old-school authorities referred to for symptoms are—

Misc. Nat. Cur., Dec. ii, ann. 6.
Ephem. Nat. Car., Cent. 10.
HOFFMANN, FR., *Med. Rat. Syst.*, ii.
LUDOVICI, *Pharmac. Med. Sec. appl.*, Gotha, 1685.
Pharmac. Wirtemb., ii.
SCHULZE, J. H., *Prælectiones in Phar.*

The 1st Edit. has 313 symptoms, this 2nd Edit. 379. In the *Chr. Kr.* there are 461.]

---

* This remedial power of the internal employment of gold in the evil effects of mercury was observed by ANT. CHALMETEUS (in *Enchiridion Chirurg.*, p. 402).

SOLUTION OF GOLD.[1]

Drawing pain in the forehead (aft. 2 h.).

A tickling itching on the forehead (aft. 1 h.).

Tearing pain in the left eye.

Redness and itching inflammation on the nose, which afterwards desquamates.

5. Red swelling of the left side of the nose; the cavity of the nose is ulcerated deep in, with a dry, yellowish scab, with sensation of internal stoppage of the nose, although the air passes readily through it.

Red swelling on and under the right nostril; in the nostril itself there is a painless ulcer-scab; it feels to him stopped up, although the air passes through it. [*Mch.*]

Externally in the upper part of the nose a burning (and somewhat itching) pain.

A crawling in the interior of the nose, as if something were running about in it.

Discharge of a greenish-yellow matter from the nose, without bad smell, for 7 days (aft. 10 d.).

10. (Ringing in the ears) (aft. 6 h.).

(After the ringing in the ears a kind of dulness of hearing, as if the ears internally were wide and hollow, owing to which nothing was heard distinctly.)

Twitching toothache sometimes on one side sometimes in the upper incisors.

Twitching toothache also in the anterior upper row of teeth. [*Mch.*]

Distension of the abdomen.

15. His breathing is very short, and as if the larynx were stopped up, for some days.

(A couple of stitches just above the heart.)

(Swelling in the wrist, without pain *per se*, only a tension on bending back the hand; on grasping, however, he has stitches in it.)

Tearing pain in the middle finger (after dinner.)

AURUM.

(Gold-leaf.)

More acute thinking faculty, and more accurate memory.*

Intellectual labours affected him much; he felt exhausted.

On stooping, vertigo, as if all turned round in a circle; on assuming an erect position it went off each time (aft. 40 h.). [*Lr.*]

* Curative action.

1 [This is called *Aurum muriaticum* in the *Chr. Kr.* It will be noticed that the usual order of the schema is departed from here, the nose coming before the ear. In the *Chr. Kr.* the usual arrangement is adopted and the signs of parenthesis omitted.]

On walking in the open-air there occurred a vertigo as if he would always fall to the left side and was intoxicated, which obliged him to go to bed, and for some time whilst lying in bed it returned on the slightest movement (aft. 43 h.). [*Lr.*]

5. In the morning, on rising, confusion of the head ; great weight in the occiput. [*Ws.*]

Confusion of the head. [*Hrr.*]

When standing he is suddenly seized with vertigo, which compels him to sit down (aft. 28 h.). [*Hrr.*]

Headache as from commencing catarrh.

Headache (increasing from morning onwards), as if the brain were bruised, which by merely thinking and reading, but especially by continued talking and writing, is increased to the extremest violence, so that the ideas become confused, and it is only by the greatest effort that anything connected can be spoken or written ; but when he ceases to speak, reflect and write, the headache always departs ; at 7 p. m. it spontaneously ceases entirely (aft. 6 h).

10. Headache, which is felt partly like bruised pain, partly in one portion of the brain, sometimes like painful pressure, sometimes like a tearing, increases from morning onwards and goes off about 3 p. m. (aft. 24 h.).

(One-sided headache like digging, boring, pecking, in the morning immediately after waking, increased by coughing and bending the head backwards.)

One-sided, sharp beating, hacking headache.

Tearing pressure in the head, here and there, especially in the forehead, with giddy feeling. [*Hrr.*]

A prickling sensation in the sinciput.

15. Headache, anteriorly in the forehead and temples, deep in the brain, a very severe tearing, which is allayed in the open air. [*Gss.*]

Aching stupefying headache, as if excited by a strong wind (aft. 11 h.). [*Lr.*]

Pressure in the left side of the forehead (aft. 1¼ h.). [*Hrr.*]

Aching tearing from the right side of the occiput to the right side of the forehead (aft. 3 h.). [*Hrr.*]

Tearing pressure in the left side of the crown, worse on movement. [*Hrr.*]

20. Tearing in the left temple. [*Fz.*]

Fine tearing in the right side of the crown (aft. 3 h.). [*Hrr.*]

Tearing pain in the left side of the crown (aft. ½ h.). [*Hrr.*]

Tearing pain in the left side of the forehead, worse on movement. [*Hrr.*]

Fine tearing in the forehead. [*Hrr.*]

Tearing cutting pain in the right side of the crown (aft. 17 d.). [*Hrr.*]

Fine tearing from the right side of the occiput through the brain to the forehead, worse on movement (aft. 1 h.). [*Hrr.*]

Tearing pressure in the right side of the occiput. [*Hrr.*]

A roaring and rushing in the head, as if he were seated beside rushing water (aft. 15 d.).

Rush of blood to the head.

30. Rush of blood to the brain (aft. $\frac{3}{4}$ h.).

Violent rush of blood in the head, on stooping, which goes off again on rising up (aft. 8 d.). [*Hrr.*]

Shooting on the frontal bone, like a slow drawing (aft. 6 h.). [*Fz.*]

A sharp stitch on the centre of the forehead, where the hair begins.

Needle-pricks on the forehead externally (aft. 24 h.). [*Hrr.*]

35. A small osseous tumour on the right side of the vertex, with boring pains *per se*, but worse when touched.

A small osseous tumour on the left side of the forehead superiorly.

Pressure on and in the left side of the forehead externally and internally (aft. 10 h.). [*Hrr.*]

Painful pressure in the temples.

Pressure on the left temple (aft 32 h.). [*Hrr.*]

40. Aching externally on the left temple, worse when touched (aft. $\frac{1}{4}$ h.). [*Hrr.*]

On lying down the cranial bones are painful as if broken to pieces, so that it took away all his vital energy.

(His head is shaken sideways and up and down.)

Feeling of weakness and aching in the eyes.

Pressure from without inwards on the left eye (aft. 8 d.). [*Hrr.*]

45. Pressive pain from above downwards on the right eyeball. [*Hrr.*]

Pressive pain from without inwards on the right eyeball, worse when touched (aft. 6 h.). [*Hrr.*]

Aching in the eyes as if a foreign body had got into it.

On looking, a sensation in the eyes as when one has been much heated, as if the blood pressed strongly on the optic nerves.

(A kind of burning in the eyes.)

50. An obtuse stitch outwards on the lower part of the left orbit.

Extreme pressure in the left orbit almost like a spasm, on its internal aspect posteriorly. [*Gss.*]

Fine tearing in the right orbit in the vicinity of the external canthus (aft. 5 h.). [*Hrr.*]

Sensation of pressing out of the left eyeball in its inner and upper angle. [*Fz.*]

Tension in the eyes which interferes with vision (aft. 1 h.). [*Hrr.*]

55. **Extreme tension in the eyes with diminution of the visual power; he cannot distinguish anything distinctly, because he sees everything double and one object seems to run into another; the tensive pain is worse when he fixes the eyes on something, and less severe when he closes them** (aft. 9 d.). [*Hrr.*]

Several single stitches in the inner canthus of the left eye and in the eyelid itself (aft. 36 h.). [*Hrr.*]

Contraction of the pupils (aft. 2, 3¾ h.). [*Lr.*]

Dilatation of the pupils (aft 3½ h.). [*Lr.*]

It seems as if the upper half of the right eye were covered by a black body, so that he can only see with the lower half objects below him, but those above remain invisible. [*Hrr.*]

60. **It seems as if a black veil were drawn over the eyes, whereby distinct vision is impaired** (aft. 6 d.). [*Hrr.*]

Sparks of fire appear suddenly before the eyes.*

A smarting pain on the left upper eyelid.

A painless smoth pimple on the right lower tarsal edge.

Swelling of the lower eyelids. [*Fr. H—n.*]

65. (Bluish internal canthus.)

The face swollen and shining, as from perspiration; the eyes as if distended and protruding.

On the right side of the face itching needle-pricks.

Drawing tearing on the left side of the face (aft. 2 h.). [*Ws.*]

In the face, on the neck, and on the chest an eruption of small pimples with purulent apices, for some hours.

70. Excessive tearing in the frontal process of the malar bone. [*Gss.*]

A tearing in the right zygomatic arch. [*Gss.*]

Aching tearing in the left external meatus auditorius (aft. ¾ h.). [*Hrr.*]

Humming before the left ear.

Crepitation in the left ear.

75. In the morning in bed roaring in the ears.

A tickling formication internally in the alæ nasi, as during coryza (aft. 2 h.). [*Lr.*]

A tickling formication internally in the alæ nasi, compelling him to scratch (aft. 2½ and 21 h.). [*Lr.*]

Sensation of stoppage of the nose as in stuffed coryza, and yet he could draw air through it very well (aft. 2½ h.). [*Lr.*]

The nasal bone of the right side and the neighbouring part of the upper jaw are painful to the touch, especially where the facial nerve comes out.

80. After walking in the open air the nose swells in the room.

Twitching on the septum of the nose from above downwards. [*Ws.*]

He cannot get air through the nose; the nostrils are ulcerated and agglutinated and painful.

The nostril appears to him to be stopped up, and yet he can get air through it. [*Fr. H—n.*]

A transient smell of brandy in the nose, with oppression of the chest.

85. (On blowing the nose he perceives a fœtid smell in the nose.)

Extremely sensitive smell; everything smells too strong (aft 48 h.).

Smarting pain in the lower part of the nose. [*Fr. H—n.*]

* Sparks of fire in the eyes are the usual prodromata of partial paralysis of the optic nerve, or obscuration of the sight by black spots always hovering before the eye. I cured one such case by means of gold.

Smarting pain in the lower part of the nose, so that tears came into the eyes, as when strong sunlight excites an inclination to sneeze, or during exalted religious sadness, or the highest degree of compassion. [*Fz.*]

Sore feeling in the nose. [*Fr. H—n.*]

90. Sore pain in both nostrils, especially on taking hold of them.[1]

Ulcerated scab in the right nostril, almost painless, yellowish, and almost dry. [*Fr. H—n.*]

Dark, brownish-red, slightly elevated spots on the nose, which are the seat of aching pain only when touched (aft. 24 h.). [*Hrr.*]

Swelling on and under the right nostril, with redness. [*Fr. H—n.*]

Both cheeks, lips, and nose are much swollen (in the morning).

95. **Swelling of one cheek** with drawing and tearing in the upper and lower jaw, and a sensation as of grumbling and hacking in the teeth, which feel longer.

Tearing pressure in the right lower jaw, especially in its ascending ramus, which goes off by pressing on it (aft. $\frac{1}{2}$ h.). [*Hrr.*]

On the outer border of the lower jaw intermittent obtuse shooting (aft. 24 h.). [*Gss.*]

In the right half of the chin a tearing. [*Gss.*]

(On the red of the under lip a burning vesicle.)

100. Dull aching pain *per se* and when swallowing in the gland beneath the angle of the lower jaw, as in a swelling of the cervical glands (aft. 3 h.).

Pain in one of the submaxillary glands as if it were swollen.

The gland beneath the ear lobe (parotid glands) is very painful when touched, like a gland pressed and squeezed between the fingers.

Tearing pressure on the right side and lower part of the neck, near the clavicle (aft. 14 d.). [*Hrr.*]

(A jerking, tearing shooting on the external cervical muscles of the left side.) (aft. 7 d.).

105. Ulcer on the gums and swollen cheeks (aft 4 d.).

Swelling of the gums on the posterior right upper molars, with aching sore pain when touched and when eating, whereby the pain extends to the two backmost molar teeth, where it becomes an obtuse tearing (aft. 14 d.). [*Hrr.*]

On chewing the upper incisors are very sensitive.

(Single stitches in the teeth.)

Sudden attack of painful loose teeth, even the incisors.

110. The molars feel on edge (aft. $\frac{1}{2}$ h.).

Twitching pain in the upper row of teeth. [*Fr. H—n.*]

An agreeable milky taste in the mouth.

Sweetness in the fore part of the tongue.

Insipid taste in the mouth.

115. Putrid taste in the mouth, when not eating, like high game.

Sometimes a sourish taste in the mouth (aft. $2\frac{1}{2}$ h.).

---

1 This symptom, though without name attached, is among the "Observations of others."

Bitter taste in the mouth with feeling of dryness (aft. 8 h.). [*Lr.*]

Pleasantly sweetish saliva collects in the mouth. [*Fz.*]

A kind of aching in the region of the palate, lasting several hours.

120. (Attacks of stretching asunder of the gullet, as if going to vomit, but without nausea.)

(Sore throat, like shooting soreness, only when swallowing) (aft. 7 d.).

(Much mucus in the fauces, for several days.)

Putrid smell from the mouth.

Smell from the mouth like old cheese.

125. Bad smell from the mouth, in the evening and at night, which he is not conscious of himself.

His food tastes well, but does not quite satisfy his appetite, and he could again eat immediately.[1]

Whilst eating the anxiety goes off. [*Fz.*]

Great thirst for six days. [*Fr. H—n.*]

Nausea in the stomach and throat. [*Hrr.*]

130. Scrobiculus cordis as if swollen; the whole epigastrium also swollen, and when pressed on, or when she laces herself tight, there is shooting there.

Pain in the stomach as from hunger.

(At noon, aching in the region of the stomach.)

Aching in the abdomen.

Aching (continued) in the subcostal region, as from flatulence, especially after taking something (food or drink), often increased by movement and walking; it goes off at last almost without any discharge of flatus.

135. Weight in the abdomen, with icy cold feet and hands.

Aching in the abdomen and heaving as though she would vomit. [*Fr. H—n.*]

Tensive pressure in the hypogastrium just below the navel and on both sides in the lumbar regions, with feeling of fulness, most severe under the navel (aft. 53 h.). [*Hrr.*]

Tensive pressure in the hypogastrium on ooth sides in the lumbar regions, but most severe just below the navel, with call to stool (aft. 6 d.). [*Hrr.*]

Single tearings in the right side of the abdomen up to beneath the ribs, as if all there were smashed, which compels him to bend double, when sitting (aft. 36 h.). [*Fz.*]

140. In the afternoon shooting in the left side of the abdomen, like stitches in the spleen.

Pinching pain in the hypogastrium, sometimes here, sometimes there (aft. 12 h.). [*Hrr.*]

Pain like contraction in the abdomen.

Flatulent colic about midnight; much flatulence is quickly developed, which cannot find an exit, and painfully rises up here and

1 This symptom also is among "Observations of others," without name attac

there, presses and resists and causes anxiety, equally felt when at rest and when moving.

Flatulent colic soon after the lightest, most moderate meal.

145. Rumbling in the abdomen.

Grumbling in the abdomen.

Grumbling and rumbling in the abdomen (aft. 1 h.). [*Hrr.*]

Grumbling in the abdomen. [*Hrr.*]

Discharge of much fœtid flatus (aft. 8 h.). [*Hrr.*]

150. Colic.* [*Ephem. Nat. Cur.*, Dec. ii, ann. 6, app., p. 6.[1]]

Pain as if bruised in the right hypogastrium, when sitting, which goes off on rising up and when he draws up the thighs (aft. 24 h.). [*Fz.*]

Pain in the groin as from a swollen inguinal gland.

Protrusion of a hernia with great pain, like cramp; flatus seems to get into the hernia.

A weakness in the groin.

155. Drawing out of the groin dowm into the thigh.

In the bend of the groin and in the tendons of the lumbar muscles a want of mobility and stiff pain when walking and spreading out the legs, as after a long journey on foot (aft. 3½ h.).

Cutting blows in both groins, during which he is obliged to draw in the abdomen and to draw up the legs. [*Ws.*]

Forcing in the right groin, in the inguinal ring, as if a hernia would protrude, when sitting; on stretching out the body; it goes off on standing up. [*Fz.*]

A twitching pinching in the left side of the pelvis, which makes him start and jump (aft. 4 h.). [*Ws.*]

160. Cramp-like pain on the inner border of the pelvis in the neighbourhood of the hip, which is increased by rubbing (aft. 36 h.). [*Ws.*]

Pinching pain on the inner side of the ischias. [*Ws.*]

Sharp stitches in the anus and rectum (aft. ¾ h.). [*Hrr.*]

Discomfort in the hypogastrium and feeling as if he wanted to go to stool, especially after a meal (aft. 36 h.). [*Hrr.*]

Every morning soft stool with some pinching.

165. Unusually copious stool, in the evening (aft. 10 h.).

Diarrhœa. [*Fr. H—n.*]

Nocturnal diarrhœa with much burning in the rectum.

Very large formed stool and hence difficult discharge of the fæces.

(Whitish-yellow stool.)

170. **Frequeut but ordinary stool** (aft. 16 h.). [*Hrr.*]

Constipation for three days. [*Gss.*]

(The quantity of urine passed is greater than the amount of fluid he has drunk.)

Constant call to urinate, whereby little, but natural urine is passed. [*Gss.*]

* From swallowing gold.

1 A casual mention of "aurea colica" as having occasionally, but rarely, oc urred. Preparation of metal not stated.

Obtuse shooting tearing in the urethra. [*Hrr.*]

175. In the morning, after rising, frequent erections and desire for coitus (aft. 16 and 40 h.).

Very much increased sexual desire, which had previously been long dormant in him.

Nocturnal erections for many successive nights.

Nocturnal erections without seminal emissions (the 1st night). [*Ws.*]

Seminal emissions for three successive nights, without subsequent weakness.

180. Nocturnal seminal emissions (the following nights). [*Ws.*]

At night seminal emission with voluptuous dreams (aft. 7 d.). [*Hrr.*]

In the night erections and pollutions. [*Gss.*]

Prostatic fluid escapes from a flaccid penis.

Shooting tearing on the glans penis, when he has a call to urinate (aft. 3 h.). [*Ws.*]

185. Needle-pricks on the point of the glans penis; each is followed instantly by a stitch over the navel towards the scrobiculus cordis (aft. 3 h.). [*Ws.*]

(Very painful twitching in the penis backwards.)

Itching on the scrotum.

Aching tensive pain in the right testicle, as from a contusion (aft. $3\frac{1}{2}$ h.). [*Lr.*]

Swelling of the lower part of the right testicle, with aching pain only when touched and rubbed, which commenced every evening about 6 p.m. and went off again about 11 o'clock (aft. 5 d.). [*Hrr.*]

190. Labour-like pains in the abdomen, as if the menses would come on.

* * *

Coryza. [*Fr. H—n.*]

In the morning on awaking dry catarrh tightly seated in the chest; he can only cough up a little viscid mucus with great effort, and this only after first getting up from bed (aft. 16 h.).

Cough. [*Fr. H—n.*]

Great tightness of chest when walking in the open air.

195. Very great tightness of chest.

Tightness of the chest; when he laughs or walks quickly he feels the chest too tight on inspiring, and it seems to him that the chest is too flat (aft. 44 h.). [*Gss.*]

Tightness of the thoracic cavity, and on inspiring obtuse stitches here and there in the chest. [*Hrr.*]

Extreme tightness of the thoracic cavity with difficulty of breathing at night (aft. 58 h.). [*Hrr.*]

Tightness of chest, also when sitting and when not moving, not allayed by any position; he always takes a deep breath, and cannot get enough air. [*Gss.*]

200. Cough on account of want of breath at night. [*Hrr.*]

Sometimes at the top of the trachea adherent mucus, which is with difficulty detached by short cough, also mucus lower down in the lung, which is expectorated in large quantity and easily; soon after this his respiration was very free, and he is wide chested (he was formerly very narrow chested).

She must sometimes take a very deep breath.

On breathing deeply and yawning, painful stitches under the ribs, whereby yawning and breathing are obstructed; this goes off on going to bed.

On inspiring sharp stitches, and (to his feelings) in the side of the bladder.

205. Frequently mucus deep in the trachea below the larynx, which, in spite of the greatest efforts, connot be coughed up. [*Gss.*]

(On expiring a rumbling in the chest down into the abdomen and groin, and after the rumbling a very rapid palpitation of the heart, with exhaustion and anxiety—hereafter slumber.)

Mucus in the fauces that can be hawked up, but that prevents him taking a full inspiration (aft. 2 h.). [*Fz.*]

Some very violent stitches in the chest, above the heart (aft. 72 h.).

Aching on the right side of the chest in the region of the fourth rib, which causes him immense anxiety. [*Fz.*]

210. Feeling of anxiety often in connexion with tightness of the thoracic cavity (aft. 3 d.). [*Hrr.*]

Palpitation of the heart (aft. $\frac{1}{4}$ h.).

Sometimes a single very strong beat of the heart.

Violent palpitation of the heart (aft. 4 d.). [*Hrr.*]

When walking the heart appears to shake as though it was loose. [*Fz.*]

215. **Obtuse cutting and shooting pain on the right side near the sternum under the last true ribs.** [*Hrr.*]

Obtuse cutting pain on the left near the sternum more severe on inspiring (aft. 9 d.). [*Hrr.*]

Obtuse stitches on both sides of the chest, with feeling of heat and oppression in the chest, increased by inspiration (aft. 2 h.). [*Ws.*]

Sharp stitches on the sternum (aft. 2 h.). [*Ws.*]

On the sternum aching, with busy anxious state of mind, as if some great happiness were about to befal him. [*Fz.*]

220. **Over the cartilages of the first three ribs on the right side a red spot, and under these cartilages, especially the second, a squeezing obtuse shooting, which sometimes lasts like a peg stuck in there, sometimes slowly declines ; but he feels little of it when walking quickly** (aft. 16 h.). [*Gss.*]

Pressure on the left side near the scrobiculus cordis, under the cartilages of the upper false ribs, more severe when expiring (aft. 7 d.). [*Hrr.*]

Pressure as from something hard on the sternum, with drawing tearing towards the shoulders. [*Fz.*]

In the morning such severe pain in the spine that he could not move a limb.

Pain in the sacrum, as from fatigue (aft. 3 h.).

225. While sitting cutting above the sacrum as if it was pressed on by something sharp. [*Fz.*]

Fine shooting tearing on the right side near the lumbar vertebræ, always removed by pressing on it (aft. 2 h.). [*Hrr.*]

Pressure on the left side near the lumbar vertebræ just above the os innominatum, and on its upper border. [*Hrr.*]

On the right near spinal column, just below the right scapula, a painful pricking as with needles (aft. ½ h.). [*Gss.*]

Tearing pain on the inner side of the scapula and beneath it, when bending the body backwards and to the left (aft. 10 h.). [*Hrr.*]

230. Tension in the nape, as if a muscle there were too short, even when not moving, worse when stooping (aft. 10 h.). [*Ws.*]

Fine stitches in the axilla. [*Ws.*]

Sore pain of the shoulders, even when not touched or moved. [*Fz.*]

Tearing tension under the axilla. [*Ws.*]

Gone-to-sleep feeling, numbness and insensibilty of the arms and thighs in the morning after waking, felt more when lying still than when moving (aft. 16 h.).

235. Tearing pressure in the middle of the anterior surface of both upper arms (aft. 15 d.). [*Hrr.*]

Fine tearing in the left upper arms, most severe when it is uncovered (aft. 3 h.). [*Ws.*]

Pressure on the under surface and in the middle of the right upper arm. [*Hrr.*]

Pressure on the left upper arm, in the periosteum (aft. 43 h.). [*Hrr.*]

Down the left arm a drawing pain lying on the bone, which goes off on moving. [*Fz.*]

240. Heaviness of the forearm when at rest, but not when moving (aft. 12 h.). [*Ws.*]

Pressure on the anterior surface of the right forearm. [*Hrr.*]

Intermittent tearing pressure on the inner surface of the left forearm (aft. 3 d.). [*Hrr.*]

Pressure on the outer side of the right forearm (aft. 12 d.). [*Hrr.*]

Cramp-like tearing deeply seated internally in the bones of the wrist, now of the right, now of the left hand, also in the right elbow-joint ; it draws from the inferior to the superior row of the carpal bones, especially observable in the night, but also during the day. [*Gss.*]

245. Tearing in the right carpal bones (aft. 8 h.). [*Hrr.*]

Tearing in the metacarpal bones and the proximal phalanx of the left little finger. [*Hrr.*]

Cramp-like pain in the metacarpal bones of the left hand, especially of the thumb, which, however, does not interfere with movement. [*Gss.*]

Itching between thumb and forefinger.

Very quick, continued, almost shooting pecking between thumb and forefinger.

250. Fine tearing in the ring and middle finger of the right hand (aft. $\frac{3}{4}$ h.). [*Hrr.*]

Fine tearing in the distal phalanx of the right thumb. [*Hrr.*]

Obtuse tearing in the finger-joints of both hands, which often extends into the limbs of both sides (aft. 5 d.). [*Hrr.*]

Tearing in the proximal joints of the fingers of the right hand (aft. 4 d.). [*Hrr.*]

Drawing in the finger-joints. [*Hl.*]

255. A fine stitch darts in a tortuous manner through the gluteal muscles of the right side in a downward direction, recurring several times (aft. 16 h.). [*Ws.*]

A kind of paralysis of the thigh ; he cannot raise it on account of stiff pain up above in the tendons of the psoas muscle.

Tearing in the thigh, like growing pain, only on moving, not when sitting (aft. 24 h.).

On walking in the open air an aching tensive pain in the muscles of the left thigh, which did not go off by touching, standing, or walking, but did so when sitting (aft. 3 h.). [*Lr.*]

Cramp-like drawing in the tendon of the psoas muscles which flexes the left thigh, down into the thigh, when sitting ; it goes off on standing up. [*Fz.*]

260. On the outside of the left thigh, in its middle, a spot which pains as if excoriated (coming on at night when lying). [*Gss.*]

Sensation in the shaft of the right femur when he throws the right thigh over the left, as if the former were broken. [*Fz.*]

When sitting, if he throws the left leg over the right, the muscles on the posterior side of the right thigh towards the hough seem to be in a twitching movement, which is not observable in aother posture or when the legs are not crossed. [*Gss.*]

Painful stiffness and paralyzed feeling of the knees when at rest and when moving.

When walking a simple pain in the right knee.

265. **Pain in the knees as if they were tightly bound**, when sitting and walking.

The right knee is weakened by walking, so that when he treads, and also after walking, in every position, a drawing pain is felt in it for a long time (aft. 24 h.). [*Gss.*]

Unsteadiness of the knees.

Aching on the left tibia when he stretches out the leg. [*Fz.*]

Above the ankles, on both sides, dull, gnawing pain, and single sharp stitches in the tendo Achillis, when at rest, which go off when moving (aft. 14 h.). [*Ws.*]

270. Tensive pressure near the right inner ankle (aft. 5 d.). [*Hrr.*]

The heels pain as if festering or as if they were filled with blood.

(Violent stitches behind the toes on the dorsum of the foot.)

(Digging pain in the place where a chilblain had been) (aft. 1 h.).

Pain as if bruised and dislocated in the proximal joint of the big toe when walking.

275. **Paralytic drawing in the right metatarsal bone of the big toe, extending to its tip.** [*Hrr.*]

Paralytic drawing in the toes of the right foot. [*Hrr.*]

Fine tearing in the toes of the right foot. [*Hrr.*]

Drawing in the toe-joints. [*Hl.*]

Pressure as from something hard in the hollow part of the sole.

280. Tearing pain on the posterior part of the right sole (aft. 30 h.) [*Hrr.*]

In the morning and all the forenoon, pain of all the joints as if beaten.

In the morning, at dawn, in bed, simple or bruised pain in all the joints, especially in the sacrum and knees, which increases the longer he lies still, whether on the back or the side, but soon goes off after getting up.

In the whole body an extermely great sensitiveness ; too sensitive to every pain ; on merely thinking of pain he imagined he felt it ; a feeling of intolerance of everything. [*Hl.*]

In the afternoon prostration and painful drawing in the blood-vessels.

285. Comfortabl feeling in the whole body.*

All his sensation are fine and acute. [*Hl.*]

Even in the worst weather he feels well and comfortable in the open air. [*Fz.*]

(Formication on the body here and there. [*Hl.*]

Itching burning radiations darting here and there, almost like stitches.

290. In the afternoon when sitting and reading he was overcome by great exhaustion, during which he fell asleep, but it was quite gone when he awoke (aft. 9½ h.). [*Lr.*]

Remarkable ebullition in the blood (aft. 24 h.), as if it boiled in the blood-vessels.

A weakness of the head combined with sopor while sitting, in the daytime.

Irresistible sleep after dinner, and during this nap he thinks a great deal (aft. 4 h.). [*Fz.*]

Frequent waking out of sleep as from fright. [*Lr.*]

295. **He moans aloud in his sleep.** [*Gss.*]

Agreeable and very rational but little remembered dreams (aft. 8 h.).

Frightful dreams.

He has frightful dreams of thieves, and cries out aloud in sleep.

Dreams of dead people.

300. He awakes in vivid dreams.

Dreams as if he should fall from a great height.

Dreams full of quarrelling.

Every night dreams and erection of the penis.

In the evening immediately after going to sleep, almost half awake, she dreamt much, as if some one were speaking to her.

305. All night long she dreamt that she was in the dark.

* Curative action.

The child slept till 3 a.m., then it became wide awake, and spoke in bold tones deliriously, with rapid utterance and red face : "Mother, thou art my gold daughter !" "What dog is that ?" "What head is that on the wall ?" "What is that running about the room ?" and her raving consisted always of questions.

Frightful dreams at night. [*Gss.*]

At night unremembered dreams. [*Lr.*]

At night vivid yet unremembered dreams. [*Lr.*]

310. All night long wide awake and sleepless, although without pains, and yet neither sleepy nor tired in the morning, as is usually the case after a sleepless night.

In the morning from 4 o'clock onwards he cannot sleep properly any longer ; he tosses about restlessly from one side to the other, because he cannot lie long in one position ; the hand on which he lies becomes soon tired ; he often wakes up. [*Gss.*]

In the morning on waking very weak.

In the morning in bed, immediately on waking, bruised headache and bruised pain in all the joints, worst when quite at rest ; immediately after getting up these pains disappear.

In the morning very tired ; her legs are painful so that she would like to lie down again.

315. Chilliness in the evening in bed ; the legs up to the knees are icy cold ; he cannot get warm all night ; sleeps in all scarcely two hours, only for half an hour at a time, during which he has anxious but unremembered dreams (aft. 16 d.).

Alternate heat and chills. [*Fr. H—n.*]

Shivering through the whole body, with goose skin on the thighs, and with shock of the brain under the frontal bone (aft. 10 h.). [*Fz.*]

In the evening, before lying down, headache, and after lying down shivering and chilliness.

Rigor in the back.

320. Sometimes chilliness betwixt the scapulæ.

(When he got into bed in the evening his soles and patellæ became cold. [*Hl.*]

In the evening in bed, before going to sleep, a febrile rigor over the whole body as if he had taken a chill in a draught of air (aft. 19 h.). [*Lr.*]

In the evening febrile rigor all over, during which the hands were cold, but the face and forehead warm, without thirst (aft. 14 h.). [*Lr.*]

At night in bed, before going to sleep, a febrile rigor through the whole body ; he could hardly get warm in bed (aft. 16 h.). [*Lr.*]

325. When he lies down in bed in the evening he is quiet, yet sleep is not to be thought of ; he thinks it is owing to the position, and he changes it ever and anon, but cannot sleep before 3 a.m. ; in the morning, waking up at 6 a.m., he is as refreshed as if he had slept sufficiently, for three successive nights. [*Hl.*]

In the evening febrile rigor over the whole body, with stuffed coryza, not followed by heat, and without thirst (aft. 14 h.). [*Lr.*]

Heat of face with cold hands and feet.

Slight transpiration at night like a vapour, and only between the thighs moisture like perspiration (aft. 10 h.)

Morning sweat all over.

330. **All day long good humour ; he was talkative and contented with himself.*** [*Lr.*]

Cheerful humour ; he was always disposed to converse with others. and was quite contented with his position.*[1]

Tolerable gaiety and agreeable comfort* (aft. 2 h.). [*Gss.*]

In the evening sometimes weeping, sometimes laughing, as if she was not quite conscious.

Trembling agitation of the nerves as if under the influence of some joyous hope (aft. 36 h.). [*Fz.*]

335. Quiet morosenese (aft. 1 h.) ; cheerfulness (aft. 3 h.) ; the two emotions afterwards alternated with one another. [*Hrr.*]

Moroseness ; he is indisposed to talk (aft. 8 h.). [*Hrr.*]

Very much given to feel offended ; the slightest thing which he thought offensive affected him deeply, and caused him to resent it. [*Hl.*]

Irascibility ; he is very excitable, and the slightest contradiction excites the utmost anger (aft. 48 h.). [*Gss.*]

Choleric.

340. He sits apart, all by himself in a corner, wrapt up in himself, as if in the deepest melancholy, when left undisturbed ; but the slightest contradiction excites the greatest **heat and anger, when he quite forgets himself, at first with quarrelling** and much talking, afterwards with few disconnected words (chiefly aft. 5 d.). [*Hrr.*]

Constant, Sulky seriousness and reservedness. [*Lr.*]

Peevish dejection ; he thinks nothing will succeed with him. [*Ws.*]

He thinks that everything happens awkwardly, or that he does everything awkwardly. [*Hl.*]

Discontent with all his circumstances ; he imagines that he finds everywhere some obstacle in the way ; at one time he thinks that this is owing to an unlucky fate, at another that he himself is to blame for it ; when the latter was the case he was particularly mortified and dejected. [*Hl.*]

345. An urging to activity, bodily as well as mental ; when he did anything, he thought he did not do it quick enough, and that he had a great deal more to do ; he could not live to his liking. [*Hl.*]

Remorse about his idleness, and yet he cannot work at anything ; it drives him out of the house, he must be always moving. [*Fz.*]

Always very restless and undecided—thought he was neglecting

* Alternating action ?

1 Though without name attached, this symptom occurs among "observations of others."

something for which he must incur reproach—without perceptible ebullition of blood ; he seemed to carry about this restlessness with him in his inmost parts ; this condition deprived him of all perseverance, all energy. [*Hl.*]

A noise before the door made him anxious ; he feared lest some one would come in ; like anthropophobia.*

Palpitation of the heart, extraordinary anxiety, wearinesr of all the limbs and drowsiness (for an hour).

350. Great anxiety that has its origin in the præcordial region ; it draws him to a place that was previously a favourite one, and drives him away again, and so from one place to another, so that he can remain long in no place. [*Fz.*]

Great weaknes and anxiety, so that he is thought to be near death. [J. H. SCHULZE, *Prælectiones in Pharm.*, Aug., p. 46.[1]]

Amid howling and crying she imagines herself to be irretrievably lost.

He imagines he has forfeited the affections of others, and this grieves him to tears. [*Fz.*]

Sad, dejected.

355. He is discontented with himself and depressed in spirits.

Melancholy ; he imagines he is unfitted for the world ; he is filled with intense delight when he thinks of death, so that he longs to die. [*Fz.*]

Contrariety of disposition.

Frequent attacks of præcordial anxiety and trembling anxiety. [*Ephem. Nat. Cur.*, Cent. 10, obs. 35.[2]]

FULMINATING GOLD.

Bellyache, especially in children, with anguish. [*Pharmac. Wirtemb.*, ii, p. 28.[3]]

Sinking of the strength, syncope, cold sweat on the limbs, violent vomiting, convulsions. [FR. HOFFMANN, *Med. Rat. Syst.*, ii, p. 287.[4]]

Violent diarrhœa. [LUDOVICI, *Pharmac. Med. Sec. appl.* Gotha, 1685, pp. 182, 188.[5]]

* Hence it was useful in cases of too great hesitancy of mind.

---

1 Not accessible.

2 No observation about gold occurs here.

3 Not accessible.

4 Statement of poisonous effects of gold. The symptoms are stated as "leading on to death."

5. Not accessible.

BELLADONNA [1]

(Atropa Belladonna).

(The freshly expressed juice of the whole plant at the commencement of its flowering, mixed with equal parts of alcohol.)

The plant gathered in the garden (on a rather dry soil and preferably on the slope of a hill) is little if at all inferior in medicinal power to the wild plant, although some physicians have asserted the contrary.

From the following completed list of the symptoms of belladonna it will readily be seen that it corresponds in similarity to a number of morbid states not unfrequently met with in life, and that hence it must frequently be homœopathically applicable for curative purposes, like a polychrest.

Those small-souled persons who cry out against its poisonous character must let a number of patients die for want of belladonna, and their hackneyed phrase, that we have well-tried mild remedies for these diseases, only serves to prove their ignorance, for no medicine can be a substitute for another.

To take an example, how often are the worst forms of sore-throat (especially those combined with external swelling) given over to death, in spite of all their employment of venesection, leeches, blisters, gargles, emollient poultices, cooling powders, sudorifics and purgatives. And yet, without all these tortures, they might have been cured in a few hours with a single minute dose of belladonna.

And what other real medicine would not be hurtful, dangerous, and poisonous in the hands of the ignorant? Certainly every powerful medicine would be so if given in unsuitable cases of disease and in disproportionately large doses—for which the so-called physician would be solely to blame. On the other hand, the most potent and energetic medicines will become the mildest by diminishing the dose sufficiently, and they will become the most curative, even for the most delicate and sensitive bodies, when they are given in appropriate smallest possible doses, and when the case of disease consists of affections very similar to what the medicine itself has shown it can call forth in healthy human beings. With such potent drugs as belladonna, we must never neglect to exercise the requisite care in the homœopathic selection. But this would never enter the head of the routine practitioner who, as is well known, is in the habit of treating all cases with a few prescriptions learned by rote.

Taught by a hundredfold experience at the sick bed during the last eight or ten years, I could not help descending to the decillion-fold

---

1 From vol. i, 3rd edit., 1830.

dilution, and I find the smallest portion of a drop* of this for a dose quite sufficient to fulfil every curative intention attainable with this medicine.

Two drops of the juice mixed with equal parts of alcohol, taken as unity (as with other vegetable juices), and shaken with 99 to 100 drops of alcohol by two downward strokes of the arm (whose hand holds the mixing phial) gives a hundredfold potentized dilution ; one drop of this shaken in the same way with another 100 drops of fresh alcohol gives the ten-thousandfold dilution, and one drop of this shaken with 100 drops of alcohol, the millionfold. And thus in thirty such phials the potentized dilution is brought to the decillion-fold, with which the homœopathic physician effects the cures he can expect to make with belladonna.

(The above is the method to be employed for the dilution and potentization of the other vegetable juices.)

Belladonna, in the small dose just described, is, if the case is homœopathically adapted, capable of curing the most acute diseases (in which it acts with a rapidity proportionate to the nature of the disorder). On the other hand, it is not less serviceable in the most chronic ailments, in which its duration of action, even in the smallest dose, amounts to three weeks and more.†

Almost all authors have asserted that vinegar is an antidote to belladonna, but that is a mere conjecture, copied in simple faith by one from another, and yet nothing is further from the truth. Repeated experience has taught me that vinegar only aggravates the ill-effects of large doses of belladonna.‡

Opium relieves the paralytic symptoms and abdominal pains caused by belladonna, but only in an antipathic and palliative way, very probably also it removes, in very small doses, the sopor caused by belladonna.

But the stupefied condition, the mania and the fury caused by belladonna, are soonest and most surely homœopathically removed by one or two small doses of *henbane*. But the intoxication by itself is best subdued by *wine*, as I have seen, and as TRAJUS and MOIBANUS long ago observed.

When small dose of belladonna, unhomœopathically selected, causes lachrymose disposition with chilliness and headache, an equally small dose of pulsatilla relieves.

But suitable help is most urgently required in cases where belladonna has been swallowed in considerable quantities, for example, in the form of its berries. In such cases relief is obtained by drinking a large quantity of strong coffee, which removes the loss of irritability and the tetanic convulsions, though it only does that antipathically. It also

* As the dose is one globule the size of a poppy seed (300 of which weigh only a grain), moistened with it, we give less than $\frac{1}{1000}$th of a drop of the decillion-fold medicinal dilution spiritualized (potentized) by succussion, for with a single drop many more than 1000 such small globules can be moistened.

† The best preventive of hydrophobia is the smallest dose of belladonna, given at first every third or fourth day, and repeated at ever longer intervals.

‡ STAPF also observed that in the violent headache from belladonna vinegar laid on the forehead increased it to such an intolerable degree that it had to be taken off.

promotes the vomiting of the berries most certainly, the fauces being at the same time irritated with a long feather in order to empty the stomach.

The erysipelatous swelling caused by belladonna are readily removed by hepar sulphuris. Camphor, too, displays much antidotal power against some of the morbid effects caused by belladonna.

The prophylactic power of belladonna (given in the smallest dose every six or seven days) discovered by me, against the true erysipelatoid smooth *scarlet fever*, as described by SYDENHAM, PLENCITZ, and others, was calumniated and ridiculed for nineteen years by a large number of medical men, who were not acquainted with this peculiar form of children's disease, and consequently mistook for it the *red miliary* (purpura miliaris, roodvonk*) that came from Belgium in 1801. This they falsely called "scarlet fever," and naturally they failed to get any result from the administration of my prophylactic and curative remedy for true scarlet fever, in this red miliary fever.† I am happy to say that of late years other medical men have again observed the old true scarlet fever. They have amply testified to the prophylactic power of belladonna in this disease, and have at last rendered me justice after having been treated so long with unmerited contempt.

* See THOMASSEN A THUESSINK, "*Over de Roodvonk*," 1816, extracted from his *Geneeskundige Waarnemingen*.

† This red miliary (roodvonk) is quite a different disease, requiring quite different treatment. Belladonna naturally does no good in it, and the ordinary routine practice allows the majority of patients to die of it. These might be all cured by the alternate administration of aconite and tincture of raw coffee—the former for the heat and increasing restlessness and agonizing anxiety, the latter for the excessive pains with the lachrymose humour. The aconite should be given in the decillion-fold dilution of the juice, and the raw coffee in the million-fold dilution ; both in the smallest portion of a drop for a dose, the one or the other, according as they are indicated, given every twelve, sixteen, or twenty-four hours. In recent times these two very different diseases (smooth scarlet fever and purple miliary) seem to have occurred complicated with one another in some epidemics ; hence in some of the patients belladonna, in others aconite, seemed to have been most useful.

[HAHNEMANN was aided in his proving of belladonna by the undermentioned disciples :—BAEHR, GROSS, HARTMANN, HARTUNG, C. HEMPEL, HERRMANN, HORNBURG, KUMMER, LANGHAMMER, J. G. LEHMANN, MOCKEL, L. E. RUCKERT, STAPF, WISLICENUS.

Symptoms have been taken from the following old-school authorities :

ACKERMANN, in *Struve's Triumph d. Heilk.*, iii. *Acta Nat. Cur.*, vol. ix. ALBRECHT, in *Commerc. lit. Nor.*, 1731.

BALDINGER, in *Neues Magazin f. Aerzte*, i. BAYLIE, *Prac. Essays on Med. Subjects*. BOUCHER, in *Journ. de Med.*, xi, Aout. BUCHAVE, in *Samml. br. Abh., f. pr. Aerzte*, xiv. BUCHHOLZ, in *Hufel. Journ.*, v. BUC'HOZ, in *Vicat, Plantes Venen. de la Suisse.*

CAMERARIUS, EL., *Obs.* ; *Med.-Chir. Wahrnehm.*, vii ; and in *Wepfer, Hist. Cic.* CARL, in *Act. Nat. Cur.*, vol. iv. *Commercium liter. Nor.*, 1731. CULLEN, *Mat. Med.*, ii.

DARIES, *Diss. de Belladonna*, Lips., 1776. DILLENIUS, in *Misc. Nat. Cur.*, Dec. iii, ann. 7, 8. DUMOULIN, in *Journ. de Med.*, xi, Aout.

EHRHARDT, *Pflanzenhistorie*, x. ELFES, in *Rust's Magazin*, vol. xxi. EVERS, in *Berliner Samml.*, iv. EVERS, in *Schmucker's Vermischten Schriften*, i.

FABER, *Strychnomania*.

G—CH, in *Hufel, Journ.*, xxii. GMELIN, EB., in *Acta Nat. Cur.*, vol. vi, app.; *Pflanzengifte*. GOCKEL, in *Frankische Samml.*, iii. GREDING, in *Ludwigii Adversaria med.* GRIMM, in *Act. Nat. Cur.*, vol. ii.

HASENEST, in *Act. Nat. Cur.*, vol. iii. HENNING, in *Hufel. Journ.*, xxi. HOCHSTETTER, *Obs. Med.*, Fft., 1674. HOFFMANN, FR., *Medicina Ration.* HORST, *Opera*, ii. HOYER, in *Misc. Nat. Cur.*, Dec. iii, ann. 7, 8. *Hufeland's Journal f. pr. Arzn.*, xvi.

JUSTI, in *Hufeland's Journ.*, vii.

LAMBERGEN, TIB., *Lectio inaug. sist. eph. pers. carcin.*, Groning., 1754. LAUNAY D'HERMONT, DE, in *Hist. de l' Acad. des Sc.* LOTTINGER, *Med.-Chir. Wahrnehm.*, Altenb., ii.

MANETTI, *Viridarium florentinum*, Florent., 1751. MAPPI, *Plant. Alsat.* MARDORF, *Diss. de Maniacis Giessensibus*, Giesae, 1691. MAY, in *Hannover. Mag.*, 1773, No. 97. *Med.-Chir. Wahrnehmungun aus verschiednen Sprachen ubersetzt*, Altenb., vii. MEZA, DE, in *Samml. br. Abh. f. pr. Aerzte*, xiv. MOIBANUS, in *Schenck*, vii. MULLER, in *Horn's Archiv.* ix. MUNCH, *Ueber die Belladonne.* MUNCH, in *Richter's Bibliothek*, v.

OLLENROTH, in *Hufel. Journ.*, vii.

PORTA, J. B. *Magia Natur.*, viii.

RAU, in *Act. Nat. Cur.*, vol. x. RAY, *Histor. Plant.*, lib. 13. REMER, in *Hufel. Journ.*, xvii.

ST. MARTIN, DE, in *Journ. de Med*, xviii Aout. SAUTER, in *Hufel. Journ.*, xi. SAUVAGES, *Nosol.*, ii. SCHAFFER, in *Hufel. Journ.*, vi. SCHMUCKER, *Chirurg. Wahrnehm.*, ii; *Vermischten Schriften.* SCHRECK, in *Commerc. lit. Nor.*, 1743. SICELIUS, *Observ.*, Dec. iv. SOLENANDER, in *Abh. der Konigl. Acad. d. Wissensch.*, Breslau, 1750. STRUVE, *Triumph der Heilk.*, i.

TIMMERMANN, *Diss. Periculum Belladonnæ.*

VALENTINI, in *Misc. Nat. Cur.*, Dec. ii, ann. 10. VICAT, *Plantes Veneneuses de la Suisse.*

WAGNER, *Misc. Nat. Cur.*, Dec. ii, ann. 10. WARE, JAMES, in *Gilbert's Annals*, 1816, xi. WASSERBERG, in *Stoll's Ratio Medendi*, iii. WEINMANN, in *Gmelin's Pflanzengifte.* WELLS, CHARLES, in *Gilbert's Annals*, 1813, ii. WETZLER, in *Annal. d. Heilkunde*, 1811, Feb. WIEDEMANN, in *Hufel. Journ.*, xxii. WIENHOLT, *Heilkr. d. Thier. Magnetismus*, i. WIERUS, *De praestig. Dæmonum*, iii.

ZIEGLER, *Beob.*, Lips., 1787.

In the *Fragmenta* there are 405 symptoms of belladonna, in the 1st Edit. 650, in the 2nd Edit. 1422, and in this 3rd Edit. 1440.]

BELLADONNA.

Vertigo. [SICELIUS,[1] *Observ.*, Dec. iv, Cas. 4.—ZIEGLER,[1] *Beob.*, Leipz., 1787, pp. 21–38.—R. BUCHAVE,[2] in *Samml. br. Abh. f. pr. Aerzte*, xiv, iv.—HENNING,[3] in *Hufel. Journ.*, xxi, i.—EB. GMELIN,[4] in *Acta. Nat. Cur.*, vi. App.]

Vertigo ; objects seem to sway hither and thither. [*Ws.*]

Whirling in the head, vertigo with nausea, as after rapid turning round in a circle, or as after the morning sleep following a nocturnal debauch. [*Hbg.*]

Whirling in the head, and at the same time a similar whirling in the pit of the stomach ; after rising it became so bad when walking, that she could not distinguish anything, everything vanished from her sight. [*Kr.*]

5. Vertigo as if all whirled round in a circle (aft. 1 h.). [*Hrr.*]

He goes round in a circle. [DE ST. MARTIN,[5] *Journal de Med.*, xviii, Aout]

Stupid and whirling in the head ; she feels better in the open air, worse in the room (aft. $\frac{1}{4}$ h.). [*Stf.*]

Attacks of vertigo, when at rest and when moving. [*Gss.*]

A giddy feeling in the whole head, like vertigo, when sitting. [*Htn.*]

10. Vertigo and trembling of the hands, so that she could not do anything with them. [BALDINGER,[6] *Neues Magazin f. Aerzte*, i, 1 St., p. 30.]

When walking he staggers, holds on to the walls, complains of anxiety and vertigo, and often talks nonsense like a drunken person. [BALDINGER, l. c.]

She rises from bed in the morning and staggers as if intoxicated, hither and thither. [GREDING, in *Ludwigii Adversar. med. pr.*, i, P. iv, p. 670[7] (14).]

Giddy swaying. [MARDORF,[8] *Diss. de Maniacis Giessensibus*, Giesæ, 1691.—LOTTINGER,[9] *Med. Chirurg. Wahrnehm.*, Altenb., ii, p. 326.—Tib. LAMBERGEN,[10] *Lectio inaug. sist. eph. pers. carcin.*, Groning., 1754.]

---

1 Not accessible.

2 Symptoms observed in whooping-cough patients to whom large doses of the extract had been administered.

3 Effects of grain doses of powdered leaves given for pemphigus.

4 Poisoning of an old man by the berries. [When the form in which the plant was taken is not mentioned, it will be understood that the berries were ingested.]

5 Poisoning of a boy of four.

6 Poisoning of four adults.

7 Greding's symptoms from vol. i of Ludwig's *Adversaria* are taken from a series of twenty-three cases, of which the first thirteen were pure epileptics and the remainder epilepto-maniacs, treated by belladonna in increasing doses of the powdered leaves. As all mental symptoms occurring in the patients of the second category must be esteemed doubtful, I have indicated them by adding to each the number of the case from which they were taken.

8 Poisoning of several persons.

9 Not accessible.

10 Symptoms observed in a patient taking an infusion of Belladonna for some mammary indurations.

Attacks of vertigo with obtuseness of senses for some minutes (aft. 12 h.).

15. All day long confusion of senses; he **knows** not what he is doing. [*Lr.*]

Obtuseness of senses.

Cloudiness of the head, with swelling of the glands in the nape (aft. 6 h.).

Intoxication.

Immediately after a meal as if intoxicated.

20. On drinking the smallest quantity of beer immediate intoxication.

Muddled head and intoxication as if from drinking wine, with bloated red face. [*Commercium liter. Nor.*,[1] 1731.]

His whole head is dazed for many days. [*Stf.*]

Muddled state as in intoxication. [HOCHSTETTER,[2] *Obs. Med.*, Fft., 1674, obs. 7.—MAY,[3] in *Hannover. Mag.*, 1773, No. 97.—SICELIUS, l. c.—DE LAUNAY D'HERMONT,[4] in *Hist. de l' Acad. des Sc.*. 1756.—ALBRECHT,[5] in *Commerc. lit. Nor.*, 1731.—BUC'HOZ,[6] in *Vicat, Plantes venen. de la Suisse*, p. 183.] [*L. Rkt.*]

Muddled state of sinciput as if an oppressive fog went hither and thither, especially under the frontal bone. [*Gss.*]

25. Muddling of the head as from much brandy and tobacco smoke. [*Hbg.*]

Muddling and confusion of the whole head, as from the disagreeable feeling of commencing intoxication. [*Gss.*]

Confusion of the head; worse during movement. [*Hrr.*]

Disinclination for all intellectual work. [*Hbg.*]

Weakness of mind and body. [*Hrr.*]

30. Weakness of mind. [WIERUS,[7] *de Praestig. Dæmonum*, iii, cap. 17.]

Stupefaction. [WAGNER,[8] *Miscell. Nat. Cur.*, Dec. ii, ann. 10, obs. 108 (11)—BUCHAVE,—WIERUS, l. c.]

Confusion of mind, [SICELIUS, l.c.]

Confusion of mind, so that he knows not whether he is dreaming or awake. [MOIBANUS,[9] in *Schenck*, vii, obs. 164.]

Confusion of the senses; sleepy and yet awake, he thinks he is dreaming, [MOIBANUS, l. c.]

35. His senses deceive him. [ACKERMANN,[10] in *Struve, Triumph der H.*, iii, p. 303.]

---

1 Same as Albrecht, *q. v.*
2 Effects of infusion in an adult.
3 Not accessible.
4 Poisoning of an adult.
5 Poisoning of two women and a boy,
6 Poisoning of a young boy.
7 Poisnning of an adult.
8 Poisoning of (1) two old women and (11) some children. [These numbers will be used to designate the subjects to whom the symptoms belong.]
9 Poisoning of a man.
10 Not accessible.

Exalted, deluded phantasy conjures up a number of beautiful pictures to her. [*Kr.*]

He imagines he sees ghosts and insects of various kinds. [MOIBANUS, l. c.]

Her nose appears transparent to her. [*Kr.*]

He imagines he sees things not present. [WIEDEMANN,[1] in *hufel. Jour.*, xxii, I.]

40. It seems to her that a spot on the left side of her head is transparent and spotted brown. [*Kr.*]

He thinks he is riding an ox. [G—CH,[2] in *Hufel. Jour.*, xvii, I.]

He does not know his own relations. [WIERUS, l. c.]

Want of consciousness ; he sat as if in a dream. [*Hbg.*]

Unconsciousness. [*Stf.*]

45. He often lay without sense, without consciousness. [*Stf.*]

Loss of consciousness and convulsion in the arm, at night. [GREDING, l. c., p. 672.]

Extreme stupefaction of the senses. [OLLENROTH,[3] in *Hufel. Jour.*, vii, 4.]

Unconsciousness. [HASENEST,[4] in *Acta Nat. Cur.*, iii, obs. 35. —GRIMM,[5] in *Acta Nat. Cur.*, vol. ii, obs. 60—(aft. 2 h,). RAU,[6] in *Acta Nat, Cur.*, x, obs. 24.—EB. GMELIN, l. c.—HOCHSTETTER, l. c.]

Unconsciousness with convulsions of the limbs. [BUCHAVE, l. c.]

50. Complete unconsciousness ; she knows nothing going on. [HENNING, l. c.]

Complete loss of reason. [SAUTER,[7] in *Huf. Jour.* xi, I, p. 125, (I).—BUCHAVE, l. c.]

Loss of reason, for some weeks. [RAU, l. c.]

Loss of reason, for some weeks. [RAU, l. c.]

Insensibility. [VICAT,[8] *Plantes veneneuses de la Suisse*, p. 181.]

Stupidity. [WAGNER, l. c. (1)]

55. During the headache her thoughts leave her ; she forgets what she thought of shortly before, and cannot recollect herself. [*Bhr.*]

Distraction of the mind ; he easily makes mistakes in his work, and forgets things that he has just undertaken to do. [*Ws.*]

He thinks now of one thing now of another ; he could not think of anything properly, and he immediately forgot all he had just thought of or read. [*Lr.*]

Impaired memory.

Very weak memory ; he forgets what he intended to do immediately, and can remember nothing.

---

1 Effects of B. when given freely to children for whooping-cough.
2 Effects of enema of infusion of leaves given for incarcerated hernia.
3 Effects of extract given for mammary scirrhus.
4 Poisoning of a young woman.
5 Poisoning of a child of three.
6 Poisoning of a man of fifty.
7 Poisoning of a child of six.—This case will be distinguised by a (I).
8 Account of general effects of leaves and berries.

60. Return of the lost memory. [GREDING, l. c., p. 650.]

He remembers long forgotten things. [WIEDEMANN, l. c.]

He remembered things that happened three years before. [*Med. chir. Wahrnehmungen aus verschiednen Sprachen ubersetzt*, Altenb., vii. p. 69.[2]]

Lively memory (curative effect) (aft. 24 h.)

Violent headache. [LAMBERGEN—GREDING, l. c., p. 669.]

65. Headache as though the brain was numb.

His whole head feels heavy, as from intoxication. [*Stf.*]

A weight in the upper part of the forehead, which causes vertigo and as it were intoxication (aft. 14 d.).

The head feels heavy as though he would fall asleep ; he is disinclined for everything.

Headache, only over the eyes, like a weight in the head, in the morning on waking, and when he touches the eyes it hurts.

70. Feeling of weight with violent aching in the whole occiput (aft. 2½ h.). [*Htn.*]

Weight of the head as if it would fall down. [*Ln.*]

In the morning headache as if something in the forehead above the eyebrows sunk down, which hinders the opening of the eyes (aft. 4 h.). [*Lr.*]

An aching feeling of weight, from the centre of the brain towards the temples, with diminution of the hearing in both ears. [*Mkl.*]

Aching in the right side of the crown, later shifting into the left side, then back again into the right. [*Mkl.*]

75. **Aching headache, especially in the forehead** (aft. 2 d.). [*Hrr.*]

Constant **dull aching headache in the side of the head** (aft. 5, 24 h.).

Painful aching feeling in the head, especially in the lower part of the forehead, just above the nose, intolerable on stepping. [*L. Rkt.*]

Headache above the orbits, as if the brain were pressed in, so that he must shut his eyes. [*Hbg.*]

Aching pain beneath the right frontal protuberance, which soon afterwards involves the whole forehead (aft. 10 m.). [*Gss.*]

80. Violent aching under the right frontal protuberance. [*Gss.*]

The aching pain under the frontal bone only occasionally declines to return again in still greater intensity. [*Gss.*]

Aching pain beneath the frontal protuberances, in teh morning soon after waking, on getting up. [*Gss.*]

Violent outward-pressing pain in left frontal protuberance. [*Htn.*]

Violent inward-pressure in the left temple, which on leaning this side of the head on something extends over the whole of the anterior half of the brain (aft. ¾ h.). [*Htn.*]

85. Violent outward-pressure in the whole of the left half of the brain, especially severe in the forehead (aft. 2½ h.). [*Htn.*]

Aching pain in the right temporal region, which on leaning the head on the hand changes into a bursting pain, and extends to the right frontal protuberance (aft. 8 h.). [*Htn.*]

---

[1] Temporary only. [2] Not accessible.

Pressure in the head, now here, now there, that each time involves large spaces. [*Hrr.*]

Aching headache in the forehead, so bad on moving that it made the eyes close, alleviated when sitting; he must lie down, whereupon it went off; on standing up it immediately returned, for two days, not aggravated either by eating or by drinking; as soon as he goes into the open air he feels as if the forehead would be pressed in, just as if a heavy stone lay on it; the third day it went off completely when sitting in the room. [*Hbg.*]

An aching deep in the brain over the whole head, whilst and after walking in the open air.

90. Headache pressing like a stone in the forehead, ameliorated by laying the head down and stooping forwards, with dilated pupils and whining ill-humor about trifles. (aft. 3 h.).

Tensive pressure in the right side of forehead. [*Hrr.*]

Tensive pressure in the left side of the crown and in the forehead (aft. 24 h.). [*Hrr.*]

Headache as if the head was screwed together from both sides and thereby became narrower. [*Bhr.*]

A constant expansion of the whole brain. [*Ln.*]

95. Violent pressing-outwards in the whole head, as though it would burst (aft. 3 h.). [*Htn.*]

Headache as if the brain would be pressed out, just above the orbits in the forehead, which hinders the opening of the eyes, and compels lying down, with extreme contraction of the pupils and very low voice (aft. 5, 24 h.).

On stooping forwards pain as if all would come out at the forehead. [*Stf.*]

Sensation as if the brain pressed towards the forehead, which immediately went off when he bent the head backwards a little (aft. 1¼ h). [*Htn.*]

On coughing the feeling of pressing asunder in the head is much more severe (aft. 3½ h.). [*Htn.*]

100. In the open air the feeling of bursting in the head is very severe, and he is afraid to cough on account of increasing the pain (aft. 4 h.). [*Htn.*]

Throbbing pressing in the left side of the occiput (aft. 5 h.). [*Htn.*]

On account of pain in the forehead he must often stand still when walking, at every step it feels as if the brain in the forehead sank and rose; this was alleviated by pressing strongly on it (aft. 6 days). [*Hbg.*]

Strong pulsation of the blood-vessels in the forehead, and pain as if the bone were raised up. [*Hbg.*]

On awaking beating of the blood-vessels in the head and in most parts of the body. [*Kr.*]

105. **Violent throbbing in the brain from before backwards and to both sides; externally it ends in painful shoots.** [*Ws.*]

Aching gnawing headache on the right side of the upper part of the head down to the ear, produced by transient gnawing pain in the hollow tooth (aft. 9 h.). [*Ws.*]

Aching shooting in the temples from within outwards (aft. ½ h.). [*Ws.*]

Cutting pressure in the temples from within outwards, always becoming more violent, extending through the brain, and there turning into severe throbbing, continuing in all positions. [*Ws.*]

Tearing preasure in the head, now here, now there, especially in the forehead and temporal region. [*Hrr.*]

110. Tearing pressure in the right temple and crown, that spreads out in various directions. [*Hrr.*]

Tearing pressure in the head here and there (aft. 5 h.). [*Hrr.*]

Drawing aching headache. [*Hbg.*]

A drawing in the head towards the forehead, as if the brain would expand. [*Ln.*]

Drawing pain from the temple to above the right orbit.

115. A drawing downwards at the temples and in the right orbit.

Boring and throbbing in the right side of the head, like that in the cheek, aggravated by every movement. [*Kr.*]

Boring and aching headache during the day on various parts, in the evening shooting. [*Kr.*]

Boring pain under the right frontal protuberance, soon after awaking in the morning. [*Gss.*]

Incessant drawing and outstretching headache, as if something rocked or swayed about in it by jerks.

120. **Jerking headache, which became extremely violent on walking quickly or going quickly upstairs, and at every step jerked downwards like a weight in the occiput** (aft. 48 h.). [*Ws.*]

The whole head is affected with shooting pain, chiefly in the forehead. [*Stf.*]

Obtuse shoots in the left temple from within outwards. [*Ws.*]

In the whole forehead slight shooting headache (aft. 1½ h). [*Stf.*]

Sharp shooting outwards in both frontal protuberances (aft. 2 h.). [*Ws.*]

125. Excessively violent headache of obtuse or aching shoots, which dart through the brain from all sides.

In the right temple violent shooting pain for a quarter of an hour (aft. 25 h.). [*Stf.*]

Some obtuse stitches in the left side of the occiput. [*Ln.*]

In the right frontal protuberance severe shooting, aggravated by stooping forwards, lessened by touch (aft. 5 m.). [*Stf.*]

Stabbing through the head as with a two-edged knife, in the evening. [*Kr.*]

130. Stabs as with a knife from one temple to the other. [*Bhr.*]

In the evening some large stitches in the occiput close behind the ear, as rapid as lightning, so that he could have cried out (aft. 6 d.)

In the right side of the head cutting stabs as with a two-edged knife which extend at one time into the sinciput, then into the crown, and then into the occiput, so that he cannot lie on either side. [*Kr.*]

Three violent strong shoots through the head from the forehead to the occiput, whereupon all the previous headache suddenly disappears (aft. $3\frac{1}{4}$ h.). [*Stf.*]

Shooting tearing in the head above the right orbit. [*Hrr.*]

135. Cutting tearing pain in the head that extends from one part to another. [*Hrr.*]

Burning tearing pain in the left frontal protuberance (aft. 4 h.). [*Htn.*]

Tearing pain in the right side of the crown, aggravated by movement. [*Hrr.*]

Tearing in the forehead externally.

Tearing in the forehead. [*Hbg.*]

140. Tearing above the eyebrows. [*Hbg.*]

Violent pains in the head of a tearing kind, in the sinciput (aft. 8 h.). [*Gss.*]

Headache on the crown, a twisting, sometimes also digging, sometimes tearing; the pain was much aggravated by external pressure; her skull appeared to her quite thin, as though it might be pressed through. [*Kr.*]

Cold feeling in the brain, in the middle of the forehead.

Drawing in the forehead. [*Kr.*]

145. Drawing pain in the frontal bone and in the nape, when at rest and when moving. [*Gss.*]

A headache apparently tearing asunder the sutures of the skull, as if a lever were inserted in order to burst open the head. [*Ln.*]

Sensation in the brain as of splashing water. [BUCHHOLZ, [1] in *Hufel. Journal*, v, 1, p. 252.]

On stooping forwards the blood rushes towards the forehead. [*Bhr.*]

On stooping the blood mounts into the head and he becomes heavy and as if giddy.

150. Ebullition of the blood to the head, without internal heat of head; when he leaned the head back it seemed to him that blood rushed in. [*Hbg.*]

Heat in the head (aft. $\frac{1}{4}$ h.). [*Stf.*]

External pain in the whole head like that from rough pulling and rumpling the hair; pain remains in the scalp. [*L. Rkt.*]

Gnawing headache externally on the frontal protuberances. [*Ws.*]

Fine shooting burning on the left frontal protuberance (aft. $\frac{1}{4}$ h.). [*Htn.*]

155. A cutting headache on the left side near the occipital protuberance. [*Gss.*]

---

1 Effects of two-grain doses of the powdered root given to a boy as prophylactic of hydrophobia.

On the right side of the head, and at the same time in the right arm, drawing pain, when at rest (after dinner). [*Hbg.*]

Very transient cramp pain on the right side of the vertex (aft. 11 h.). [*Ws.*]

Cramp pain on the root of the nose. [*Ws.*]

Severe cramp pain on the frontal protuberance, that extends downwards over the zygoma to the lower jaw. [*Ws.*]

160. External feeling of contraction of the frontal and eye muscles. [*Ln.*]

Scratching itching on the forehead (aft. 1 h). [*Ws.*]

A painful boil on the temple.

Red painless pimples break out on the temple, on the right corner of the mouth, and on the chin ; on scratching bloody water exudes (aft. 13 h.). [*Lr.*]

Swelling of the head. [*Kr.*—MUNCH,[1] *On Belladonna*—HORST,[2] *Opera*, ii, p. 488.]

165. Great swelling of the head and redness all over the body.* [MUNCH,[1] in *Richter's Biblioth.*, v, p. 387.]

Falling out of the hair, for an hour (aft. 24 h.).

The hairs, which were previously idioelectric, are no longer so (aft. 24 h.).

The external head is so sensitive that the slightest touch, even the pressure of the hair, causes her pain. [*Kr.*]

Restless expression. [BOUCHER,[3] in *Jour. de Med.*, xxiv, 310.]

170. Distorted features. [BOUCHER, l. c.]

Paleness of face. [SICELIUS, l. c.]

Pale face with thirst. [GREDING, l. c., p. 650.]

Pale face with increased appetite. [GREDING, l. c., p. 650.]

Sudden paleness of face for a considerable time. [GREDING, l. c., p. 677 (16).]

175. Often extreme pallor of face, instantaneously changing into redness of face, with cold cheeks and hot forehead.[4] [GREDING, l. c., p. 662.]

Hot feeling in face without external redness (aft. 8 h.). [*Ws.*]

Burning hot feeling in the whole face, without redness of cheeks and without thirst, with moderately warm body and cold feet (aft. 4 h.), [*Htn.*]

Creeping hot feeling in the face beneath the skin (aft. ¼ h.). [*Ws.*]

Burning heat over the face, without thirst (aft. 10 h.). [*Lr.*]

180. Unusual redness of the face. [*Ln.*]

Great redness and heat in the face, without perspiration (aft. 24, 30. h.). [*Mkl.*]

* In two days.

1 Effects of large doses (gr. 4—14) of the powdered root given as prophylactic of hydrophobia.

2 Poisoning of an adult by inspissated juice.—The head, he says, "swelled to double its size"

3 Poisoning of five children.—It is only the eyes which are said to be distorted.

4 Occurring during a succession of epileptic paroxysms.

Very red, hot face, with icy-cold limbs. [*Stf.*]

Glowing redness of face, with violent indescribable pains in head [*Stf.*]

Heat and redness only on the head.

185. Perspiration only on the face.

Rush of blood to the head, red cheeks. [BUCHAVE, l. c.]

Great heat and redness of the cheeks. [BUCHAVE, l. c.]

Face very swollen and hot. [BUCHAVE, l. c.]

Redness and heat in the whole face, as if he had drunk much wine. [*Hbg.*]

190. Heat in the face all day, as if the blood had mounted to the head from drinking wine (aft. 12 h.).

Blood-red face. [SAUTER, l. c. (1).]

Swollen skin of face, as if an eruption were going to break out. [SAUTER,[1] l. c. (11).]

Face bluish-red, with great heat of the body, in the evening. [WIEDEMANN, l. c.]

Scarlet redness of the face and chest during sleep. [SCHAFFER,[2] in *Hufel. Journ.*, vi.]

195. Scarlet redness of the skin of the body, especially of the face, with marked activity of the brain. [WETZLER,[3] in *Annalen der Heilkunde*, 1811, Febr.]

Dark-red spots on the face, resembling the rash of scarlet fever, with full pulse. [WIEDEMANN, l. c.]

Along with sudden rigor great dulness of head and sight, red eyes, and swollen face covered with very small, unequal, dark-red spots, especially on the forehead. [GREDING, l. c., p. 685 (19).]

In the morning on awaking a small bluish-red spot on the left cheek, which gradually enlarges until the bluish-red swelling involves the whole cheek, with burning and shooting in the actual red part, and boring and throbbing in the whole cheek, much aggravated by movement; after some days the other cheek swelled, and the swelling lasted eight days. [*Kr.*]

Red swollen face. [MAY, l. c.]

200. Red swollen face with staring eyes. [JUSTI,[4] in *Hufel. Journ.*, vii, 4, p. 65.]

Swollen face.

The face was red and swollen, but the rest of the body pale. [GRIMM, l. c.]

Swelling of the cheeks, with burning pain. [*Fr. H—n.*]

Hard large swelling on the face about the nose and eye, with swelling of the parotid gland on the opposite side, lasting five days. [GREDING, l. c., p. 668.]

205. Swelling of the left cheek about the nose and eye, which comes

---

1 Effects of large doses of powdered leaves given in fully-developed hydrophobia. Symptoms from this source will be distinguished by a (11).

2 Effects of B. given to children for whooping-cough.

3 Not accessible.

4 Effect of a single full dose given to an adult as prophylactic of hydrophobia.

on in the afternoon, increases the following day with heat, and lasts five days. [GREDING, l. c., p. 667.]

Swollen face. [MUNCH, l. c.]

Swelling of the face, and especially of the lips. [LAMBERGEN,[1] l. c.]

An uninterrupted quivering (and winking) of both eyelids. [*Ln.*]

All day long an uninterrupted trembling and quivering of the right upper eyelid, that at last becomes painful. [*Htg.*]

210. Expanded eyelids, eyes standing wide open.

Throbbing pain in the lower eyelids towards the inner canthus, with great inflammatory swelling at that point, with much lachrymation, for half an hour (aft. 32 h.). [*Mkl.*]

The eyes close and become watery. [*L. Rkt.*]

Heaviness in the eyes, especially the upper lid. [*L. Rkt.*]

After waking in the morning, the eyes again close involuntarily; she cannot keep them open until she gets up. [*Kr.*]

215. **Itching stitches in the inner canthi which only leave off for a short time on rubbing** (aft. 1 h.). [*Ws.*]

The inner canthus of the left eye is very painful, even when lightly touched. [*Gss.*]

Smarting in both eyes. [*Hbg.*]

Involuntary lachrymation of the eyes.

Salt water runs constantly out of the eyes. [*Hbg.*]

220. Lachrymation of the eyes. [*Mkl.*]

Dryness of the eyes (of the nose, mouth, pharynx). [WASSERBERG,[2] in *Stoll, Ratio Medendi*, iii, p. 403.]

Burning dry feeling in both eyes, alternately worse in one or the other (aft. 7 h.). [*Mkl.*]

Pain and burning in the eyes. [GREDING, l. c., p. 644.]

Increased heat and hot feeling in the eyes. [*Mkl.*]

225. Feeling of heat in the eyes; it is as if they were enveloped in a hot vapour.

Photophobia; he avoids looking into the light. [JUSTI, l. c.]

Burning of the eyes, accompanied by painful itching; but both cease when the eyes are pressed upwards (aft. 28 h.). [*Mkl.*]

In the morning the white of the eye is red-streaked, with aching pain.

Inflammation of the eyes; injection of the veins of the white of the eye, with a tickling sensation.

230. Inflammation of the eyes; the conjunctiva is traversed by red blood-vessels, with shooting pain; the eyes water. [*Hbg.*]

Shooting in the eyes towards the interior. [*Kr.*]

Yellowness of the white of the eye.

In the morning the eyes are quite sealed up with matter. [*Mkl.*, *Kr.*]

Swelling and purulent inflammation of the left punctum lachrymale,

---

1 In connection with S. 367.

2 Proving on self. The observer adds, after "eyes," "with burning in these and in the lids."

at first with burning pain, afterwards with aching pain, for three days (aft. 4 d.). [*Mkl.*]

235. A general aching in both eyes, as if hard spring water had got into the eyes. [*Ln.*]

When she closes the eyes, an aching pain deep in the eyeball. [*Stf.*]

A cloudy aching comes in the right orbit and goes from that alternately into the forehead and back again. [*Gss.*]

Aching and watering of the eyes, especially in the morning. [*F. H—n.*]

Creeping aching pain in the eyes, as if they were full of sand; she must rub them (aft. 1 h.).

240. Aching in the eyes, as if sand had got into them (aft. 2½ h.). [*Lr.*]

Aching in the eyes, as from a grain of sand. [GREDING, loc. cit., p. 650.—*Mkl.*]

Pain in the orbits; sometimes it is as if the eyes were torn out, sometimes (and this more persistently) as though they were pressed into the head, to which a pain is superadded, that presses from the forehead upon the eyes. [*Gss.*]

A tearing in the eyes proceeding from the inner canthi. [*L. Rkt.*]

Drawing pain under the left eye upwards.

245. Contracted pupils, difficult to dilate.

Very contracted pupils all day; they only dilate in the evening. [*Stf.*]

Contracted pupils (aft. 10 m.). [*Gss.*]

Contrcted pupils (aft. 1¼ h.). [*Ws.*]

Contracted pupils (aft. 2½ h.). [*Lr.*]

250. The dilatation of pupils commenced after half an hour, and then increased gradually. [*Gss.*]

Dilated pupils after 3½ hours. [SAUTER, l. c (1).—*Ln.*]

The pupils are very dilated in the evening, even when the light is held close to the eye (aft. 12 h). [*Gss.*]

Dilated pupils (aft. 14, 15 h.). [*Lr.*]

The pupils are more dilated, from the third day onwards. [*Stf.*]

255. Dilated immovable pupils. [MAY, l. c.]

Extremely dilated pupils. [BOUCHER, l. c.]

A small white pustule in the left, extremely dilated pupil. [*Hbg.*]

Extremely dilated pupils (from laying a fresh belladonna leaf on an ulcer beneath the eye). [RAY, *Histor. plant.*, lib. 13, cap. 23.]

Sometimes complete loss of, sometimes merely diminished, vision, with enormously dilated and quite immovable pupils. [ELFES, in *Rust's Magaz.*, vol. xxi, pt. 3.]

260. Complete dilatation of the pupil of the right eye and blindness for three weeks (from the juice of the plant injected into the eye). [DARIES, *Diss. de Belladonna*, Lips., 1776., pp. 34, 35.]

Obscuration of vision from dilated pupils. [BUCHAVE, l. c.]

Obscuration of vision, with extremely dilated pupils. [GREDING,[1] l. c., vol. ii, p. 324.]

---

1 From three cases of jaundice treated by belladonna.

Blindness, the pupil of the right eye extremely dilated and incapable of contracting. [GREDING, l. c., p. 662.]

Great dimness of vision. [JUSTI, l. c.]

265. Before the eyes, as if dim, dark, and black (aft. 1¼ h.). [*Stf.*]

Blindness. [HASENEST,[1] *Acta Nat. Cur.*, vol. iii, obs. 35.]

Amaurosis for three days ; he cannot read print. [HASENEST, l. c.]

He awakes blind. [EL. CAMERARIUS,[2] in his *Obs.* and in *Wepfer, Hist. Cic.*]

The eyes are blind and stand open. [EL. CAMERARIUS, l. c.]

270. Extreme weakness of sight. [OLLENROTH, l. c.]

Transient blindness, with headache. [GREDING, l. c., p. 679 (17).]

Dimness of vision, alternating with convulsions in hands and feet, dulness of head and weariness of limbs. [GREDING, l. c., p. 683 (18).]

Dimness of vision, dryness of mouth, and pain in belly. [GREDING, l. c., p. 606.]

Dulness of sight for three hours. [GREDING, l. c., p. 679 (17).]

275. Along with dulness of sight trembling in all the limbs. [GREDING, l. c., p. 643.]

Long-sightedness (presbyopia), as in old age. [LOTTINGER, l. c.]

He only sees distinctly distant objects and perfectly parallel rays (*e. g.* a star in the sky) (from bellodonna juice injected into the eye). [CHARLES WELLS, in *Gilbert's Annals*, 1813, pt ii, p. 133, and JAMES WARE, ibid., 1816, pt. xi.]

Long-sightedness, as in old age (presbyopia) ; he can only read large print. [LAMBERGEN, l. c.]

Mist before the eyes, blindness [SAUTER, l. c. (1).—BUCHHOLZ, l. c.]

280. As if mist were before the eyes, obscuration. [*Ln.*]

On reading he cannot perceive anything in the book except the white border, which surrounds black letters transformed into rings. [MOIBANUS,[3] in *Schenk*, vii, obs. 164.]

Feeling as if he could see nothing, and yet he saw when he tried to see anything, and strained the eyes to do so. [*L. Rkt.*]

The letters tremble and quiver, of a golden and blue colour, when reading. [BUCHHOLZ, l. c.]

Before the eyes a large, bright coloured ring round the candle, particularly of a red colour ; sometimes the flame seems to be quite dissipated in rays (aft. 15 h.). [*Mkl.*]

285. Before the eyes she sees flames, when she lays her hand on the swollen cheek, and the air appears to be misty. [*Kr.*]

She sees on the ceiling of the room a white star as large as a plate, and light silver clouds pass over it from left to right—several times and in various places. [*Kr.*]

Large bright sparks from the eyes.

He sees sparks before the eyes. [ZIEGLER, l. c.]

---

1 Poisoning of a young woman.
2 Poisoning of four children.
3 Poisoning of a man.

On moving the eyelids he sees sparks, as from electricity. [ZIEGLER, l. c.]

290. Sees objects double. [HENNING,—SICELIUS, l. c.—*Stf.*]

He sees nothing at all near, and everything double at a distance. [*Stf.*]

He sees objects multiplied and dark. [SAUTER, l. c. (11).]

He sees objects inverted. [HENNING, l. c.]

Feeling in the eyes as if they stood farther out. [*Stf.*]

295. Projecting eyes, with dilated pupils (aft. 6 h.). [*Mkl.*]

Staring eyes. [MULLER,[1] in *Horn's Archiv,* ix.]

Bold look. [DUMOULIN,[2] in *Jour. de Med,* xi, Aout.]

The eyes are projecting and sparking. [GRIMM, l. c.]

Glittering (glassy) eyes. [ZIEGLER, l. c.]

300. The eyes are very animated, with fully dilated pupils (aft. 20 h.). [BOUCHER, l. c.]

The eyes are red, glittering (glassy), and roll about in the head. [SAUTER, l. c. (II).]

The eyeballs rool about in a circle spasmodically. [BOUCHER, l. c.]

The eyes are distorted. [GREDING, l. c., p. 657.]

Spasms of the eyes, distorting them. [SCHRECK,[3] in *Commerc. lit. Nor.*, 1743.]

305. Eyes and hands are in constant spasmodic movement. [BOUCHER, l. c.]

Unsteadiness of head and hands (aft. 6 h.)

The eyes are distorted, with redness and swelling of face. [BUCHAVE, l. c.]

Squeezing pressure on the left zygoma. [*Ws.*]

A tearing and drawing under the right zygoma (aft. $\frac{1}{4}$ h.). [*Gss.*]

310. Pressure under the right zygoma. [*Gss.*]

When chewing, in the right maxillary joint a violent shooting, extending into the ear, which continues after chewing, but more as a twitching (aft. 1 h.). [*Stf.*]

Fine stitches in the cavity of the maxillary joint (aft. 1 h.). [*Ws.*]

Stitches from the upper jaw into the inner ear.

Stitches in the parotid gland.

315. Violent stitch in the right parotid gland, extending to the auricle, when it terminates in a crampy pain (aft. 2 h.) ; next day the same about the same hour (aft. 26 h.).

Tearing pain on the posterior side of the cartilage of the left ear. [*Ws.*]

Tearing pressure on the lower half of the cartilage of the right ear. [*Hrr.*]

Tearing in the right auricle, which extended backwards. [*Hbg.*]

Tearing downwards **in the inner and outer ear.**

320. Tearing pain in the right auricle, and downwards in the whole side of the face (aft. 24 h.).

Stitches in the external meatus auditorius. [*L. Rkt.*]

---

1 Not accessible.

2 Poisoning of two little girls.

3 Fatal poisoning of a boy of three.

Pinching in the ears, first in the right, then in the left, immediately after the hiccup. [*Kr.*]

A disagreeable aching in the meatus auditorius, as if a finger were bored in. [*Ln.*]

Feeling in the external meatus auditorius, as if some one pressed upon it. [*L. Rkt.*]

325. A very disagreeable feeling in the right ear, as if it were forcibly torn out of the head. [*Gss.*]

Alternately out-tearing and in-pressing pain in the ears and temples, alternating with a similar pain in the orbits. [*Gss.*]

Earache in the left ear (aft. 5 d.). [*Hbg.*]

Sharp blows in the inner ear, with squeezing, like earache. [*Ws.*]

Near the right ear boring pain. [*Kr.*]

330. Aching tearing behind the right ear (aft. ½ h.). [*Htn.*]

Behind the left ear to the neck the muscles are painful, as if they were strongly pressed, the same in the frontal muscles. [*Hbg.*]

A flying stitch darts from the ear into the chin (aft. 1 h.). [*Ws.*]

Stitches in the inner ear, with impaired hearing in it.

Stitches in the inner ear during eructation from the stomach with the taste of food (aft. 12 h.).

335. Drawing pain from the ears to the nape. [*Hbg.*]

Violent pressure on the mastoid processes below the ear. [*Gss.*]

Cutting blows through the mastoid process inwards (aft. 12 h.). [*Ws.*]

Purulent discharge from the ears for twenty days. [*F. H—n.*]

Increased sensitiveness of the auditory organ. [SAUTER, l. c. (11).]

340. First a noise like trumpets and drums in the ears and like roaring (immediately); afterwards humming and buzzing, worst when sitting, better when standing and lying, still better when walking.

Noises in the ears. [VICAT, l. c., p. 181.]

Rushing noise in the ears, vertigo, and dull bellyache. [GREDING, l. c., p., 658.]

Wind rushes out of the ears. [GREDING, l. c., p. 658.]

In the morning, immediately after waking, a fluttering and bubbling before the ears.

345. Deafness, as if a skin were stretched before the ears.

Difficulty of hearing.[1] [GREDING, l. c., p. 694 (23).]

On the root of the nose a couple of small red lumps, paining like a fester, but only when touched (aft. 16 d.). [*Ws.*]

Pimples break out on the cheeks and nose, rapidly fill with pus, and become covered with a scab.

Very cold nose.[2] [GREDING, l. c., p. 664.]

350. Smell before the nose like rotten eggs for a quarter of an hour (aft. 4 h.). [*Lr.*]

Aching pain in the nasal bones. [*Gss.*]

In the nose above the alæ pain as if bruised on touching it externally.

---

1 Immediately after a severe epileptic paroxysm.

2 Continuing during seven days of mania.

Too sensitive sense of smell; the odour of tobacco smoke and soot is intolerable to him (aft. 1 h.).

Nose-bleeding (immediately).

355. Nose-bleeding at night.

Nose-bleeding in the morning.

Painful drawing over the left half of the nose. [*Hbg.*]

Creeping in the point of the nose, that goes off on rubbing. [*Ws.*]

Fine stitches in the point of the nose from the evening onwards through the night.

360. Sudden redness of the point of nose, with burning sensation.

A very painful left nostril, that is plugged up with matter in the morning (aft. 6 weeks). [*Stf.*]

Under the nose fine stitches (aft. ½ h.). [*Ws.*]

Great swelling of the upper lip; it is stiff on opening the mouth.

Painful ulcerous state of the nostrils at the side where they unite with the upper lip.

365. **The nostrils and the angles of the lips are ulcerated, but neither itch nor are painful.**

Drawing in the upper lip followed by red swelling. [*Kr.*]

Abscess of the upper lip, causing painful swelling, with fever, headache, and loss of appetite, ending in free discharge of pus.[1] [LAMBERGEN, l. c.]

A white-headed pimple under the left ala nasi, without pain.

Ulcerated angle of the mouth, exactly where the two lips unite, with uncommon tearing pains round about, even when at rest and *per se* (aft. 5 h.).

370. Sore feeling in the corners of the mouth, as if they would become ulcerated (aft. 5, 6, 7 days). [*Stf.*]

Small pimples, one on the upper lip near the right ala nasi, covered with a scab, another under the border of the lower lip and on the inner skin of the lower lip, all with smarting pain as from salt water. [*Hbg.*]

Small pale-red pimples at the corners of the mouth without sensation; they soon go off without suppurating. [*Hrr.*]

On the upper lip a pimple, with creeping sensation when let alone, but with itching shooting when touched.

In the corner of the lips an ulcer with red border and eroding itching.

375. On the lower external lip-edge burning pain and small vesicles (aft. 24 h.). [*Stf.*]

The lips, especially the upper lip, crack in the middle on sneezing and coughing.

A pimple on the border of the lip, equidistant from the middle and the corner, which becomes transformed into an ulcer covered by a scab, and pains like an inflamed part.

Spasmodic movements of the lips. [MULLER, l. c.]

The right corner of the mouth is drawn outwards.[2] [GREDING, l. c., p. 662.]

---

1 Filled up from Hahnemann's abbreviations.

2 See note to S. 175.

380. A spasm draws the mouth awry (risus sardonicus). WEINMANN, in *Gmelin's Pflanzengifte*, p. 296.]

Mouth drawn awry by spasms [DE ST. MARTIN, l. c.]

Bloody foam before the mouth (shortly before death). [*Commerc. lit. Nor.*, 1731.]

Bloody foam before the mouth, shaking of the head, and grinding of the teeth from early morning till noon. [GREDING, l. c., p. 691 (22).]

Pimples betwixt lips and chin, filled with pus, with burning smarting pain, especially painful at night (aft. 6 days). [*Stf.*]

385. A pimple with smarting eroding pain externally, below and to the side of the lip.

A pimple on the side of the chin, with itching shooting, but more shooting than itching ; this sensation is removed by scratching.

Several small pimples on the chin.

A number of small miliary papules on the chin, with burning pain on touching them (aft. 3 d.). [*Hbg.*]

Sharp stitches on the chin (immediately). [*Ws.*]

390. A nestling spasm-like feeling in the chin.

Trismus ; impossibility of opening the jaws on account of painful stiffness of the chewing muscles (by day).

Closure of the jaws, trismus. [HASENEST—MAY, l. c.]

She clinched her teeth together so that they could not be separated, though great force was employed, with twitchings in all the limbs and chilliness. [MUNCH, in *Richter's Bibliothek*, v, p. 566.]

She bit her teeth so tightly together that a tooth had to be broken out in order to introduce fluids. [BALDINGER, l. c.]

395. Stitches and tension in the lower jaw towards the ear. [*L. Rkt.*]

She feels as if the lower jaw were drawn backwards ; pushing it forwards causes great pain, biting causes horrible pains. [*Kr.*]

At the angle of the lower jaws a red boil, which is hard and not painful unless pressed on, which causes shooting pain.

On the lower border of the right lower jaw sharp stitches. [*Ws.*]

Throbbing on the lower border of the lower jaw (aft. ½ h). [*Ws.*]

400. In the lower jaw (in the glands ?) (a jerking drawing ?) pain that darted in rapidly and quickly went off. [*Stf.*]

Swollen cervical glands, which are painful at night ; on swallowing they do not hurt. [*Bhr.*]

Stitches in a gland at a side of the neck.

On the left side of the neck, in the cervical muscles, a cramp-like tensive sensation, even when not moving (aft. ¼ h.). [*Htn.*]

Her head is drawn backwards ; it buries itself at night deep in the pillow. [*Bhr.*]

405. Stiffness of the neck, so that he cannot lay the head sideways. [*Kr.*]

Stiffness of the nape. [*Bhr.*]

Drawing in the cervical muscles. [*Hbg.*]

In the right cervical muscles drawing aching pain. [*Hbg.*]

Fine stitches in the pit of the throat. [*Ws.*]

410. Aching sensation on the left side of the larynx, which is increased by external pressure (aft. ½ h.). [*Htn.*]

Feels the beating of the cervical arteries. [*Kr.*]

Aching pain in the nape close up to the occiput, which is not altered by movement (aft. 3 h.). [*Htn.*]

Violent stitches in the nape often renewed, in the region of the second and third cervical vertebræ, on holding up the head (aft. ¾ h.). [*Htn.*]

Violent grinding of the teeth. [MUNCH, l. c.]

415. Grinding of the teeth with much foam before the mouth of the smell of rotten eggs. [GREDING, l. c., p. 692 (22).]

Grinding of the teeth and convulsion of the right arm. [GREDING, l. c., p. 687 (20.).]

Grinding of the teeth with copious flow of saliva from the mouth. [GREDING, l. c., p. 653.]

Extremely painful swelling of the gums on the right side, with fever and chilly feeling. [GREDING, l. c., p. 686 (20).]

Vesicle on the gums beneath one of the front teeth, with pain as if burnt.

420. The gums on being touched pain as if ulcerated.

Heat in the gums; itching and throbbing in them.

Very tiresome itching on the gums, with pains in the throat. [BALDINGER, l. c.]

The gum at a hollow tooth bleeds (aft. 6 d.). [*Ws.*]

On sucking with the tongue at the hollow teeth, blood flows out of them, without pain. [*Ws.*]

425. A drawing in the upper front molars of the right side, remaining the same under all conditions. [*Gss.*]

Tearing pain in a lower hollow tooth and in the sound molar next it; the contact of air or of food increases the pain horribly (aft. 4 d.). [*Hrr.*]

Toothache more drawing than shooting.

Toothache with drawing in the ear.

He wakes up after midnight with violent tearing (?) in the teeth.

430. By the contact of the open air a uniform simple toothache, like the pain of excoriation (aft. ¼ h.).

Not while eating, but only several minutes after eating the toothache comes on, increases gradually to a high degree, and declines equally gradually; it does not come on after drinking.

Toothache in the evening after lying down and during intellectual work; a dull pain in the nerve of the roots of the teeth, almost like the pain of excoriation, and when worse like a continual cutting.

Toothache; sharp drawing from the ear downwards into the hollow teeth of the upper jaw, where the pain became boring, slighter whilst eating, more severe after eating, never quite leaving off by day, but worst at night and completely hindering sleep (after drinking coffee it changed to a dull jerking and boring). [*Hpl.*]

Dull drawing in right upper row of teeth all night; the pain prevented sleep; the painful part was somewhat swollen (with burning pain) and hot to the touch ; sometimes painful jerks in the teeth. [*Hbg.*]

435. A fine shooting pain in an upper hollow molar all day, allowing him but little sleep at night, followed by swelling of cheek.

(A transient digging toothache.)

(The incisors feel too long.)

Teeth painful on biting as if the roots were festering and would break off.

Single, very painful twitches or throbs in the root-nerves of one or several teeth.

440. In the mouth a feeling of increased space, just as if the tongue was further down than usual. [*Kr.*]

Feeling as if the tongue were asleep, dead and numb, in the morning. [*Kr.*]

Feeling of coldness and dryness in the fore half of the tongue. [*Kr.*]

The whole tongue is painful, especially when touched. [*Stf.*]

Cracked, white furred tongue, with great secretion of saliva. [*Hbg.*]

445. On the middle of the white furred tongue severe smarting pain, as from a vesicle (aft. 3 d.). [*Stf.*]

On the tip of the tongue a feeling as if a vesicle were there which has burning pain on being touched, for two days. [*Hbg.*]

The lingual papillæ are bright red, inflamed, and much swollen (aft. 3 d.). [*Stf.*]

Trembling of the tongue. [WEINMANN, l. c.]

Stammering of the tongue. [RAU, l. c.]

450. **Stammering weakness of the organs of speech, with perfect consciousness and dilated pupils** (aft. 2, 3 h.).

He stammers like a drunken person. [BUCHAVE, l. c.]

Transient speechlessness (aphonia). [SAUVAGES, *Nosol.*, ii, 2, p. 338.]

Paralytic weakness of the organs of speech.

Speechlessness ; they emit no sound (aphonia).[1] [WAGNER, l. c. (1).]

455. Dumbness. [HASENEST, l. c.]

Difficult speech, difficulty of breathing, and great prostration, after the anxiety.

Speaking is very difficult for him ; his voice is piping.

Very low voice, with headache, as if the brain would be pressed out, just over the orbits, in the forehead, which prevents the eyes being opened, and compels him to lie down, with extreme contraction of the pupils.

Tongue covered with much viscid, yellowish-white mucus. [JUSTI, l. c.]

460. Viscid mucus in the mouth. [*Mkl.*—GREDING l. c., p. 648.]

Viscid saliva hangs in long strings out of the mouth. [GREDING, l. c., p. 687.]

---

1 In the original, "stupidæ atque *aowvol.*"

Great flow of saliva. [OLLENROTH, l. c.]

Ptyalism.

Soreness inside the cheek ; the opening of the salivary ducts is as if eroded.

465. He often spits out viscid mucus. [GREDING, l. c., p. 684 (19).]

He has much mucus in the mouth, especially in the morning after rising, sometimes of a putrid taste. [*Hrr.*]

The saliva in the throat was inspissated, viscid, white, and adherent to the tongue like glue, so that she must always take some liquid into the mouth. [SICELIUS, l. c.]

Slimy mouth, with the feeling as if he had a bad smell from the mouth, as when the stomach is deranged.

In the morning the mouth is full of mucus ; he must wash it out from time to time ; after eating the mucus disappears.

470. **Slimy mouth in the morning on awaking, with aching headache (both lasting but a short time.)**

In the morning on awaking he smelt very badly out of the mouth.

Great feeling of dryness in the mouth, with very irritable humour ; yet the mouth and tongue look moist.

Great feeling of dryness in the mouth ; there was very little viscid mucus on the tongue, and the lips were hot and their skin peeled off.

Viscid mucus in the mouth and dry feeling. [*Hrr.*]

475. Dryness in the mouth. [ZIEGLER, l. c.]

Great feeling of dryness in the moist mouth, with stickiness and great thirst. [*Stf.*]

Great dryness in the throat. [CULLEN,[1] *Mat. Med.*, ii, p. 307.]

Dryness in the mouth with thirst. [*Ln.*]

Aridity of the mouth, as if the inner skin had been removed by something acrid. [LOTTINGER, l. c.]

480. Dryness of the mouth that can scarcely be got rid of. [DE MEZA,[2] in *Samml. br. Abh. f. A.*, xiv, 3.]

Dryness in the throat. [WIENHOLT,[3] *Heilkr. d. Thier. Magnetismus*, i, p. 310.]

Feeling of excessive dryness in the mouth, and yet the tongue was always moist. [*Stf.*]

Excessive dryness of the mouth that caused constriction in the throat. [*Stf.*]

His fauces and pharynx were constricted on account of the extreme dryness of the mouth ; there was not a trace of mucus there, and only moderate thirst, still he could swallow milk. [*Stf.*]

485. Dryness in the mouth, the fauces, and the nose. [BUCHAVE—LAMBERGEN, l. c.]

He cannot swallow on account of dryness of mouth, fauces, and nose. [BUCHAVE, l. c.]

---

1 Effects of infusion in a sufferer from cancer of lip.

2 Effects of a five-grain dose of the powdered leaves in a case of mammary tumour.

3 Not accessible.

Throwing up of blood, seemingly proceeding from the fauces.* [CULLEN, l. c.]

Flow of blood from mouth and nose.[1] [WAGNER, l. c. (11).]

Scraping scratching on the palate, occurring by itself. [*Ws.*]

490. On the palate all as if raw and sore, especially painful when touched with tongue and on chewing, as though denuded of skin (aft. 6 days, lasting several days). [*Stf.*]

Pains in the throat. [BALDINGER, l. c]

Fine tearing on the inner surface of the angle of the left side of the inferior maxilla, on the left tonsil and behind it, unaltered by touching ; violent tearing on swallowing (aft. 2 d.). [*Hrr.*]

Dryness in the fauces and burning on the tongue. [OLLENROTH, l. c.]

Burning sensation in the fauces. [HENNING, l. c.]

495. Though the mouth is sufficiently moist there is violent burning in the throat, which is not alleviated by drinking, but is transiently ameliorated by a little sugar. [*Bhr.*]

Long-continued burning pain in the fauces ; food and drink burn in the mouth like alcohol. [REMER,[2] in *Hufel. Jour.*, xvii, 2.]

Inflammation of throat and fauses. [RAU, in *Acta Nat. Cur.*, vol. x, p. 90—GOCKEL, in *Frankische Samml.*, iii, p. 44.[3]]

Constant urging and need to swallow ; he felt as if he must choke if he did not swallow.

Sore throat ; stitches in the pharynx and pain as from internal swelling, only felt when swallowing and on turning the neck, as also when touching the side of it, but not when at rest or when talking.

500. The throat is swollen internally. [RAU, l. c.]

The throat is sore on swallowing and spitting out ; a sensation as from swelling, more on the felt side. [*Kr.*]

Pain in the throat and bellyache. [GREDING, l. c., p. 652.]

Sore throat becoming worse every hour, heat, scratching, constriction and sore feeling. [*Kr.*]

Difficult and painful swallowing. [VICAT, l. c.]

505. A violent shooting pain in the throat on swallowing and breathing. [*Stf.*]

Stitches in the throat on the left side, equally bad whether swallowing or not. [*Htn.*]

Inflammation of the tonsils, which after 4 days pass into suppuration, during which he cannot swallow a drop. [GREDING, l. c., vol. ii, p. 321]

* This terminated fatally. Even after death the bodies of those poisoned by belladonna showed bleeding from nose, mouth, and ears ; they became, either only in the face, or on one side of the body, or all over, blackish-violet, or covered with gangrenous spots ; the epidermis soon became detached, the abdomen swollen, and within twelve hours they became decomposed, as testified to by EB. GMELIN and FABER.

---

1 When throwing up the berries from the operation of an emetic.

2 Effects of full doses of powdered root in a case of melancholia.

3 Poisoning of a child of five.

Difficult deglutition. [MAY,—GREDING, l. c., p. 694.]

Impeded swallowing.

510. Painless inability to swallow.

Impeded swallowing. [REMER, l. c.—GREDING, l. c., p. 648.]

Great constriction of the gullet. [CULLEN, l. c.]

Transient but frequently recurring contraction of the œsophagus, more on swallowing than at other times, each time followed by a scratching pain in the region of the epiglottis as if there was something raw and sore there. [*Ln.*]

Sore throat; when swallowing scraping in the palate and as if rubbed raw there.

515. Throat affection; narrowing (contraction) of the gullet, whereby swallowing is impeded (aft. 3 h.).

Painful narrowing and contraction of the gullet; on making the preparatory movements to swallow it feels tense and stretched although nothing is swallowed; when actually swallowing it is not more painful; even when quite the feeling of narrowness in the throat is painful (aft. 60 h.). [*Ws.*]

On swallowing, a feeling in the throat as if all were too narrow there, as if contracted, as though nothing could get rightly down (aft. 2 h.). [*Stf.*]

She could not swallow solid food. [SICELIUS, l. c.]

He chews the food without being able to swallow it, because the throat appears to him to be contracted. [BALDINGER, l. c.]

520. In her unconscious state she often pushes her finger deep down her throat, scratches her gums, and presses her neck with both hands. [BALDINGER, l. c.]

He swallows water with the greatest difficulty, and can only get down an extremely small quantity. [EL. CAMERARIUS, l. c.]

Horror of all fluids, so that she makes frightful faces at them. [BALDINGER, l. c.]

Liquid poured out makes her furious. [BALDINGER, l. c.]

Inability to swallow. [DE LAUNAY D'HERMONT, l. c.—MANETTI,[1] *Varidarium florentium*, Florent., 1757.]

525. Paralytic weakness of the internal parts of the mouth [LOTTINGER, l. c.]

Something rose from the abdomen and pressed in the throat, with retching, but without nausea and without vomiting. [*Stf.*]

Lost taste. [LOTTINGER, l. c.]

Insipid taste in the mouth. [*Hbg.*]

Spoilt taste in the mouth. [GREDING, l. c., p. 657.]

530. Disgusting taste in the mouth, with clean tongue.

Corrupted taste of the saliva. [VICAT, l. c.]

Putrid taste in the mouth, when she had eaten.

Putrid taste in the mouth as from putrid meat, two hours after eating (aft. 8 h.). [*Mkl.*]

Putrid taste comes up from the fauces, also when eating and drinking, although food and drink have their proper taste. [*Ws.*]

---

1 Poisoning of a puppy by the juice of the berries.

535. A sickly sweet taste in the mouth. [*Hbg.*]

Sticky taste in the mouth.

Salty sourish taste in the mouth. [*Stf.*]

Salt taste of the food, as if it were all salted (aft. 25 h.). [*Stf.*]

At the commencement of the meal proper taste of the food, but all at once everything tasted partly too salt, partly like nothing and insipid, with feeling in the throat (pit of the throat) as if the ingesta would be thrown up again. [*Stf.*]

540. Bread smells and tastes sour to him.

Bread tastes sour to him.

The bread tastes sour to her. [*Hbg.*]

Disgust at milk, which at other times she generally drank and with relish ; it has a disgusting very repulsive smell and (sourish-bitter) taste to her, which, however, goes off on continuing to drink. [*Stf.*]

In the evening the bread and butter, at least the last portion of it, tastes very sour, whereupon generally some heartburn ensued, which lasted two hours (for eight successive evenings) (aft. 4 d.).

545. (Bitter taste of bread and apples, in the evening.)

Coffee is repugnant to her. [*Bhr.*]

Disgust at camphor. [*Bhr.*]

Hunger, but no inclination for any kind of food. [*Hbg.*]

Repugnance to food. [GRIMM,—LOTTINGER, l. c.]

550. Complete repugnance to all food and drink, with quick weak pulse. [GREDING, l. c., p. 677 (16).]

Total loss of appetite.[1] [LAMBERGEN, l. c.]

Want of appetite, with headache. [GREDING, l. c., p. 659.]

Diminished appetite ; animal food is especially repugnant. [*Ws.*]

Dislike to beer.

555. Dislike to acids.

Long-continued **repugnance to food.**

No appetite ; he loathes everything.

(He gets a longing for one thing or another ; but when he partakes of it he does not relish it.)

After smoking tobacco all appetite goes.

560. Anorexia, with empty feeling and hunger ; on commencing to eat he relishes the food and eats as usual. [*Hrr.*]

Increased appetite (curative action.)

Appetite for water-soup and bread and butter, but for nothing else. [*Kr.*]

After eating but little, a peculiar contracting feeling in the stomach. [*Mkl.*]

After eating cough and great thirst. [GREDING, l. c., p. 665.]

565. Immediately after a meal as if intoxicated (aft. $6\frac{1}{2}$ h.). [*Lr.*]

After eating violent pinching below the navel, close beneath the abdominal integuments (aft. $2\frac{1}{2}$ h.). [*Htn.*]

After taking beer, internal heat. [*Ws.*]

No desire for drinks ; adipsia.

Adipsia. [*Hrr.*]

---

1 In connection with S. 367.

570. Desire for drinks without thirst; he hardly brought the cup to his mouth when he set it down again (aft. 8 h.). [*Lr.*]

Astonishing thirst in the evening with watery taste, but all drinks disgusted her. [*Kr.*]

Strong thirst for cold drinks, without heat (aft. 7 h.). [*Lr.*]

At noon, violent thirst (returning several days at the same time). [*Kr.*]

Eructation with the taste of the ingesta.

575. Bitter eructation after eating.

Frequent eructation from the stomach. [*Ln.*]

Eructation with loss of appetite. [GREDING, l. c., p. 679 (17).]

Eructation and vertigo. [GREDING, l. c., p. 673 (15).]

Ineffectual desire to eructate.

580. **Half suppressed, incomplete eructation.**

Putrid eructation. [GREDING, l. c., p. 657.]

Burning, sour eructation, whereby also corrosive sour fluid came into the mouth with a kind of retching. *Stf.*]

Heartburn (when smoking tobacco); there long remains a scratching burning smarting sensation at the entrance to the gullet, and chiefly at the upper border of the larynx (aft. 2 h.).

Flow of water into the mouth, in the evening, for half an hour. [*Kr.*]

585. Nausea and inclination to vomit **in the throat** (not in the pit of the stomach), sometimes with bitter eructation, in the evening. [*Stf.*]

After breakfast, squeamishness.

In the forenoon, frequent attacks of nausea (aft. 72 h.).

Inclination to vomit while walking in the open air.

Nausea in the stomach. [*Hrr.*]

590. Disgust with inclination to vomit, especially when he is about to eat. [SICELIUS, l. c.]

Frequent disgust and retching. [GREDING, l. c., p. 645.]

Nausea, inclination to vomit, and such great thirst that she must drink enormous quantities of water. [BALDINGER, l. c.]

Vomiting in the evening. [GREDING, l. c., p. 650.]

Vomiting, vertigo, and flying heat. [GREDING, l. c., p. 643.]

595. Vomiting and profuse sweat. [GREDING, l. c., p. 675 (16).]

Excessive vomiting. [GOCKEL, l. c.]

Vomiting of mucus about noon. [GREDING, l. c., p. 672.]

Bilious, slimy vomiting. [DE MEZA, l. c.]

Vomiting of undigested food partaken of twelve hours previously. [GRIMM, l. c.]

600. Vomiting (aft. 6 h.), and immediately afterwards sleep for several hours. [EL. CAMERARIUS, l. c.]

Inclination to vomit, ineffectual retching. [MAY, l. c.]

He yawns and retches till he is blue in the face, whilst he stretches one hand over the head, but with the other strikes his abdomen irrepressibly. [GREDING, l. c., p. 668.]

Ineffectual effort to vomit. [*Hbg.*]

He awakes thrice about midnight; he heaves thrice as if to vomit, but without result, with the sweat of anxiety.

605. Ineffectual effort to vomit, empty retching.

He cannot vomit, want of irritability of the stomach. [MAY, l. c.]

Fourteen grains of tartar emetic do not make him vomit, he does not even feel sick after taking it. [BALDINGER, l. c.]

Several times violent hiccup. [*Ln.*]

Violent hiccup that jerked her upwards, whereupon she became deaf until the next attack. [*Kr.*]

610. Violent hiccup about midnight. [GREDING, l. c., p. 653.]

Something intermediate between eructation and hiccup.

Hiccupy eructation ; a spasm compounded of eructation and hiccup.

At night eructation, with profuse sweat. [GREDING, l. c., p. 669 (14).]

After hiccup convulsions of the head and limbs, then nausea and weariness. [GREDING, l. c., p. 672 (14).]

615. Hiccup, with convulsion alternately of the right arm and left leg, followed by great thirst, with redness and heat of head. [GREDING, l. c., p. 670 (14).]

Painless throbbing and beating in the pit of the stomach.

Violent pains in the region of the scrobiculus cordis. [WAGNER, l. c. (11).]

Hard pressure in the stomach, especially after eating (aft. 24 h.). [*Hrr.*]

(At night periodical pain in the scrobiculus cordis, with trembling.)

620. When he has eaten he has stomachache.

An aching in the scrobiculus cordis, partly gnawing.

(Aching, shooting pain in the left side under the ribs.)

Fulness under the short ribs ; on stooping the pit of the stomach feels full, and there is blackness before the eyes (aft. 4 d.).

Violent stomachache after a meal, and also later after that time (aft. 5 h.). [*Hrr.*]

625. **Painful aching in the pit of the stomach only when walking ; it forces him to walk slowly** (aft. 48 h.). [*Ws.*]

Under the sternum air seemed to have accumulated, which went off by rumbling in the belly, whereupon the nausea became always more intense. [*Kr.*]

Spasm in the stomach.[1] [MANETTI, l. c.]

Spasm in the stomach like cramp. [EL. CAMERARIUS, l. c.]

Long-lasting spasm in the stomach every time during dinner.

630. After a scanty meal a peculiar contractive feeling in the stomach. [*Mkl.*]

After lying down in bed in the evening, distended epigastrium, with tensive pain in the stomach.

Contractive pain in the scrobiculus cordis. [*Mkl.*]

Burning in the stomach.[2] [HENNING, l. c.]

Stitches in the scrobiculus cordis. [*Hbg.*]

---

1 In a puppy, from juice forced into the stomach. The full symptom reads—"profound convulsion of the stomach, like hiccup, lasting for half an hour."

2 Every time she took a dose. So also in S. 494.

635. Stitches in the scrobiculus cordis.
Horrible, shooting cutting pain in the scrobiculus cordis, which forces the body to bend backwards, and compels him to hold his breath.
Inflammation of the stomach.[1] [GOCKEL, l. c.]
Inflammation of the upper part of the duodenum.[1] [GOCKEL, l. c.]
Burning in the abdomen. [ALBRECHT, l. c.]
640. Constant bellyache. [GREDING, l. c., p. 644.]
Bellyache, constipation, diuresis, with eructation and inclination to vomit. [GREDING, l. c., p. 666.]
(After drinking milk, bellyache, some stitches.)
(Cutting in the belly, in the evening, some hours before going to sleep.)
Bellyache, spasmodic tension from the chest to low down in the hypogastrium, which does not permit the slightest movement (aft. ½ h.).
645. Bellyache and leucorrhœa. [GREDING, l. c., p. 672 (14).]
In the evening pressure in the abdomen as from a stone, with pains in the loins. [GREDING, l. c., p. 681 (18).]
Bellyache, as from a hard weight, only when walking and standing, always going off when sitting.
Quite low down in the hypogastrium pressure as from a heavy weight.[2] [GREDING, l. c., vol. ii, p. ii, p. 323.]
In the right groin, in the inguinal ring, on sitting stooping forwards, a sensation as if a hard body pressed out, but the part is not hard to the touch (aft. 6 d.). [*Ws.*]
650. On sitting bent forwards a sensation in the right groin as if a hard body pressed out. [*Stf.*]
In the hypogastrium, immediately below the navel, sensation as if the bowels were forcing outwards, most felt when standing (aft. 6 d.). [*Ws.*]
When pressing on the pit of the stomach he has an out-pressing pain in the side of the abdomen.
Inflation of the abdomen.[3] [GOCKEL, l. c.]
Distended, but not hard nor painful abdomen. [BOUCHER, l. c.]
655. Distended, hard abdomen. [JUSTI, l. c.]
Along with sensation of distension of the abdomen a constrictive bellyache below the navel, which comes by jerks, and compels him to bend himself forwards (aft. 4 h.).
Abdomen tense round about the ribs. [EL. CAMERARIUS, l. c.]
A distension of the abdomen, with rumbling or rolling in the bowels on the left side. [*Ln.*]
A drawing-in of the abdomen, with pressive pain (when lying). [*Hbg.*]
660. Squeezing, constrictive pain in the bowels deep down in the

1 Ascertained *post mortem*.
2 Taking the place of a pain in the hypochondrium, back, and loins, which he had before beginning the medicine.
3 After death. It is described as "extraordinary and preternatural."

hypogastrium, alternating with obtuse stitches or jerks towards the perinæum (aft. 36 h.)

A constriction of the abdomen about the umbilical region, as if a knot or lump would be formed. [*Ln.*]

In the morning, immediately after getting out of bed, a violent tensive aching pain in the whole hypogastrium, but especially in the pubic region ; it is as if the hypogastrium (rarely the epigastrium) were spasmodically constricted, sometimes as if it were distended (though not actually distended) ; pains that gradually increase and gradually decline (aft. 24 h.). [*Gss.*]

A contraction of the abdomen in the umbilical region. [*Ln.*]

Squeezing and gripping round about the navel, so that he must bend forwards. [*Hbg.*]

665. Contractive pain in the abdomen ; she must bend forwards on account of the pain.

Bellyache, as if a part in the abdomen were grasped with the nails, a gripping, clutching, clawing.

A squeezing together in the umbilical region, worse at noon and in the afternoon.

When walking, great clawing together in the right side of the belly, besides sharp shooting from there up through the right side of the chest and out at the axilla. [*Ws.*]

An extremely painful clawing together in the umbilical region, coming from the sides and uniting in the navel. [*Stf.*]

670. Pinching bellyache, whereby he is compelled to sit with his body bent together, with ineffectual call to diarrhœa and subsequent vomiting.

Pinching in the bowels. [*Hbg.*]

Pinching in the side of the abdomen, the hepatic region, so that when he wished to rise up from his seat he could not do so on account of the pain. [*Hbg.*]

Pinching across the epigastrium and downwards as if in the colon. [*Mkl.*]

Violent pinching deep in the abdomen, which is much aggravated by drawing in the belly and by bending the upper part of the body over to the left side (aft. 6 h.). [*Htn.*]

675. Great stitches in the inguinal glands.

Fine stitches in the left groin. [*Mkl.*]

Obtuse stitches in the right side of the abdomen at the last ribs. [*Ws.*]

Violent shooting as with a blunt knife between the right hip and the navel (aft. 12 h.). [*Gss.*]

From the umbilical region round over the left hip to the lumbar vertebræ a shooting cut, as if in a single thrust, in which latter region it terminated, and where it was most painful (aft. $\frac{3}{4}$ h.). [*Gss.*]

680. Obtuse knife-thrusts on the left side below the navel. [*Gss.*]

An aching, shooting pain in the umbilical region (aft. 24 h). [*Ln.*]

Early in bed, in the left side of the abdomen on which he is lying quietly, an aching cutting, which goes off as soon as he turns on the other side (aft. 11 d.). [*Ws.*]

Violent cutting pressure in the hypogastrium, sometimes here, sometimes there (aft 1 h.). [*Hrr.*]

Cutting in the whole of the hypogastrium, but more violent in the left side. [*Gss.*]

685. Itching stitches at the navel, which go off by rubbing (aft. 1 h.). [*Ws.*]

Anxious heat in the abdomen, in the chest, and in the face, with stuffed nose. [*Ws.*]

Heat from below upwards, so that the sweat of anxiety broke out, followed by nausea combined with frightful anxiety, until the nausea went always further down. [*Kr.*]

Painfulness of the whole abdomen, as if all were sore and raw, lasting long (aft. 1 h.). [*Stf.*]

Violent reiterated rumbling in the bowels. [*Gss.*]

690. Loud rumbling in the abdomem, with the feeling as if all there were mixed up together (aft. $\frac{1}{4}$ h.). [*Stf.*]

A rumbling and pinching in the abdomen. [*Ln.*]

Very frequent discharge of flatus almost without smell. [*Ln.*]

Frequent discharge of inodorous flatus.

During a motion of the bowels, shivering.

695. During a motion of the bowels a shudder ran over the child.

On straining at stool feeling in the abdomen as if diarrhœa were coming on, with internal heat in the abdomen (aft. 1 h.). [*Ws.*]

Pappy stool mixed with mucus. [*Hbg.*]

Heat of head, alternating with diarrhœa. [GREDING, l. c., p. 672 (14).]

Diarrhœa, inclination to vomit, and stomachache. [GREDING, l. c., p. 672 (14).]

700. Curdled, yellow, somewhat mucous stool.

(Motions of a very sour smell.)

Stools as white as chalk.[1] [WEINMANN, l. c., p. 138.]

Green stools.[2] [GREDING, l. c., vol. ii, p. 320.]

Green stools, with diuresis, and yet sweat at the same time.[2] [GREDING, l. c., vol. ii, p. 319.]

705. Several watery stools immediately after profuse sweat. [JUSTI, l. c.]

At first soft diarrhoeic stool, **but afterwards frequent urging to stool, whereby very little or nothing at all comes away.** [*Ws.*]

Uncommonly diminished stool, only small evacuations occur for several days. [*Hbg.*]

Urging to stool, which comes away thinner than usual, but in sufficient quantity. [*Hrr.*]

Frequent thin stools, with tenesmus ; he felt a frequent desire to go, he must go to stool every quarter of an hour (aft. 48 h.).

---

1 Not found.

2 During recovery from jaundice.

710. He has a constant desire to go to stool.

Straining at stool; a scanty diarrhœic motion comes away, and is immediately followed by very much increased straining (aft. 3 h.). [*Stf.*]

Frequent urging to stool, without any, or with only a very scanty and hard motion. [*Hrr.*]

Tenesmus and bellyache. [FABER,[1] *Strychnomania*, p. 13, obs. 5.]

Ineffectual urging to stool.

715. After ineffectual urging to stool, vomiting.

A kind of tenesmus, a constant pressure and forcing towards the anus and genitals, alternating with painful contraction of the anus (aft. 12 h.).

Pressure in the rectum towards the anus. [*Mkl.*]

Constipation. [FR. HOFFMANN,[2] *Medicina ration.*, p. 273.]

After a confined motion distension of the abdomen and heat of head. [GREDING, l. c., p. 673 (14).]

720. He cannot strain at stool. [*Fr. H—n.*]

Contractive pain in the rectum, then sore pain in the epigastrium, followed by rapid discharge of slimy diarrhœa, at last empty straining.

Severe itching, and at the same time constrictive sensation in the anus. [*Gss.*]

Itching in the lower part of the rectum.

Violent, sudden, painful itching in rectum, and anus.

725. Itching externally at the anus (while walking in the open air).

A pleasant tickling in the lower part of the rectum.

Single, rapid, great stitches in the rectum (when moving) (aft. 3 h.).

Hæmorrhoidal bleeding for several days.

Involuntary discharge of the stool, temporary paralysis of the sphincter ani. [DUMOULIN, l. c.]

730. Involuntary discharge of the excrements. [GREDING, l. c., p. 690 (22).]

Small, rapid, involuntary stools.

Suppressed evacuation of stool and urine for ten hours.

Suppressed evacuation of stool and urine, with extraordinary perspiration. [BALDINGER, l. c.]

Difficult micturition.

735. Suppressed urine.[3] [DE LAUNAY D'HERMONT, l. c.—SICELIUS, l. c.]

Retention of the urine, which only passes by drops. [LOTTINGER, l. c.]

Frequent call to pass urine. [GREDING, l. c., p. 658.]

Frequent call to urinate, but the urine passed in strikingly small quantity, though of natural colour. [*Gss.*]

Frequent urging to urinate, with scanty discharge of urine (aft. 1 h.). [*Lr.*]

---

1 General account of effects of B.

2 Statement of effects of soporifics in general (including opium.)

3 We can say nothing about Sicelius, but de Launay d'Hermont's symptom is only "difficult micturition."

740. Incessant urging to urinate. [BUCAVE, l. c.]
Yellow, turbid urine. [ACKERMANN, l. c.]
Clear, lemon-coloured urine. [JUSTI, l. c.]
Golden-yellow urine. [*Hbg.*]
Bright yellow, clear urine (aft. 4 h.).
745. (Whitish urine.)
Urine with white, thick sediment (aft. 12 h.).
Urine turbid, like yeast, with reddish sediment.
Frequent micturition. [*Hbg.*]
Frequent micturition of copious urine. [SAUTER, l. c. (11).]
750. Flow of urine (enuresis[1]). [SAUTER (11), l. c,—GREDING, l. c., pp. 644, 648, 650, 652, 675, 686]
Frequent micturition of copious, pale, thin watery urine. [GRIMM, l. c.]
Discharge of a quantity of watery urine, with perspiration. [BAYLIES, *Pract. Essays on Med. Subjects*, p. 37.]
Along with discharge of a large quantity of urine, and with increased appetite, he is quite cold to the touch. [GREDING, l, c., p. 694 (23).]
At night diuresis, with profuse sweat. [GREDING, l. c., p. 689 (22).]
755. Along with constant diuresis profuse night sweat. [GREDING, l. c., p. 689 (21).]
Diuresis, thirst, and obscuration of vision in the morning. [GREDING, l. c., p. 970 (14).]
Diuresis, with perspiration, good appetite and diarrhœa. [GREDING, l. c., p. 667.]
Diuresis, with profuse sweat. [GREDING, l. c., p. 684 (19).]
Diuresis, diarrhœa, and appetite. [GREDING, l. c., p. 661.]
760. Urine more copious than the drink taken would warrant. [HORST, l. c.]
Diuresis on the occurrence of the catamenia. [EVERS, in *Schmucker's Vermischten Schr.*, i, p. 185.[2]]
Involuntary discharge of urine. [BOUCHER, l. c.]
Involuntary discharge of urine, temporary paralysis of the neck of the bladder.[3] [DUMOULIN, l. c.]
During profound sleep (by day) his urine escaped.
765. He cannot retain his urine.
Sensation of winding and turning in the bladder, as from a large worm, without urging to pass water.
In the night obtuse pressure in the vesical region.
Immediately after making water a smarting sensation on the outer border of the prepuce.
In the anterior part of the glans penis an itching tickling like the bite of a flea. [*Hbg.*]
770. Before falling asleep in the evening in bed tearing upwards in the left spermatic cord several times repeated. [*Mkl.*]

---

1 This is what we now call "diuresis."
2 From a case of serous apoplexy, in which B. was given.
3 See S. 729.

The prepuce is retracted behind the glans, whence he has a disagreeable sensation in the exposed glans (aft. 4 h.). [*Mkl.*]

A long stitch along the urethra, which commenced at the bulbous portion of the urethra, and extended to its orifice, whilst walking (aft. 3 h.). [*Htn.*]

A violent forcing and starining towards the genitals, as if all would fall out there ; worse when sitting bent foward and when walking, better when standing and sitting upright (aft. 10 h.). [*Stf.*]

When not passing water obtuse stitches in the urethra, behind the glans, especially when moving.

775. Whilst passing water drawing in the spermatic cord.

Discharge of prostatic fluid from flaccid penis.

On the glans penis a soft painless pimple.

Sweat on the genitals at night.

Great stitches in the drawn-up testicles (aft. 12, 18, 30 h.).

780. **Nocturnal emission of semen, with flaccid penis.**

Two seminal emissions in one night.

At every step violent stitches in the pubic region, as if in the internal genital organs (aft. 10 h.). [*Stf.*]

Nocturnal seminal emission without lascivious dreams (the first night). [*Lr.*]

Indifferent at the thought of the difference of the sexes ; he cannot summon up any lascivious, lustful thoughts ; the sexual desire in the imagination is as if extinct.

785. The most voluptuous pictures and stories excite neither his imagination nor his genital organs ; he remains indifferent to them (aft. 20 h.).

Before the catamenia weariness, bellyache, want of appetite, and dimness of vision. [Greding, l. c., p. 679 (17).]

During the catamenia perspiration on the chest, yawning, and rigor running over the back. [Greding, l. c., p. 671 (14).]

During the catamenia cardiac anxiety, [Greding, l. c.]

During the catamenia great thirst. [Greding, l. c., p. 672 (14).]

790. During the catamenia a cramp-like tearing, sometimes here and there in the back, sometimes in the arms.

Appearance of the catamenia.

Catamenia four days too soon.

Increased menses.[1] [Lambergen, l. c.]

Increase and delay of the menses to the thirty-second, thirty-sixth, and forty-eighth day. [Greding, in several places.]

795. (In the morning a pressing as if all would be forced out at the genitals (with distension of the abdomen) ; after the pressing the abdomen contracted, and white mucus escaped from the vagina.)

Ill-smelling metrorrhagia. [Evers,[2] in the *Berliner Samml.*, iv.]

Leucorrhœa and colic. [Greding, l. c., p. 672 (14).]

* * *

---

1 Curative effect.

2 Not found.

Repeated sneezing. [*Ln.*]

The nose is sometimes stuffed, sometimes water flows from it. [*Bhr.*]

800. **Catarrh, or cough with coryza.**

Fluent coryza only in one side of the nose and out of one nostril.

Coryza, with stinking odour in the nose as of herring-pickle, especially on blowing the nose. [*Kr.*]

Hoarseness. [VICAT, l. c.]

Rough, hoarse voice.

805. Noise and rattling in the bronchial tubes. [RAU, l. c.]

Every inspiration excites irritation to (dry) tussiculation.

For several successive days, about noon, violent cough, with discharge of much viscid saliva. [GREDING, l. c., p. 691 (22).]

Fit of coughing, followed by heat. [*Kr.*]

Nocturnal cough, which often wakes her out of sleep, after which she immediately falls asleep again. [*Kr.*]

810. Fit of coughing, as from inspiring dust, wakes her up at night, with expectoration of mucus. [*Hbg.*]

(In the forenoon) severe dry cough, as if some foreign substance had fallen into the trachea, with coryza (aft. 3 h.). [*Lr.*]

In the evening, after lying down in bed, an itching tickle in the back part of the larynx, exciting to irresistible, dry, short cough.

It is as if something lay in the scrobiculus cordis, which always excites coughing.

He has a tightness in the chest like dry catarrh, exciting him to dry cough.

815. Oppression in the chest (in the upper part of the trachea); he expectorates something like old catarrhal mucus, of purulent appearance (in the morning in bed and after getting up) (aft. 16 h.).

Cough commences in the evening (about 10 o'clock), and comes every quarter of an hour and oftener, of three or four impulses.

Cough with taste of blood in the mouth.

In the morning on coughing expectoration of bloody mucus.

(Cough hollow and scraping.)

820. Violent cough during sleep, with grinding of the teeth (aft. 10. h.).

Cough with needle-pricks in the side under the left ribs (aft. 6 h.). [*Lr.*]

When coughing a violent aching pain in the nape as if it would break (aft. 3½ h.). [*Htn.*]

Dry tussiculation whereby the throat is scraped. [*Stf.*]

Oppression of the chest. [SCHMUCKER,[1] *Chirurg. Wahrnehm.*, ii.]

825. Difficult breathing. [RAU, l. c.]

(When coughing the child strains much, and is peevish.)

(Before every fit of coughing the child became quiet, and just before the cough came it cried.)

(The attacks of coughing ended in sneezing.)

---

1 Observation on a patient.—In original, "viel Angst und Beklemmung."

(When coughing the stomach turns over as about to vomit, even when it is empty.)

830. Very difficult respiration.[1] [DE LAUNAY D'HERMONT, l. c.]

Violent, small, frequent, anxious respirations (aft. 18 h.). [GRIMM, l. c.]

A pressure in the cardiac region, which stops the breath and causes anxiety.

Pressure on the chest (it affected the heart).

She felt at the heart (the scrobiculus cordis) like cardiac oppression; she could not breathe properly; at the same time nausea, which rises up to the throat, as if she must vomit, and so cardiac oppression and nausea in fits about every seven minutes (aft. $\frac{1}{4}$ h.). [*Stf.*]

835. After drinking (coffee) short breathing (in the afternoon) (aft. 3 d.). [*Hbg.*]

Whilst walking frequently an oppression in the scrobiculus cordis, a kind of spasmodic feeling, that comples him to breathe deeper (aft. 1 h.). [*Htn.*]

Over the chest violent oppression as if it was forced inwards from both sides (aft. 5 h.). [*Htn.*]

Tightness of chest. [VICAT, l. c.]

In the evening in bed a very oppressed feeling in the chest, which is not removed by voluntary coughing; he could only draw his breath wit h difficulty, just as if the phlegm in the wind-pipe hindered him; at the same time a burning in the chest (aft. 60 h.).

840. Sometimes he breathed, sometimes he seemed to have fetched his last breath, in four recurring attacks during a quarter of an hour. [EL. CAMERARIUS, l. c.]

Burning in the right side of the chest. [*Hbg.*]

Heat rises suddenly from the abdomen into the chest and goes off very rapidly (aft. $\frac{1}{2}$ h.). [*Ws.*]

Stitches in the sternum when coughing and when yawning.

Whilst walking fine stitches under the clavicle from before backwards (aft. 4 d.). [*Ws.*]

845. Fine stitches in the left side of the chest from the sternum to the axilla, aggravated by movement, without reference to breathing. [*Ws.*]

Fine shooting pain in the chest. [GREDING, l. c., pp. 661, 681.]

On the right side of the chest a deeply penetrating and enduring stitch, without reference to breathing (aft. 72 h.). [*Ws*]

Stitches in the side of the chest under the right arm, which impede respiration, in the evening.

In the right side, stitches here and there under the skin, to a certain extent externally.

850. Stitches in one of the breasts (aft. 3 h.).

Painful stitches on the left side of the chest, without relation to breathing. [*Ws.*]

Stabs of short duration, as from a blunt knife under both last

---

1 No such symptom found in d'Hermont's narrative. He expressly says, "la respiration etoit *libre.*"

ribs, near the ensiform cartilage, and above the false ribs (aft. 8 m.). [*Gss.*]

Shooting pinching pain in the chest on both sides of the upper part of the sternum. [*Ws.*]

Intermitting aching cutting on the right side of the chest, without reference to inspiration or expiration (aft. ½ h.). [*Ws.*]

855. Continued aching shooting in the left costal cartilages, becoming still more violent and passing into an almost burning sensation on expiration (aft. 3 h.). [*Htn.*]

Sharp pressure from within outwards in the region of the sixth true rib (aft. ¼ h.). [*Ws.*]

A sharp pressive pain in the sternum, immediately above the ensiform cartilage. [*Gss.*]

An aching pain under the right nipple. [*Gss.*]

Aching pain in the chest and between the shoulders.

860. **Aching pain in the chest with short breath, at the same time between the shoulders, when walking and sitting.** [*Hbg.*]

Aching squeezing pain in the left and right breast. [*Hbg.*]

A throbbing pain under the sternum above the scrobiculus cordis. [*Gss.*]

Aching in the right side of the chest, which causes anxiety.

Great restlessness and throbbing in the chest.

865. (When at rest, palpitation of the heart, as if the shock went up to the throat, worse on moving, with difficult slow breath.)

When she goes upstairs the heart clucks, a kind of palpitation. [*Stf.*]

A corroding gnawing pain under the last right cartilages of the ribs (aft. 2 h.). [*Gss.*]

Painful blisters containing water on the sternum.[1] [LAMBERGEN, l. c.]

The chest and thighs covered with very small dark-red irregular spots. [GREDING, l. c., p. 685 (19).]

870. In an unimpregnated woman, milk comes into the breasts and flows out ; on the left breast there appeared small, scattered pimples, which cause creeping itching, which is relieved by rubbing.

The ischia are painful ; she feels as if she had no flesh there, but she is better when sitting on a hard than on a soft seat. [*Kr.*]

A dark (mist-like), painful drawing in the whole extent of the pelvis, but this pain wanders alternately from the sacrum to the os pubis. [*Gss.*]

Spasmodic sensation in the left lumbar region. [*Hbg.*]

Extremely painful cramp-pain in the sacrum and coccyx ; he can only sit for a short time, becomes quite stiff from sitting and on account of the pain cannot rise up again ; he cannot even lie comfortably, it often wakes him up at night, and then he turns on the other side with violent pains ; he cannot lie at all on the back ; he gets most relief from standing and walking about slowly, but he cannot walk quickly (for 8 days). [*Ws.*]

---

1 Probably the effect of long-continued wet dressings on the mamma.

875. When he rises up after sitting, he gets a pain at the border of the ilium over the hips, as if a sharp body was cutting its way outwards. [*Ws.*]

Rheumatic pain in the back. [GREDING, l. c., p. 674 (15).]

At the left side of the spinal column, below the false ribs, aching pain. [*Hbg.*]

Gnawing in the spinal column and cough.

Shooting and gnawing pain in the spinal column.

880. In the vertebræ, stabbing from without inwards as with a knife. [*Kr.*]

In the right side of the back and spinal column, pain as if dislocated.

Cramp-like aching sensation in the middle of the spinal column, which becomes tensive when he tries to straighten his back (aft. ½ h.). [*Htn.*]

The back, especially the scapulæ, is covered with large red pimples; the whole skin looks red, and pains, whed touched, as if excoriated, but in the apices of the pimples the pain is fine shooting (aft 10 d.). [*Ws.*]

Pain in the head extending into the scapulæ. [GREDING, l. c., p. 656.]

885. Boil on the shoulder.

Aching pain under the left shoulder-blade, more towards the outer side. [*Gss.*]

Drawing pressure between the right scapula and the spinal column. [*Hrr.*]

Pain between the scapulæ as from a sprain.

Violent drawing between the scapulæ down the spinal column, in the evening.

890. Cramp-pain, almost like pinching, between the right scapula and the spinal column. [*Ws.*]

(A tickling itching on the left scapula.) [*Ln.*]

Itching shooting on the right scapula, causing her to scratch. [*Ws.*]

Shooting itching on the scapulæ, that goes off on scratching. [*Ws.*]

Fine stitches on the right scapula. [*Ws.*]

895. Repeated shoots as from electricity, from the left scapula towards the right (aft. 1 h.). [*Mkl.*]

Shooting aching on the top of the left shoulder (aft. 3 h.). [*Htn.*]

Painful stiffness between the scapulæ and in the nape on turning the neck and head hither and thither, in the morning (aft. 16 h.).

Externally on the neck aching pain, on bending the head back and on touching the place.

Glandular swellings on the nape with cloudiness of head (aft. 6 h.).

900. Pimples break out on the nape and arm, rapidly fill with pus, and become covered with a scab.

Painful swelling of the left axillary gland (aft. 5.).

Swelling of the affected arm and foot. [MUNCH, in *Richter's Bibliothek.* v, p. 558.]

A stretching and wrenching of the upper extremities. [*Ln.*]

Rheumatic pains of the arm combined with formication, followed next day by spasm of the arm. [GREDING, l. c., p. 671 (14).]

905. Arm as if numb and painful. [SAUTER, l. c. (11).]

Swelling of the arm. [MUNCH, l. c.]

Great feeling of exhaustion in the arms, still more in the hands, as if she must allow them to hang. [*Stf.*]

Heaviness in both arms.

Heaviness of the left arm.[1] [GREDING, l. c., p. 694 (23).]

910. Paralysis of the right arm.[2] [GREDING, l. c., p. 662.]

A heaviness and paralysis of the upper extremities, most of the left arm. [*Ln.*]

Weakness, like paralysis, first in the right upper arm, afterwards also in the forearm (aft. 5 h.). [*Mkl.*]

Paralytic aching in the left upper arm, with paralytic feeling and weakness in the whole of the left arm. [*Hrr.*]

Paralytic drawing aching, with weakness in the right upper and forearm (aft. 4 d.). [*Hrr.*]

915. **Paralytic tearing aching on the anterior surface of the left upper arm** (aft. 5 d.). [*Hrr.*]

Cramp of the right arm, with grinding of the teeth. [GREDING, l. c., p. 687 (20).]

(Painful) twitching in the arms, more in the right than the left. [*Stf.*]

He raises the right arm involuntarily and without knowing it above the head. [GREDING, l. c., p. 692 (22).]

A downward-drawing in the muscles of the right upper arm, and when it got down it then twitched several times back in the region of the right elbow-joint upwards towards the shoulders, and then it ceased for a time.

920. Convulsive shock of the arms as from the most violent shivering.

Spasmodic shocks of the arms. [GREDING, l. c., p. 644.]

Continual inward-twisting (intorsio) of the arms and hands.[3] [BOUCHER, l. c.]

She occasionally stretched out her arms and hands, as if she would clutch something. [BOUCHER, l. c.]

A violent outward-stabbing pain, as with a blunt knife, under the head of the humerus. [*Gss.*]

925. In the right arm on which she had not lain (about 3 a.m.) a stiffness (she could not bend it), with a feeling as if it were shorter than the other, and tearing pain in it). [*Stf.*]

---

1 Relieved by venesection.

2 See note to S. 175.

3 The original is simply "contorsions continuelles."

Drawing pain in the inside of the left upper arm.. [*Hbg.*]

Tearing pain in the humerus. [*Hbg.*]

Bruised pain in the upper arms (aft. 6 h.). [*Ws.*]

Tearing pain in the humerus.

930. A slow running upwards on the left arm, as when a fly creeps on the skin, frequent rubbing does no good.

A pimple on the left arm, below the elbow-joint, dark red, without sensation or suppuration, paining like a sore on being touched (aft. 9 d.). [*Hrr.*]

Below the right elbow a pimple, touching it causes shooting pain. [*Ws.*]

(The elbow pains on being moved and touched, as if burnt.)

A rumbling in the left arm in the bend of the elbow, as if water or a heavy fluid coursed through the blood-vessels. [*Hbg.*]

935. Cutting pain in the left elbow-joint internally, when walking. [*Ws.*]

Sharp stitches externally on the left elbow-joint (aft. 72 h.). [*Ws.*]

Paralytic drawing pain in the elbow.

Paralytic drawing pain in the elbow and fingers of the left hand. [*Hbg.*]

Fine stitches on the left forearm (aft. 24 h.). [*Ws.*]

940. Obtuse shooting in the middle of the internal portion of the forearm which becomes gradually worse, and at length very violent. [*Gss.*]

Cutting tearing in the lower muscles of the right forearm (when at rest) (aft. $5\frac{1}{2}$ h.). [*Htn.*]

Cutting tearing in the lower muscles of the left forearm (aft. $\frac{3}{4}$ h.). [*Htn.*]

Paralytic tearing in the bones of the wrist. [*Hrr.*]

Shooting tearing in the metacarpal bones of the left hand. [*Htn.*]

945. Tearing ache in the metacarpal bones and the distal joint of the left index. [*Hrr.*]

Frequent cold perspiration of the hands.

The backs of both hands are covered with small, red spots, which rapidly disappear. [*Ws.*]

Swelling of the hands. [WIENHOLT, l. c., p. 310.]

Great swelling of the hand. [MUNCH, l. c., p. 390.]

950. Feeling of stiffness on the right hand and fingers; she could not bend them. [*Stf.*]

He cannot turn the hand freely on its axis (*e. g.* when dropping a fluid out of a phial), he can only do it by jerks, just as if there was a deficiency of synovia in the wrist-joint; but this impeded movement is painless (aft. 4 h.).

Painful drawing in the proximal phalanges of the left middle finger, as if in the periosteum [*Hrr.*]

Paralytic tearing in the middle-joint of the right index. [*Hrr.*]

The distal joint of the middle finger feels stiff, and on bending it has simple (sore ?) pain.

955. Tearing cutting in the muscles of the right little finger. [*Htn.*]

Sharp stitches in the metacarpal bone of the thumb (aft. 1 h.). [*Ws.*]

The points of the fingers of the left hand pain as if pinched. [*Hbg.*]

Along with chilliness of the body stitches out at the finger-points, chiefly when grasping.

In the point of the middle finger, feeling as if something were stuck in and had caused ulceration, worst when touched. [*Ws.*]

960. On the finger a blister with painful inflammation. [LAMBERGEN, l. c.]

A pustule breaking out close to the nail of the right index exuded much fluid. [GREDING, l. c., p. 673 (15).]

The fingers are easily dislocated.

On the inside of the thigh, sore pain.

Pain of the thighs and legs as if generally bruised, and as if brittle, towards the shafts of the bones fine shooting and gnawing, besides severe tearing in the joints ; the pain mounts gradually from the ankles to the hips, when seated compelling the feet to be constantly moved and shifted ; relieved by walking (aft. 4 h.). [*Ws.*]

965. In the legs sometimes weariness, with drawing pain in them.

A kind of stretching ; he is compelled to stretch out the legs (aft. 11 d.).

When walking, weight in the thighs and legs, along with stiffness of the knee-joints (aft. 12 h.). [*Ws.*]

Increased[1] weight of the thighs and legs (and discharge of yellow nasal mucus with increased thirst). [GREDING, l. c., vol. ii, p. 321.]

Paralytic drawing in the right thigh and leg. [*Hrr.*]

970. Paralysis of the lower extremities, she must lie down, with nausea, trembling, anxiety and vertigo. [BALDINGER, l. c.]

Temporary paralysis of the lower extremities.[2] [DUMOULIN, l. c.]

Cramp-pain in the gluteal muscles with tension, on bending the body. [*Ws.*]

On the right hip three or four violent stitches when at rest and when moving. [*Stf.*]

On the right hip-joint cold feeling (rapidly passing off) (aft. 1 h). [*Ws.*]

975. Pain in the left hip with limping. [GREDING, l. c., p. 687 (20).]

When she lies on the right hip she has pain in the left, but if she lies on the left the pain goes off (aft. 8, 9 d.).

On walking a paralytic tension in the hip-joints as if they were dislocated. [*Ws.*]

Cutting, jerking tearing in the posterior muscles of the left thigh when sitting (aft. $\frac{3}{4}$ h.). [*Htn.*]

---

1 "Increased," *i. e.* only an aggravation of a symptom she had before beginning the medicine.

2 See SS. 729, 763.

Cutting shooting in the external muscles of the right thigh, just above the knee, only when sitting (aft. $2\frac{1}{4}$ h.). [*Htn.*]

980. In the thighs extreme heaviness and stiffness when walking. [*Kr.*]

Heaviness in the thighs even when sitting. [*Hbg.*]

A pain drawing outwards towards the skin at a small spot on the inner surface of the left thigh (aft. 1 h.). [*Gss.*]

Hard pressure in the middle of the anterior surface of the right thigh. [*Hrr.*]

A knife-stab in the middle of the thigh more towards the posterior side (immediately after a meal). [*Gss.*]

985. A fluctuating throbbing pain on the upper and inner part of the left thigh (aft. 29 h.). [*Gss.*]

Tingling buzzing sensation above the right knee when sitting (aft. $\frac{1}{4}$ h.). [*Htn.*]

Cramp-like pain in the right knee, near the patella, towards the outer side, when sitting. [*Htn.*]

Violent pains in the knee. [*Stf.*]

On moving, the outer hamstring of the left knee feels tight and as if too short, alternating with a similar feeling in the inner hamstring, but it is always worst in the outer. [*Mkl.*]

990. In the right popliteal region pinching and aching pain. [*Hbg.*]

Obtuse stitches in the left popliteal region (aft. $\frac{1}{4}$ h.). [*Gss.*]

A twitching in the right popliteal region (aft. 4 h.). [*Ln.*]

Trembling of the knees. [MULLER, l. c.]

A disagreeable feeling in the joints of the lower extremities. especially the knees, as if they would bend beneath him, especially when walking and chiefly when descending.

995. A twitching in the popliteal region upwards into the muscles of the thigh.

A clucking in the foot as if drops fell in it (aft. 54 h.).

Very rapid clucking in front of the left knee, when sitting (immediately). [*Ws.*]

Needle pricks under the left patella, when sitting. [*Gss.*]

Aching shooting in the right petella, when sitting (aft. $3\frac{1}{2}$ h.). [*Htn.*]

1000. When treading with the left foot painful stitches shoot up to the knee (aft. 38 h.). [*Ws.*]

Cutting drawing on a small spot on the feet, that spread from below upwards, first through the legs and thighs, then through the sacrum up to the shoulders. [*Kr.*]

Paralytic weariness in both legs. [*Mkl.*]

On going upstairs weariness of the legs, especially of the calves. [*Stf.*]

In the legs a drawing-up sensation, externally only crawling, internally innumerable stitches. [*Ws.*]

1005. In the leg pain as if it were squeezed and a commotion (dull tearing) and working in it, especially at night, relieved by hanging down the leg freely (aft. 10 h.).

A burning tearing up the legs through the inner surface of the popliteal region.

Trembling heaviness of the legs.

Dull tearing in the legs. [*Hbg.*]

The foot was so painful that she had to keep the limb horizontally extended and immovable.[1] [LAMBERGEN, l. c.]

1010. Painful feeling of weight of the right leg on crossing it over the left leg (4 hours). [*Htn.*]

A drawing heaviness of the legs.

Tearing pain in the tibia.

Feeling in the right leg like growing pain, a stiff feeling combined with heaviness. [*Htn.*]

Drawing tearing pain in the right tibia with an out-pressing sensation in it (aft. 4 h.). [*Htn.*]

1015. Sharp shoots in the left calf which come from below upwards. [*Ws.*]

Cramp in the calf on bending the leg, in the evening in bed, which goes off on stretching out the leg (aft. 72 h.).

Tearing pressure in the middle of the inside of the leg, without reference to movement or touching. [*Hrr.*]

On the left tibia in front an aching when standing. [*Hbg.*]

Sweat on the feet without warmth when sitting. [*Hbg.*]

1020. Eroding itching on the feet and dorsum of the feet. [*Hrr.*]

Obtuse stitches on the dorsum of the left foot, when sitting, not affected by external pressure. [*Ws.*]

On walking in the open air tension in the right ankle-joint.

On walking and bending the foot pain in the metatarsal bones as if sprained.

Tearing pain in the metatarsal bone of the big toe.

1025. Cramp in the sole of the foot, in the evening, in bed, on drawing up the knees.

Burning and digging in the soles of the feet. [*Kr.*]

Violent itching of the feet.

Creeping upwards in the feet (aft. 20 h.).

Swelling of the feet.

1030. Heat especially in the feet.

In the soles of the feet boring, digging pain (aft. several h.).

Shooting pain in the soles of the feet (aft. ½ h.).

Bruised pain in the ball of the heel when treading.

A kind of painless drawing or running from the heel to the toes, round about the ankle (aft. 30 h.).

1035. Boring or tearing stitches in the tendo Achillis.

(When walking) tearing in the sole of the left foot, mingled with stitches, for a quarter of an hour. [*Mkl.*]

Tension on the sole of the right foot about the heel, which then changed into tensive pressure; on pressing on it the pain goes off for some time (aft. ¼ h.). [*Hrr.*]

1 In connection with S. 1044.

Complaint about very painful cramp in the left arm and in the back, which in the evening extends as far as the thighs. [GREDING, l. c., p. 652.]

In the evening she wished to stretch herself, but could not do it for pains. [*Kr.*]

1040. Usually when the pain had reached its climax it disappeared suddenly, and in an instant there occurred instead a pain at another part. [*Gss.*]

Painful sensitiveness of the skin at the least touch. [*Kr.*]

Crawling itching all over the body, flying about, now here, now there. [*Ws.*]

Red scaly eruption on the lower parts of the body, extending to the abdomen. [ZIEGLER, l. c.]

On the planter surface of the foot, and on the shin bone, blisters filled with water, that readily burst. [LAMBERGEN, l. c.]

1045. When walking, at every second or third step, a stitch in the affected part extending into the head, just as when one pricks oneself unexpectedly ; not when sitting.

(The parts where the shooting pain had been are very painful to external touch.)

Boring pain in the glands.

Gnawing pain in the affected part (aft. 1 h.).

The external application of belladonna makes the part sensitive to the open air.

1050. Cold, painful, long-continued lumps and swellings (apparently secondary action).

Tearing itching here and there, especially after lying down in bed in the evening ; after rubbing the tearing pain alone remains, but more severe.

Ulcer is painful almost only in the night (from 6 p.m. to 6 a.m.) burning, as if something would press out, and the part were as if paralysed and stiff (aft. 48 h.).

(Ulcer covered with a black crust like coagulated blood.)

Ulcer exudes almost nothing but bloody ichor.

1055. Ulcer is painful on being touched, almost burning pain (aft. 4 h.).

In the ulcer violent itching (aft. 1 h.).

In the ulcer cutting pain when at rest, and tearing pain on moving the part (aft. 20 h.).

Round about the ulcer sore pain (aft. 4 h.).

(Soreness in the bends of the joints.)

1060. **Suddenly attacking, horrible crampy pain on one side of the chest, one side of the abdomen, in one loin, or in one elbow, especially during sleep, whereby he is forced to bend the painful part inwards and to crouch together** (aft. 8, 16, 30 h.).

(A drawing pain in the feet going upwards to the scapulæ, and thence into the fingers, lastly into the teeth, which thereby are set on edge and become loose.)

(Drawing pain in all the limbs.)

In the evening in bed itching stitches here and there in the skin, as if from fleas.

In the afternoon especially (about 3 or 4 o'clock), all the ailments are worse ; in the forenoon they are more tolerable.

1065. Violent spasmodic laughter.

Slight convulsive movements of the limbs. [DUMOULIN, l. c.]

Convulsive movement of the limbs. [RAU, l. c.—GREDING, l. c., p. 671.]

Subsultus tendium. [ELFES, l. c.]

Twitching in the limbs. [ZIEGLER, l. c.]

1070. After a slight vexation the most violent spasms, which urged him to run against the walls. [*Stf.*]

Convulsions of the limbs with hiccup. [GREDING, l. c., p. 671 (14).]

During startings of the limbs, weariness and anxiety.[1] [GREDING, l. c., p. 672 (14).]

Convulsions. [EB. GMELIN, *Pflanzengifte*, l. c.]

Convulsive momentary stretching out of the limbs on awaking.

1075. Repeated convulsions and cruel spasms, especially in the flexor muscles. [GRIMM, l. c.]

Severe jerks and very loud raving. [BALDINGER, l. c.]

Epileptic convulsions. [WAGNER, l. c., (1).]

Horrible convulsions resembling epilepsy. [GRIMM, l. c.]

Convulsions, distortions of all muscles. [DE ST. MARTIN, l. c.]

1080. Convulsions of all the limbs. [MUNCH, l. c.]

In the intervals, when free from convulsions, he utters the loudest cries, as if he suffered great pains. [GRIMM, l. c.]

Head and trunk drawn quite back to the left side, so that he could not walk.[2] [GREDING, l. c., p. 662.]

Insensible, with rattling breathing and twitching in face and hands. [BALDINGER, l. c.]

At one time amazing distortion of the limbs, at another complete immobility. [EL. CAMERARIUS, l. c.]

1085. Loss of all sensation ; stiffness of the lower extremities ; excessive distention of all the blood-vessels of the skin, with uncommonly red, swollen face, extremely full and rapid pulse and profuse sweat. [BALDINGER, l. c.]

Frequent stiffness and immobility of the limbs ; for example, he could not move the left foot. [*Stf.*]

Stiffness of all the limbs under the guise of a feeling of weariness.

Stiffness of the whole body.[3] [EHRHARDT, *Pflanzenhistorie*, x, p. 126.]

Spasmodic stretching of the limbs with distortion of the eyes. [GREDING, l. c., p. 664.]

1090. In the morning weary and restless in the limbs on account of pains, she wanted always to change the position of her limbs. [*Kr.*]

---

1 This would be better stated—"After heat and redness of the face, with great thirst, she had lassitude, anxiety, and slight startings of the limbs."

2 See note to S. 175.

3 Poisoning of a boy of seven.

Great restlessness in all the limbs so that he could not remain still. Unsteadiness of head and hands.

Bodily restlessness ; he was compelled to move the whole body hither and thither, especially the hands and feet ; he cannot remain long in any position, sometimes he lies, sometimes sits, sometimes stands, and he always changes his position in one way or another [*Hrr.*]

Trembling with convulsive shock.

1095. Trembling in all the limbs, inability to walk, distended vessels all over the body, and disagreeable irritating sensation in the throat, for several days. [BALDINGER, l. c.]

Trembling at the heart, in the forenoon.

Trembling and weariness of the limbs. [GREDING, l. c., p. 644.]

Weariness of the limbs. [SICELIUS, l. c.]

In the evening so tired, he can scarcely walk (aft. 50 h.).

1100. Lassitude in all the limbs and disinclination for work. [*Gss.*]

Disinclination and horror of work, of movement (aft. 1, 5 h.).

Heaviness of the hands and feet. [*Bhr.*]

Weakness of the body. [WIERUS, l. c.]

Sinking of the strength. [WAGNER, l. c. (1).]

1105. Great weakness. [CARL, *Acta. Nat. Cur.*, iv, obs. 86.[1]]

Weariness all day through, and sleep in the afternoon. [*Hbg.*]

Especially in the evening very faint, and at the same time shortness of breath.

General weakness.

Weak uncertain gait, the knees are inclined to bend beneath him ; he cannot walk.

1110. Frequently recurring short attacks of great weakness ; all feels too heavy to her, and drags her downwards as though she would sink together. [*Bhr.*]

Paralytic-like weakness of all the muscles of the upper and lower extremities (aft. 6 d.). [*Hbg.*]

Paralytic-like weakness of all the muscles, especially of the legs.

Paralysis, at one time in this, at another in that part.[2] [GREDING, l. c., p. 703.]

Paralysis of the right arm and right leg.[2] [GREDING, l. c., pp. 661, 663.]

1115. The left side, especially the arm and leg, are quite paralysed.[2] [GREDING, l. c., p. 662.]

Attacks of syncope. [GREDING, l. c.]

Apoplectic state.[3] [WAGNER, l. c. (11).]

He lay for four days, without eating anything and motionless, like a corpse. [J. B. PORTA, *Magia Natur.*, viii.]

Lethargic, apoplectic state ; for a day and night they lay without

---

1 Symptoms produced by a decoction of the root in a sufferer from rheumatic gout.
2 See note to S. 175.
3 After epileptic convulsions.

motion in any limb ; on being pinched they opened their eyes, but emitted no sound. [WAGNER, l. c., (1).]

1120. Soporose state. [HASENEST, l. c.]

Very deep slumber.

Deep sleep. [DILLENIUS,[1] *Misc. Nat. Cur.* Dec. iii, ann. 7, 8, obs. 161.]

Deep sleep for twenty-four hours. [WIERUS, l. c.]

Very deep sopor, with subsultus tendium, pale cold face, cold hands, and hard, small, rapid pulse. [MAY, l. c.]

1125. Stupefaction that compels him to sleep in the forenoon ; he slept profoundly for an hour and a half ; on awaking great hunger, with severe burning heat and dryness in the mouth, without thirst ; thereafter when coughing foul breath, smelling of human excrement. [*Htg.*]

Before midnight restless sleep ; the child tosses about, kicks, and speaks crossly in its sleep.

Immediately on falling asleep he dreams.

After long sleep great thirst. [GREDING, l. c., p. 684 (19).]

Sleep full of dreams ; she is occupied with many people ; she wants to go away, but does not go so far as that. [*Kr.*]

1130. She dreams to an uncommon extent, but tranquilly, of home occupations. [*Stf.*]

Very profound sleep, without many dreams, until towards morning (aft. 5 d.). [*Hbg.*]

Night sleep with unremembered dreams ; he fell asleep sooner than usual and woke earlier, and not without refreshment, which, however, always after a few hours gave place to the lassitude in the limbs that was always present at other times. [*Gss.*]

He dreams of danger from fire, and wakes in consequence (aft. 54 h.).

Frightful dreams vividly remembered.

1135. At night very stupefied sleep, anxious dreams of murderers and highwaymen ; he once heard himself call out loudly, but without thereby coming to his senses. [*Mkl.*]

In the evening frequent starting up out of sleep on going to sleep ; the feet were jerked upwards and the head forwards. [*Ws.*]

Intolerable sleep on account of horribly increased pains and frightful dreams.

He starts up and wakes, just when about to fall asleep.

Full of affright and terror she awakes at night ; it seemed to her as if there was something under her bed that made a noise ; she had dry heat on waking.

1140. She started in otherwise quite sleep, as though she were falling deep down, whereupon she gave a violent start. [*Stf.*]

In his sleep he starts up in a fright and wakes. [*Hbg.*]

Anxiety prevents sleep.

Nocturnal sleeplessness on account of anxiety, with drawing pain in all the limbs.

---

1 Poisoning of a mother and six children by the berries.

Fright in a dream, whereon he wakes, and there is sweat on the forehead and pit of the stomach.

1145. He is constantly wakened up out of sleep by frightful dreams and twitchings. [ZIEGLER, l. c.]

In his stupefied sleep he opens his eyes, gazes wildly about him, and then falls again into snoring sleep. [BALDINGER, l. c.]

At night he had dreams that tired his mind very much, and in the morning he was quite weary when he ought to get up. [*L. Rkt.*]

At the time of going to sleep he knew not whether he was dreaming or waking. [*Hbg.*]

Vivid, but unremembered dreams. [*Lr.*]

1150. Lying in bed in the evening it seems to him that he is swimming away with his bed; for ten successive evenings, immediately after lying down, he seems to swim in his bed. [*Fr. H—n.*]

In the morning he cannot rouse himself out of sleep; on awaking he is very cross. [*Ws.*]

Singing and talking loudly in sleep.

She sleeps much, and even when the cough wakes her, she falls asleep again immediately, and yet in the morning she is giddy and tired. [*Kr.*]

Frequent waking out of sleep, and though he turns first on one side and then on the other, he can get no rest and cannot go to sleep again. [*Lr.*]

1155. At night, sleeping or waking, interrupted breathing; inspiration and expiration last only half as long as the pause before taking the new inspiration; the expiration came in jerks, and was louder than the inspiration; the inspiration lasted only a little longer than the expiration.

(When asleep suffocating snoring during inspiration.)

Frequent waking out of sleep at night, just as if he had slept enough (the first night). [*Lr.*]

Vain efforts to sleep. [GRIMM, l. c.]

He cannot sleep at night; the delusion that he had to do something necessary keeps him from sleeping.

1160. Very little sleep. [*Ln.*]

Sleeplessness for several days. [HOYER,[1] in *Misc. Nat. Cur.*, Dec. iii, ann. 7, 8, obs. 176.]

Constant drowsiness, with inclination to stretch out the limbs, in the evening from 5 to 9 o'clock (aft. 11 h.). [*Mkl.*]

(Sleeplessness, with alleviation of the pains, at night.)

Sleeplessness.

1165. Constant confusion, with sleepiness (aft. 4 h.). [*Gss.*]

Drowsiness (aft. $\frac{1}{2}$ h.).

Towards evening, in the twilight, sleepiness with yawning, but in the morning feeling of not having slept enough.

On awaking from sleep headache and great exhaustion.

In the morning on awaking headache only over the eyes, like a weight in the head, and touching the eye causes pain.

---

1 Poisoning of an old woman by the berries.

1170. In the morning very tired and giddy. [*Kr.*]
Drowsiness perceived immediately after waking. [*Gss.*]
Dozing. [SAUVAGES, l. c.—VALENTINI,[1] *Misc. Nat. Cur.*, Dec. ii, ann. 10, obs. 118.]
A sort of coma, with small, weak, irregular pulse. [BOUCHER, l. c.]
Drowsiness, with restlessness. [MARDORF, l. c.]
1175. Great drowsiness. [SICELIUS, l. c.]
Afternoon attack of frequent stretching and yawning, during which the eyes fill with tears (aft. 48 h.).
Frequent yawning. [EB. GMELIN, l. c.]
Yawning like an intoxicated person. [MARDORF, l. c.]
Frequent yawning as if he had not slept enough (aft. $2\frac{1}{4}$ h.). [*Lr.*]
1180. Feverish movements. [ZIEGLER, l. c.—SAUVAGES, l. c.]
Feverish movements every other day. [SAUTER, l. c. (11).]
Fever after every dose. [LENTIN,[2] *Beobacht.*, p. 81.]
Evening fever.[3] [G—CH, l. c.]
Violent thirst (aft. 30 h.).
1185. Violent thirst after midnight and in the morning.
Anxious thirst. [GRIMM, l. c.]
Very troublesome thirst. [MAY, l. c.]
Excessive thirst for cold water (aft. 4 h.). [EL. CAMERARIUS, l. c.]
Tormented by burning thirst and heat in all parts ; she longs for drink from time to time, but rejects it when offered to her. [GRIMM, l. c.]
1190. After the perspiration at first induced has diminished, the thirst increases and the appetite falls off. [GREDING, l. c., p. 650.]
At night much thirst and dryness of the mouth.
Thirst, frequent micturition, and dimness of vision in the morning. [GREDING, l. c., p. 670 (14).]
In the morning great thirst. [*Hbg.*]
Great thirst, frequent micturition, profuse sweat. [GREDING, l. c., p. 690 (22).]
1195. She is deathly pale, quite lifeless, and cold as snow. [*Kr.*]
In the morning, icy-cold hands, with confusion of the head and lachrymose humour.
Coldness of the whole body, with pale face.
Cold feet, with heat in the internal ear, in the evening.
Cold feet, with swollen red face and rush of blood to head.
1200. Coldness of the whole body, especially of the feet. [*Hbg.*]
Cold hands and feet, with rather profuse cold perspiration of the feet (aft. 10 h.). [*Mkl.*]
Cold hands and feet. [*Ln.*]
An unusual cold feeling in the legs, chiefly in the feet (aft. 5 h.). [*Ln.*]
Chilliness. [MUNCH, l. c.]

---

1 Same narrative as that of Mardorf (*q.v*).
2 Effects of B. administered for mammary scirrhus.
3 Not found.—The whole history related by G—ch embraces a few hours only.

1205. A violent chill seizes her in the back and scrobiculus cordis, or in both arms at once, and thence spreads all over the body. [*Bhr.*]

(Chilliness after evening.)

In her sleep she is chilly and feels the coldness while asleep; she is also cold on awaking.

Chilliness, especially on the arms, with goose-skin, on undressing; at the same time redness and heat of ears and nose.

Chill and rigor with goose-skin even when close to the warm stove (aft. 1 h.). [*Mkl.*]

1210. Febrile chill with fine shooting pain in the chest. [GREDING, l. c., p. 661.]

As soon as a cold wind plays on her she immediately shivers; otherwise she feels better in the open air. [*Kr.*]

Over-sensitiveness to cold air. [SAUTER, l. c. (11).]

Frequent yawning and then chill over the body, but only running over the skin externally, in the evening. [*Bhr.*]

Rigor over arms and abdomen, not on the head (aft. 2 h.).

1215. Immediately after noon slight rigor with dimness of vision. [GREDING, l. c., p. 685 (19).]

Rigor over one arm. [*Hbg.*]

Rigor over the abdomen. [*Hbg.*]

Febrile rigor and cold hands. [*L. Rkt.*]

Towards evening fever; shaking rigor jarks her up in bed, after two hours heat and general perspiration, without thirst either during the rigor or the heat.

1220. In short fits rigors run down the back, not followed by heat. [*Ws.*]

Very small, slow pulse. [*Hbg.*]

Fever: in the morning febrile chill, followed by slight heat. [GREDING, l. c., p. 644.]

Fever: **chilliness running all over the body** (aft. 1 h.)—**four hours afterwards hot feeling and heat, especially of the face.** [*Hrr.*]

Fever: at night febrile chill, which was soon succeeded by heat of the body, and frequent micturition and weariness of the limbs; the following night a double febrile attack of the same kind, with vertigo and thirst. [GREDING, l. c., p. 643.]

1225. Fever: cold rigor through the body; in the afternoon heat spreads over it. [*Hbg.*]

Fever: in the evening on undressing some chilliness over the body, then heat on the whole of the left side of the body.

(Fever: after the chill feels well for several hours, then sweat only on the face, the hands (?), and the feet (?) before the heat comes; no sleep during the heat, almost complete absence of thirst during the chill, and none at all during the sweat and heat; only during the sweat on the face some headache, but none during the chill or heat.)

(Fever: first putrid taste in the mouth, then heat of the face and hands; after the disappearance of the heat the pain increased.)

Frequently during the day repeated febrile attacks, shaking rigor followed by general heat and sweat all over the body, without thirst either in the chill or the heat.

1230. Fever : along with external coldness there is inward burning heat.

Fever : alternations of chill and heat. [*Bhr.*]

Fever : Sudden alternations of heat and chill, both without thirst, with drowsiness by day (aft. 12 d.). [*Ws.*]

Several febrile attacks in one day, in which the heat followed the chill in from a few minutes to half an hour, always without thirst in the chill and heat, and generally with confusion of the head. [*Hrr.*]

Fever : in the evening, in bed, chill, then heat ; the chill spread from the sacrum, ran up over the back, and down again to the thighs. [*Kr.*]

1235. Strong, quick pulse. [*Ln.*]

Large, full, slow pulse.

Very small, quick pulse.

Large quick pulse, accelerated by ten beats. [*Gss.*]

Violent heat. [RAU, l. c.]

1240. Burning skin. [EL. CAMERARIUS, l. c,]

Very great heat all over, with delirium. [*Commerc. lit. Nor.*, 1731.]

Burning heat externally and internally [VICAT, l. c.]

Inward burning. [CARL, l. c.]

General dry heat on the extreme ends of the feet and hands with adipsia and paleness of face, for twelve hours.

1245. Internal heat, burning in the gastric region. [HASENEST, l. c.]

Internal heat ; everything she takes seems too cold. [*Kr.*]

Acute fever, burning fever.[1] [DE LAUNAY D'HERMONT, l. c.]

Burning fever (causus) (aft. 12 h.). [DE ST. MARTIN, l. c.]

Burning heat of the body and greatly swollen blood-vessels of the skin, with rage. [BALDINGER, l. c.]

1250. Along with great heat, swelling of the external blood-vessels of the body, with unquenchable thirst. [BALDINGER, l. c.]

Swollen cutaneous veins. [*Hbg.*]

The blood-vessels of the limbs are distended, the arteries of the neck in particular beat so that the lower jaw, when the mouth is a little open, at every beat strikes against the upper jaw, and thus a slight chattering of the teeth arises, at the same time warmth and warm feeling all over the body, but especially on the head. [*F. H—n.*]

In the morning on waking a beating of the arteries in the head, and in all parts of the body. [*Kr.*]

At night, particularly towards morning, he is too hot in bed, and yet he dare not uncover himself ; the uncovered parts pain as from a chill.

1255. Great heat of the body, more violent and more frequent pulsations

---

1 This represents, in the original—"the skin was dry and burning, and the pulse small, wiry, hard, and extremely frequent."

of the arteries, especially of the temporals, with stupid feeling of the head, followed by profuse sweat. [GREDING, l. c., ii, 2, p. 319.]

Daily after dinner great heat of body, especially of the head, so that the face becomes occasionally very red. [GREDING, l. c., i, p. 665.]

Daily about noon (for twelve days) sudden heat of head, and redness of face, with great dimness of vision and much thirst, for an hour. [GREDING, l. c., p. 670 (14).]

Feeling of heat, with heat of the whole body, especially in the face, which was red and perspiring, with confusion of head (aft. 4 h.). [*Hrr.*]

(In the evening heat on the hands and feet, but not on the arms and legs.)

1260. Slight movement (walking) causes heat of the body.

Redness and heat of face, with great thirst. [GREDING, l. c., p. 672 (14).]

Inflammation of the surface of the whole body. [SAUVAGES, l. c.]

Redness of the whole body. [MUNCH, l. c.]

Redness of the whole body, with quick pulse. [BUCHAVE, l. c.]

1265. Heat of the whole body, with violet-redness of all the skin. [WIEDEMANN, l. c.]

Great swelling of the fece, and intense heat, which at times extends over the whole body. [BUCHAVE, l. c.]

The whole body is swollen, burning hot, and red. [SAUTER, l. c. (1).]

Speedy death, and a universal gangrene throughout the whole body, which in a short time became black throughout, and so flaccid that the cuticle adhered to the surgeon's hands. [MAPPI, *Plant. Alsat.*, p. 36[1].]

Sudden inflammations. [MARDORF, l. c.]

1270. Very transient inflammations (phlogoses) and tightness of the chest. [GREDING, l. c., p. 648.]

Redness and swelling of the affected part. [SAUTER, l. c. (11).]

Prickling, stinging sensation all over the skin, especially on the soles of the feet. [SAUTER, l. c. (11).]

Creeping sensations. [GREDING, l. c., p. 672 (14).]

Itching of the whole body and eruption of red fleabite spots (aft. 4 h.). SAUTER, l. c. (11).]

1275. Chest and abdomen are covered with small, red, somewhat elevated, painless spots, that often disappear and then suddenly re-appear, with general redness of the skin. [*Ws.*]

Acute, erysipelatous fever, accompanied by the inflamed swellings, even passing into mortification.

Inflamed red and variously shaped patches on the skin ; scarlet-red spots over the body (which itch ?) (aft. 16 h.).

Blood-red spots all over the body, especially on the face, neck, and chest. [SAUTER, l. c. (11).]

Measly cutaneous eruption. [BUCHAVE, l. c.]

1280. Dark red, scarlatina-like spots all over the body, with small,

1 From drinking a large quantity of the juice mixed with wine.

quick pulse, tightness of chest, violent cough,[1] raving, increased memory, rubbing of the nose and dilated pupils. [WIEDEMANN, l. c.]

Scarlatina rash (the first days). [STRUVE,[2] *Triumph d. Heilk.*, i, p. 64.]

Eruption on the skin of bullæ, which exude a quantity of limpid or creamy lymph, and therewith such intense pain that the patient, though accustomed to suffering, cannot refrain from lamentations and tears. [LAMBERGEN, l. c.]

Great heat (immediately) and then very profuse sweat. [GREDING, l. c., ii, 2, p. 320.]

Heat of the body with sweat (aft. 2 h.). [*Ln.*]

1285. Sweat (after several hours). [ACKERMANN, l. c.]

He perspires, on slight movement, all over, chiefly on the face, down the nose.

He feels very hot ; he perspires all over, but without thirst.

He perspires freely all over when walking in the open air (in the wind) and at the same time gets bellyache, just as if he had got a chill.

Night-sweat, which has a burnt odour.

1290. Profuse night-sweats, which do not weaken him. [ACKERMANN, l. c.]

Night-sweat. [*Hbg.*]

Morning sweat. [ZIEGLER, l. c.]

Profuse sweat. [EVERS, in *Schmucker's verm. Schriften*, i, p. 185. GREDING, l. c., p. 652.]

Cold sweat on forehead (aft. 1 h.). [*L. Rkt.*]

1295. **Every night profuse sweat.** [GREDING, l. c., in various places.]

Night sweat during sleep, after midnight.

Waking immediately after midnight in perspiration (he cannot go to sleep again) ; the sweat continues while he is awake (aft. 54 h.).

(During sleep at night no perspiration, but he perspires in his day sleep.)

Sweat while asleep. [BUCHAVE, l. c.]

1300. Sweat all over the body during sleep. [SAUTER, l. c. (11).]

Sweat all over from 4 p.m. to midnight, then sleep during the sweat. [SAUTER, l. c. (11).]

Profuse sweat with diuresis. [ZIEGLER, l. c.—GREDING, l. c., pp. 688, 689 (21, 22).]

Very profuse, long-continued sweat, which stains the linen dark. [GREDING, l. c., p. 667.]

Sudden breaking out of general sweat, which disappears as suddenly. [*L. Rkt.*]

1305. Sweat as soon as he covers himself with the bed-clothes, especially on the upper parts. [*Hbg.*]

It is only the parts that are covered with the bed-clothes that perspire, in the evening.

Quite early in the morning (about 2 or 3 a.m.) after awaking,

---

1 This was the previously existing whooping-cough, increased in violence.

2 Not accessible.

perspiration when the arms are covered, which goes off when he uncovers them.

In the morning, intermitting sweat, that rose from the feet up into the face, where it was particularly profuse; but immediately afterwards she got cool again. [*Kr.*]

During the febrile heat there occurs general perspiration when the hands are covered by the bed-clothes, but when she uncovers them general chilliness.

1310. Trembling. [HORST.—DE LAUNAY D'HERMONT.—EB. GMELIN, l. c.]

He readily starts, especially when any one approaches him. [*L. Rkt.*]

By day, great anxiety; she cannot rest anywhere; she feels as if she should run away.

Great anxiety about the præcordia. [WAGNER, l. c. (1).]

Very anxious and fearful. [*Mkl.*]

1315. Anxiety in the cardiac region (aft. 3 h.). [*Ln.*]

Anxiety, during the menses. [SCHMUCKER, l. c.—LAMBERGEN, l. c.]

Frequent groaning (grunting) especially in the morning, without being able to tell why, or what pain makes him do so.

Grunting and groaning at each expiration.

Grunting and groaning in sleep.

1320. Sighs.[1] [EB. GMELIN, l. c.]

Groaning alternating with hopping and dancing. [MARDORF, l. c.]

With a sudden cry he trembles in hands and feet. [GREDING, l. c., p. 644.]

Much anxiety, and an hour afterwards perspiration. [HENNING, l. c.]

Events which hitherto he had hoped for with pleasure, now appear to him in an anxious light; they appear to him frightful and horrible. [*L. Rkt.*]

1325. In the momentary intervals, when free from fury, complaints of intolerable anxiety, so that she wished to die. [BALDINGR, l. c.]

About noon and evening, præcordial anxiety, headache, redness of face and bitterness of mouth. [GREDING, l. c., p. 671 (14).]

Anxiety and restlessness. [EB. GMELIN, l. c.]

Restlessness. [BOUCHER, l. c.]

Great restlessness, she cannot remain long seated in one place; she is driven all about. [*Kr.*]

1330. Continual turning about of the whole body, as in chorea. [BOUCHER, l. c.]

Incessant movement of the body, especially of the arms, with unaltered pulse. [BOUCHER, l. c.]

Great movement hither and thither in bed. [BOUCHER, l. c.]

Unconnected talking in the evening. [ACKERMANN, l. c.]

Raving, delirium. [ZIEGLER.—MAY.—EL. CAMERARIUS.—*Med. Chirurg. Wahrnehm.*, vii.—EB. GMELIN.—BUC'HOZ, l. c.]

---

1 Immediately before death.

1335. Continual delirium. [HORST, l. c.]

After eating the delirium is allayed. [*F. H—n.*]

He makes preparations to go home.[1] [GREDING, l. c., p. 688 (21).]

He is delirious, and cries out in his dreams that he must go home, because everything is on fire there. [GREDING, l. c., p. 688 (21).]

Raves about wolves being in the room ; at the same time full pulse. [G—CH, l. c.]

1340. Delirious talk about dogs surrounding him. [HUFELAND, *Jour.*, xvi.]

He is beside himself, raves, talks much about dogs, his arm and face swell. [MUNCH, l. c.]

At night he talks nonsense, by day he is sensible. [GREDING, l, c., p. 676 (16).]

Nocturnal delirium, which is allayed by day. [GREDING, l. c., p. 655.]

At one time he is delirious, at another he answers sensibly and bemoans himself. [EL. CAMERARIUS, l. c.]

1345. Delirium in recurring paroxysms.[2] [ALBRECHT, l. c.]

He murmurs as in sleep. [HASENEST, l. c.]

She talks nonsense and extreme folly. [GRIMM, l. c.]

Foolish chatter. [BOUCHER.—EL. CAMERARIUS (aft. 6 h).—BUCHAVE, l. c.—GREDING, l. c., p. 650.]

She chatters nonsense with great rapidity. [SAUTER, l. c. (1).]

1350. Chattering like a mad person, with staring, protruding eyes. [BUCHAVE, l. c.]

Chattering, lascivious.[3] [GREDING, l. c., p. 663.]

After the chattering fit speechlessness. [BUCHAVE, l. c.]

Gay mania. [SAUVAGES, l. c.]

Sits unoccupied behind the stove ; she tries to compose songs, and sings aloud songs of a gay, though nonsensical character ; sometimes she whistled, but would neither eat nor drink ; at the same time she neither heard nor saw anything, with paleness of face and sweat on the forehead. [*F. H—n.*]

1355. He sings and trills. [*Med. Chir. Wahrnehm.*, vii.]

Excessively gay disposition, he is disposed to sing and whistle (evening) (aft. 13 h.). [*Ws.*]

Involuntary, almost loud laughter, without having any laughable thoughts. [*L. Rkt.*]

He smiles for a long time to himself. [GREDING, l. c., p. 650.]

Frequent laughter. [GREDING, l. c., p. 651.]

1360. Laughing and singing she touches surrounding objects all day. [GREDING, l. c., p. 690 (22).]

She bursts out in loud laughter, sings, and touches things near her. [GREDING, l. c., p. 679 (17).]

Loud laughter. [GRIMM.—DUMOULIN.—HOCHSTETTER, l. c.—*Med. Chirurg. Wahrnehm.*, vii.]

---

1 See next symptom.

2 Not found.

3 See note to S. 175.

Uncontrollable loud laughter. [CARL, l. c.]

Unrestrainedly and exuberantly merry, inclined to scold without cause, and to insult in a laughing humour. [*Htg.*]

1365. Excessive gaiety after supper, the vital powers extraordinarily increased for a quarter of an hour, followed by drowsiness. [*Mkl.*]

Ridiculous grimaces; she takes hold of those about her, at one time she sits, at another she acts as if she were washing, at another as if counting money, at another as if she were drinking. [HASENEST, l. c.]

At one time he displays laughing madness, at another he talks sensibly (aft. 1, 16 h.).

He does foolish, ridiculous tricks (aft. ½, 6, 8 h.).

Various gesticulations. [HOCHSTETTER, l. c.]

1370. Insanity. [HOCHSTETTER, l. c.]

Insanity; they strip themselves, run about the streets in their shirts, gesticulate, dance, laugh loudly, chatter nonsense, and do foolish things. [DILLENIUS, l. c.]

He walks lifting his feet high, as if he must step over things in his path, like a drunken person. [SICELIUS, l. c.]

Violent shaking of the head. [GREDING, l. c., p. 653.]

Great shaking of the head, foam before the mouth, and lost consciousness. [GREDING, l. c., p. 673 (14).]

1375. She claps her hands above her head, with a short, very violent cough that threatens to suffocate her, at night. [GREDING, l. c., p. 691 (22).]

He claps his hands, wags his head from side to side, and viscid saliva hangs down in long strings from his lips. [GREDING, l. c., p. 691 (22).]

She distorts her facial muscles in a horrible way, protrudes her tongue to its full extent, clacks with her tongue, and retches as though she would vomit, in fits. [GREDING, l. c.]

At one time he grasps hastily at those near him, at another he shrinks back in affright. [SAUTER, l. c. (11).]

Weeping. [DUMOULIN, l. c.]

1380. Very excited humour, she is always disposed to weep. [*Bhr.*]

While walking, in the open air she is overcome by lachrymose anxiety; she is weary of life, and wishes to go into the water to drown herself.

Lachrymose fearfulness (aft. ⅛ h., aft. 2, and within 8 h.).

At first piteous weeping, which then passes into impatient and impassioned howling (with chilliness) (aft. 1 h.).

Violent weeping, whining, and howling without cause, combined with fearfulness (aft. 2 to 8, aft. 8 to 12, rarely aft. 12 to 20 h.).

1385. Weeping and excessive crossness on awaking from sleep.

Depression, unhappiness. [BOUCHER, l. c.]

He gets up at night and walks up and down buried in thought. [GREDING, l. c., p. 682 (18).]

Indisposed, indifferent to everything, defective activity of body and mind. [*Mkl.*]

Hourly alternation of weeping and cross humour.

1390. Excessive indifference, for hours; one might take her life, she would not stir. [*Kr.*]

Apathy; nothing can make an impression on her; after some days very sensitive cross humour; she has no pleasure in anything.

Cheerless, peevish, disinclined for everything.

Whining peevishness about trifles, with headache like pressure from a stone.

Disinclined to speak. [*Hrr.*]

1395. He wishes for solitude and quiet; all noise and visits from others are repugnant to him. [*Hrr.*]

Silent moroseness (aft. 8 h.), two days afterwards ordinary humour, but the following day again morose. [*Hrr.*]

Very morose and serious. [*Hbg.*]

He was cross about one thing and another.

Very irritable humour with great dryness in mouth.

1400. Great irritability and acuteness of the senses; everything tastes and smells stronger; the sense of touch, the sight, and the hearing are more acute, and the humour is more mobile and the thoughts more active (aft. 3 h.).

Peevishness, nothing was right for him; he was angry with himself. [*Fr. H—n.*]

Very excited; she soon loses her temper and then begins to weep. [*Bhr.*]

He is easily excited to anger, even by trifles. [*Hrr.*]

They stammered out violent language. [DUMOULIN, l. c.]

1405. Delirium either in recurring paroxysms or continued; it was at first merry, but afterwards changes into fury. [VICAT, l. c.]

Howling and crying out about trifles, which becomes worse when spoken to kindly, with pupils that easily dilate and very readily contract.

Violent inclination to quarrel, which cannot be soothed.

Delirium with wildness. [HOYER, l. c.]

Fury. [VALENTINI.—WIERUS.—SCHRECK, l. c.]

1410. Fury; the boy does not know his parents.* [SOLENANDER,[1] in *Abhand. der Konigl. Acad. d. Wissench.*, Breslau, 1750, p. 364.]

She tosses wildly about in bed (aft. 10 h.). [SAUTER, l. c. (1).]

She tears her night-dress and bed-clothes. [SAUTER, l. c. (1).]

He strikes his face with his fists. [GREDING, l. c., p. 664.]

Maniacal fury with violence.

1415. Fury, with gnashing of the teeth and convulsions. [MAY, l. c.]

In place of eating what he desired he bit the wooden spoon to pieces, gnawed the dishes, and growled and barked like a dog. [MUNCH, in *Richter's Biblioth.*, v, p. 564.]

Madness, in which the patient was often very merry, sang and cried out, then again spat and bit. [ELFES, l. c.]

* From a single berry.

1 Same case as that of Wierus. The symptom is made up of SS. 1409 and 42.

She does nonsensical things, tears her clothes to rags, picks up stones from the ground and pelts those around her with them (aft. 2 h.). [Sauter, l. c. (1).]

Fury ; he injures himself and others and strikes about him. [Greding, l. c., p. 664.]

1420. He tries to bite those about him at night. [Greding, l. c., p. 682 (18).]

Fury ; she clutches those about her by the hair. [Mardorf, l. c.]

Along with burning heat of the body, with open, staring, and fixed eyes, such fury that she must constantly be held fast in order to prevent her attacking others, and when thus held so that she could not move she spat constantly at those about her. [Baldinger, l. c.]

After sleep excessive moroseness ; he bites those about him. [Buchave, l. c.]

He bites at everything near him. [Munch, l. c.]

1425. Inclination to bite those about him. [Dumoulin, l. c.]

Inclination to tear everything about her to pieces. [Dumoulin, l. c.]

He tears to pieces everything about him, bites, and spits. [Sauter, l. c. (11).]

Throws off the bed-clothes in his madness. [Eb. Gmelin, l. c.]

Tries to jump out of bed. [Eb. Gmelin, l. c.]

1430. So anxious and distracted that she apprehends the approach of death.[1] [Timmermann, *Diss. Periculum Belladonnæ.*]

He fears death is nigh. [Eb. Gmelin, l. c.]

Fearful mistrust.

Fearful madness ; he is afraid of an imaginary black dog, of the gallows, &c (more frequently in the first 12 hours, more rarely in the following hours).

Madness ; he thinks that his living body is putrifying.

1435. He tries to run away. [Sauter, l. c. (11).]

He makes an excuse and runs out into the open fields. [Munch, l. c.]

She tries to strangle herself, and begs those about her to kill her, for this time she must die. [Greding, l. c., p. 690 (22).]

She begs those around her to kill her. [Greding, l. c., p. 692 (22).]

Throws herself down from a height (in delirium). [Buch'oz, l. c.]

1440. Throws herself into the water. [Sauter, l. c. (1).]

---

1 This symptom cannot be found in Timmermann's treatise.

BISMUTHUM.[1]

(Bismuth, Wismuth.)

(This brittle, easily melted, reddish-white metal is dissolved in a sufficient quantity of nitric acid to saturation, the perfectly limpid solution is dropped into a considerable quantity of pure water—from 50 to 100 parts—and well stirred; the precipitated white sediment (oxyde of bismuth), after standing a couple of hours, is freed from the superincumbent fluid by carefully decanting; then, again, as much pure water mixed with a few drops of potash is poured on it, and the sediment well stirred through it. The precipitate, after standing for some hours, is freed from the superincumbent water by decanting, and the sediment is completely dried on blotting-paper, on which other blotting-paper is laid, and weights laid on it, until all moisture is removed. When perfectly dried this is the oxyde of bismuth, one grain of which is triturated for an hour with a hundred grains of milk-sugar in a porcelain mortar, what adheres to the bottom of the mortar being frequently scraped up with a bone spatula. Of this hundredfold powder-attenuation one grain is again triturated with a hundred grains of milk-sugar in the same manner for an hour, so that $\frac{1}{10000}$th of a grain of oxyde of bismuth is contained in each grain of this powder; a very small portion of a grain of this is the dose employed for homœopathic use.)

THE few symptoms recorded below of the pure effects of bismuth on the healthy human body, which I should like to see increased will teach us useful homœopathic employment of it in important morbid states. Among others they—*e. g.* Symp. 32 and 53—show how the commendations of oxyde of bismuth in a kind of stomach-ache and gastralgia, by ODIER, CARMINATI, BONNAT, and others, are solely based on homœopathy, though this was unknown to them, and also that the power of oxyde of bismuth in palpitation, warranted by ODIER, rests only on the peculiar property possessed by this drug, of exciting strong and peculiar palpitation of the heart in the healthy (see Symp. 56); not to mention other indications for its use.

But as these qualities of our oxyde of bismuth are purely homœopathic, we see, at the same time, how improperly these and other physicians acted in administering in such cases such large doses of it—1, 2, 6, up to 12 grains for a dose, two, three, and four times a day—thus, in their ignorance, running the risk of injuring their patients.

As has been said, and the most careful observations prove it, where bismuth is indicated in similar and other cases, a single dose of the smallest possible part of a ten-thousandfold attenuation prepared in the manner described above fulfils the object perfectly.

[HAHNEMANN was assisted in this proving by F. HARTMANN, C. T. HERRMANN, C. F. LANGHAMMER.

No symptoms are derived from old-school sources.

The 1st edit. had only 7 fewer symptoms than are in this 2nd edit.]

---

1 From vol. vi, 2nd edit., 1827.

In the morning, long continued dizziness.

Vertigo ; sensation as if the brain whirled round in a circle (aft. 1 h.). [*Hrr.*]

Vertigo : sensation as if the front half of the brain whirled round in a circle, several times a day, for several minutes at a time. [*Hrr.*]

Confusion of the head. [*Hrr.*]

5. The head is extremely heavy (aft. 1 h.). [*Hrr.*]

Violent aching heavy pain in the forehead, especially above the root of the nose and in both temples, when sitting (aft. 3½ h.). [*Htn.*]

Pressure and feeling of weight in the forehead, more severe when moving. [*Hrr.*]

Pressure and feeling of weight in the occiput, more severe when moving. [*Hrr.*]

Hard pressure from within in both temples, unaffected by movement or touching (aft. 2½ h.). [*Hrr.*]

10. **Dull, aching drawing in the head, here and there,** worse on moving. [*Hrr.*]

Dull aching drawing in the head, here and there. [*Hrr.*]

Obtuse cutting pain in the brain, which commences over the right orbit and extends to the occiput (aft. 3 d.). [*Hrr.*]

Boring pain outwards, now in the right, now in the left, frontal protuberance, sometimes in both at once (aft. 9 h.). [*Htn.*]

Tearing pressure in the right temple internally, but more externally, increased by pressing on it. [*Hrr.*]

15. Twitching tearing pain in all the left occipital bone, more violent close to the parietal bone (aft. 2½ h.). [*Htn.*]

A burning, contractive pain in the head, especially in the forehead and eyes.

A constant digging and boring, as with a blunt instrument, in the forehead, **eyes,** and nose down to its tip—an alternate contraction and expansion.

Tearing pain in the forehead, over the right internal canthus of the eye and posteriorly in the orbit (aft. 24 h.). [*Hrr.*]

Pressure on the right eye-ball from before backwards and from below upwards (aft. 10 h.). [*Hrr.*]

20. **Mucus in both canthi** (aft. 8½, 10 h.). [*Lr.*]

Earthy complexion, blue borders round the eyes ; the features are quite disfigured, as if he had been very ill. [*Hrr.*]

Drawing pressure in the external meatus auditorius of the left ear (aft. 24 h.). [*Hrr.*]

Tearing pressure in the external cartilage of the ear, which went off by pressing on it (aft. 4 d.). [*Hrr.*]

Pressure on the right zygomatic arch regularly recurring at short intervals, unaffected by touch. [*Hrr.*]

25. Gums swollen, with sore pain—the whole of the interior of the mouth is painful as if excoriated.

A drawing aching in the molar teeth, from the back to the front ones, with drawing pain in the cheeks.

In the evening tongue furred white, without heat or thirst (aft. 7, 12 h.). [*Lr.*]

In the morning, taste of blood ; the mucus hawked up is tinged with blood.

Metallic sweetish sour taste on the back part of the tongue. [*Hrr.*]

30. **In the evening great thirst for cold drinks, without heat** (aft. 6, 12 h.). [*Lr.*]

Nausea in the stomach, he feels as though he would vomit—especially severe after a meal. [*Hrr.*]

Pressure in the stomach, felt particularly after a meal. [*Hrr.*]

Loud rumbling in the right side of the abdomen, when standing (aft. 2 h.). [*Lr.*]

Rumbling in the hypogastrium, without sensation. [*Hrr.*]

35. Painless rattling in the hypogastrium. [*Hrr.*]

Frequent discharge of flatus. [*Hrr.*]

Discomfort in the hypogastrium with pressure here and there (aft. 8 h.). [*Hrr.*]

Pinching pain in the hypogastrium, here and there (aft. 7 h.). [*Hrr.*]

Pinching pressure here and there in the hypogastrium with rumbling and rattling. [*Hrr.*]

40. **Pinching pressure in the hypogastrium, and rumbling with urging to stool—sensation as if he must go to stool.** [*Hrr.*]

In the evening straining at stool, without being able to pass anything (aft. 13 h.). [*Lr.*]

He must frequently pass urine, and every time in large quantity ; the urine is watery (aft. 12.). [*Hrr.*]

Aching pain in the right testicle, worse when touched (aft. 2 h.). [*Hrr.*]

At night emission of semen without voluptuous dreams. [*Lr.*]

* * *

45. Oppression of the chest.

A hot burning contraction of the chest, so that he can with difficulty breathe and speak.

Cough which disturbs him at night in his sleep, with much expectoration—also as much coughing by day.

Pain in chest and back, a boring and burning.

Fine shooting in the sternum, in its middle, not affected by inspiration or expiration (aft. 8 h.). [*Htn.*]

50. Tearing around and near the left nipple (aft. 2 d.). [*Hrr.*]

Pressive pain, sometimes greater, sometimes less, in the right side of the chest, near the sternum, on a small spot, unaffected by inspiration or expiration (aft. 4 h.). [*Htn.*]

Hard pressure near the left nipple inwards towards the sternum. [*Hrr.*]

Squeezing pressive pain in the region of the diaphragm, transversely through the chest, when walking (aft. 2 h.). [*Htn.*]

Fine tearing stitches in the region of both nipples (as if superficialy in the lungs and at the same time in the pectoral muscles), sometimes more severe on inspiring and expiring. [*Hrr.*]

55. (Pinching stitches in the region of both nipples, unaffected by inspiration and expiration). [*Hrr.*]

Strong beating of the heart. [*Hrr.*]

Obtuse shooting tearing in the region of the last rib. [*Hrr.*]

Intermittent stitches on the last false ribs of the left side, where they are attached to the spinal vertebræ. [*Hrr.*]

When sitting, pain in the left side of the back, as from prolonged stooping (aft. 8 h.). [*Lr.*]

60. Sharp pressure on the upper border of the right scapula and the clavicle. [*Hrr.*]

Tensive pressure on the right side of the neck, near the cervical vertebræ, when moving and when at rest (aft. 3 h.). [*Hrr.*]

Sensation of muscular twitchings in the right side of the neck. [*Hrr.*]

Aching tearing in the right shoulder-joint. [*Hrr.*]

In the anterior muscles of the left upper arm, a contractive spasmodic pain, during complete corporeal rest (aft. 24 h.). [*Lr.*]

65. A (spasmodic) contractive tearing in the muscles of the right arm (aft. 14 h.). [*Lr.*]

Paralytic pressure on the front of the right upper arm. [*Hrr.*]

Hard pressure on the left forearm, more towards the inferior and outer part. [*Hrr.*]

Paralytic tearing pressure on the right forearm, towards the outside, sometimes more above, sometimes more below, which went off on moving and touching. [*Hrr.*]

Paralytic weariness and weakness in the right arm. [*Hrr.*]

70. Cutting tearing in the inferion muscles of the right forearm (aft. 12 h.). [*Htn.*]

A vibrating pain in both bones of the left forearm, as if bruised (aft. 13 h.). [*Htn.*]

Paralytic tearing pressure on the right forearm, particularly severe in the bones of the wrist (aft. 1 h.). [*Hrr.*]

Tearing in the right wrist bones, which went off by movement. [*Hrr.*]

Trembling of the hands, observed when eating.

75. Sensation of weakness in the hand, as if he could not hold the pen, and trembled (aft. 8 h.). [*Htn.*]

Acute tearing pain about the right external protuberance of the wrist extending into the muscles of the hand, worst in the protuberance itself (aft. 11 h.). [*Htn.*]

Violent tearing pain in the bones of the left wrist (aft. 1½ h.).
Tearing in the metacarpal bones of the right fore and middle fingers (aft. 11 h.). [*Hrr.*]

Itching tearing pressure on the inner protuberance of both wrist, which induces scratching. [*Hrr.*]

80. Fine tearing in the proximal joints of the little finger. [*Hrr.*]

Aching tearing in the tips of the ring and little fingers of the right hand. [*Hrr.*]

Fine tearing in the finger-tips of the right hand, especially under the nails (aft. 3 d.). [*Hrr.*]

Intermittent fine tearing in the ball of the left thumb (aft. 2 h.). [*Hrr.*]

Intermittent hard pressure above the left knee-joint, on the lower part of the thigh, towards the outside, unaltered by touching or moving. [*Hrr.*]

85. Drawing from the middle of the calf and the front of the left leg, extending down into the foot. [*Hrr.*]

Itching erosion near the tibiæ and on the dorsum of both feet, near the ankle-joint, which becomes worse by scratching; he must scratch till the blood comes. [*Hrr.*]

Drawing on the right outer ankle, that went off on moving. [*Hrr.*]

Tearing pain under the right outer ankle, which always ended behind on the tendo Achillis (aft. 9. h.). [*Hrr.*]

Aching tearing between the two last metatarsal bones of the left foot close to the toes, whilst sitting (aft. 10 h.). [*Htn.*]

90. Fine tearing in the left heel. [*Hrr.*]

Tearing pain on the right heel, near and on the tendo Achillis (aft. 5 h.). [*Hrr.*]

Aching tearing in the point of the right big toe. [*Hrr.*]

Fine tearing in the proximal phalanges of the left toes. [*Hrr.*]

Exhaustion and relaxation. [*Hrr.*]

95. Whilst working a great desire to sleep overcomes him; he reads, but knows not what; he must lie down, when he immediately fell asleep and had confused dreams, in the forenoon. [*Hrr.*]

In the morning, some hours after getting up, extreme drowsiness; but after dinner, when in his healthy days he sometimes had a nap, he could not fall asleep, for several days. [*Hrr.*]

In the evening, during slumber, violent starting, as if he were falling (aft. 14½ h.). [*Lr.*]

At night, frequent waking up out of sleep as from fright. [*Lr.*]

At night, vivid anxious dreams. [*Lr.*]

100. **At night, sleep disturbed by voluptuous dreams, without, but oftener with, seminal emissions.** [*Lr.*]

He lies on his back at night. [*Lr.*]

At night frequent waking with weariness. [*Lr.*]

Flying heat all over the body, especially on the head and chest, without chilliness either before or afterwards, in the morning soon after rising (aft. 24 h.). [*Hrr.*]

Restless crossness ; everything is repugnant to him. At one time he sits, at another he lies, sometimes he walks about, but remains only a very short time in one position, because it immediately becomes disagreeable to him. [*Hrr.*]

105. Ill-humour all day ; he was very quite and would not speak ; in the evening more cheerful. [*Lr.*]

He is sullen and discontented with his condition and complains about it (aft. 24 h.). [*Hrr.*]

He commences first one thing then another, but only remains for a short time at one thing. [*Hrr.*]

Solitude is intolerable to him. [*Hrr.*]

BRYONIA ALBA.[1]

(White Briony.)

(The juice expressed from the fresh root dug up before the flowering time, is mixed with equal parts of alcohol, and, for homœopathic use, is diluted and potentized as directed in the introduction to pulsatilla, up to the thirtieth potency.)

The duration of the action of a somewhat large dose of this vegetable juice can be perceived for a couple of weeks.

The similarity of its effects to many of the symptoms of rhus toxicodendron cannot fail to be noticed; in the preface to the latter medicine I have sufficiently dwelt upon this. At the same time bryonia affects the disposition quite differently, its fever consists chiefly of chilliness, and its symptoms are mostly excited or aggravated by corporeal exertion, although its alternating effects, when the symptoms are relieved by movement, are not very rare.

Hence, when using broynia in diseases, there occur cases where the remedy, although chosen as homœopathically as possible and given in sufficiently small dose, does not render adequate service in the first twenty-four hours. The reason of this is that only one, and that the wrong series, of its alternating actions corresponded. In such cases a fresh dose administered after twent-four hours effects amelioration by the production of the opposite alternating actions. (The same happens with respect to all drugs, a second dose given immediately and quickly after the first one partially destroys the action of the first dose.) This happens with only very few other medicines having alternating actions (*vide* the preface to ignatia), but it occurs not rarely with bryonia.

When it has been really wrongly selected and was not truly homœopathic, the bad effects are generally removable by rhus, or, according to circumstances, by some other medicine corresponding more exactly to the bad effects produced, such as camphor.

From the rich treasury of symptoms it causes in the healthy human body, a number of artificial morbid states may be put together, of which we may happily avail ourselves for the homœopathic relief of many ailments of daily occurrence, especiatly certain fevers, and some kinds of the so-called abdominal spasms of the female sex. Hence its remedial powers are of great extent.

In severe acute diseases, with great excitement, the most serviceable dose is a very high attenuation, one higher than I have previously used, to wit, a very small globule of the decillionfold potency. The more or less strong olfaction of a globule the size of a mustard seed moistened with this attenuation acts more gently and certainly, and is equally

1 From vol. ii, 3rd edit. 1833.

efficacious in its effects upon the vital force—so amenable to accurately selected homœopathic remedies—which has been appointed by the wise Creator for bringing about the cure.

[The following assisted HAHNEMANN in his proving of bryonia :—FRIED. HAHNEMANN, HERRMANN, HORNBURG, MICHLER, E. F. RUCKERT, STAPF,

The only reference to another authority is in Symptom 682 where the name NICOLAI appears, but without any reference to enable us to identify him.

The 1st edit. gives 510 symptoms, the 2nd and 3rd 781.]

BRYONIA.

Vertigo.

Vertigo, as if he were whirled round, or as if everything whirled round him, when standing.

In the head a dull, giddy confusion, [*Mch.*]

A kind of vertigo as if he were intoxicated, and as if the blood rushed violently towards his head. [*Hrr.*]

5. He feels as if intoxicated, he is disposed to lie down. [*Fr. H—n.*]

Vertigo as soon as he rose from his seat ; all turned round about him ; after walking for some time this went off.

Vertigo as if from intoxication, all day (aft. 8 d.).

Staggering in the morning. [*Fr. H—n.*]

Vertigo, with feeling of heaviness, he felt as if all whirled round him in a circle. [*Hrr.*]

10. Vertigo and fullness in the head. [*Hbg.*]

Giddy, as if whirling, when she sits up in bed, and nausea in the centre of the chest, as if about to faint.

In the evening (aft. 8 p.m.) such vertigo when standing that he staggered backwards, and would have fallen backwards.

When he attempts to walk he staggers as if he would fall backwards.

When walking staggering to either side, as if he could not stand firmly (aft. 48 h.).

15. After moving, when standing, she sways to one side.

In the morning, on rising from bed, so giddy and whirling, as if all went round in a circle in his head.

All day long giddy in the head and weak in the limbs.

He can hardly turn his head on account of a feeling of fullness in it. [*Hbg.*]

In the region of the crown and forehead dull movements in the head, which causes vertigo and cessation of thought. [*Mch.*]

20. Rather dizziness in the head than vertigo.

So weak in mind that his thoughts leave him, as if he were about to faint, at the same time heat of face, chiefly when standing.

Illusion of the mind ; her own head seems to her much too heavy. [*Fr. H—n.*]

Stupid in the head, with striking forgetfulness. [*Fr. H—n.*]

She did not rightly know what she was doing (in the room), worse when lying, for twenty-four hours (immediately) [*Fr. H—n.*]

25. She did not know what she was doing, and let everything fall out of her hands (in the room). [*Fr. H—n.*]

The head is stupid, thinking difficult. [*Hrr.*]

He wishes for things that are not present.

He wishes for things immediately, and then will not have them.

Want of memory, forgetfulness (aft. 4 h.).

30. His head felt very heavy.

Excessive heaviness of the head (frequently, and aft. 4 d.). [*Hrr.*]

Great heaviness of the head and pressure of the whole brain forwards.

Stupefaction of the head.

Head feels empty (aft. 1 h.). [*Hrr.*]

35. Dulness in the head until he goes to sleep.

In the morning the headache commences not on awaking, but on first opening and moving the eyes.

In the morning on awaking the head is dull and painful, as if he had been drinking and dissipating the previous evening; he is unwilling to get out of bed.

(On treading a pressure in the head.)

In the occiput obtuse pain. [*Hbg.*]

40. Dull aching in the occiput. [*Rkt.*]

Throbbing headache in the forehead, so that he must lie down. [*Fr. H—n.*]

Digging pressure in the front part of the brain, with pressing towards the forehead, especially violent when stooping or walking quickly ; a walk tires him very much (aft. 24 h.). [*Hrr.*]

A pain in the forehead, aching so much that he can hardly stoop. [*Hbg.*]

Pressure from within outwards above the left orbit, in the brain, which passed into a pressure from above inwards in the eyeball (aft. 3 d.). [*Hrr.*]

45. Aching pain in the head, mainly on one side, together with tiresome aching feeling in the eye of that side (afternoon). [*Rkt.*]

An obscure compression in the head, in the forehead above the eyes.

First the blood mounted to the head, then ensued a compression from both temples.

Sensation as if the head were compressed from both ears.

Compressive pain at both sides of the head. [*Hbg.*]

50. Headache : a compression with jerks in the brain, like beating of the pulse.

In the morning, before day-break, pain as if the head were bound round, with weight in it, mingled with stitches ; on account of pain she could not raise her eyes, and when she stooped she could not rise up again (aft. 60 h.).

Violent headache, like great heaviness in it, as if it inclined to all sides ; with pressure in the brain outwards, and great desire to lie down (immediately).

Headache, after a meal, and when walking an outward pressure in the forehead.

Headache as if all would come out at the forehead.*

55. **Headache when stooping as if all would fall out at the forehead.†**

When sitting (stooping) and reading, giddy heaviness in the head, which is allayed by raising up the head.

Headache only when stooping, a pressing out at the forehead, mingled with stitches.

In the head an aching as if the brain were full and pressed asunder, chiefly when sitting.

An out-pressing pain in both temples.

60. Headache as if something pressed the skull asunder.

In the morning, in bed after awaking, when lying on the back, headache in the occiput, which extends to the shoulders, like a weight which presses on a sore place.

Semilateral headache: a (digging) pressure on a small spot of the right half of the brain, as from a kind of digging or tearing along the bones of the upper and lower maxillæ, stands in connexion with a painful submaxillary gland (aft. 30 h.).

Headache: in the morning after rising a twitching drawing in the bones of the cheeks and jaws.

Twitching tearing from the right malar bone up to the right temple externally, more violent when touched. [*Hrr.*]

65. Tearing pain in the left side of the head (aft. 24 h.). [*Fr. H—n.*]

(Tearing pain over the forehead then tearing in the cervical muscles, then tearing in the right arm.)

While walking in the open air a stitch in the head through the temple.

Anteriorly in the forehead single stitches, with dulness of the head. [*Hbg.*]

Shooting in the head from the forehead to the occiput.

70. A whirling sensation in the right side of the forehead, and a stitch in the left side of the forehead.

More twitching than throbbing pain in the head, with hot face.

In the right side of the head a throbbing, which can also be felt externally by the hand.

In the morning, on waking, headache on the crown, a painful throbbing.

In the forehead and occiput pain, a hollow throbbing (aft. 2 h.).

75. A throbbing headache, which includes the eyes, so that she cannot see well; on moving the beating in the head is quicker, she imagines she hears it.

In the head a chirping as from grasshoppers.

* Comp. 395.

† The sensation of asunder-pressing corresponds almost completely with that of compression 46, 47, 48, 50. 51, as it is felt by the brain enclosed in the unyielding skull; the organic sense cannot then distinguish whether the pain is owing to the great distension or from the resistance of the skull, and yet both are to blame for it.

A clucking in both temples.

Pain on the temple, as if someone pulled him by the hair there.

On the top of the head a spot, the size of half-a-crown, with burning pain, which is not painful when touched.

80. The head is especially painful when touched, chiefly on the sinciput. for twenty-four hours. [*Fr. H—n.*]

Sore feeling on one side of the occiput when touched. [*Hbg.*]

A smarting erosion on the occiput (at night).

In the morning great greasiness of the hair of the head, the head itself is cool; the hands became quite greasy on combing the hair (afr 10 h.).

On combing out the hair great itching on the head.

85. (A painful throbbing in all parts of the face, which is also felt under the fingers when touched.)

Itching needle-pricks in the right frontal muscle. [*Hrr.*]

A tension in the frontal muscles beneath the skin, on moving the eyes.

Heat in head and face, with redness.

Great heat in head and face. [*Hbg.*]

90. Flying heat over the face. [*Hbg.*]

A tension in the skin of the face, on moving the facial muscles.

Red spot in the face and on the neck (for two days).

Paleness of the face for twenty-four hours. [*Fr. H—n.*]

Red, hot, soft swelling of the face. [*Fr. H—n.*]

95. Swelling of the left side of the face, more down along the nose, with some pain in it (during the diarrhœa). [*Fr. H—n.*]

Great swelling of the upper half of the face, especially a great swelling under the eyes and over the root of the nose, with swelling of the eyelids; he could not open the left eye for four days (aft. 3 d.). [*Fr. H—n.*]

Contractive pain in the right palpebral muscle. [*Hrr.*]

Redness and swelling of the eyelids, with aching in them, for three days (aft. 3 d.). [*Fr. H—n.*]

In the left lower eyelid a pimple the size of a pea, painful when touched, for sixteen days (aft. 24 h.). [*Fr. H—n.*]

100. Soft boil at the inner canthus of the left eye; from time to time much pus escapes from it, for ten days (aft. 6 d.). [*Fr. H—n.*]

In the morning on waking he can scarcely open the eyes, they are stuck together by a purulent mass. [*Hrr.*]

Pain as from a burn above the left eye and on the left side of the nose, which is somewhat allayed by pressing on it. [*Fr. H—n.*]

Pain like burning out at the left eye (aft. 24 h.). [*Fr. H—n.*]

Aching in the eyes, with burning itching sensation in the eye-lids. [*Hbg.*]

105. Aching in the eyes for sixteen successive days. [*Fr. H—n.*]

Pressure on the right eyeball, more from above downwards (aft. 3 d.). [*Hrr.*]

A fine throbbing in the right eyeball. [*Fr. H—n.*]

Frequent lachrymation of the eyes. [*Hrr.*]

A dimness of vision of the left eye, as if it were full of water.

110. In the morning weakness of vision ; when she attempted to red all the letters ran together.

(*Presbyopia*) : she could see at a distance, but not near (aft. 24 h.).

The lower eyelid sometimes red and inflamed, the upper quivers.

In the left inner canthus raw pain and soreness.

In the morning the eyelids as if gummed together, somewhat red and swollen, and with pain as if rubbed and heated.

115. In the morning, on awaking an aching in the eye, as if pressed on by the hand, or as if in a room full of smoke.

In the morning the integuments of the eyes are swollen **and as if gummed up with matter.**

Swelling of the lower eyelid, internally aching pain ; eyes gummed up in the morning.

Smarting in the eyes, as if sand (?) were in them, which compels rubbing.

In the afternoon sensation in the right eye, as if a grain of sand were in it.

120. In the forenoon sudden swelling of one eye with pain, without redness ; matter exudes, and the conjunctiva is dark red and swollen.

The eyes water in the air

On the border of the left upper eyelid an itching mingled with burning and tearing.

Itching in the left outer canthus mingled with some smarting, not removed by rubbing (aft. 6 h.).

The eyes full of tears and the eyelids itch, as if something were healing ; he must rub.

125. A small tetter on the right cheek (aft. 4 d.). [*Fr. H—n.*]

Swelling of the right cheek close to the ear, with burning pain (aft. 4 d.). [*Fr. H—n.*]

Painful pressure under the right malar bone, removed by external pressure (aft. 1 h.). [*Hrr.*]

Pinching pressure in the cavity of the joint of the right jaw, increased by movement. [*Hrr.*]

Ringing before the left ear, as of small bells (aft. 1 h.). [*Fr. H—n.*]

130. In the meatus auditorius a contractive pain, which at first went off by clearing away the wax with the finger, but always came back again, with hardness of hearing. [*Mch.*]

Sensation in the external meatus as if a finger were pressed upon it, which is increased by bending down to read. [*Rkt.*]

Obtuse pain round about the left ear. [*Hbg.*]

Pain like a burning out at the left ear (aft. 6 h.). [*Fr. H—n.*]

Burning in the lobe of the ear. [*Hbg.*]

135. Hard boil behind the ear, which often changes its size (aft. 24 h.). [*Fr. H—n.*]

Boil-like swelling in front of the ear, which after twelve hours burst, discharged, and formed a yellow scab. [*Fr. H—n.*]

Humming before the right ear.

Sensation as if the ears were stopped up, and no air could penetrate into them.

When he walks in the open air, and after his walk comes into the house, he feels stitches, now in one, now in the other ear.

140. Blood comes out of the ears.

Violent aching on the right concha.

(Ulcerated concha.)

A frequent formication and tickling in the septum of the nose, especially when blowing the nose.

On the left side of the tip of the nose a swelling, with twitching pain in it, and, on touching it, as if it were going to gather.

145. An ulcer inside the left nostril with smarting pain.

Swollen nose with epistaxis for several days (aft. 5 d.). [*Fr. H—n.*]

Epistaxis on three successive days (the 10th, 11th, and 12th d.). [*Fr. H—n.*]

Epistaxis, several times a day, for fourteen days. [*Fr. H—n.*]

Epistaxis (aft. 10, 16 d.). [*Fr. H—n.*]

150. Epistaxis from the right nostril (aft. 9 d.). [*Fr. H—n.*]

Daily profuse epistaxis (aft. 14 d.). [*Fr. H—n.*]

First epistaxis and then ulcerated nostrils (sore nose).

Epistaxis (aft. 48, 72 h.).

In the morning after rising, epistaxis for a quarter of an hour.

155. Epistaxis in sleep, about 3 a.m., so that he is woke up by it. (aft. 4 d.).

Epistaxis without having previously stooped.

(A pimple on the chin, which causes shooting pain when touched.)

Drawing, with pressure in the throat up to the ear. [*Hbg.*]

Pain in the posterior part of the throat, felt when moving. [*Hbg.*]

160. Tensive stiffness of the left side of the neck. [*Hbg.*]

Rheumatic stiffness in the side of the neck towards the nape. [*Hbg.*]

Tension in the nape on moving the head. [*Hbg.*]

On the left side of the nape and neck, of the facial and masseter muscles, sore pain on moving, which rendered turning the head and chewing difficult and almost impossible (aft. 24 h.). [*Hbg.*]

Itching needle-pricks on the neck (especially when he has walked quickly) which cause him to scratch; they are removed by scratching (aft. 24 h.). [*Hbg.*]

165. Chap in the lower lip [*Fr. H—n.*]

Burning in the lower lip. [*Hbg.*]

On the lower lip small ulcerated fissures, which cause burning pain when touched. [*Fr. H—n.*]

On the right commissure of the mouth, and more on the lower lip, a small elevation, which from time to time bleeds profusely, for six days. [*Fr. H—n.*]

A vesicle on the red part of the lower lip with burning pain.

170. Eruption below the left commissure of the lips with smarting pain.

Eruption on the lower lip beyond the red part, with itching smarting pain as from salt.

Between the under lip and gum a shooting, very acute twitching (in the morning in bed), as in cancer of the lip.

Toothache, twitching and shooting in the teeth towards the ear, which compelled her to lie down.*

In the evening, in bed, twitching toothache, now in the upper, now in the lower molars (for an hour); when the pain was above, and the point of the finger was applied there, the pain suddenly ceased and went into the opposite lower tooth (aft. 5 d.).

175. Twitching toothache during the (accustomed) tobacco-smoking (aft. 1 h.).

Drawing, sometimes twitching toothache in the molars of the left upper jaw, only during and after eating, at the same time the teeth felt too long and as if they waggled to and fro (aft. 6 h.). [*Hrr.*]

Drawing pain in the molars of the upper and lower jaw (aft. 24 h.). [*Hrr.*]

Looseness of all the teeth observable when touching them and biting.

Pain in a molar tooth only when chewing.

180. When at rest, and especially in bed, a horrible toothache, which is alleviated by chewing. [*Hbg.*]

Toothache on taking something warm into the mouth.

While eating there occurs a tearing shooting toothache (that extends down into the cervical muscles), which is especially aggravated by warmth.

Pain as if the tooth were screwed in and then raised up (which is only relieved for an instant by cold water, but is better by walking in the open air); at the same time tearing in the cheek and pinching in the ears, at night until 6 a.m.

Toothache; on opening the mouth the air entering causes pain.

185. Toothache after midnight (about 3 a.m.) as if an exposed nerve in a hollow tooth were painfully affected by cold air penetrating to it; the pain is increased to an intolerable degree by lying on the unaffected side, and only goes off when lying on the cheek of the affected side.

On drinking cool liquid a sore pain comes into the tooth.[1]

The gums are painful as if sore and raw, with painful loose teeth.

In the morning after waking sensation as if all the molars were too long; they could be moved to and fro by the fingers so loose were they; she could bite nothing with them, and when she bit with

* There are several symptoms caused by bryonia which compel the person to lie down; comp. 285, 479, 631, 708, or, at least, to sit down, 296, and several that are increased by walking and standing, *e. g.* 308; but, on the other hand, the alternating action, where the symptoms are relieved by movement, and cannot bear quiet lying and sitting, is much more frequent with bryonia.

1 This symptom is given here as it stands in the 2nd edit. In the 3rd the transcriber has introduced a superfluous "not" that destroys the sense of the symptom.

them there was pain as if the teeth fell out, for fifteen hours (aft. 48 h.). [*Stf.*]

The teeth appear to him to be too long. [*Fr. H—n.*]

190. Spongy gums.

Simple pain of one of the submaxillary glands, as if from being pinched (aft. 12 h.).

Painful stiffness of all the cervical muscles on movement, and roughness in the throat on swallowing.

Sensation on the lower jaw as if there were a node on the bone, with tensive pain on turning the head (aft. 61 h.). [*Stf.*]

Red miliary eruption on the neck. [*Fr. H—n.*]

195. Rough scrapy feeling in the throat (aft. 5 h.). [*Hbg.*]

He feels as if swollen at the back of the throat, and as if he had a severe catarrh, which makes talking difficult. [*Hbg.*]

Round the neck a smarting itching eruption, especially after the sweat.

In the inside of the throat shooting on pressing it from the outside and on turning the head.

Shooting in the throat when swallowing.

200. Pressure in the œsophagus as if he had swallowed a hard angular body.

She cannot get the food and drink down; she has a choking in the œsophagus.

(Sensation when swallowing, as if the throat were swollen internally or were full of mucus, which cannot be got rid of by hawking.)

Sore-throat: dry and raw in the throat during empty swallowing; on drinking this sensation goes off for a short time, but soon recurs; it is worst in the warm room.

In the evening dry feeling at the back and upper part of the throat (aft. 48 h.).

205. Dry feeling, not on the tongue, but above on the palate.

Blisters on the border of the tongue anteriorly, which smart and burn. [*Fr. H—n.*]

Dryness in the mouth, so that the tongue sticks to the palate. [*Fr. H—n.*]

Dryness in the mouth without thirst. [*Hbg.*]

In the morning dry feeling in the mouth (aft. 48 h.). [*Mch.*]

210. The interior of the mouth feels to him dry, without thirst.

Dry feeling only inside the upper teeth.

Much thirst by day, without heat.

Violent thirst for twenty two days. [*Fr. H—n.*]

Thirst, especially in the morning. [*Fr. H—n.*]

215. Violent thirst, day and night. [*Fr. H—n.*]

After eating great thirst, for sixteen days. [*Fr. H—n.*]

The saliva runs out at the corners of the mouth involuntarily.

Spitting much saliva. [*Fr. H—n.*]

Collection of much soapy frothy saliva in the mouth. [*Hbg.*]

220. Tongue furred very white.

Insipid, disgusting taste in the mouth (aft. 5 d). [*Mch.*]
Sweetish, disgusting taste in the mouth. [*Fr. H—n.*]
Insipid, sickly taste in the mouth; he has almost no taste.
Insipid taste and sickly feeling in the mouth.

225. Sweetish, qualmish taste in the mouth.
She has no taste of the food; but when not eating her mouth is bitter.
Everything tastes bitter, he cannot get down the food.
After dinner a bitter taste remained constantly at the back of the palate.
In the morning sickly, bitter taste in the mouth.

230. In the morning when fasting taste in the mouth as from decayed teeth or putrid flesh (aft. 12 h.).
With tolerably clean tongue a nasty taste in the throat, as when one's breath smells; the taste is like the smell of stinking flesh; whilst eating she feels nothing of it.
He has a fœtid smell from the mouth.
Late in the evening there comes a rancid, smoky taste in the throat.
Anorexia without bad taste (aft. 3 h.).

235. Spoilt appetite. [*Hbg.*]
Want of appetite (for 10 d.). [*Fr. H—n.*]
The stomach is empty; he has hunger without appetite. [*Hrr.*]
In the morning when fasting voracious hunger, with want of appetite. [*Hbg.*]
Hunger, with anorexia. [*Mch.*]

240. Constant nausea, and immediately afterwards voracious hunger (aft. some h.). [*Fr. H—n.*]
In the morning voracious hunger, with thirst and flying heat (aft. 30, 72 h.). [*Mch.*]
Great hunger for fourteen days. [*Fr. H—n.*]
Excessive hunger for six days. [*Fr. H—n.*]
Voracious hunger, without appetite.

245. Voracious hunger, lasting into the night.
He has hunger, and eats, but he does not relish food.
He has no appetite for milk; but when he takes it the appetite for it comes, and he commences to relish it.
He longs for many things which he cannot relish.
The food smells good, but on commencing to eat her appetite goes off.

250. Appetite for wine.
Appetite for coffee.
Great longing for coffee (aft. 5 h.). [*Fr. H—n.*] [*Mch.*]
Frequent eructation of nothing but air.
After eructation hiccup, without having previously taken any food

255. After eructation hiccup for a quarter of an hour (aft. 48 h.).
Violent hiccup.
Violent eructation after a meal, from morning till evening.

Eructation, with taste of food.

Drinks do not cause eructation, but the smallest quantity of food does, but only of air, without bad taste.

260. (Eructation, with burnt taste in the mouth and mucus in the throat.)

With every eructation a shooting pain.

(A burning almost uninterrupted eructation, which makes his mouth rough and prevents his tasting of food.)

After eating an acrid dry taste, with persistent dryness in the front part of the mouth, without thirst; the lips are dry and chapped.

In the evening after lying down bitter taste in the mouth.

265. Eructation after eating, at last bitter eructation.

After a meal bitter eructation.

Without eructation there comes a bitterness up into the mouth with sickness.

He eructates acidity, and sourish water collects in the mouth.

In the morning, after an anxious dream, sickness without being able to vomit, and frequent empty eructation.

270. Nausea in the evening before going to sleep.

Frequent, sometimes sourish eructation after eating. [*Hrr.*]

Nausea, lasting 24 hours, with running of much water from the mouth (aft. 5 m.). [*Fr. H—n.*]

Nausea, especially when smoking tobacco (in one accustomed to it). [*Hbg.*]

Sickness (immediately). [*Mch.*]

275. Several times vomiting of yellow and green mucus. [*Fr. H—n.*]

immediately after midnight he wakes with nausea; he must vomit food and bile.

She has rising of food which comes into the mouth by a kind of belching.

Eructation of the contents of the stomach, with hardly any effort to vomit.

After eating food that he relished sickness and loathing.

280. She vomits solid food but not fluids.

Early every morning, two hours after rising, nausea for half an hour, with accumulation of water in the mouth.

In the evening nausea, and then flow of a quantity of water from the mouth (water-brash).*

Nausea, sickness, without having eaten anything (aft. 1 h.).

In the morning, on awaking, nausea, sickness.

285. (Vomiting of blood and lying down.)

In the morning (about 6 a.m.) vomiting of a bitter, musty, and putrid fluid, the taste of which remains in her mouth.

After drinking (in the afternoon) qualmish and sick.

In the evening vomiting of mucus (aft. 5 h.).

In the evening (6 p.m.) retching of water and mucus, like water-brash; it rose up in his chest, and at the same time the whole body was cold.

* Comp. 402.

290. Painful sensation in the œsophagus, rather low down, as if it were constricted there.

In the morning she brings mucus up from the stomach by a kind of belching.

(Cough, especially after eating.)

(A quarter of an hour after each meal headache, which then goes off gradually, but is renewed after the next meal.)

After every meal distension of the abdomen.

295. Cutting, as with knives, in the region of the scrobiculus cordis (aft. 1 h.).

Immediately after the (evening) meal violent aching in the scrobiculus cordis when walking, at last pressure on the bladder and perinæum to an intolerable degree ; it went off on sitting (aft. 12 h.).

Stomachache as soon as he has eaten anything, and even while eating.

After eating pressure in the stomach ; it was as if a stone lay there and made him cross.

After eating pressure in the stomach. [*Hbg.*]

300. Pressure in the stomach when walking. [*Hbg.*]

Pinching in the scrobiculus cordis (aft. 12 h.). [*Mch.*]

Sensation in the scrobiculus cordis as if it were swollen. [*Hbg.*]

Under the scrobiculus cordis a very disagreeable feeling, like swelling. [*Hbg.*]

Heat in the abdomen (and all the interior of the body). [*Hbg.*]

305. Aching and pinching in the hypogastrium. [*Hrr.*]

Loud rumbling in the abdomen for fourteen days. [*Fr. H—n.*]

Loud rattling in the abdomen, especially in the evening in bed, for eighteen days. [*Fr. H—n.*]

A squeezing and aching in the abdomen in the umbilical region, when walking and standing.

Contractive pain in the stomach, some hours after eating.

310. After a meal contractive pain in the stomach, then cutting in and over the scrobiculus cordis, eructation, heat rising up, nausea and vomiting only of the food that has been eaten (aft. 48 h.).

Hard swelling about the navel and under the hypochondria.

Sudden ascites ; he cannot get his breath and must sit down (aft. 18 h.).

Excoriation in the overlapping folds of the abdomen, in the iliac region.

Tensive pain in the hepatic region.

315. Buring pain in the abdomen, in the hepatic region (aft. 8 h.).

Pain in the abdomen as though he would vomit (aft. 5 d.)

Pain in both sides of the abdomen like stitches in the spleen.

First tearing and drawing in the abdomen, especially on moving, then shooting, especially during an evacuation of the bowels, and chiefly in the evening.

Violent cutting stitches in the abdomen from below upwards, as high as the stomach (after drinking a cup of warm milk, in the afternoon); the pain compelled him to bend double, and disappeared after a motion of the bowels.

320. Around the navel a painful twisting with stitches.

Bellyache combined with anxiety, that impedes his breathing; it was relieved by walking.

Flatus passes in the night, not without previous loud rumbling and noise.

After the (evening) meal, flatulent colic with a pressure in the region of the cæcum.

Pains in the abdomen as if he had been purged, or as if hæmorrhoids would come on.

325. After dinner spasmodic pains in the abdomen.

Rumbling in the bowels and sensation as if he would be purged.

Bellyache as if diarrhœa was about to come on, for an hour and a half (aft. 5 m.). [*Fr. H—n.*]

Horrible cutting in the bowels (in the forenoon) as if she would have dysentery, without evacuation of the bowels.

When walking in the open air a pressure on the navel, as from a button.

330. (Sensation as if a lump lay deep in the abdomen.)

In the abdomen and in the umbilical region a griping and pinching as after a chill, for several days, and (aft. 3 d.) after the bellyache a copious thin evacuation by stool.

Very ill-smelling, frequent stools, preceded by cutting in the abdomen.

Distended abdomen; there is always a rumbling in the abdomen and bellyache (cutting in the bowels), and yet constant constipation; sensation as if something stuck in his abdomen.

Bellyache during the stool, as from constriction and pinching together with the hand.

335. Causes open bowels.

Stool twice daily; after some days constipation.*

Brown, frequent, thin stools in an infant at the breast.

Frequent stools (aft. 48 h.).

Very big formed fæces passing with difficulty.

340. Diarrhœa (aft. 3 d.).

Diarrhœic stool (aft. 28 h.). [*Hbg.*]

Loose evacuations without suffering (aft. 24, 30 h.). [*Mch.*]

Diarrhœa for four successive days, once every three hours, so quick that he cannot retain it; the following twelve days the ordinary stool passed with equally unexpected rapidity. [*Fr. H—n.*]

Diarrhœa for two days, which made her so weak that she had to keep her bed (aft. 3 d.). [*Fr. H—n.*]

345. Diarrhœa mostly in the morning. [*Fr. H—n.*]

Diarrhœa, especially at night, and with every evacuation burning in the anus (aft. 7 d.). [*Fr. H—n.*]

Diarrhœa which smelt strongly of decayed cheese. [*Fr. H—n.*]

Thin, bloody stool (aft. 24 h.). [*Fr. H—n.*]

* Bryonia seems more frequently in its primary action to keep back the stool, and its secondary action, in which it does the opposite, is rarer; hence, when its other symptoms indicate it, it can cure constipation permanently, which few medicines besides nux-vomica and opium can do.

Diarrhœa preceded by cutting in the abdomen (aft, 44, 72 h.).

350. After hard stool long-continued burning in the rectum.

Very costive motion, with pressing out of the rectum, which, however, soon returned of itself; thereafter diarrhœic stool with fermentation in the abdomen. [*Fr. H—n.*]

Very hard stool.

Soft stool, with burning sharp pain in the anus.

Itching, jerk-like, coarse stitches from the anus up into the rectum.

355. (Nocturnal diarrhœa.)

Burning and cutting before the urine comes (aft. 3 d.). [*Fr. H—n.*]

The urine is hot as it passes. [*Fr. H—n.*]

Pain in the abdomen when urinating.

Sensation when urinating as if the urinary passages were too narrow.

360. He must get up several times at night to pass water.

He had great urging to urinate; he must get up at night to urinate.

Although the bladder was not full he had such urging to make water that he was hardly able to retain it for an instant (aft. 12 h.).

When he has urinated the neck of the bladder contracts, and yet he feels as if some more urine wanted to pass.

He cannot retain his urine long; when he has the desire to urinate and does not immediately respond to it, he feels as if the urine passed involuntarily (and yet when he looks he finds that none has come away.)

365. When moving there often pass unconsciously some drops of hot urine.

After urinating he feels in the bladder as if he had not passed all the urine, and some drops pass away involuntarily.

Urging to urinate and frequent discharge of urine when walking in the open air (aft. 6 h.).

A pain compounded of itching, burning, and shooting in the anterior part of the urethra, when not urinating.

Burning in the urethra.

370. (An aching pain in the urethra.)

(A drawing and tearing in the forepart of the urethra, when not urinating.)

Some stitches in the testicles (immediately) when sitting.

On the border of the prepuce a shooting, burning itching.

The glans penis is covered with miliary rash which itches.

375. Swelling of the left labium majus, on which a black, hard pustule comes, resembling a small button, without pain and without inflammation.

Very distended abdomen; she has great uneasiness there, and such pinching as though the catamenia were coming on.

The menses come on eight days too early. [*Fr. H—n.*]

The menses come on fourteen days too early. [*Fr. H—n.*]

The menses appeared slightly three weeks too soon. [*Fr. H—n.*]

380. The menses occur within a few hours, sometimes eight days too soon.*

(Increase of the leucorrhœa.) [*Fr. H—n.*]

* * *

In the morning, violent sneezing (aft. 18 h.).

In the morning violent sneezing and yawning (aft. 48 h.).

Frequent sneezing, especially when he passes his hand over the forehead.

385. Some hoarseness and only one tone of the voice when walking in the open air.

A kind of hoarseness, and at the same time disposition to perspire.

Voice rough and hoarse (aft. 4 h.). [*Hrr.*]

Hoarseness for twenty-one days. [*Fr. H—n.*]

Fluent coryza for eight days. [*Fr. H—n.*]

390. Severe fluent coryza, so that he talked through his nose, at the same time continual chilliness, for eight days. [*Fr. H—n.*]

Severe fluent coryza with much sneezing, for eight days (aft. 48 h.). [*Fr. H—n.*]

Severe coryza with pain in the forehead. [*Fr. H—n.*]

Severe coryza without cough (aft. 36 h.).

Violent, rather stuffed coryza (aft. 48 h.).

395. Severe coryza, with shooting headache, as though all would come out at the forehead, especially on stooping† (aft. 70 h.).

Viscid phlegm in the fauces that was detached by hawking. [*Hbg.*]

Dry cough.

Dry cough as it were from the stomach, preceded by a crawling and tickling in the scrobiculus cordis.

Cough from a constant crawling up in the throat; phlegm is then ejected.

400. Cough with expectoration (immediately). [*Fr. H—n.*]

Cough with expectoration, in the forenoon, for four successive days (aft. 34 h.). [*Fr. H—n.*]

Continual, dry cough, especially in the morning, during which water runs out of his mouth, like water-brash.‡

(Nausea excites him to cough.)

When coughing vomiting of food.

405. When coughing a long-continued stitch deep in the brain on the left side.

A dry, hacking cough ; single, spasmodic severe blows against the upper part of the wind-pipe, which seems to be covered with dry, firm mucus ; even tobacco-smoke excites it.

Irritation to hacking cough ; it seems as if some mucus were in the wind-pipe ; when he has coughed for some time he feels a pain there compounded of soreness and pressure ;

* This is primary action, hence bryonia will often be a powerful stopper of metrorrhagia.

† Comp. 54, 55.

‡ Comp. 282.

the pain becomes more violent by speaking and smoking tobacco (aft. 4 h.). [*Hrr.*]

When he comes from the open air into the warm room he has a feeling as if vapour were in the wind-pipe, which compels him to cough ; he feels as if he could not breathe in air enough (aft. 2 h.). [*Hrr.*]

Viscid phlegm in the wind-pipe that is detached by frequent hacking cough. [*Hrr.*]

410. In the morning in bed a severe cough, that lasted a quarter of an hour, and brought away much mucous expectoration.

In the morning he has oppression of the chest ; he feels as if clogged with mucus in the chest, and it is not readily detached.

In the throat scraping, painful, hacking cough, as from roughness and dryness of the larynx, in the evening after lying down in bed.

A hacking dry cough striking against the top of the wind-pipe.

He coughs up small lumps of coagulated blood (aft. 3 h.).

415. He coughs and hawks yellow mucus from the fauces.

When coughing shooting in the throat internally.

When coughing stitches in the last rib.

When coughing stitches in the sternum ; he must support the chest with his hand ; stitches also when merely touching it.*

When coughing he sneezes twice.

420. When coughing he has heaving as if he would vomit, without nausea.

When coughing pain in the scrobiculus cordis.

When coughing it goes through his whole head.

When coughing it always goes into the head like a pressure.

Immediately before a fit of coughing frequent gasping for air, quick spasmodic breathing, as if the child could not get its breath, and on that account could not cough ; a kind of suffocative attack, followed by cough ; particularly after midnight.

425. Aching in the scrobiculus cordis, which oppresses her chest.

An extraordinary warmth in the region of the scrobiculus cordis makes her breathing short with a kind of aching pain.

Burning pain in the right side of the chest (aft. 8 h.).

Impeded respiration.

The breathing is made short ; he must expire more quickly.

430. Tightness of chest (aft. 1 h.).

An attack of stitch in the side and oppression of the chest for twelve hours.

Tightness of chest ; she felt a need to breathe deeply (as if her chest were stopped up and she could not get air), and when she tried to breathe deeply she had pain in the chest, as if something were stretched out which opposed itself to stretching.

Anxiety in the morning which proceeded from the abdomen, as if a purgative had been taken, and as if the breath were too short.

Rapid, anxious, almost impossible breathing on account of

* Comp. 512, 535, 601.

stitches in the chest, first under the scapulæ, then under the pectoral muscles, which hinder breathing and compel him to sit up; then stitches in the crown of the head.

435. Aching all over the chest (aft. 24 h.).

On the sternum superiorly pressure as with the hand; she fancies she cannot walk in the open air without pain there.

In the middle of the sternum aching pain, also when breathing, with icy-cold feet.

On the chest an aching, as if it were oppressed with phlegm, and on inspiring some shooting in the sternum, which seems to be alleviated by eating.

Heaviness in the chest and heaviness in the body, which went off by eating.

440. On breathing deeply stitches in the side on the ribs, in jerks, which went off in the open air.

On inspiring a stitch from the upper part of the chest through to the scapula.

On inspiring the curves of the ribs towards the back are the seat of tensive pain, which on breathing more deeply increases to an obtuse stitch, especially under the scapulæ, and mostly on stooping forwards.

In the evening (6 p.m.) shooting in the chest with oppression.

A momentary stitch in the left clavicle, followed by a simple pain (afterwards there was only simple pain).

445. On turning in bed, stitch in the chest on the side on which he is not lying.

In the lower part of the right side of the chest shooting and beating like a pulse.

A shooting pressing from within outwards in the chest.

On the slightest breath a stitch as if in an ulcer, which lasts as long as the respiration, on a small spot beneath the sternum, which smarts like an ulcer even when touched,* but still more on raising the right arm, in the morning (aft. 24 h.).

Pain on the ensiform cartilage on touching it, as if blood were extravasated, in the evening.

450. Pain all over the chest, with oppression, which goes off on discharging flatus, in the evening (9 p.m.).

An attack as if the ailment rose up and took away breath and speech.

A grasping together of the chest near the sternum.

Pain in the chest close above the scrobiculus cordis, squeezing, worst when she sits on a chair and stoops, and when she lies in bed upon the side.

Palpitation of the heart, for several successive days (aft. 12 h.). [*Fr. H—n.*]

455. **Internal heat in the chest.** [*Hbg.*]

Heat in the chest and face. [*Hbg.*]

Sensation as if all were loose in the chest and fell down into the abdomen. [*Hbg.*]

* Comp. 418, 512, 535, 602.

Squeezing pressure behind the sternum, aggravated by expiration and inspiration (aft. 5 d.). [*Hrr.*]

Great swelling of the anterior of the chest externally. [*Hbg.*]

460. In an indurated nipple single slight electric-like shocks for two and a half hours, after which all traces of the induration were gone (aft. 5 h.). [*Stf.*]

Sharp outward shooting pain under the right nipple, in the cavity of the chest, only on expiring. [*Hrr.*]

(A stretching over from the short ribs.)

Tension in the chest when walking.

On the right side of the nape towards the shoulder painful stiffness of the muscles when moving the head.

465. A pain in the nape where it joins the occiput, like combined pain and weakness, as if the head were weak.

Pain in the nape as after a chill.

Aching between the scapulæ and opposite them in front of the chest, when sitting, which went off by walking.

Burning under and between the scapulæ. [*Mch.*]

Painful pressure on the top of the right shoulder, worse on being touched; on breathing deeply an obtuse shooting there which extends backwards and outwards into the shoulder-joint (aft. 10 h.). [*Hrr.*]

470. A spasmodic pain between the scapulæ, almost like shuddering.

Shooting in the lumbar vertebræ. [*Hbg.*]

Shooting pain in the sacrum and back, at night for six hours (aft. 70 h.). [*Fr. H—n.*]

Sacral pains which interfere much with walking. [*Fr. H—n.*]

Burning in the back. [*Mch.*]

475. A contractive pain across the whole back, as if it were firmly bound with bands, almost like cramp (in the afternoon from 4 to 8 p.m.) (aft. 48 h.).

A drawing down the back when sitting, which goes off by movement.

Painful shooting twitching close to the spine on both sides, when sitting, especially in the morning and evening.

Bruised pain in the sacrum when sitting, worst when lying, little felt when moving.

He can neither bend nor stoop for pain in the back and lumbar vertebræ, a tearing, more felt when standing than when sitting, but not when lying.

480. A couple of coarse stitches, like knife-stabs, in the hip.

A crawling running, as of a mouse, from the axilla to the hip.

Obtuse stitch over the shoulder, towards the arm. [*Hbg.*]

In the upper arm, especially on raising it, a kind of stitches. [*Rkt.*]

(A quivering and twitching in the deltoid muscle.)

485. A drawing through the shafts of the arm-bones, like a thread, extending into the tips of the fingers.

An aching on both humeri which prevents him falling asleep in the evening.

A nervous tearing in the interior of the arms downwards.

Sweat in the axillæ.

Pain on raising the arm in the region of the acromion process, as from dislocation (aft. 3 h.).

490. Swelling of the right upper arm to the elbow.

Stitches in the right elbow-joint. [*Hbg.*]

Swelling on the elbow-joint and somewhat above and below it to the middle of the upper and fore-arm and on the feet, for three hours. [*Hbg.*]

Tearing pain on the internal surface of the forearm, from the elbow in a line to the wrist-joint (aft. 5 d.). [*Hrr.*]

Red miliary eruption on the upper side of the forearm. [*Fr. H—n.*]

495. (Violent shooting and formication in the left arm.)

Shooting in the point of the elbow, with drawing in the tendons, extending into the hand ; the shooting is aggravated by bending the elbow.

(In the hand formication, as if gone asleep.)

Shooting pains in the joints of the hands and heaviness of them. [*Hbg*]

He cannot grasp firmly with the hands. [*Hbg.*]

500. Trembling of the hands and distended veins thereof. [*Hbg.*]

In the wrist joint pain as if sprained or dislocated at every movement (aft. 24 h.).

Fine shooting in the wrist, when the hand becomes warm and when at rest ; but it does not go off by movement.

About midnight an inflammation of the back of the hand, with burning pain.

Hot feeling in the palms of the hands and the forearms ; she must lie out of bed in the morning ; after some hours cold feeling in them.

505. Stiffness and numb feeling in the palms of the hands.*

Jerking tearing in the joints between the metacarpus and fingers, or in the last finger-joints, lasting a short time. [*Rkt*]

Involuntary twitching of the fingers of both hands on movement. [*Hbg.*]

In the fingers shooting pains when writing. [*Hbg.*]

(Falling asleep of the fingers of both hands up to the wrists.)

510. Feeling of paralysis in the fingers.

(In the ball of the thumb pain like shooting and cramp.)

Somewhat hot, pale swelling of the distal joint of the little finger ; there are shoots in it on moving the finger and pressing on it.†

A papule between the right thumb and index, which causes shooting pain when touched.

In the root of the little finger pain as if there were matter in it.

515. Bruised pain of the sacrum and thighs.

* Comp. 576

† Comp. 448, 535, 602.

A pain comes by jerks like cramp into the sacrum when sitting and lying.

The sacrum pains as if bruised when lying on it.

Pain in the hip-joint, like jerks or blows, when she lies or sits ; it is better when walking.

When walking bent forwards shooting pain from the hip-joint into the knee.

520. Pain in the trochanter, startling shooting on making a false step ; when at rest throbbing therein ; the part hurts very much when touched.*

Unsteadiness in the thighs and legs, and staggering when going downstairs (aft. 20 h.).

In the hips obtuse shooting pain. [*Hbg.*]

Itching on the hips and thighs (aft. 48 h.). [*Fr. H—n.*]

Tearing pain in the right thigh when moving. [*Fr. H—n.*]

525. **Great weakness in the thighs ; he can hardly go upstairs ; less when going downstairs.** [*Rkt.*]

Vacillation of the thighs, especially on going up and downstairs (aft. 2 d.). [*Fr. H—n.*]

Great weakness in the thighs, observable even when sitting (aft. 8 h.). [*Rkt.*]

Drawing in the thighs as if the catamenia were about to come on.

In the morning, in bed, the thigh becomes stiff, like cramp.

A stitch in the upper and anterior part of the thigh.

530. Bruised pain in the middle of the thigh, and beating as with a hammer on the same spot when sitting.

When sitting and at night when lying cramp in the knee and sole of the foot.

On going downstairs pain as if the patellæ would break.

On going upstairs the legs are weak.

Tensive, painful stiffness of the knees.

535. Under the knee a pustule, which only hurts and shoots when touched.

A (tearing and) burning in the right knee.

The patellæ are painful as if they had been beaten loose.

An itching, as if something were healing, in the hough, and sweat on that part at night.

Stitches in the knees when walking. [*Hbg.*]

540. Fine, flying stitches in the knee-joints only when moving. [*Rkt.*]

Dry eruption on and in the houghs, which itches in the evening, looks red, and after scratching causes stinging pain. [*Fr. H—n.*]

Weakness, especially in the knee-joints. [*Hbg.*]

Weakness, especially in the knee-joint (immediately). [*Mch.*]

The knees totter and bend under him when walking. [*Hbg.*]

545. **The legs are so weak that they can scarcely support him on beginning to walk, and even when standing.** [*Hbg.*]

Swelling of both legs (aft. 40 h.). [*Fr. H—n.*]

* Comp. 601, 602.

On the outside of the left calf bruised pain on moving and turning the foot, as also on touching ; when quite at rest numb feeling on the part for many days (aft. 12 h.). [*Hbg.*]

Swelling without redness of the lower half of the legs, with the exception of the feet, which are not swollen. [*Hbg.*]

Violent drawing pain in the leg, especially the calf, for an hour, followed by sweat (aft. 4 d.).

550. Drawing pain in the shafts of the bones of the legs.

(Eruption exuding moisture on the thighs.)

A tearing, twitching pain in the upper half of the tibia.

A twitching in the leg at night ; by day a twitching like an electric shock.

Sudden swelling of the legs.

555. In the morning cramp in the left calf (aft. 12 h.).

At night, when lying in bed, cramp in the feet, in the dorsum of the feet and heels (aft. 6 h.)

At night cramp in the calf (a contractive tension) which went off by movement.

Stitch-like tearing from the feet up to the houghs, less when at rest than when moving. [*Hbg.*]

Pressure on the inner border of the left foot (aft. 1 h.). [*Hrr.*]

560. Tearing in the dorsum of the right foot the first night. [*Fr. H—n.*]

Hot swelling of the foot (aft. 8 h.).

Hot swelling of the instep, with bruised pain when the foot is stretched out ; the foot feels tense on treading, and on touching it pains as if gathering and as if ulcerated.

(White pustules on the foot, with pain in them like a bad ulcer, the foot became red, and he could not walk for pain.)

Along with the swelling of the feet tearing in the tibiæ and heaviness in the arms.

565. In the evening the feet feel tense and swollen.

In the ankle-joint tension on moving.

In the dorsum of the foot tensive pain, even when sitting.

On two nights, immediately after lying down, felling as if a hook penetrated the heel ; obtuse stitches rapidly following one another, for a quarter of an hour.

In the morning, in bed, needle-pricks in both heels, which went off after rising.

570. Pain in the feet as if sprained.

Shooting in the feet. [*Hbg.*]

In both soles such violent shooting that she could not tread, with tension in the ankle-joints ; neither could she lie on account of tension and shooting. [*Fr. H—n.*]

Single stitches into the toes. [*Hbg.*]

In the hollow part of the sole stitches on treading.

575. Knife-stabs in the left sole.

In the hollow of the soles when treading pain as though they were numb* and tense.

* Comp. 505.

Sensation of heaviness in the feet and numb feeling in them, as if they were swollen.

Shooting and aching in the ball of the big toe, also pain there as if frost-bitten.

The corn, hitherto painless, aches and pains, worst when treading, but also when at rest.

580. Corns pain as if sore on the slightest touch, even of the bed-clothes.

In the right toe-ball a shooting pain, more when sitting, less when walking.

In the toe-balls of both feet a shooting, with great feeling of heat towards evening ; he must take off his shoes.

The (hitherto painless) corn has burning shooting pain when touched ever so gently ; but this pain ceased immediately on applying strong pressure.

Pain on the left toe-ball as if bruised.

585. Bruised pain of the arms and legs, even when lying, and worse when sitting than when walking ; when lying he must always change the position of the limbs on account of this pain ; but wherever he placed them it appeared to him better to lay them somewhere else.

Every part of the body when grasped pains as if bruised or gathering, especially in the scrobiculus cordis, and particularly in the morning.

All the body is painful, as if the flesh were loose, for sixteen days. [*Fr. H—n.*]

All the limbs are as if bruised and paralysed (in evening), as if he had lain on a hard couch (aft. 4 h.).

A painless drawing to and fro in the affected part.

590. Uneasy aching drawing pain in the periosteum of all the bones, as in the commencement of intermittent fever, in the forenoon (aft. 24 h.).

A pressing in the whole body, especially on the chest.

Severe drawing through all the limbs.

It is intolerable to him to keep the affected part still, he moves it up and down.

A visible twitching in the arms and legs when sitting, by day.

595. When the pain declines the part trembles and the face becomes cold.

Stitches in the affected part.

Pricks all over the body, as with pins.

On a slight mental emotion (on laughing) there suddenly occurs a shooting (itching) burning all over the body as if he had been whipped with nettles or had nettlerash, though nothing is to be seen on the skin ; this burning came on afterwards by merely thinking of it, or when he got heated.

Burning itching and persistent stitches on various parts, in the evening after lying down in bed (aft. 2 h.)

600. Stitches in the joints when moving and touching them.

Stitches that make her start in the affected part.*

* Comp. 520.

Shooting in the affected parts when pressing on them.*

(A painful beating in the arteries throughout the body.)

(Itch-like eruption only on the joints—on the inside of the wrists, on the bend of the elbow and on the outer side of the olecranon process, also on the outer side of the knee more than on the hough.)

605. Miliary rash on the arms, on the anterior part of the chest, and above the knees, which becomes red in the evening, itches and burns before she lies down in bed; in bed, however, when she becomes warm, the rash and itching disappear.

Papules comes on the abdomen and hips, which burn and itch, and when she scratches they feel sore.

Yellowness of the skin of the whole body, also of the face (aft. 12 d.). *Fr. H—n.*]

Red elevated miliary eruption all over the body, in a mother and her sucking infant; in the latter it appeared after two days, in the mother after three days. [*Fr. H—n.*]

Eruption on the abdomen and on the back up to the nape and on the forearms, which burns and smarts before midnight and in the morning. [*Fr. H—n.*]

610. Eruption all over the body, especially on the back to over the throat, itching so violently that he would like to scratch all to pieces.

In the evening griping and itching on the legs, about the knees and on the thigh; after scratching or rubbing there appear small, red, elevated papules, which cause a burning pain; when the papules are developed all the itching ceases.

Immediately before going to sleep, by day or in the evening, on various places of the soft parts of the body, a tearing itching, or, rather, digging, itching-burning stitches.

A tickling itching (by day) on the arms, hands, and feet, with miliary papules.

Red round spots, like lentils and larger, on the skin of the arms, without sensation, which do not disappear by pressing on them.

615. Red, small spots on the skin of the arms and legs, which cause pain as from stinging nettles; when pressed they disappear for an instant.

An excoriated, painless part commences to burn violently.

Tearing pain in the ulcer.

(The ichor of an ulcer stains the linen blackish.)

The ulcer feels chilly, and is painful, as if exposed to excessive cold.

620. In the morning, after rising, a smarting pain in the region of the scab (of the ulcer), which increases when he stands, is relieved when sitting, and disappears during moderate exercise.

In the region of the scab a throbbing, which is nearly shooting (after dinner).

He disliked the open air, though he was formerly fond of it. [*Fr. H—n.*]

In the room he felt too anxious, but better in the open air. [*Fr. H—n.*]

* Comp. 418, 448, 512, 535.

General weakness. [*Hbg.*]

625. Weakness in the lower extremities, which compelled him to sit down. [*Hrr.*]

Weak, lazy, tired and sleepy. [*Fr. H—n.*]

She is weak, the arms and legs are painful; when she works a little, the arms are like to sink down, and when she goes upstairs she can scarcely get on.

When walking, especially after rising from a seat and on commencing to walk, want of firmness in all parts of the body, as though all the muscles had lost their power; on walking further this is relieved (aft. 48 h.).

She feels weakest when walking in the open air.

630. When walking in the open air he feels qualmish and sick, the legs are so feeble and he is so weak in the head, that he feels as if he would fall; he pants and there comes a warmth into the chest which goes to the head; in the room this went off, but returned in the open air.

During a walk in the oppen air she was not tired, but as soon as she came into the room she was immediately so tired that she must sit or lie down.

On the slightest exertion the strength is immediately gone.

Heaviness and weariness in all the limbs; she can scarcely move her feet from heaviness, when walking.

Weariness of the feet, as if she had been running a great way.

635. On rising after a meal his feet feel enormously heavy.

Exhaustion.

Very feeble when sitting, less so when he walks.

He thinks he is better when he is lying.

In the morning he cannot get out of bed, and (without being exhausted) would like to remain long in bed.

640. Great exhaustion on awaking from sleep.

Soon after waking from his (mid-day) sleep he feels more poorly, all his morbid symptoms are in increased degree, and he is out of spirits.

One night he sleeps soundly till the morning, and remains sleepy all day, the next he sleeps uneasily, and the following day is wide awake.

On rising from bed he has an attack of faintness, with cold sweat and rattling in the abdomen.

Very much disposed to yawn (gapish), **frequent yawning all day.**

645. Frequent yawning. [*Hbg.*]

Constant yawning before dinner, with great thirst. [*Rkt.*]

Stretching and extending the limbs (in the afternoon). [*Rkt.*]

Drowsiness immediately after eating. [*Hbg.*]

Great drowsiness, also by day, for several successive days. [*Fr. H—n.*]

650. Constant inclination to sleep for three days. [*Fr. H—n.*]

So sleepy, he would like to sleep all day, for thirteen successive days. [*Fr. H—n.*]

Great drowsiness by day and great desire for the mid-day sleep; and when he woke from this all his limbs were as if asleep.

By day, when alone, great drowsiness.

(Tired, and yet he cannot sleep; when he wants to go to sleep he loses his breath.)

655. She tosses about with her hands and feet till 1 a.m., as from anxiety; she lies as if deprived of reason, with cold sweat on the forehead, and groans; thereupon exhaustion came on.

He cannot lie in bed in the morning, everything he lies on hurts him.

At night in bed restlessness; he is late of falling asleep, and does not sleep soundly.

She tosses about in bed at night till 1 a.m., she cannot fall asleep on account of anxious feeling of heat, and yet she has no heat perceptible externally.

Sleeplessness on account of agitation in the blood and anxiety (he must get up out of bed); the thoughts crowded on one another, without heat, sweat, or thirst.

660. Immediately after lying down in the evening in bed sensation of heat and external heat all over, without thirst, all night long; he turns from one side to the other, but cannot expose any part without immediately getting violent bellyache, a pinching shooting, or a shooting pinching, such as occurs from flatulent spasm here and there, with sleeplessness on account of a great flow of thoughts; in the morning this condition is allayed, but no flatulence is observed.

Sleeplessness at night on account of agitation in the blood; he tosses about in bed.

For several nights he cannot sleep for heat; the bed-clothes are too hot for him, and on throwing them off he becomes too cool, but without thirst and almost without sweat.

He could not go to sleep rightly, a warmth and agitation in the blood kept him awake till 12 o'clock.

He cannot get to sleep at night before 2 a.m., and must toss about in bed like a child that has become restless; in the morning after awaking he is still very sleepy.

665. She does not get to sleep until about 4 a.m., and then dreams of dead people.

The child cannot go to sleep in the evening, cannot get any rest; it gets out of bed.

Sleeplessness before midnight.

He cannot get to sleep before midnight on account of a frequent shuddering sensation that runs over one leg or arm, followed by some perspiration.

In the evening in bed, after a short sleep, she wakes up; she has a twisting about in the scrobiculus cordis, she becomes sick and like to be suffocated, she must sit up.

670. Moaning in sleep about 3 a.m.

In the evening before going to sleep she starts up in affright.

Starting on going to sleep in bed everyeve ning.

Starting up in sleep so as to wake.

He starts up from an anxious dream and howls aloud.

675. On awaking he cannot get rid of his dream ; he continues to dream though awake.

She awakes every hour during the night, and remembers what she has dreamt, and when she falls asleep again she dreams another equally vivid dream which she remembers equally well on awaking.

Very restless at night ; about 3 a.m. anxious dreams ; she cries out aloud in sleep.

Dreams causing anxiety.

He dreams when awake that he wishes to smash some one's windows.

680. Restless sleep with confused dreams ; he tosses from one side to the other. [*Hbg.*]

Restless sleep full of thoughts. [*Mch.*]

Somnambulic state, sleep-walking. [NICOLAI . . .]

Stool passes involuntarily at night in sleep. [*Fr. H—n.*]

Dreams full of quarrelling and vaxatious things.

685. **Dreams all night very vividly of anxious and careful attention to his business.**

In his dreams he is occupied with household affairs.

In her dream at night she gets up and goes to the door as if she would go out.

(He makes motions of his mouth in his sleep as though he were chewing.)

Wakened up out of sleep he talks nonsense.

690. Nocturnal delirious talking.

In the morning, at break of day, delirious chattering of business to be done, which ceases when the pain commences.

Before midnight (about 10 p.m.), along with great heat of the body and perspiration (without thirst), a delirious, frightful delusion, as if attacked by soldiers, so that he was on the point of running away (by throwing off the clothes and getting cool the delirium was allayed).

Towards evening, in sleep, the mouth was drawn to and fro, the eyes were opened and distorted, and she talked nonsense, as though she were awake, she spoke distinctly, but hurriedly, as if she imagined that strange persons were about her ; she looked freely about her, talked as to strange children, and wanted to go home.

Waking up early at night.

695. He sleeps only before midnight, and then no longer, remains wide awake, but feels great weariness when lying, which increases in the legs after getting up, but then soon goes off again.

Sleep does not refresh him ; on awaking in the morning he is still quite tired ; the weariness goes off in getting up and dressing.

She sleeps all day, with dry intense heat, without eating or drinking, with twitching in the face ; she passes her stools involuntarily six times under her ; they are brown and very fetid.

In the afternoon shivering, then heat, at the same time with chilliness ; the chilliness was in the chest and arms (and yet the arms and chest were warmer than usual), the heat was in the head, with pulsating throbbing pain in the temples, which was worse in the evening; shivering, heat and chilliness were unaccompanied by thirst.

After the midday siesta he is chilly and dazed in the head.

700. He must drink frequently at night (aft. 30 h.).

In the morning on awaking, headache.

On awaking, chilliness

(At night the hands and feet are as if dead (insensible), asleep, icy cold, and cannot be warmed.)

He feels cold all down his right side.

705. Chilliness in the arms.

Chilliness all over, all the first day.

Chilliness in the open air. [*Fr. H—n.*]

Violent rigor throughout the body, as in ague, which compels her to lie down, with shooting pain in the left side, above the hip, as if a suppurating ulcer there would contract, but without thirst or subsequent heat (aft. 48 h.). [*Stf.*]

Rigor all over the skin.

710. Rigor towards evening.

In the evening, after lying down, **chilliness in bed.**

Chilliness in the evening before lying down.

Much shivering.

Chilliness in, and dread of, the open air.

715. After a walk in the open air she gets chilly in the room; she did not feel chilly in the open air.

During a sudden general heat, feeling of chilliness (aft. ½ h.).

Great thirst (he must drink much cold fluid) with internal heat, without being hot to the touch externally. [*Hbg.*]

Great thirst. [*Hbg.*]

Thirst without external heat. [*Hbg.*]

720. **Sensation of heat in the face with redness of it and thirst** (aft. 3 h.). [*Hrr.*]

Flying heat. [*Hbg.*]

Heat in the interior of the body (especially in the abdomen). [*Hbg.*]

In the evening heat in the external ear, followed by shivering and rigor in the thighs (aft. 4 h.).

Fever: lying down, chilliness, yawning, nausea; then perspiration without thirst, from 10 p.m. till 10 a.m.

725. Fever: in the forenoon heat (with thirst); after some hours (in the afternoon) chilliness without thirst with redness of face and slight headache.

At every movement and every noise she is attacked with sudden dry heat.

Heat only in the lower extremities, in frequent fits; she feels as if she got into hot water.

In the evening, hot red cheeks and rigor all over, with goose-skin and thirst.

First thirst (aft. 1 h.), then adipsia, with cold hands and feet (aft. 4 h.).

730. In the evening her throat is full of mucus and she gets thirsty.

Violent thirst.

Great thirst.

Strong thirst; she can and must drink much at a time, and the drink does not oppress her.

In the morning, on rising, great thirst.

735. The thirst is increased by drinking beer.

Only internal heat with insatiable thirst.

An extraordinary warmth in the region of the scrobiculus cordis makes her extremely thirsty (but not the dryness in the throat).

Heat without thirst.

Heat on the body without thirst.

740. In the morning several times dry heat all over.

At night a dry heat.

In the morning he has heat in the head; the head feels warm.

In the forenoon heat in the head; it appeared to come out at the forehead.

Towards evening heat of the face.

745. A red, round, hot spot on the cheek, over the zygoma.

Internally great warmth; the blood seems to burn in the blood-vessels.

Red urine.

He easily broke out into perspiration on the least exertion, also at night.

He perspires all over when walking in the cool air.

750. Warm perspiration in the palms.

Towards morning perspiration, especially in the feet.

Morning sweat.

An anxious perspiration preventing sleep. [*Fr. H—n.*]

He perspires while eating. [*Fr. H—n.*]

755. He perspires on the slightest exertion. [*Fr. H—n.*]

Profuse perspiration of the whole body, also of the head, when lying in bed.

Perspiration which looked like oil when wiped off, by day and night. [*Fr. H—n.*]

Very profuse warm perspiration over the whole body; even the hair was dripping wet. [*Fr. H—n.*]

Profuse nocturnal sweat from 3 p.m., for twenty successive nights. [*Fr. H—n.*]

760. Profuse perspiration for six successive nights. [*Fr. H—n.*]

Some perspiration towards morning after waking.

Sour smelling, profuse sweat during a sound sleep at night.

In the night (about 3 a.m.) he has thirst before the sweat, then for four hours perspiration of a sweetish-sour smell, before this ceased headache came on compounded of aching and drawing, which after getting up changed into emptiness of the head.

He woke suddenly at night (about 3 a.m.) and fell into a slight transpiration, which lasted till morning, during which he lay most easily on the back, and only slumbered a little, with dryness of the mouth in front and of the lips. without thirst (aft. 8 h.).

765. In bed slight transpiration from evening till morning, during which he only sleeps from 12 till 3 o'clock.

Raving about business for an hour (aft. ½ h.).

He attempted several times to escape from bed. [*Fr. H—n.*]

Hesitation ; apprehensiveness (aft. 18 h.).

Anguish in the whole body, that always drove him about, and wherever he came he had no rest.

770. **Anxiety ; he is apprehensive about future.** [*Hrr.*]

Very irritable disposition, disposed to starting, fear, and crossness.

Very cross and inclined to anger.

First dejection of spirits, lastly (aft. 5 d.) cheerfulness. [*Mch.*]

Dejection of spirits. [*Hbg.*]

775. Much weeping for a day and a half. [*Fr. H—n.*]

Disposition at once angry, cross and lachrymose.

Cross ; imagined she could not finish the work ; she always took hold of the wrong thing and constantly wished to take something else ; then a pressing aching headache in the forehead.

Ill-humoured and disposed to scold. [*Hbg.*]

Morose ; looking at everything with ill-will. [*Hbg.*]

780. Too busy ; she wishes to undertake and to work at too many things (aft. 20 h.).

(Extreme ill-humour ; indisposed to think ; fatigue of the mental powers.)

CALCAREA ACETICA.[1]

(*Acetate of Lime.*)

Experience, and experience alone, but not baseless conjecture, can and dare pronounce respecting the power of drugs to effect alterations in the health of human beings.

From the earliest times it has been firmly accepted as a maxim in ordinary medicine, that calcareous substances introduced and taken into the human body are useless and powerless. It was, no doubt, conceded that they absorbed and neutralised morbid acids present in the stomach, but even in such cases the calcareous neutral salt thence resulting was held to be unmedicinal.

In the ordinary condition of the stomach there is no free acid in the gastric juice, and likewise none in many of its morbid states, and hence pure calcareous earth, considering its nature, may perhaps not be a medicine capable of altering the health of human beings; but the inference from this as to its non-medicinal character in a state of solution, without an appeal to experience on the subject, is like all inferences *a priori* in medicine, which are not based on facts, to say the least, extremely premature and dogmatic, like most of those in ordinary medicine.

Some cases of great disturbance of the health following the ingestion of pure carbonate of lime in persons who were manifestly suffering from morbid acidity in the stomach induced me to institute experiments with it in a dissolved state, and I found it possessed of great medicinal power, as the following symptoms show.

In order to obtain pure calcareous earth dissolved in pure acetic acid, I boiled crude, well-washed oyster shells for an hour in pure spring water, then broke them into fragments without using any metal instrument, and dissolved these fragments in distilled vinegar, which I heated up to the boiling point in a porcelain vessel until complete saturation was gradually effected. The filtered solution was evaporated to one fifth in a similar vessel, and with this fluid neutral salt, without the addition of alcohol, the following experiments were made.

It has a dark-yellow colour, and after a time precipitates a dark coloured glutinous substance, whereby the solution obtains a lighter yellow colour. The addition of some alcohol, about half as much by measure as the quantity of the solution, preserves the preparation from becoming mouldy, and makes it fit for medicinal use.

A drop of this is not seldom a too large homœopathic dose. Ten to twelve globules the size of poppy seeds moistened with it are usually sufficient for a full dose.

---

1 From vol. v, 2nd edit., 1826.

Frequent very small doses of camphor allay the action of this medicine when it acts too violently in irritable subjects.

[HAHNEMANN was assisted in this proving by FRANZ, HARTMANN, LANGHAMMER, and WISLICENUS.

No symptoms are taken from old-school authorities.

The 1st Edit. has 255 symptoms, all "observations of others." This 2nd Edit. has 270, 236 only being observations of others, while 34 are HAHNEMANN'S own. In the *Chr. Krank.* the symptoms of *calc. acet.*, reduced to 253, are incorporated with those of *calc. carb.*, but distinguished by a sign.]

CALCAREA ACETICA.

Vertigo, as if the body did not stand firm (aft. 6 h.). [*Ws*]

Attack of stupefying vertigo, the head tended forwards to the left side when at rest and when moving (aft. $\frac{3}{4}$ h.). [*Lr.*]

Slight transient giddiness in the head (aft. $\frac{1}{4}$ h.). [*Htn.*]

When walking in the open air vertigo, he inclined to fall to the right side (aft. 2 h.). [*Lr.*]

5. Headache as from much rapid turning round—as if stupid in the head, from 3 a.m. till 4 p.m. (aft. 25 d.).

Every time he stooped sensation on the right side of the head, as if pains in the head commenced (aft. $6\frac{1}{2}$ h.). [*Htn.*]

Aching stupefying pain in the forehead, as in vertigo, when at rest and when moving (aft. $1\frac{1}{4}$ h.). [*Lr.*]

In the left side of the occiput jerking pressing outwards, which extended to the nape (aft. 14 h.). [*Htn.*]

Aching pain in the forehead, especially over the left eye-brow, when walking in the open air (aft. 3 h.). [*Lr.*]

10. Violent pressing outwards in the whole of the left half of the brain (aft. 12 h.). [*Htn.*]

Aching pain darting rapidly through the occiput, which only goes off gradually (aft. $3\frac{1}{2}$ h.). [*Htn.*]

Pressive pain in the right temple, close to the eye, as if something hard pressed upon it (aft. $5\frac{1}{2}$ h.). [*Htn.*]

After stooping for some time, when standing, heavy headache, with pressure outwards in the whole forehead, but especially over the left eye (aft. $5\frac{1}{2}$ h.). [*Htn.*]

Aching pressing pain in the whole head, especially in both temples (aft. 9 h.). [*Htn.*]

15. Drawing aching headache in the left side of the occiput, with stiff sensation in the nape. [*Fz.*]

Drawing aching headache in the left palpebral region. [*Fz.*]

In the right side of the occiput an outward pressing pain (aft. $\frac{1}{2}$ h.). [*Htn.*]

When reading obfuscation of the whole head, with aching stupefying pain in the forehead like a vertigo, which deprived him of his mental powers ; he must stop reading, and knew not where he was (when sitting) (aft. $4\frac{1}{2}$ h.). [*Lr.*]

Aching pain in the right frontal protuberance, which extended to the right eye, and caused it to close involuntarily (aft. $1\frac{1}{2}$ h.). [*Htn.*]

20. In the morning after rising from bed, aching stupefying pains in the whole head, as if he had not yet slept enough, or had been revelling all night (aft. 14 h.). [*Lr.*]

Violent out-pressing, aching pain in the left temporal region (aft. $13\frac{1}{2}$ h.). [*Htn.*]

Whilst reading, when sitting, aching stupefying pain in the forehend, such as one gets in a violent wind (aft. 29 h.). [*Lr.*]

Sensation in the occiput as if it were pressed asunder from time to time (aft. $9\frac{1}{2}$ h.). [*Htn.*]

Aching stupefying headache, which involves especially the whole forehead, when at rest and when moving. [*Lr.*]

25. Drawing headache in the right side of the forehead, over the eye and in the occiput, on straining the thinking power (aft. 2 h.). [*Fz.*]

Obtuse pressive darts into both temples (aft. 24 h.). [*Ws.*]

When walking obtuse pressive darts, especially in the left side of the forehead, going off during the walk (aft. 27 h.). [*Lr.*]

The head is very heavy, in both temples he has strong jerks, and the whole head is painful when he stoops, but this goes off on rising up again (aft. $9\frac{1}{2}$ h.). [*Htn.*]

On the top of the head in the region of the crown strong throbbing, like that of an artery, with cutting blows outwards (aft. 10 h.). [*Ws.*]

30. Aching drawing, sometimes tearing headache, sometimes in the forehead, sometimes in the occiput, sometimes in the temples, which goes off by applying pressure, and disappears on straining the thoughts (aft. 3 d.). [*Fz.*]

When standing, regularly recurring out-boring knife thrusts in the left temporal region, which were only alleviated by touching, but which immediately disappeared on sitting down (aft. $\frac{3}{4}$ h.). [*Lr.*]

Violent stitches by jerks through the whole left half of the brain, which are often renewed, and then leave there an asunder-pressing sensation (aft. 3 h.). [*Htn.*]

Intermittent boring knife thrusts in the left temple, going off on touching (while sitting) (aft. 8 h.). [*Lr.*]

Pulsating stitches in the left side of the crown (aft. some m.). [*Ws.*]

35. When sitting boring stitch-like pain in the left side of the forehead, which goes off immediately on touching, walking, and standing (aft. $12\frac{1}{2}$ h.). [*Lr.*]

Intermittent needle pricks in the left side of the forehead in all positions (aft. 7, 27 h.). [*Lr.*]

In the open air he is quite well, but as soon as he enters a room the headache recurs with increased severity, and he is very cross and unwilling to speak. [*Fz.*]

Aching stupefying pain on the right side of the forehead above the eyebrow, which is particularly aggravated by stooping (aft. 50 h.). [*Lr.*]

Fine stitches on the crown, externally (aft. 7 h.). [*Ws.*]

40. Itching formication on the hairy scalp, not removed by rubbing (aft. 10 h.). [*Ws.*]

Tickling itching on the hairy scalp, which compels scratching, during which the roots of the hairs are painful when touched, for half a day (aft. $4\frac{1}{4}$ h.). [*Lr.*]

Boring stitches in the middle of the forehead, just as if it penetrated into the brain (aft. 3 h.). [*Ws.*]

On touching the occiput sore pain on the left side, as if the part were gathering (aft. 32 h.). [*Lr.*]

The whole of the scalp is painfully sensitive, especially on moving the frontal muscles to and fro (aft. $1\frac{1}{2}$ h.). [*Ws.*]

45. Drawing and aching in the temporal bone. [*Fz.*]

Aching drawing headache in the right temporal muscles, and pressure on the upper row of teeth ; both go off as long as he presses on the temple, and instead thereof there occurs aching pain in the forehead (aft. 2 d.). [*Fz.*]

In the evening drawing aching pain in the temporal muscle. [*Fz.*]

Cramp-like pain in the right temple (aft. 6 h.). [*Ws.*]

Cramp-like pain in the left temporal region (aft. 8, 14 h.). [*Lr.*]

50. After a meal drawing aching pain about the temples (aft. 2 d.). [*Fz.*]

Pressive sensation in the left temporal bone as if it were pressed in, at once internally and externally (aft. $7\frac{1}{2}$ h.). [*Htn.*]

On moving the lower jaw digging stitches in the left temple, near the superciliary arch (aft. 5 h.). [*Lr.*]

Suppurating pimple above the left eyebrow (aft. 5 h.). [*Lr.*]

Boring stitch on the upper border of the orbit, from within outwards (aft. 5 h.). [*Ws.*]

55. Dilated pupils (aft. $1\frac{1}{4}$ h.). [*Lr.*]

Contracted pupils (aft. 25, 26 h.). [*Lr.*]

Shooting in the internal and external canthi [*Fz.*]

Violent tearing stitches in the right eye as if it were inflamed (aft. 4 h.). [*Fz.*]

Itching stitches in the internal canthi, which go off by rubbing (aft. $\frac{1}{8}$ h.). [*Ws.*]

60. **Burning sensation in the left upper eyelid, towards the inner canthus** (aft. $6\frac{1}{2}$ h.). [*Ws.*]

Mucus in the canthi, for two days (aft. 10 h.). [*Lr.*]

On moving the eyelids he notices stickness of them, with aching in the outer canthi (aft. 55 h.). [*Lr.*]

On awaking from sleep the eyes were closed up with mucus (aft. 24 h.). [*Lr.*]

Tickling itching on the right outer canthus, which compels rubbing (aft. 25 h.). [*Lr.*]

65. Fine formication under the eye and on the side of the nose under the skih. [*Ws.*]

Fine twitching on the upper border of the orbit down to the nose (aft. $\frac{3}{4}$ h.). [*Ws.*]

Long-sightedness*; he could see all objects distinctly at a concider-able distance all day long (aft. 28½ h.). [*Lr.*]

Slight whirring in both ears, with confusion of the whole head (aft. ½ h.). [*Ws.*]

Cramp-feeling on the back of the left concha (aft. 9 h.). [*Htn.*]

70. Twitching in the cartilage of the ear (aft. 48 h.). [*Ws.*]

A boil under the lobe of the ear, on account of which, when chewing, there is tensive pain in the maxillary joint.

Sensation in the right ear as if something were pushed before the membrana tympani, without diminution of the hearing (aft. 15 h.). [*Lr.*]

Stitches in the ears.

Throbbing on both malar bones like the pulsation of an artery (aft. 6 h.). [*Ws.*]

75. Tensive sensation in the right cheek as if it were swollen (aft. 2 d.). [*Fz*]

In the middle of the cheek a painless pimple that exuded moisture after scratching it, and left behind it a greenish scab (aft. 48 h.). [*Lr.*]

Dull pain in the fleshy parts of the left ceek (aft. 2¼ h.) [*Lr.*]

Gnawing pain at the root of the nose (aft. 1 h.). [*Ws.*]

Illusion of smell; in the nose he perceived a smell as of rotten eggs or gunpowder (aft. 1 h.). [*Lgh.*]

80. Aching pain in the right upper jaw when chewing (aft. 3 h.). [*Htn.*]

Violent tearing in the right upper jaw (aft. 9 h.). [*Htn.*]

Itching formication on the upper lip, under the septum nasi, which goes off on rubbing, but immediately reappears in another place close by (aft. 1 h.). [*Ws.*]

Roughness and dryness of the lips, especially of the upper lip, as if it would chap (aft. 49 h.). [*Lr.*]

Under the right commissure of the mouth a large exuding scab, for many days (aft. 14 d.).

85. **Tickling itching on the border of the left lower jaw which forces him to scratch** (aft. 10 h.). [*Lr.*]

Swelling of the submaxillary gland, with aching feeling in it. [*Fz.*]

Gnawing toothache in the right upper molars, as if they would become hollow, in all positions (aft. 6 h.). [*Lr.*]

Boring sensation in the upper gums, on the right side, followed by swelling of them, with aching drawing in the right temporal muscle (aft. 3 d.) [Fz.]

Stitches in the teeth.

90. Toothache: fine shooting in the gums of the whole upper jaw (aft. 2¼ h.). [*Lr.*]

Sensation of roughness and soreness of the tongue, which is covered with white fur (aft. 1 h.). [*Lr.*]

Heat in the mouth, burning on the tongue, and painful vesicles on it.

* In a very short-sighted person; curative reaction of the organism.

The back of the palate is rough and scrapy; this excites coughing, but is not removed by coughing (aft. 12 h.). [*Ws.*]

Sore-throat: violent stitch on the right and upper part of the œsophagus when not swallowing (aft $\frac{3}{4}$ h.). [*Htn.*]

95. In the morning much hawking up of mucus.

Swelling of the left cervical gland under the angle of the jaw, as large as a pigeon's egg, with shooting pain on the left side of the throat when swallowing.

Dryness in the mouth, with feeling of an excessive quantity of mucus at the back of the pharynx, observable when swallowing (aft. $1\frac{3}{4}$ h.). [*Lr.*]

Dryness in the mouth as from chalk (aft. 1 h.). [*Fz.*]

Collection of saliva in the mouth; he could not swallow down the saliva fast enough (aft. $1\frac{1}{2}$ h.). [*Lr.*]

100. Qualmishness and accumulation of saliva in the mouth (aft. 3 h.). [*Lr.*]

Milk tastes sour and is repugnant to him (aft. $\frac{1}{2}$ h.). [*Htn.*]

Milk tastes well to him (aft. 3 h.). [*Htn.*]

Food has too little taste; meat especially is not relished. [*Fz.*]

After a meal the headache is always increased, and even while eating it comes on with great sensitiveness of the teeth when chewing, as if they were loose and bent over. [*Fz.*]

105. **Great thirst and desire for cold drinks, particularly for fresh water; he must drink much cold water**, for eight hours (aft 8, 10, 55 h.). [*Lr.*]

Frequent empty eructation (aft. $\frac{1}{2}$, 1 h.). [*Lr.*]

Sourish eructation (aft. $\frac{1}{2}$ h.). [*Lr.*]

Constant sourish eructation. [*Htn.*]

Disgusting sourish eructation (aft. 1 h.). [*Lr.*]

110. **Frequent hiccup** (aft. $\frac{1}{4}$, $3\frac{1}{2}$, 10, 28, 34 h.). [*Lr.*]

Severe hiccup for a quarter of an hour (aft. 5 h.). [*Ws.*]

Nausea and inclination to vomit; he thought he must vomit (aft. $1\frac{1}{4}$ h.). [*Lr.*]

He felt as if he must vomit; he has eructations, and the water flows into the mouth, with a kind of vertigo in the head (immediately). [*Htn.*]

When sitting great anxiety, which appeared to come from the stomach, with hot burning in the abdomen, which all goes off immediately when standing or walking (aft. 26 h.). [*Lr.*]

115. Long stitches in the right side under the ribs (aft. $13\frac{1}{2}$ h.). [*Htn.*]

Tensive oppressive pain in the whole subcostal region, and in the scrobiculus cordis (aft. 19 h.). [*Htn.*]

Pinching nipping sensation in the whole subcostal region, which extends to the sternum, there becomes fine shooting, and excites eructation (aft. $\frac{3}{4}$ h.). [*Htn.*]

Dull pinching choking sensation just under the scrobiculus cordis (aft. $\frac{1}{4}$ h.). [*Htn.*]

Anxiety in the scrobiculus cordis (aft. 6 h.). [*Ws.*]

120. Violent pinching pains in the epigastrium and chest, which end here and there in a small stitch (aft. ½ h.). [*Htn.*]

A stitch that gives a shock from the hepatic region into the chest (aft. 10 h.). [*Fz.*]

Pinching sensation on a small spot, somewhat below the navel, which on rubbing with the finger changes into a clucking (aft. 2½ h.). [*Htn.*]

Tearing in the abdominal muscles, increased by inspiration (aft. 2 h.). [*Ws.*]

In the abdominal muscles under the ribs a number of needle-pricks from within outwards, especially on inspiring (aft. 5 h.). [*Ws.*]

125. Frequent formicating, upward-pushing and loud rumbling in the right side of the abdomen, as from accumulated flatulence, which also came away (aft. ¼ h. [*Lr.*]

Audible bubbling in the right side of the abdomen, as if diarrhœa would come on (aft. 3½, 5 h.). [*Lr.*]

Loud rumbling and grumbling in the abdomen as from emptiness (aft. 1½, 28 h.) [*Lr.*]

In the right lumbar region a cutting, out-pressing pain, which goes off for a short time when touched, but returns immediately. [*Fz.*]

Sore pain on both sides of the groin, as if a glandular swelling would occur there, especially perceptible when walking; a small elevation of the gland can be felt there (aft. 10 h.). [*Lr.*]

130. Tearing pain in the inguinal glands when sitting and walking (aft. 9 h). [*Fz*]

Pinching, almost spasmodic, pain in the abdominal integuments of the right groin on a small spot, only painful when speaking and pressing with the finger on it (aft. 8 h.). [*Htn.*]

Aching tensive sensation in the left inguinal region (aft. 8 h.). [*Htn.*]

Swelling of the glands in the left groin (aft. 22 d.).

Tension in the inguinal glands, also when sitting (aft. 40 d.).

135. Pinching bellyache low down in the hypogastrium in the region of the bladder, frequently recurring, whereupon some flatus always passes (aft. ¼ h.). [*Htn*]

Frequent noiseless discharge of flatus (aft. 1 h.). [*Lr.*]

During the evacuation of the stool, a tenesmus at the end of the rectum, and loud grumbling and rumbling in the abdomen. [*Ws.*]

Diarrhœa three or four times a day, for many days, not weakening.

Frequent evacuation of hard, pappy, and thin motions during the day, without suffering; but the following two days, constipation.* [*Lr*]

140. The second day he has no stool. [*Fz.*]

* 139 to 143. As acetate of lime excites and frequently causes with such certainty stools and urine in the primary action, and that without pain in the bowels (the sensation in the rectum, S. 137, excepted), the homœopathic physician will know how to employ it usefully.

Stool first thin, then crumbly, without pain in the bowels (aft. 5½ h.). [*Htn.*]

Frequent urging to urinate with copious discharge of urine (aft. 1, 4 h.). [*Lr.*]

Frequent urging to urinate with scanty and very scanty discharge of urine (aft. 26 n.). [*Lr.*]

(The urine after standing looks cloudy, like muddy water.) [*Ws.*]

145. An acute tug in the orifice of the urethra.*

Tickling itching at the end of the glans penis, compelling rubbing (aft. 10 h.). [*Lr.*]

Itching tickling on the prepuce, compelling rubbing (aft. 9 h.). [*Lr.*]

Along with the tensive pain in the left groin, the left testicle is drawn spasmodically, and with pain, like aching, up to the abdomen, and is also painful when touched.

The first night two seminal emissions with voluptuous but unremembered dreams. [*Htn.*]

150. Two seminal emissions in one night without voluptuous dreams. [*Lr.*]

Seminal emission the first night. [*Fz.*]

(At first it increases the leucorrhœa.)

Discharge of blood from the womb, for some days, like menses, not weakening, in an old woman who had not menstruated for years (aft. 7 d.).

* * *

Frequent sneezing, without coryza. [*Lr.*]

155. Coryza with painful sensitiveness of the nose and internal heat in the head (aft. 72 h.). [*Ws.*]

Fluent coryza with much sneezing (aft. 27 h.). [*Lr.*]

Fluent coryza with headache† (aft. 5 d.).

Stuffed coryza with frequent sneezing (aft. 52 h.). [*Lr.*]

Severe stuffed coryza with pains in the head (aft. 32 d.).

160. **Tickling irritation in the trachea causing short cough** (aft. 2½ h.). [*Lr.*]

On expiration loud rattling in the wind-pipe, as in children whose chest is full of mucus, for a quarter of an hour (aft. 37 h.). [*Lr.*]

Obtuse blows from the posterior wall of the thoracic cavity up to between the shoulders, synchronous with the heart's beats, with great anguish (aft. 8 h.). [*Ws.*]

Difficult inspiration and great anxious tightness of chest, like tension on the lower part of the chest, so that it took away his breath, to suffocation, for an hour ; when moving and when sitting (aft. 30 h.). [*Lr.*]

Anguish in the chest, as if it were too tight ; his breath is short, particularly when sitting, and he feels an aching pain in the whole chest, especially on inspi-

* From a dose of powdered oyster shells in acidity of the stomach.

† Both removed immediately by smelling at a solution of camphor.

ration ; the heart beats anxiously and tremblingly. [*Ws.*]

165. Itching stitches on the chest, worst when expiring, going off by rubbing (aft. 46 h.). [*Ws.*]

At every beat of the heart a broad stitch upwards in the pectoral muscles (aft. 10 h.). [*Ws.*]

Shooting drawing pain in the region of the heart (aft. 9½ h.). [*Ws.*]

The whole chest is painfully sensitive on touching and on inspiration. [*Ws.*]

Gnawing pain on the left side of the chest, as if externally on the ribs and sternum, only slightly aggravated by inspiring (aft. 1 h.). [*Ws.*]

170. In the last false ribs a cutting pain from within ontwards, increased by inspiring (aft 3 h) [*Ws*]

Sharp stitches in the left side under the axilla out of the chest, worst when inspiring (aft. 2 h.) [*Ws*]

Sharp stitches in the right side of the chest from within outwards, independent of inspiration (aft. 7 h.). [*Ws.*]

Severe stitches out of the thoracic cavity through the spinal column, out between the shoulder-blades (aft. ½ h.) [*Ws.*]

Twitching shooting on the sacrum and at the same time on the leg above the ankle-joint (aft. 2 h.). [*Ws.*]

175. On walking in the open air, frequent needle-pricks in the middle of the spine, almost making him cry out, somewhat diminished by standing (aft. 30 h.). [*Lr.*]

Sharp stitches inside the scapula (aft ½ h.). [*Ws.*]

Severe stitches in both axillæ (aft. 7 h.). [*Ws.*]

Twitching in the shoulder and arm.

In the right shoulder-joint, a pressive pain, only when at rest, not on moving or raising the arm.

180. Fine twitching in the left upper arm (aft. ¼ h.). [*Ws.*]

Cramp-like pains, quite superiorly in the muscles of the upper arm (when walking in the open air) (aft. 29 h.). [*Lr.*]

Tearing stitch in the muscles of the upper arm (when sitting) (aft. 36 h.). [*Lr.*]

Tearing twitching in the upper arm (aft. 7 h.). [*Ws.*]

Cramp-like tearing in the muscles of the right upper arm (when sitting) (aft. 2 h.). [*Lr.*]

185. Fine needle-pricks in the muscles of the left forearm near the wrist-joint (aft. 3 h.). [*Lr.*]

Twice, cramp-like tearing in the muscles of the left forearm (aft. 40 h.). [*Lr.*]

Cramp-like pain on the outside of the left and right forearms, near the wrist joint (aft. 1¼, 13, 29 h.). [*Lr.*]

Cramp-pain on the forearm in front of the elbow-joint (aft. 1 h.). [*Ws*]

Boring needle-pricks in the muscles of the left forearm, near the wrist-joint (aft. 1 h.). [*Lr.*]

190. Tearing stitches in the muscles of the left forearm (aft. 37 h.). [*Lr.*]

Tearing stitch-like pain in the muscles of the right forearm (aft. $1\frac{1}{2}$ h.). [*Lr.*]

Tearing pressure in the muscles of the left forearm, when at rest and when moving (aft. 3 h.). [*Lr.*]

When walking painful pressure in the muscles of the left forearm, which goes off immediately on touchiug, standing, and sitting (aft. $\frac{1}{4}$ h.). [*Lr.*]

Dislocation pain on the outer border of the left forearm, near the wrist-joint, worse when at rest than when moving (aft. 4 h.). [*Lr.*]

195. Sharp stitches in the external protuberance of the wrist (aft. 1 h.). [*Ws.*]

Shooting crawling on the wrist-joint (aft. 10 h.). [*Ws.*]

Tickling like needle-pricks in the right palm, exciting scratching (aft. 12 h.). [*Lr.*]

Tickling itching in the right palm, compelling scratching (aft. 30 h.). [*Lr.*]

Itching tickling on the outer border of the left palm, near the little finger, compelling scratching (aft. $5\frac{1}{2}$ h.). [*Lr.*]

200. Cramp-like pain near the proximal joint of the right forefinger (aft. $2\frac{3}{4}$ h.). [*Lr.*]

Cramp-like pain betwixt the proximal joints of the third and fourth fingers of the right hand (aft. 7 h.) [*Htn.*]

Tickling itching on the outer border of the proximal phalanx of the forefinger, exciting scratching (aft. 4 h). [*Lr.*]

Tearing in the knuckles of the fingers (aft. 28 d.).

Pinching on the upper and anterior border of the os ilii. [*Ws.*]

205. Cutting pain in the acetabulum of the hip-joint (when sitting) (aft. 3 h.) [*Ws.*]

Pinching twitching on the posterior aspect of the hip-joint, more severe when at rest than when moving (aft. $\frac{1}{2}$ h.). [*Ws.*]

When walking drawing dislocation pain in the hip-joint (aft. 4 h.). [*Fz.*]

Tearing in the hip-joint and about the anterior crest of the ilium, extending into the groin, when moving. [*Fz.*]

When standing and walking a cramp-like needle-prick in the muscles of the right thigh, which went off on sitting down (aft. $\frac{3}{4}$ h.). [*Lr.*]

210. Tearing pain on the inner side of the thigh, when moving, [*Fz.*]

Shooting aching on the inner side of the left thigh (when sitting) (aft. 3 h.). [*Htn.*]

Sharp stitch above the left knee on its outer side (aft. 5 h.). [*Ws.*]

Tearing stitches above the knee on the inner side of the thigh when sitting (aft. 12 h.). [*Fz.*]

Sharp stitches in the right knee-joint (aft. 4 h.). [*Ws.*]

215. Swelling of the knees.

Under both patellæ an inflamed swelling.

When walking in the open air bruised pain close under the patella (aft. 13 h.). [*Lr.*]

When sitting dislocation pain on the left patella, which went off on touching, walking, and standing (aft. 12 h.). [*Lr.*]

Drawing, cramp-like pain on the patella (aft. 2 d.). [*Fz.*]

220. When lying the lower extremities, especially the legs, are painful, as if bruised. [*Fz.*]

Cramp-like pain close to the shaft of the tibia (when sitting) (aft. 36 h.). [*Lr.*]

Tearing twitching on the front of the leg, under the knee (when at rest). [*Ws.*]

Intermittent pressive pain on the calf. [*Fz.*]

Aching pain on the left tibia, near the ankle-joint, when walking in the open air (aft. 52 h.). [*Lr.*]

225. Bruised pain on the legs as if fatigued ; he must often change his position. [*Ws.*]

Swelling of the feet (for 11 d.).

(Burning of the feet in the evening.)

✓ **When sitting and standing intermittent cramp-like needle-pricks in the toes of the right foot, which go off when walking** (aft. $\frac{1}{2}$ h.). [*Lr*]

Violent stitch in the right little toe, which seems to be outside the toe (aft. 14 h.). [*Htn.*]

230. Painful cramp in the soles of the feet and the toes, only at night (aft. 11 d.).

Painful cramp in the soles on bending forwards the foot, as when drawing on boots.

Cramp in the soles of the feet after walking a little time, which is relieved by walking longer, but goes off when sitting.

In the soles of the feet severe tearing.

Cramp-like pain in the middle of the left sole, more towards its outer border (aft. $5\frac{1}{4}$ h.). [*Htn.*]

235. Sharp stitches in the proximal joint of the big toe when at rest (aft. 24 h.). [*Ws.*]

After working in water and washing, aggravation of the symptoms.

Itching all over the body, also by day (aft. 5, 23 d.).

Brings on itching in a spot where there was a tetter a year previously (aft. 5 d.).

Frequent yawning, as if he had not slept enough (aft. 56 h.), [*Lr.*]

240. Towards evening great drowsiness and crossness. [*Fz.*]

In the morning great drowsiness and crossness, with aching pain all over the forehead (aft. 2 d.). [*Fz.*]

Frequent waking up from sleep, with tossing about ; he imagines he is lying upside down in bed (aft. 23 h.). [*Lr.*]

Frequent waking from sleep as from being disturbed (aft. 20 h.). [*Lr.*]

At night he is very restless, frequently wakes up, speaks aloud in his sleep, but in the morning knows nothing about it. [*Htn.*]

245. Restless sleep ; almost all night long he cannot go to sleep, and while tossing about he gradually perspired all over the body (aft. 10 h.). [*Lr.*]

Frequent waking from sleep, as if he had already slept enough (aft. 67 h.). [*Lr.*]

Long profound sleep in the morning, with many vivid dreams about innocent events of long ago. [*Ws.*]

Vivid dreams full of strife and quarrelling. [*Lr.*]

Dreams of a horrible frightful character. [*Lr.*]

250. Vivid, confused, unremembered dreams. [*Lr.*]

Febrile rigor all over the body, with frequent yawning, without thirst, and not followed by heat (aft. $2\frac{1}{2}$ h.). [*Lr.*]

Febrile regor all over the body as if he had caught cold (aft. $\frac{3}{4}$ h.). [*Lr.*]

Febrile rigor oll over the back (aft. 25 h.). [*Lr.*]

Febrile rigor all over the body, with cold hands and warm face (aft. 48 h.). [*Lr.*]

255. **Febrile rigor all over the body, with warm forehead, hot cheeks, and icy cold hands, without thirst** (aft. 2 h.). [*Lr.*]

Evening fever : externally he was chilly with internal heat and great thirst ; even in bed he was chilly and at the same time he perspired, but he could not get warm ; at last profuse sweat till morning (aft. 10 h.).

At night much heat and short breath.

In the evening on lying down, external heat, with internal chilliness (aft. 72 h.). [*Ws*]

Glowing heat and redness of the whole face, with hot forehead and cold hands, with great thirst, for several hours (aft. 12 h.). [*Lr.*]

260. **Morning sweat every day** (aft. 7 d.).

Not without inclination to work, but indifferent to all external things ; sunk in thought about the present and future. [*Lr.*]

Very grave and full of care ; busied with the present and the future ; he becomes sad almost to tears. [*Lr.*]

Anxious disposition as it something evil had happened or he had to fear reproaches ; at the same time, however, persistent inclination to work. [*Lr.*]

Very sad humour, as if he had to expect bad news (aft. 14 h.). [*Lr.*]

265. Morose, cross, very peevish, also very indifferent to the most important things ; he did everything unwillingly and as if forced to do them. [*Lr.*]

Whenever he sits idle and quiet, he becomes sleepy and cross, and everything is distasteful to him. [*Fz.*]

All day long peevish and cross, but at last crotchetty and talkative (aft. 39 h.). [*Lr.*]

He is not disposed to speak, but not ill-humoured (aft. 6½ h.). [*Htn.*]

He is more cheerful and would like to be in company and speak with people (aft. 10 h.). [*Htn.*]

270. The first part of the day anxious, then cheerful, and at last contented with himself (aft. 62 h.). [*Lr.*]

CAMPHORA.[1]

[The alcoholic solution of the almost crystalline substance resembling a solidified æthereal oil, derived from the camphor-tree, *Laurus camphora*, L.]

I give here the symptoms hitherto observed from camphor, not as a complete list of all the effects to be expected from it, but only as a commencement thereof, so that at some future period the remainder of its effects may be added to this list.

From the earliest times this medicine has been blindly used and improperly employed in large and massive doses, so that its true action has never been ascertained, nor could it be ascertained, as it has almost always been given only along with several other drugs, either mixed up with, or administered at the same time with it, and moreover, and this is the worst, it has only been employed amid the tumult of the symptoms or diseases. For the pure effects of it, observed by ALEXANDER,* are very meagre and confined to mere general expressions.

The action of this substance is very puzzling and difficult to determine, even in healthy organisms, because, its primary action more often rapidly alternates and becomes mixed up with the reactions of the life (secondary action) than is the case with any other medicine, so that it is frequently hard to distinguish what is to be ascribed to the reaction of the body, and what to the alternating action of the camphor in its primary action.

But, at all events, commencement of a pure proving of it must be made, and as such I offer the following symptoms.

In its curative action camphor is just as puzzling and wonderful, for it removes the violent effects of very many, *extremely different*, vegetable medicines (and even those of the animal drug cantharides and of many mineral and metallic drugs), and hence it must have a sort of general pathological action, which, however, we are unable to indicate by any general expression ; nor can we even attempt to do so for fear of straying into the domain of shadows, where knowledge and observation cease, whilst imagination deceives us into accepting dreams as truth ; where we, in short, abandoned by the guiding of plain experience, grope about in the dark, and with every desire to penetrate into the inner essence of things, about which little minds so presumptuously dogmatize, we gain nothing by such hyperphysical speculations but noxious error and self-deception.

* WILL. ALEXANDER, *Medical Essays and Observations*, 1755.

1 From vol. iv. 2nd edit., 1825.

Camphor, as I can testify from experience, removes the too violent action of very many drugs, whether unsuitably employed or given in too large doses, but generally only in the primary action, as a kind of contrarium, as a palliative. For this purpose it must be given very frequently, but in very small doses—when requisite every five to fifteen, or when there is great urgency every two or three minutes, about one drop of the saturated alcoholic solution (one eighth of a grain) shaken up in half an ounce of water until dissolved, or by means of olfaction of a saturated alcoholic solution of camphor every three, four, six, ten, fifteen minutes.

One grain of camphor (dissolved in 8 drops of alcohol) combines with 400 grains of tepid water, and when shaken becomes completely dissolved, contrary to the assertion in almost all works on materia medica that it is quite insoluble in water.

I have not found camphor suitable as an antidote to the violent effects of ignatia.[1]

The rapid exhaustion of its action and the quick change of its symptoms render it incapable of curing most chronic diseases.

That cutaneous inflammation, which spreads in a radiating manner, is bright red, the redness disappearing for an instant when pressed with the finger, commonly called *erysipelas* (rose), when it arises from internal causes is always only a single symptom of the disease. Now, as camphor when applied externally excites a kind of erysipelas, so, in acute diseases accompanied by erysipelas, it is useful as an external application, if the other symptoms of the internal malady are present among the symptoms of camphor.

When the influenza endemic in Siberia comes among us, as it does occasionally, when the hot stage has already commenced, camphor is of service, only as a palliative certainly, but an invaluable palliative, seeing that the disease is one of short duration. It should be given in frequent but ever increasing doses, dissolved in water as above described. It does not shorten the duration of the disease, but renders it much milder, and hence it conducts the disease innocuously to its termination. (On the other hand, nux vomica, in a single dose, and that the smallest possible, will often remove the disease homœopathically in a few hours.)

When dangerous effects ensue from a large dose of camphor, opium is useful as an antidote ; and, on the other hand, camphor is a prompt antidote in opium poisoning ; thus each of these substances removes the effects of the other. It is therefore astonishing how opium and camphor have hitherto been given in combination in one prescription !

[In this proving HAHNEMANN was assisted by FRANZ, HERRMANN, STAPF, WISLICENUS.

The following old-school authorities are quoted :

ALEXANDER, *Experim. Essays.*

BREYNIUS and PAULINUS, in *Murray's App. med.*

COLLIN, *Observat. circa morbos.* CULLEN, W., *Mat. Med.*, ii.

GEOFFROY, *Matiere medic.*, iv. GRIFFIN, *Diss. de Camphoræ viribus*, Edin.

---

1 In the preface to *Ignatia*, camphor is said to be the antidote to some of its effects.

HEBERDEN, *Medic. Transact.*, i. HERGT, in *Hufel. Journ.*, xxvii. HOFFMANN, FR., *Diss. de usu int. Camph.*, 1714. HUFELAND, *Journal fur pract. A.*, i.

KOOLHAAS, in *Med. Not. Zeit.*, 1799.

LOSS, *Obs. med.*

MEZA, DE, *Compend. med. pract.* MURRAY, *Appar. med.*

ORTEL, *Med. pract.*

POUTEAU, *Melanges de Chirurgie.*

QUARIN, *Method med. febr.*

SOMMER, in *Hufel. Journ.*, vii. SPONITZER, in *Hufel. Journ.*, v.

TODE, in *Acta Haffn.*, iv.

UNZER, *Med. Handbuch*, ii.

WHYTT, *Works.*

In the *Frag. de vir.* Camphor has 147 symptoms, in the 1st Edit. 344, and only one additional symptom in this 2nd Edit.]

CAMPHORA.

He staggers to and fro when walking, and must catch hold of something in order to stand firmly. [*Ws.*]

He rubs his forehead, head, chest, and other parts, knows not what is the matter with him; he leans against something, his senses leave him, he slips and falls to the ground stretched out quite stiffly, the shoulders bent back, the arms at first somewhat bent, with hands directed outwards and somewhat flexed, spread-out fingers, afterwards all parts stretched straight out and stiff, with head bent over to one side, with stiff open lower jaw, with incurved lips and gnashing teeth, closed eyes and incessant twitchings of the facial muscles, coldness all over, and breathlessness for a quarter of an hour (aft. 2 h.). [*Ws.*]

Vertigo. [UNZER,[1] *Med. Handbuch*, ii, 25.—ALEXANDER,[2] *Experiment. Essays*, p. 227.—COLLIN,[2] *Observat. circa morbos*, pt. iii, p. 148.]

Vertigo, he must hold on by something, he felt as if he could not stand firmly. [*Hrr.*]

5. Intoxication. [COLLIN, l. c.—GRIFFIN,[2] *Diss. de Camphoræ viribus*, Edin.—DE MEZA,[3] *Compend. Med. prac.*, p. 3.]

Heaviness of the head with vertigo, the head sinks backwards (aft. 10 m.) [*Hrr.*]

Giddy heaviness of the head (aft. ½ h.). [*Hrr.*]

When walking he staggers as if drunk. [*Hrr.*]

Vertigo recurring at different times. [GRIFFIN, l. c.]

10. Frequent short attacks of vertigo. [HUFELAND,[4] *Jour. fur pract. A.*, i, p. 428.]

Confusion of the head with perfectly clear consciousness. [*Sft.*]

Want of memory.[5] [ALEXANDER.—UNZER, l. c.]

After the attack of tetanus with unconsciousness and vomiting, complete want of recollection, like loss of memory (aft. 3 h.). [*Ws.*]

---

1 Not accessible.

2 Proving with large doses.

3 Not accessible.

4 From large doses in rheumatic patients.

5 With Alexander, this describes the state of his mind after recovering consciousness.

The senses vanish (aft. a few m.).

15. Loss of consciousness.

His senses leave him. [ALEXANDER, l. c.]

Heaviness of the head. [GEOFFROY,[1] *Matie're medic.*, iv, p. 30.]

Headache. [HUFELAND, l. c.]

For several successive days headache after rising in the morning. [*Fz.*]

20. Severe headache. [UNZER, l. c.]

Throbbing headache.

Aching feeling in the head. [*Stf.*]

Aching tearing headache.

Headache like bruised feeling or soreness of the brain.

25. Headache as from constriction of the brain.

Aching in the occiput. [*Stf.*]

In the evening, aching headache over the left eye (aft. 9 h.). [*Fz.*]

Throbbing shooting headache in the forehead, which lasts all night, with general dry heat, but without thirst.

In the temples, throbbing aching. [*Stf.*]

30. Transient headache, as if the brain were compressed from all sides, but only felt in semi-consciousness when he pays no attention to his body ; when, however, he becomes conscious of his pain and thinks of it, it immediately disappears (aft. 4½ h.). [*Fz.*]

Pressure in the middle of the forehead (aft. 3½ h.). [*Hrr.*]

Obtuse headache over the frontal bone, with inclination to vomit.

Headache pressing from within outwards (immediately). [*Ws.*]

Tearing pressure in the right temple (aft. 1 h.). [*Hrr.*]

35. Tearing aching and pressing outwards in the left side of the forehead (aft. 7½ h.). [*Hrr.*]

Headache : cutting blows dart through the forehead and temples to the middle of the brain, returning after short pauses, immediately after lying down (aft. ½ h.). [*Ws.*]

Violent single shoots in the right half of the brain (aft. 4 h.).

Cutting pressure from the left side of the occiput to the forehead (aft. ½ h.). [*Hrr.*]

Tearing shooting headache in the forehead, and pressive on the upper part of the frontal bone (aft. 4 h.). [*Fz.*]

40. Fine tearing in the head, especially in the forehead (aft. 7 h.). [*Htn.*[2]]

Fine tearing in the right temple and forehead (aft. 1¾ h.). [*Hrr.*]

A constrictive pain in the base of the brain, especially in the occiput and above the root of the nose, which continues without intermission, during which the head is leant to one side or the other ; a pain that is much aggravated by stooping low, lying down, or external pressure—with coldness of hands and feet, hot forehead, and waking slumber.

---

1 General statement from authors.

2 Probably a misprint for *Hrr.*, as Hartmann does not appear as one of the provers.

Fine tearing pain in the left side of the forehead and left side of the occiput (aft. ½ h.). [*Hrr.*]

Heat in the head and tearing headache, transient in character, and going off by pressing on it (aft. 11 h.). [*Fz.*]

45. **Rush of blood to the head** (aft. 6 h.).

Extraordinary rush of blood to the head.* [WHYTT,[1] *Works*, p. 646.—MURRAY,[2] *Appar. Med.*, iv., p. 584.]

The head is drawn spasmodically towards the shoulder† (aft. some m.).

(Fatal) inflammation of the brain. [QUARIN,[3] *Method. med. febr.*, p. 57.]

Paleness of the face.

50. Very pale face, with eyes at first closed, afterwards open and staring, with eye-balls directed upwards (aft. 2 h.). [*Ws.*]

Very red face. [QUARIN, l. c.]

Spasmodic distortion of the facial muscles, with foam before the mouth.‡ [ORTEL,[4] *Med. pract. Beob.*, i, 1, Lpz., 1804.]

Pressure on the right palpebral muscle (aft. ¾ h.), [*Hrr.*]

Staring inflamed eyes. [QUARIN, l. c.]

55. He stares at every one with an astonished expression, without consciousness (aft. 2 h.). [*Ws.*]

Sensation of tension in the eyes (aft. ¾ h.). [*Hrr.*]

In the outer canthus of the eye a smarting (aft. ½ h.).

Frequent twitching in the outer canthus of the eye (aft. 28 h.). [*Fz.*]

Visible twitching and quivering of the upper eyelid (aft. 36 h.). [*Fz.*]

60. Smarting itching in the eyelids. [*Stf.*]

Smarting and shooting in the eyelids (aft. 5 h.). [*Fz.*]

* The preliminary vertigo and the unconsciousness from a strong dose, along with the coldness of the rest of the body (see note to 47, 304, 311 to 313), seems to be the primary action of camphor, and points to a diminished flow of blood to parts at a distance from the heart; on the other hand, the rush of blood to the head, the heat of the head, &c., are only a secondary action or reaction of the life in the same degree of intensity as was the previous opposite state, the primary action above mentioned. Just so, rapidly occurring, slight inflammation may therefore sometimes be removed by the palliative refrigerant effect of the primary action of camphor given internally, but long-standing inflammations cannot be so removed. The prolonged, or frequently repeated administration of camphor, is not unfrequently followed by obstinate inflammations of the eyes, which are of long duration, like every secondary action or reaction of the organism (comp. 283 to 292 and 297) I will not deny that the external application of camphor acts homœopathically in acute cases of ophthalmia but I will not venture to say that this is my experience, as I never treat such cases by external remedies.

† From a large dose given to a child, which caused loss of consciousness and deathly coldness of all parts of the body.

‡ From several grains of camphor injected into the median vein.

1 Effect of thirty grains.

2 General statement from authors. Here he is merely quoting Whytt.

3 Occasional effects of large doses in fever patients. Query always, how much is fever and how much camphor?

4 Not accessible.

The eyelids are studded with many red spots (aft. 24 h.). [*Ws.*]

The eyes water in the open air. [*Stf.*]

In the white of the right eye a couple of red spots, without pain (aft. 24 h.). [*Ws.*]

65. Out-pressing pain in the right eyeball on moving it (aft. 2 h.). [*Fz.*]

Sensation in the left eyeball like pressure and blows from behind upon it (aft. 2½ h.). [*Fz.*]

Inflammation of the eyes (aft. 10 h.).

The eyeballs are turned upwards.

Distorted eyes. [ORTEL, l. c.]

70. Staring, distorted eyes.

Contracted pupils.

Extremely contracted pupils (aft. 35 m.). [*Hrr.*]

Dilated pupils (aft. 5 h.).

Obscuration of the sight. [WHYTT,—UNZER, l. c.]

75. **Sensation as if all objects were too bright and shining** (aft. 5 h.).

Wonderful figures hover before his eyes. [UNZER, l. c.]

He cannot bear the light (aft. ½ h.).

Feeling of heat in the lobes of the ears. [*Stf.*]

Redness of cheeks and lobes of the ears.

80. Hot, red ear-lobes. [*Stf.*]

Ringing in the ears.[1] [ALEXANDER, l. c.]

A kind of tearing in the left ear (aft. 1 h.).

In the left meatus auditorius externus a dark red abscess, larger than a pea; on touching it he felt a shooting pressure (aft. 12 h.); **it suppurated after 36 hours.** [*Hrr.*]

In the anterior angle of the nostrils a shooting pain, as if the part were ulcerated and raw (aft. 2 h.).

85. Painful looseness of the teeth (aft. 10 h.).

The teeth feel too long, with a toothache apparently proceeding from swelling of the submaxillary glands.

Toothache: transient cutting blows dart through the gums at the roots of the incisors and canine teeth* (aft. ¼ h.). [*Ws.*]

Dry feeling on the back of the tongue, like scraping, with much saliva. [*Stf.*]

Constant collection of saliva in the mouth (aft. ½ h.). [*Hrr.*]

90. **Collection of saliva in the mouth, which is sometimes slimy and viscid** (aft. 1½ h.). [*Hrr.*]

Foam appears in front of the mouth (aft. a few m.).

A dry scraping sensation on the palate. [*Stf.*]

Single coarse stitches in the palate (aft. 4 h.).

A chilly sensation rises into the mouth and along the palate (aft. 4 to 6 h.). [*Fz.*]

95. Disagreeable warmth in the mouth. [ALEXANDER, l. c.]

* From the smell.

1 Just before losing consciousness.

Violent burning on the palate down into the œsophagus, that urges him to drink, but is not allayed by any amount of drinking* (immediately). [*Ws.*]

Sensation of heat in the mouth and stomach. [MURRAY, l. c.]

In the morning, bad smell from the mouth, which he is himself aware of (aft. 20 h.).

Closure of the jaws (trismus).

100. (Nocturnal) sore-throat *per se*, and still more when swallowing, as if the gullet were sore and excoriated, with sensation in the throat as from partaking of something rancid.

Eructation and bringing up of the contents of the stomach.

After a meal frequent and almost constant empty eructation (aft. 3 h. and later). [*Hrr.*]

Pleasure in drinking, without thirst.

The first 24 hours, adipsia. [*Ws.*]

105. The first 36 hours, adipsia. [*Hrr.*]

Increased taste of all food; the beef-tea tastes too strong (aft. 2 h.).

The taste in the mouth is in itself correct, but everything he eats, and even the (accustomed) tobacco smoking, tastes bitter (aft. 13 h.). [*Fz.*]

Tobacco has a disagreeable bitter taste (aft. 2¾ h.). [*Fz.*]

Dislike to the (accustomed) tobacco smoking; although it does not taste ill, tobacco is repugnant to him, and causes him to vomit.

110. Food tastes bitter, meat more so than bread, with eructation during and after eating, tasting of camphor (aft. 4 h.). [*Fz.*]

Frequent ejection of watery saliva. [*Stf.*]

Nausea. [GRIFFIN,—ALEXANDER, l. c.]

Nausea with flow of saliva. [*Stf.*]

Nausea and inclination to vomit, which always goes off after an eructation (aft. ¼ h.). [*Fz.*]

115. After several attacks of inclination to vomit, short attacks of vertigo. [HUFELAND, l. c.]

At the commencement of the vomiting, cold sweat, especially in the face. [*Ws.*]

Bilious vomiting, tinged with blood. [GRIFFIN, l. c.]

In the scrobiculus cordis, feeling as if it was distended and bruised, with fulness in the abdomen (aft. 25 h.). [*Fz.*]

Pain in the stomach.

120. Pain in the gastric region. [HUFELAND, l. c.]

Aching pain in the scrobiculus cordis or in the anterior part of the liver.

Contractive pain under the short ribs extending into the lumbar vertebræ.

Aching pain in the hypochondria (aft. 1 h.).

Manifest coolness, especially in the scrobiculus cordis [Fr. HOFFMANN, *Diss. de usu int. Camph.*, 1714, p. 20.]

125. Cold sensation in the epigastrium and hypogastrium (aft. ¼ h.). [*Hrr.*]

* From the smell.

Violent burning heat in the epigastrium and hypogastrium (aft. 4 h.). [*Hrr.*]

Burning heat in the hypogastrium (aft. 1¼ h.). [*Hrr.*]

Burning in the stomach. [WHYTT,—UNZER,—GRIFFIN, l. c.]

First discharge of much flatus, and after several hours, pressure in the abdomen, in the morning, as from distension with flatulence.

130. Flatulent sufferings in the abdomen.

The digestion is impeded [W. CULLEN,[1] *Arzneimittell.*, ii, p. 331.]

Cutting colicky pain, at night (aft. 5.).

Feeling of hardness and weight in the abdomen above the navel. [*Stf.*]

In the whole right side of the abdomen, as far as the hepatic region and chest, drawing bruised pain, more internally than externally, especially when inspiring (aft. 3½ h.). [*Fz.*]

135. Pinching pain in the hypogastrium, especially the umbilical region (aft. 7½ h.). [*Hrr.*]

In the right side of the hypogastrium a shooting drawing heaviness, which is still more distinctly felt on pressing on it. [*Fz.*]

Hard pressure in the left side of the hypogastrium (aft. 1 h.). [*Hrr.*]

Drawing in the left side of the hypogastrium with a tensive bruised sensation (aft. 12 h.). [*Fz.*]

Burning shooting on a spot the size of the hand, below the anterior crest of the ilium towards the groin. [*Fz.*]

140. Aching on the left side of the pubes at the root of the penis, in the groin, when standing (aft. 10 h.). [*Fz.*]

Itching formication in the right groin, which goes off on rubbing it (aft. ¼ h.). [*Ws.*]

Out-pressing on the pubes in the groin, at the root of the penis, as if a hernia would come out (aft. 12 h.). [*Fz.*]

Ascites of short duration. [HERGT,[2] in [*Hufel. Journ.*, xxvii, I, p. 151.]

Urging to stool: the stool is of the ordinary character, but little is passed, whereupon there is again great urging with the evacuation of a still smaller quantity (aft. 1 h.). [*Hrr.*]

145. Urging to stool (aft. 4 h.). [*Hrr.*]

The first day two stools after some pinching in the abdomen, the second day no stool, the third day rather hard and difficult stool. [*Fz.*]

Constipation.

The excrements are passed with difficulty, not without exertion of the abdominal muscles, just as if the peristaltic movement of the bowels were diminished, and at the same time the rectum were contracted (aft. 24 h.).

Obstinate constipation of the bowels.[3] [ALEXANDER, l. c.]

150. The rectum is as if contracted, swollen and painful when flatus is expelled.

1 From forty grains taken by a female maniac. This symptom not found.

2 From three grains twice daily.

3 Alexander simply states that he was "extremely costive at stool the day after" swallowing the dose.

Soreness in the rectum. [*Stf.*]

Greenish-yellow turbid urine of a mouldy smell (aft. 10 h.). [*Ws.*]

He passes turbid urine, which on standing becomes quite turbid and thick, of a whitish-green colour, without depositing a sediment. [*Hrr.*]

Red urine.

155. Red urine.[1] [*Fr. Hoffmann*, l. c.]

In the first hours, little urine and without suffering, but after several hours (in the afternoon) when urinating a smarting pain, for several days, in the posterior part of the urethra, and after urinating pressure in the vesical region, like a fresh call to urinate. [*Fz.*]

Diminished power of the bladder ; although there is no mechanical obstruction the urine passes very slowly out of the bladder when urinating (aft. 20 h.).

Thin stream of the urine discharged.

The urine passes in a very thin stream, as in stricture of the urethra (aft. 2½ h.). [*Hrr.*]

160. Retention of urine with urging to urinate and tenesmus of the the neck of the bladder.

Retention of the urine the first twelve hours, with constant pressure in the bladder and call to urinate, during which nothing passed ; but after twenty-four hours, frequent urination in the ordinary quantity, therefore on the whole increased quantity of urine discharged, but after forty-eight hours more frequent and more copious urination. [*Hrr.*]

In the first ten hours, no urine is passed. [*Ws.*]

Strangury almost immediately. [HEBERDEN,[2] *Medic, Trans.*, i, p. 471.]

Involuntary urination after great urging to urinate.

165. Almost involuntary urination, and after urinating pain in the urethra, like a contraction from before backwards.

Painful urination.

Scalding urine.

Shooting itching on the inner surface of the prepuce. [*Hrr.*]

(A contractive sensation in the testicles.) [*Stf.*]

170. The first two days, weakness of the genital organs, and loss of sexual desire. [*Ws.*]

The first two days, relaxation of the scrotum, deficiency of erection of the penis, loss of sexual desire, but after 48 hours much stronger erections than in ordinary times.* [*Hrr.*]

Tendency to nocturnal seminal emissions.

* The loss of sexual desire, erections, and seminal emissions, is, as is obvious from these observations, only primary action of camphor, and hence it only acts in a palliative manner when we attempt to combat with it inordinate sexual desire, erections, and the frequent nocturnal seminal emissions which have lasted long ; there follows then an increase of the malady by the opposite reaction of the organism (secondary action). (Comp. 173.)

---

1 "Very rarely," the author says.

2 Effects of large doses in patients.

For several nights, seminal emissions (aft. 60 h.). [*Fz.*]

Exalted sexual desire. [BREYNIUS and PAULINUS, in *Murray's Appar. Med.*, iv., p. 518.]

175. Sexual ecstasy. [KOOLHAAS,[1] in *Med. Nat. Zeit.*, 1799.]

Impotence in the male. [LOSS,[2] *Obs. Med.*, p. 314.]

A kind of violent labour pains, as if during parturition.* [HEBERDEN,[3] l. c.]

* * *

In the morning, on rising (and in the evening on going to sleep ?), discharge of thin nasal mucus, without sneezing and without true coryza (aft. 18 h.).

Coryza (aft. 10 h.).

180. Stuffed coryza.

Deep and slow respiration.

Oppressed, anxious, panting respiration. [ORTEL, l. c.]

Heavy, slow, difficult breathing (aft. $1\frac{1}{4}$ h.). [*Hrr.*]

Almost complete suspension of the respiration.

185. The breathing almost entirely ceases.[4] [CULLEN, l. c.]

On the sternum superiorly, pressure as from a weight. [*Fz.*]

Pressure on the sternum when standing (aft. 27 h.). [*Fz.*]

Soft pressure internally on the chest under the sternum, with difficult inspiration, and a chilling sensation, which rose out of the chest into the mouth (aft. 29 h.). [*Fz.*]

Mucus in the wind-pipe, which makes the voice not clear, and is not removed by hacking cough and hawking.

190. Pain in the trachea and bronchial tubes, most when coughing, but also by clearing the throat and hawking.

Complaint of a constrictive feeling in the larynx, as from sulphur fumes. [ORTEL, l. c.]

Feels as if he would be suffocated, and the larynx constricted. [SOMMER,[5] in *Hufel. Jour.*, p. 87.]

Suffocating tightness of the chest, as if it arose from a pressure in the scrobiculus cordis (aft. 1 h.).

Stitches in the left side of the chest when walking (aft. $\frac{1}{2}$ h.). [*Fz.*]

195. Painful sensation in the chest like stitches. [*Stf.*]

Shooting in the chest and tussiculation, as if caused by a cutting, chilling sensation deep in the trachea (aft. 2 h.). [*Fz.*]

The stitches in and on the chest became every day stronger. [*Fz.*]

Palpitation of the heart.

After a meal he feels and hears the beating of his heart against the ribs (aft. $4\frac{3}{4}$ h.). [*Fz.*]

* In a widow.

1 Not accessible.

2 From continual smelling of camphor in a man, æt. 40.

3 From forty grains given in enema. Nothing is said about the patient being a widow.

4 In original—"the breathing seems to have almost entirely ceased."

5 From gr. viij to xij given in lead-colic.

200. Fine shooting in the nipples (aft. 2 h.).

Fine tearing pain on the right side near the nipple down towards the pelvis (aft. 4½ h.). [*Hrr.*]

Tearing pressure on the anterior border of the scapula, which interferes with the movement of the arm (aft. 32 h.). [*Fz.*]

Drawing painful stitches through the scapulæ and between them, extending into the chest, on moving the arms, for two days (aft. 24 h.) [*Fz.*]

Tearing pain in the nape on bowing the head (aft. 2 h.).

205. Repeated painless drawing in the cervical vertebræ when moving. [*Stf.*]

When walking in the open air, painful drawing and stiff feeling on the side of neck and down the nape (aft. 5 h.). [*Fz.*]

Tensive pain in the nape and posterior cervical muscles, increased by every movement and by turning the neck (aft. 15 h.). [*Hrr.*]

Stitches in the nape, near the right shoulder, on moving (aft. 1½ h.). [*Fz.*]

Pressure on the top of the shoulder (aft. 2 h.). [*Fz.*]

210. Convulsive circular movement (rotation) of the arms.

Tearing pressure posteriorly in the middle of the right upper arm. [*Hrr.*]

Twitching fine tearing from the middle of the inner surface of the left upper arm to the middle of the forearm (aft. ¾ h.). [*Hrr.*]

Painful pressure in the right elbow-joint, worse on leaning on it, whereby the pain extends into the hand (aft. 1½ h.). [*Hrr.*]

Stitches in the forearm (aft. 1¾ h.). [*Fz.*]

215. Tearing pressure on the left radius, a little above the wrist-joint (aft. 7 h.). [*Hrr.*]

Painful pressure on the inner surface of the left forearm (aft. 1¾ h.). [*Hrr.*]

Tearing pressure on the inner surface of the left forearm (aft. 1¾ h.). [*Hrr.*]

Constantly increasing itching combined with pricking pain on the back of the hand and the knuckles of the fingers, going off on scratching (aft. 4½ h.). [*Fz.*]

Itching on the knuckles of the fingers and between them (aft. 25 h.). [*Fz.*]

220. In the distal joint of the thumb, on moving it, a pain as if sprained (aft. 20 h.).

Itching in the palm of the hand (aft. 5 h.). [*Fz.*]

Drawing in the glutæus maximus at its attachment to the crest of the ilium, as if it would lame the thigh. [*Fz.*]

Difficulty of moving, and fatigue of the thighs.

Drawing bruised pain in the thighs, after walking (aft. 5 h.). [*Fz.*]

225 **In the right thigh and on the inside near and below the patella, drawing bruised pain ; he fears that the leg would bend forwards under him.** (aft. 4¼ h.). [*Fz.*]

Tearing in the thighs (aft. 28 h.). [*Fz.*]

The thighs at the back above the houghs are painful, as after a long journey on foot. [*Fz.*]

When sitting with the knee flexed the leg goes to sleep, with cold feeling (aft. 21 h.)

Shooting on the right patella, when sitting (aft. 1 h.). [*Fz.*]

230. Tearing on the knees under the patella, worst when walking (aft. 6 h.). [*Fz.*]

Cracking and creaking in the joints of the loins, knees, and ankles.

Staggering, weariness, and heaviness of the lower extremities (aft. 1 h.). [*Hrr.*]

The knees seem to him to bend forwards, and are as if bruised (aft. 26 h.). [*Fz.*]

Aching drawing under the patella, on the inside of the knee (aft. 30 h.). [*Fz.*]

235. Great feeling of weakness of the legs when walking; the thighs are as if bruised and stiff. [*Stf.*]

Heaviness of the legs, as from a weight hanging in the knee-joints and drawing them down. [*Hrr.*]

Pressure in the middle of the inner surface of the left leg. [*Hrr.*]

Pressure on the left leg above the ankle and more posteriorly. [*Hrr.*]

In the morning on treading and walking, pain in the ankle-joint, as from having made a false step or sprained the part (aft. 18 h.).

240. Under the right ankle when standing, an aching drawing pain between the ankle and the tendo Achillis, which becomes tearing on moving the foot (aft. $4\frac{1}{2}$ h.). [*Fz.*]

Trembling of the feet.

Trembling staggering and unsteadiness of the feet.

Drawing cramp pain on the dorsum of the foot, especially when moving. [*Fz.*]

Tearing pressure on the dorsum of the right foot. [*Hrr.*]

245. **Tearing cramp-pain on the dorsum of the foot up along the outside of the calf to the thigh** (aft. 13 h.). [*Fz.*]

Tearing anteriorly in the tips of the toes and under the nails of the left foot, when walking (aft. 10 h.). [*Fz.*]

Sore pain on the knuckles of the toes and in the corns (aft. 26 h.). [*Fz.*]

Most of the pains of camphor are when moving. [*Fz.*]

Discomfort in the whole body (aft. 3 h.). [*Hrr.*]

250. Indescribable discomfort in the whole body (aft. $\frac{1}{2}$ h.). [*Hrr.*]

Most of the pains from camphor were, on the first day, only present in a state of half attention to himself—hence also when going to sleep, tearing in various parts of the body—and they went off, especially the headache, as soon as he became aware that he had pains and paid attention to them; on the other hand, he could, the following day, cause pains by force of imagination, or, rather, he felt them only when giving great attention to himself, hence he felt best when he did not think of himself. [*Fz.*]

Rheumatic shooting pains in all the muscles, especially between the scapulæ.

Pain in the periosteum of all the bones.

Difficulty of moving the limbs.

255. Paralytic relaxation of the muscles.

In the evening, after lying down in bed, an itching here and there in the body (aft. 6 h.).

Violent itching.* [SPONITZER, in *Hufel. Journ.*, v. pp. 518, 545.]

Erysipelatous inflammation.†

Erysipelas.‡ [SPONITZER, l. c.]

260. Syncopal stupefaction of the senses. [UNZER, l. c.]

Insensibility. [CULLEN, l. c.]

He beats his breast and falls into a faint (aft. ½ h.). [CULLEN, l. c.]

Out-stretching tetanus with unconsciousness for a quarter of an hour, then sinking down in a relaxed state of the whole body, so that he can scarcely be kept in the erect position, for a quarter of an hour, after which consciousness returns on vomiting (aft. 2½ h.). [*Ws.*]

Extreme weakness. [DE MEZA, l. c.]

265. Unusual sinking of the forces,[1] with yawning and stretching. [ALEXANDER, l. c.]

Relaxation and heaviness of the whole body (aft. 25 m.). [*Hrr.*]

Frequent yawning [*Stf.*]

Yawning and sleep. [GRIFFIN, l. c.]

Drowsiness.

270. Drowsy fatigue: he felt as if he would fall asleep (aft. 1 h.). [*Hrr.*]

Sopor. [ALEXANDER, l. c.]

Sopor and talking nonsense.[2] [FR. HOFFMANN, l. c.]

Sleeplessness. [GEOFFROY, l. c.]

(In sleep the inspiration is shorter than the expiration.)

275. During sleep he mutters and sighs.

Talking in a low voice during sleep all night.

Snoring in sleep during both inspiration and expiration.

During slumber with closed eyes, objects present themselves to his fancy, which seem to him at one time too thick, at another too thin, changing as rapidly as the pulse goes (aft. 2 h.).

Dreams about schemes to be carried out. [*Fz.*]

280. Spasms. [COLLIN, l. c.]

Convulsions.[3] [QUARIN,—ALEXANDER, l. c.]

* From the external application.
† From camphor applied externally.
‡ From the external application.

---

1 In the original, "unusual lassitude and depression of spirits."
2 Quoted from authors only to question it.
3 In Alexander's case, during loss of consciousness.

Violent convulsions. [TODE,[1] in *Acta. Haffn.*, iv, 4.]
Trembling. [ALEXANDER,—UNZER, l. c.]
Small, hard, and always slower and slower pulse.

285. Small slow pulse, 60 beats per minute (aft. $\frac{1}{2}$ h.). [*Hrr.*]
Pulse slower by 3 beats. [ALEXANDER,—GRIFFIN, l. c.]
Pulse slower by 10 beats. [HUFELAND.—ALEXANDER, —CULLEN, l. c.]
Weak, small pulse.[2] [HOFFMANN, l. c.]
Very weak, scarcely perceptible pulse. [CULLEN, l. c.]

290. Full, quick pulse.
Pulse gradually increasing in rapidity. [GRIFFIN, l. c.]
On continuing to take larger doses[3] the pulse beame quicker by 10 to 15 beats, and tense. [HUFELAND, l. c.]
After leaving off the gradually increased doses of camphor, the pulse increased in rapidity for several (nearly ten) days without increase of the temperature of the body. [HUFELAND, l. c.]
Pulse increased by twenty-three beats (aft. 3 h.). [ALEXANDER, l. c.]

295. Quicker pulse. [MURRAY,—HOFFMANN, l. c.]
Full, irritable pulse. [HUFFLAND, l. c.]
Very quick pulse. [QUARIN, l. c.]
Disposition to inflammations. [GEOFFROY, l. c.]
He is over sensitive to cold air.

300. He easily takes cold, and then there ensues either rigor or cutting in the abdomen, with diarrhœic discharges of blackish-brown or black fæces like coffee grounds.
Chilliness (after 10 h.).
Shivering, chilliness and occurrence of goose-skin all over the body for an hour (immediately). [*Fz.*]
Frequent chilliness in the back. [*Stf.*]
Shivery feeling, shivering with goose-skin ; **the skin of the whole body is painfully sensitive and the slightest touch is painful.**

305. Slight shivering with pale face. [GRIFFIN, l. c.]
Heat in the head and sensation in it as if sweat would break out, whilst a shudder goes over the limbs and abdomen (aft. 3 h.).
Chilliness on the cheeks and in the back. [*Stf.*]
Chilliness over the whole body (aft. $\frac{1}{4}$ h.). [*Hrr.*]
Rigor and chattering of the teeth. [ORTEL, l. c.]

310. **The body is quite cold all over.**
Coldness of the body with paleness. [CULLEN, l. c.]
After a meal coldness and drawing through the whole body, with cold arms, hands and feet (aft. $4\frac{3}{4}$ h.). [*Fz.*]
Coldness for an hour, with deathly pallor of the face.* [POUTEAU,[4] *Melanges de Chirurgie*, 184.]

* From 60 grains.

---

1 From five grains in commencing fever. 2 Not found.
3 By "large doses" gr. xl—lx are meant.
4 In a woman, three weeks after labour.—The sixty grains were given for colic.

(Fever : great chilliness with chattering of the teeth and much thirst, and after the chill he immediately falls asleep, but the sleep is often interrupted, almost without the least heat following.)

315. Cold sweat.

Profuse cold sweat. [ORTEL, l. c.]

In the evening, great feeling of coldness over the whole body and headache as if the brain was contracted, with aching above the root of the nose (aft. 12 h.). [*Fz.*]

Chilliness on the whole body (aft. $2\frac{1}{2}$ h.) ; then (aft. $1\frac{1}{2}$ h.). increased warmth of the whole body. [*Hrr.*]

Chilliness in the back intermingled with warmth as if sweat would break out. [*Stf.*]

320. Along with cold hands, hot sensation in the face (aft. $1\frac{1}{2}$ h.). [*Fz.*]

Heat on the head, hands and feet, without thirst.

Increased warmth of the whole body with redness of the face (aft. $\frac{3}{4}$ h.). [*Hrr.*]

Agreeable warmth through the whole body (after 3 h.). [*Fz.*]

Heat on the whole body, which increased to the greatest height when walking (aft. 5 h). [*Hrr.*]

325. Heat with trembling. [ALEXANDER.—UNZER, l. c.]

Sopor and squeezing (contractive) headache, great heat of the whole body with distended blood-vessels, very rapid breathing, and bruised pain in the back, but without thirst and with clean taste.

Great heat[1] (after some time). [HOFFMANN, l. c.]

Sweat (with odour of camphor). [MURRAY, l. c.]

Warm sweat on the forehead and palms.

330. Warm sweat all over the body.

Feeling of dryness in and on the body, especially on the head and in the bronchial tubes (aft. 2 h.).

Very dry skin, even in bed, with good appetite. [HUFELAND, l. c.]

Trembling movement of the heart. [ORTEL, l. c.]

Anxiety.

335. Very great anxiety. [HOFFMANN, l. c.]

She tosses about anxiously in bed, with constant weeping. [HUFFLAND, l. c.]

The ideas become confused ; delirium. [DE MEZA, l. c.]

Talking nonsense. [HUFELAND, l. c.]

He talks nonsense and undertakes nonsensical things. [UNZER, l. c.]

340. Rage, with foam before the mouth.[2] [ALEXANDER, l. c.]

All external things are repugnant to him, and excite in him a repellent crossness.

The boy crawls into a corner and howls and weeps ; he takes offence at everything one says to him, as if he thought he was being ordered about, and he thinks he is insulted and affronted.

The pain disappeared, but this condition supervened. On recovering from it, she was well.

1 Quoted from authors only to question it.

2 During unconsciousness.

Quarrelsomeness, insists he is right.
He is hasty and does things in a hurry.

345. The first day the disposition was lazy and unhappy during the cold and rigor ; after twenty-four hours, however, the disposition became ever better and better, even during the pains. [*Fz.*]

CANNABIS SATIVA.[1]

(*Hemp.*)

(The fresh expressed juice of the tops of the flowering male or female hemp-plant, mixed with equal parts of alcohol, and after standing some time the clear supernatant fluid decanted off.)

Hitherto only the seeds, generally (rubbed up with water) as emulsion, or as decoction, have been used with advantage in the inflammatory stage of gonorrhœa, and in ancient times (by DODONÆUS, SYLVIUS, HERLIZ) in some kinds of jaundice. In the former case the homœopathic reason for its utility is evident from the peculiar similar morbid states observed in the urinary organs after the administration of hemp to healthy persons, although no physician ever recognized this. The plant itself has only been used as a domestic remedy, but it was much employed in Persian country inns in order to relieve the fatigue of pedestrian travellers (CHARDIN, *Voyage en Perse*), for which it is truly homœopathic as the following cannabis symptoms (269 to 275) demonstrate.

But we may employ the juice of hemp for curative purposes of much more importance in various diseases of the genital organs, of the chest, of the organs of the senses, &c. for which the following observations present the homœopathic indications.

For a long time I employed the undiluted alcoholic tincture of cannabis, in the dose of the smallest portion of a drop; but the higher and the very highest yet made dilution and potency ($\overline{X}$) of it develops the medicinal powers of this plant in a much greater degree.

[HAHNEMANN's fellow-provers of cannabis were—FRANZ, GROSS, FR. HAHNEMANN, HEMPEL, HUGO, STAPF, TRINKS, HARTLAUB, and WAHLE.

A few symptoms were taken from the following old-school sources :

HALLER, in *Vicat, Mat. Med.*

MORGAGNI, *De Sed. et Causis Morb.*

NEUHOLD, in *Act. Nat. Cur.*, iii.

OLEARIUS, *Oriental. Reisebeschreib.*

RAMAZZINI, *Diatribe de Morb. Artif.*

The 1st Edit. has only 69 symptoms, the 2nd Edit. has 308, this 3rd Edit. 330.]

CANNABIS.

Vertigo when standing and dizziness. [*Gss.*]
Vertigo when walking, as if he would fall sideways (aft. 1 h.). [*Ho.*]
Whirling and stupid in the head (immediately). [*Gss.*]
Giddy and dull in the head. [*Ws.*]

1 From vol. i, 3rd edit., 1830.

5. Attacks of vertigo. [NEUHOLD,[1] in *Act. Nat. Cur.*, iii, p. 150, *et seq.*]

Confusion and dulness of the head. [*Stf.*]

Hesitation and unsteadiness of the mind ; overpowering vividness of the thoughts that arise. [*Hl.*]

Wanting in reflective power, deficient in imagination, spiritless. [*Stf.*]

The thoughts seem to stand still ; he stares before him ; he feels as if his mind were occupied by elevated contemplations, but he does not know what they are ; with a slight feeling of aching pain on the parietal bone. [*Fz.*]

10. He can, no doubt, think of one thing and another, but the ideas remain stationary, as if they stood still, and he looks long at the object on which he was going to work. [*Fz.*]

He often makes mistakes in writing. [*Stf.*]

Agreeable warmth in the brain. [*Fz.*]

Quivering as if in the blood of the head, chest, and stomach.

Great rush of blood to the head.

15. Rush of blood to the head, which causes an agreeable warmth in it, but with aching pain in the temples. [*Fz.*]

Throbbing pain that extends forwards into the right temple ; at the same time a warmth about the head ; the cheeks are red and hot ; in the warmth the nausea increases. [*Ts. Hb.*]

Violent pains in the head. [NEUHOLD, l. c.]

Very penetrating headache. [NEUHOLD, l. c.]

Uninterrupted headache all day. [*Fz.*]

20. Constant pain on the top of the head, as if a stone lay on it. [*Fz.*]

Confusion of the head ; it is heavy and she feels a painful pressure on the forehead and eyelids, so that they are like to close. [*Gss.*]

Pressure under the frontal protuberance too deep through the brain into the occiput. [*Gss.*]

When leaning the head against the wall an aching on the opposite side internally in the head. [*Gss.*]

Pressure in the temples. [*Ho.*]

25. Aching pain in the right occipital bone. [*We.*]

Tension first in the occiput then in the sinciput, lastly **in the temples** (aft. ½ h.). [*Ho.*]

On moving the head a painful sensation in the head and nape. [*Stf.*]

Drawing pain in the occiput towards the ears. [*Stf.*]

Painful constriction of the sinciput. [*Gss.*]

30. **The sinciput is compressed from the borders of the orbits to the temples ; not relieved by stooping.** [*Gss.*]

Below the left frontal protuberance a beating outwards, immediately followed by stupefying pressure on that part. [*Gss.*]

On a small spot of the parietal bone (afterwards on other parts

1 Effects of effluvia of hemp, before being dried.

of the head also) a cold feeling as if a drop of cold water fell on it [*Gss.*]

A creeping in the skin of the hairy scalp.

A kind of tickling spasm in the temples (aft. $\frac{3}{4}$ h.). [*Ho.*]

35. Feeling as if the eyebrow were pressed down. [*Gss.*]

Tearing pressure on the upper eyelid. [*Gss.*]

Alternate dilatation and contraction of the pupils in one and the same light (aft. 1 h.). [*Ho.*]

Weak feeling in the eyes, and weakness of vision ; distant and near objects are indistinct (aft. $1\frac{1}{2}$ h.). [*Ho.*]

The cornea of the eye becomes opaque ; pannus.

40. A circle of white flaming zig-zags on the right side of the field of vision ; so that he can see objects only partially and indistinctly. [*Gss.*]

Cataract.[1] [NEUHOLD, l. c.]

Pressure outwards at the back of the eyes (aft. $\frac{3}{4}$ h.). [*Ho.*]

Sensation of spasmodic drawing in the eyes (aft. $\frac{3}{4}$ h.). [*Ho.*]

Slight palpitation on many parts of the face, especially in the muscles of the left cheek. [*Gss.*]

45. Paleness of the face [MORGAGNI,[2] *De Sed. et Causis Morb.*, Epist. x, art. 13.]

Drawing pressure on the left zygoma. [*Gss.*]

Itching here and there in the face.

Formication, itching, and smarting as from salt, in the face.

Large lumps on the nose surrounded by red swelling, like acne.

50. Itching swelling on the ala nasi (aft. some h.).

Dryness in the nose.

Stupefying pressure as with a blunt point on the root of the nose. [*Gss.*]

Warm sensation in the nose as if it would bleed. [*Fz.*]

Epistaxis to syncope.[3] [NEUHOLD, l. c.]

55. Epistaxis.

Roaring before the ears.

Sensation as of a skin drawn before the ears. [*We.*]

Instantaneous pain as if the auricle were drawn out of the head. [*Gss.*]

Acute twitching pain in the right membrana tympani extending to the shoulder. [*We.*]

60. Sore pain in the external aural cartilage, which he might have somewhat pressed as he lay at night in bed. [*Gss.*]

Tinnitus aurium. [NEUHOLD, l. c.]

A throbbing in the ear. [*Stf.*]

---

1 The original is "suffusiones oculorum," and occurs in a list of the observed effects of hemp. Though technically this phrase *may* mean cataract (as in Celsus, seventh book, vii, 13, 14), yet it seems unlikely that the author means to hazard in this manner so startling an assertion as that hemp can cause it.

2 Cases of disease occurring in adult male hemp-dressers, but not adduced as results of their occupation. This is merely a statement that the man was pale, but otherwise in good health.

3 From the odour alone.

In the ear a throbbing forcing pain that extends almost into the cheek, goes off immediately on stooping and recurs on rising up again (aft. 3 h.). [*Stf.*]

Stitches in the external meatus when chewing. [*Gss.*]

65. Fine stitches from within outwards in the left ear. [*Ws.*]

Pain behind the right ear as if a blunt point were violently thurst in. [*Gss.*]

Large sharp stitches on the mastoid process. [*Gss.*]

Stupefying compressive pain on the left side of the chin, in which the teeth of that side participate. [*Gss.*]

Cramp-like pain in the teeth on the left side of the lower jaw. [*Fz.*]

70. Fine pecking in the left ramus of the lower jaw, on the cessation of which a drawing always ensues. [*Gss.*]

A darting and fine pecking in several teeth at the same time. [*We.*]

Eruption on the red part of the lips and on the corner of the mouth.

Pinching aching in the cervical muscles over the throat. [*Gss.*]

Speech is difficult.[1] [MORGAGNI, l. c., Epist. xv, art. 6.]

75. Altered speech, more a clangour than a human voice.[2] [MORGAGNI, l. c., Epist. vii. art. 13.]

He could not speak properly ; at one time words failed him, at another the voice itself (for 4 hours) ; towards evening the attacks recurred, at one time there was a stream of eloquence, as if forced from him, at another a stoppage in his discourse, so that he sometimes repeated the same word ten times in succession in one breath, sometimes anxiously recalling his whole thought he was annoyed that he could not repeat it in the same words. [*Fz.*]

The speech is given out with extraordinary anxiety and agony on account of pain in the back. [*Fz.*]

In the morning burning dryness in the palate.

A burning in the throat.[3] [MORGAGNI, l. c., Epist. xv, art. 6.]

80. Dryness in the mouth ; the saliva is viscid, at the same time want of thirst especially in the evening, and hot hands. [*Stf.*]

On partaking of food that he relishes highly, there occurs, when he is nearly satiated, a transient sickness up in his throat. [*Gss.*]

Belching of a bitter-sour acrid fluid. [*Gss.*]

Without nausea or retching, a tasteless water rises up in his throat and wind-pipe so that he always chokes in swallowing. [*Gss.*]

Eructation of a bitter-sour fluid into the mouth. [*Gss.*]

85. **Eructation of nothing but air.** [*Gss.*]

A choking sensation always rises up in the throat, as from acidity of the stomach. [*Gss.*]

A choking in the scrobiculus cordis rises thence up into the throat. [*Gss.*]

---

1 In subject of S. 223, *q. v.*
2 Local effect.
3 See note to S. 74.

Nausea ; she heaves as though she would vomit. [*Ts. Hb.*]

Vomiting of a slimy bitter-tasting water ; at the same time a scraping in the throat, followed by stupid feeling and confusion of the head in the occiput. [*Ts. Hb.*]

90. Green bilious vomiting.[1] [MORGAGNI, l. c., Epist. vii, art. 13.]

She became anxious and apprehensive in the scrobiculus cordis, with oppression of the breathing and palpitation ; warmth rises up to the throat and stops the breath, as if something stuck in the wind-pipe, with flying heat. [*Gss.*]

Fulness in the abdomen, compelling him to breathe deeply.

Cardialgia. [NEUHOLD, l. c.]

Pinching in the scrobiculus cordis. [*Gss.*]

95. Cutting in the scrobiculus cordis. [*Gss.*]

After stooping a cutting above and across the stomach. [*Fz.*]

Uninterrupted obtuse shooting in front, just below the ribs near the scrobiculus cordis, which only varies in degree ; by moving the body forwards or backwards it is alleviated for an instant, but soon returns. [*Gss.*]

On the left side, near the xiphoid cartilage, burning shooting pain. [*We.*]

In the left side, just under the ribs, an obtuse shooting when breathing and when not breathing. [*Gss.*]

100. At various times several attacks of the most violent stomach pains, with paleness of the face and perspiration on the face, pulse almost extinct, and rattling respiration like that of a dying person.[2] [MORGAGNI, l. c., Epist. xxiv, art. 13.]

The stomach is extremely painful to the touch, as if ulcerated ; but it goes away on eating. [*Fz.*]

He feels as if he had caught cold in the stomach ; in the forenoon especially he has working round in the bowels and pinching, but without diarrhœa.

Several mornings, from 8 to 10 a.m., sensation under the navel as if he had caught cold ; a working round in his abdomen, but without diarrhœa.

Just above the navel pinching (after a meal). [*Gss.*]

105. Pinching throughout all the abdomen. [*Gss.*]

In the epigastrium anxious beating, like strong pulse beats. [*Gss.*]

On the right near the navel pain like a beating there from within outwards. [*Gss.*]

In the left side under the last ribs, towards the back, there is a beating outwards as with a small hammer. [*Gss.*]

110. On the left near the navel, and at the same time behind near the spine, pain as if the parts were seized by pincers and compressed. [*Gss.*]

All the bowels pain as if bruised. [*Fz.*]

---

1 Local effect. See S. 226.

2 Subject of S. 218, 219, 224, 307. Heart found much enlarged post mortem.

In the abdomen shaking of the bowels on moving the arms violently, as if the bowels were quite loose. [*Fz.*]

An almost sore itching for several hours at the navel, where, after rubbing, there is acute sore pain.

Tickling sensation on the integuments of the hypogastrium (aft. ½ h.). [*Ho.*]

115. Shudder in the abdomen, as from the movement of cold water therein (aft. 8 m.). [*Ho.*]

In the side of the abdomen an out-stretching. [*Fz.*]

In the right hypochondrium a painful hard swelling.[1] [MORGAGNI, l. c., Epist. xxiv, art. 13.]

Encysted abdominal tumour, without swelling of legs or feet.[2] [MORGAGNI, l. c., Epist. x, art. 13.]

Abdomen and chest are externally painful.[3] [MORGAGNI, l. c., Epist. xv, art. 6.]

120. Drawing pain from the renal region to the inguinal glands, with anxious sick feeling in the scrobiculus cordis.

In the renal region pain as if ulcerated *per se*, and on touching. [*Fz.*]

In the side of the abdomen, just under the ribs, sharp blows. [*Gss.*]

Flying, pinching stitches in the abdomen. [*Gss.*]

A working round in the abdomen, and then in the left side obtuse stitches up into the ear. [*Gss.*]

125. Flatulence sticks in the epigastrium and hypogastrium until the evening with colicky pains. [*We.*]

Painful jerks dart round about in the abdomen from one place to another, as if something alive was in it ; at the same time a drawing from the left hip-bone over to the right and thence into the knee ; but the pain remains all the time in the hip, and assumes the character of tearing blows. [*Gss.*]

In the evening in bed she has obtuse stitches in both sides of the abdomen, they then spread up the back, and there are similar stitches between the scapulæ, they then return into the sides of the abdomen. [*Gss.*]

Painful blows above the bend of the left groin. [*Gss.*]

Needle prick on the right side of the mons veneris. [*We.*]

130 In the bend of the groin at first some twitching blows, he then feels the region of the inguinal ring as if stretched, and the inguinal ring itself as if pressed out. [*Fz.*]

In the inguinal ring an out-pressing and pain, as if all were ulcerated there. [*Fz.*]

Every morning discharge of much almost inodorous flatus. [*Gss.*]

Colicky pains in the epigastrium, followed by a diarrhœic stool and a sore pain in the anus. [*We.*]

---

1 Liver found diseased post mortem.

2 Subject of S. 217, found post mortem to be due to spinal incurvation. This symptom occurred eight days before death. Morgagni says only "abdomen universum tumere." After death much turbid fluid was found in the peritoneu .

3 See note to S. 74.

The first five days normal stool, the following two days quite constipated. [*Gss.*]

135. In the rectum and sacrum a pressing as if all the bowels descended and would be pressed out, when sitting. [*Fz.*]

At the anus a sensation as if something cold dropped out on the skin. [*Fz.*]

Contractive pain at the anus ; at the same time she feels as if the thighs were drawn together, so that she must close them. [*Gss.*]

Itching in the perinæum.

Urging to urinate, with aching pain.

140. Turbid white urine.

Urine reddish and turbid.

Difficulty in urinating ; paralysis of the bladder.*[1] [MORGAGNI, l. c., Epist. x, art. 13.]

Urine full of flocci, as if pus were mingled with it. [*Fr. H—n.*]

Diuresis ; he must urinate frequently at short intervals, when a large quantity of urine resembling water is discharged (immediately). [*Gss.*]

145. A tearing as if in the fibres of the urethra, as it were in the form of a zig-zag. [*Hl.*]

Itching, tickling stitches in the anterior part of the urethra. [*We.*]

Burning shooting in the posterior part of the urethra during the passage of the urine (aft. 10 h:) [*Ho.*]

Whilst urinating pain from the mouth of the urethra going backwards, burning smarting, posteriorly more shooting.

Simple, but violent burning in the anterior part of the urethra during the flow of urine.

150. Burning in the mouth of the urethra while urinating.

Burning while urinating, but especially immediately afterwards.

Burning during, but especially after urinating, worst in the evening.

Whilst urinating, from the glans penis to the back part, a pain at first burning, and after urinating smarting pain.

Even when not urinating some burning pain in the anterior part of the urethra, which obliges him to be almost continually trying to pass water, even when there is no more urine in the bladder.

155. Shooting smarting pain when passing water, when not urinating a smarting pain.

When not urinating pressure as if to make water, especially in the anterior part of the urethra.

Stitches along the urethra when not urinating.

When standing twitching stitches in the posterior part of the urethra.

Burning throughout the urethra, but only at the beginning and the end of micturition. [*Fr. H—n.*]

160. Anteriorly in the orifice of the urethra, very fine shooting pecking when not urinating. [*Fz.*]

* The urine could at first only be passed by means of the catheter, but afterwards not even by this instrument, because it gets stopped up by mucus and pus.

1 In subject of S. 118, eight days before death, after paraplegia had lasted some time.

Cutting pain in the anterior part of the urethra when urinating. [*Fz.*]

Watery mucous discharge from the urethra. [*Fr. H—n.*]

Painless discharge of a clear transparent mucus from the urethra (prostatic fluid ?) without erection. [*Fz.*]

The orifice of the urethra is stuck together by a fluid which becomes visible when pressed. [*Hl.*]

165. The whole penis is somewhat swollen, without actual erection. [*Fr. H—n.*]

The urethra is as if inflamed, and painful in its whole length when touched; during erection there occurs tensive pain.

Stream of urine spread out.

Frequent erections of the penis; afterwards stitches in the urethra.

Frequent erections by day, only when sitting, not when walking.

170. When coughing erections of the penis, then pain in the urethra.

Painless discharge of mucus from the urethra (a kind of gonorrhœa ?).

Swelling of the glans and penis; a kind of erection without sensation. [*Fz.*]

Coldness of the genitals with warmth of the rest of the body (the same day, and lasting three days). [*Hl.*]

Disinclination for coitus. [*Fr. H—n.*]

175. Swelling of the right and lower side of the prepuce. [*Fr. H—n.*]

Swelling of the frenum and of the prepuce, especially where the frenum ends. [*Hl.*]

Pleasant itching on the border of the prepuce and at the orifice of the urethra. [*We.*]

Disagreeable itching on the right side of the prepuce at its anterior border, more internally, but pleasant during and after scratching. [*Fr. H—n.*]

An itching under the prepuce and at the frenum, with some redness and moisture behind the corona glandis. [*Hl.*]

180. Eroding burning and shooting in the external parts of the prepuce, and in the urethra at the corona glandis. [*Fz.*]

The whole of the prepuce is dark red, hot, and inflamed. [*Fr. H—n.*]

Soreness on the border and on the inside of the prepuce. [*Fr. H—n.*]

Constant burning on the whole of the prepuce and glans, for four days; on applying cold water there occurred soreness. [*Fr. H—n.*]

The border of the prepuce is excoriated. [*Fr. H—n.*]

185. The glans itself is dark red, as dark red as the prepuce itself. [*Fr. H—n.*]

The skin of the glans is covered with lentil-sized, bright-red spots, brighter than the glans itself. [*Fr. H—n.*]

The whole penis pains when walking as if excoriated and as if scalded (he must tie it up in an upright position). [*Fr. H—n.*]

Round about the back of the corona glandis an exudation and moisture like gonorrhœa preputialis. [*Fr. H—n.*]

On the right near the penis pain like penetrating blows, when at rest and when moving. [*Gss.*]

190. When standing, a tensive pain in the spermatic cord, and contraction of the scrotum, with a contractive feeling in it.

When standing a pressive feeling in the testicles, a tugging in them.

Swelling of the prostate gland.

The sexual desire is much excited, but sterility is caused. [OLEARIUS,[1] *Oriental. Reisebeschreib.*, p. 529.]

Excites the sexual desire in human beings and in animals. [HALLER, in *Vicat,*[2] *Mat. Med.*]

195. Profuse menstrual flux (from external application). [NEUHOLD, l. c.]

Premature labour (in the eighth month) accompanied by frightful convulsions.[3] [NEUHOLD, l. c.]

* * *

Dryness and dry feeling in the nose (aft. 5 d.).

Dry feeling and heat in the nose.

Sneezing and feeling of stuffed coryza, and yet he can breathe through the nose. [*We.*]

200. In the morning, viscid mucus sticks in the lower part of the wind-pipe ; coughing and hacking cannot reach it, and he strains much to detach a little, which, however, does not come into the mouth, and which he must swallow ; after the coughing and hacking there remains a scraping feeling down along the wind-pipe, as if it was raw and excoriated there ; at length the mucus detaches itself spontaneously and he must repeatedly hawk it up. [*Gss.*]

In the morning she has scraping in the chest as from salt ; she must hack and swallow what she hawks up because it will not come into the mouth. [*Gss.*]

About the seventh day the previously viscid phlegm detaches itself easily in the morning, and the previous difficulty of breathing (as if a weight lay on the chest) was immediately relieved. [*Gss.*]

Oppression of the breathing from a tensive aching pain in the middle of the sternum, which is also painful to the touch ; at the same time sleepiness.

Inspiration is difficult ; it is as if a weight lay on her chest. [*Gss.*]

205. She is oppressed on the chest and has a feeling of anxiety in the throat ; she must breathe deeply. [*Gss.*]

Violent pinching together under the sternum, in the lower part of the chest, whereby the breathing is not impeded ; on bending back it goes off, and is worst when stooping forwards and then worse when inspiring. [*Gss.*]

In the left side of the chest, without oppression of the breathing, a pushing with intermittent obtuse stitches—a kind of pressing inwards. [*Gss.*]

---

1 General statement of effects ; but C. Indica is probably intended.

2 General statement of effects.

3 From lying all day on fresh hemp. Preceded by S. 18.

In both sides of the chest blows or knocks, which recur frequently and at the same time impede respiration, but are most painful in the region of the heart.

On corporeal exertion and stooping, a couple of violent blows at the heart, as if it would fall out ; at the same time a warmth about the heart (aft. 48 h.).

210. A beating in her left side on the ribs. [*Gss.*]

An out-hammering under a costal cartilage near the sternum. [*Gss.*]

Digging under the top of the sternum, without oppression of the breathing. [*Gss.*]

Drawing pain at the left last rib. [*Fz.*]

Shooting in the external thoracic integuments. [*Fz.*]

215. Cutting over the external thoracic integuments. [*Fz.*]

Tensive oppression of the left half of the chest, with slight jerking, palpitation of the heart and anxiety. [*Gss.*]

At the xiphoid cartilage an elevation and a node, which grew for two years painlessly and then caused difficulty of breathing.[1] [MORGAGNI, Epist. x, art. 13.]

Beating of the heart at a low place.[2] [MORGAGNI, Epist. xxiv, art. 13.]

Pain in the cardiac region.[3] [MORGAGNI, l. c.]

220. Tightness of chest. [RAMAZZINI,[4] *Diatribe de morb. artif.*, Cap. 26.]

Difficult breathing, without expectoration.[5] [MORGAGNI, l. c., Epist. vii, art. 18.]

Very much impeded respiration. [MORGAGNI, l. c., Epist. xv, art. 6.]

Orthopnœa ; he could only breathe with his neck stretched upwards, with whistling in the wind-pipe, and great distension of the abdomen.[6] [MORGAGNI, l. c.]

On lying down, difficult respiration.[7] [MORGAGNI, l. c., Epist. x, art. 13.]

225. Six or seven times inflammation of the chest and lungs.[8] [MORGAGNI, Epist. vii, art. 13.]

Inflammation of the lungs with vomiting of a green bilious matter,[8] [MORGAGNI, l. c.]

Inflammation of the lungs with incoherent talking.[8] [MORGAGNI, l. c.]

---

1 See note to S. 118.

2 Rather, "the pulsations of the heart are felt below the natural limits." See note to S. 100.

3 See note to S. 100.

4 Affections of workers in hemp *and linseed* ; therefore mere local and mechanical irritations.

5 Subject of S. 225. Being tired with carrying a burden, had S. 309 and 228, and came into hospital with this dyspnœa. Died of phrenitis. See Hahnemann's note to S. 330.

6 A man convalescing from acute fever, "after irregularities in food and drink and continual handling of hemp," had this symptom with S. 222, 74, 79, 119, 229.

7 See note to S. 100.

8 Local effect.

Pain like needle-pricks on the left nipple.[1] [MORGAGNI, l. c.]

Expiration caused him to cough.[2] [MORGAGNI, Epist. xv, art. 6.]

230. Sometimes tussiculation proceeding from the pit of the throat, when a cool, salt fluid is felt deep back in the throat. [*Stf.*]

Constant cough. [RAMAZZINI, l. c.]

Dry, very violent cough. [NEUHOLD, l. c.]

On the coccyx, pressure as with a blunt point. [*Gss.*]

On the left near the coccyx in the bone, a pain as if this part was forcibly pressed against a hard body. [*Gss.*]

235. On the lower dorsal vertebræ of the thorax a heavy pressive and fine shooting pain (for 50 days), which sometimes extended to the loins or to the scapulæ.[3] [MORGAGNI, Epist. x, art. 13.]

Slowly intermitting obtuse stitches on the left side of the back, under the last rib. [*Gss.*]

Pain in the middle of the back as if pinched with forceps, which extended forwards towards the abdomen. [*Fz.*]

The pain in the back often takes away his breath. [*Fz.*]

On the right near the scapula, itching fine stitches, that go off after scratching. [*Gss.*]

240. Burning under the right scapula. [*Fz.*]

On the lowest part of the nape, stabbing as with a knife. [*Fz.*]

Drawing upwards in the nape on the cervical vertebræ. [*Fz.*]

Drawing from the nape to the ear, rather cramp-like and external. [*Gss.*]

Tearing pressure on the top of the shoulder in fits. [*Gss.*]

245. On pressing between the head of the clavicle and the head of the humerus a severe pain, that radiated down into the fingers. [*Gss.*]

On extending the arm, sensation in the shoulder, as if it was bruised. [*Fz.*]

Cramp-like, intermitting contraction of the right hand. [*Gss.*]

(Wrist-joint as if dead ; he could not move it.)

Cramp-like contraction of the metacarpal bones. [*Gss.*]

250. Obtuse stitch inferiorly in the palm over the bones of the wrist. [*Gss.*]

Coldness and cold feeling of the hands. [*Ho.*]

Cramp in the joint of the thumb when writing. [*Fz.*]

Formication as if asleep in the tips of the fingers, and as if they were numb (immediately after taking the drug). [*Hl.*]

A sudden paresis of the hand ; when eating he could not hold the fork with the fingers ; the whole hand trembled on taking hold of anything ; there was a kind of helplessness and painful powerlessness in it. [*Stf.*]

255. Eruption of pimples on the buttock and thigh ; small white vesicles with large, red, smooth areola, which burn like fire, especially when lying on them or touching them ; they leave brownish-red spots after two days, which are very painful when touched. [*Fz.*]

---

1 See note to S. 221.
2 See note to S. 223.
3 See note to S. 118.

On the right hip a cramp-like, twitching, strangling pain, almost making him cry out.

In the flesh of the upper part of the thigh, near the groin, acute sharp needle-pricks [*Gss.*]

A shudder passes over the thighs (immediately). [*Gss.*]

Shudder on the right thigh, like goose-skin. [*Fz.*]

260. Painless cramp-sensation at the back of the right thigh, as if a muscle were beginning to twitch. [*Fz.*]

Constant aching anteriorly in the middle of the thigh, when sitting. [*Gss.*]

A shudder often runs over the legs from below upwards. [*Gss.*]

Prickling burning on the left knee in fits. [*Gss.*]

Cramp in the calf when walking.

265. When walking a drawing like cramp in the popliteal space, which spreads up along the inner muscles of the thigh. [*Fz.*]

Snapping of the patella on going upstairs. [*Fz.*]

The right leg is first difficult to move, then paralysed, so that the power of movement more than the sensibility is awanting.[1] [MORGAGNI, l. c., Epist. x, art. 13.]

Burning in the right tibia when standing. [*Fz.*]

Painful live blood on the back of the foot. [*Gss.*]

270. Painful stretching tension on the arch of the foot. [*Gss.*]

Drawing hither and thither in the left foot from the toes to the ankle. [*Gss.*]

Drawing and aching in the heel, when sitting. [*Fz.*]

Drawing in the ball of the right big toe. [*Fz.*]

Shooting itching in the ball of the left big toe. [*Fz.*]

275. On moving, rheumatic drawing in the periosteum of the shafts of the bones of all the limbs, as if they were bruised. [*Fz.*]

Here and there in the flesh a superficial pinching, as if the part were grasped by the fingers. [*Gss.*]

Tearing contractive pressure on the left knee, in the forehead, and on several other parts of the body. [*Gss.*]

A very tiresome fine pricking, as with a thousand needle points, all over the body, so that he cannot bear it, at night in bed, when he gets into a perspiration from warm covering; it first commences in a few places, and when he then scratches and it leaves off for a short time, it then spreads over many other parts; at the same time he has g eat cardiac anxiety, and the sensation as if he were repeatedly sprinkled with hot water; it goes off when he removes the bed-clothes. [*Gss.*]

Tearing blows, and tearing, deeply-penetrating pricks on several parts, especially on the limbs. [*Gss.*]

280. Hysterical fits.[2] [NEUHOLD, l. c.]

Tetanic spasms of the upper extremities and of the trunk from time to time, which lasted a quarter of an hour, and during which

1 See note to S. 118.

2 "In those predisposed to them," Neuhold says.

vomiting of yellow fluid or some confusion of the mind ensued.*[1] [MORGAGNI, l. c., Epist. x, art. 13.]

After a meal he is weary and lazy; everything, even speaking and writing, affects him. [*Gss.*]

After a meal her feet are very heavy. [*Gss.*]

Immediately after a meal he is weary in every limb, and feels in the left side under the short ribs a tearing pressing; pressing upon it causes pain in the part. [*Gss.*]

285. Lazy and indolent throughout the body. [*Fr. H—n.*]

He is lazy and weary, yawns much and stretches himself as if he would go to sleep. [*Gss.*]

Great exhaustion after slight movement; after going upstairs he lay for a long time quite exhausted on the sofa before he could again move freely and speak. [*Stf.*]

She feels ill all over the body, cannot remain up, must lie down from weariness and heaviness of the limbs. [*Ts. Hb.*]

He fears he will fall to the ground so suddenly does weakness arise, particularly in the lower extremities; he staggers on the slightest movement of the body, but he seems to possess more firmness when walking (aft. 3 h.). [*Fz.*]

290. **Exhaustion**, giving way of the knees, and sensation like dull pain in them (aft. 1 h.). [*Ho.*]

Powerlessness of the body.[1] [MORGAGNI, l. c., Epist. x, art. 13.]

Incessant yawning for a quarter of an hour (aft. 1½ h.). [*Ho.*]

Drowsiness by day. [*Stf.*]

Irresistible drowsiness, in the forenoon.

295. Drowsiness all day. [*Fz.*]

Sleeplessness.[2] [MORGAGNI, Epist. xv, art. 6.]

Sleeplessness after midnight.

Restless sleep.

He wakes at night out of slumber with horrible dreams, and cannot remember where he is.

300. (Extraordinary fear of bed, in which, however, he lies down after all.) [*Fz.*]

At night, restless sleep, frequent waking, confused, sometimes anxious dreams, pollutions and after them sleep of exhaustion. [*Fz.*]

Dreams of misfortunes happening to others.

Dreams of disagreeable and frightful character, in which he is unsuccessful in everything, which causes him great anxiety. [*Gss.*]

He has every night confused dreams, which are, however, remembered after awaking. [*Gss.*]

305. Very vivid dreams of a horrible character, whereby, however, he

* Then ensued paralysis and death. Post-mortem examination showed pus in the kidneys, thickened lining membrane of the bladder, distension of the blood-vessels of the diaphragm, water in the convolutions of the brain, none in the cavities.

1 See note to S. 118.

2 In subject of S. 223. Much serum found in brain post mortem.

does not feel anxious, but always retains a sort of presence of mind. [*Gss.*]

In the morning after waking from an almost unbroken sleep, he is more weary than when he lay down the night before. [*Gss.*]

Very small pulse [1] [MORGAGNI, l. c., Epist. xxiv, art. 13.]

Slow, scarcely perceptible pulse. [*Ho.*]

Rigor. [2] [MORGAGNI, l. c., Epist. vii, art. 13.]

310. Fever, rigor with the most extreme thirst, and after drinking shivering, at the same time cold hands, knees and feet; therewith hurried disposition, trembling, contortion of the face; sometimes lachrymose, sometimes joyful, sometimes furious disposition; everything annoyed him, so that he got in a furious passion over it: during the rigor, some warmth in the back and feet, which perspired, but did not feel warm to the touch. [*Fz.*]

Chill with thirst, not followed by heat, and without perspiration, in the afternoon (after 52 h.).

The whole body is cold, but the face grows always warmer and warmer. [*Ho.*]

Warmth and feeling of warmth of the face. [*Ho.*]

Perspiration on the forehead and neck, at night.

315. Shudder passing over the trunk with a sensation of a certain discomfort, in short attacks. [*Gss.*]

Shudder runs over all the body, comes also on the head and draws as it were the hairs together. [*Gss.*]

Chilly for several hours (immediately). [*We.*]

He is cold to the feeling in the limbs and has rigor. [*Gss.*]

Ebullition of blood. [NEUHOLD, l. c.]

320. Nothing gives him pleasure; he is indifferent to everything. [*Fz.*]

Disposition in the forenoon dejected, in the afternoon cheerful.

Sadness.

Cheerfulness as from intoxication (aft. 1 h.). [*Ho.*]

Wavering and uncertain humour. [*Hl.*]

325. Mind anxious.

Apt to start at a slight noise (aft. 1¼ h.). [*Ho.*]

Peevish especially in the afternoon. [*Fr. H—n.*]

Sometimes gay, sometimes grave mania. [3] [MORGAGNI, l. c., Epist. vii, art 13.]

Very vexed and angry about trifles. [*Stf.*]

330. Sometimes furious mania, so that he spat in the faces of those around him.* [MORGAGNI, l. c.]

* After a poultice on the head, convulsions, subsultus tendinum, death. Post-mortem examination showed purulent deposits and pus in the lungs, pleuritis, and diaphragmitis, firm clots in the cavities of the heart.

---

1 See note to S. 100.
2 See note to S. 221.
3 In subject of S. 221.

CAPSICUM ANNUUM.[1]

(The ripe seed-capsules along with the seeds reduced to powder and digested in alcohol, in the proportion of 20 grains of the powder to 400 drops of alcohol, without heat, for a week, the mixture being shaken twice daily to form a tincture, twenty drops of which contain one grain of capsicum-powder.)

In both the Indies where "Spanish pepper" (*Piper Indicum sive Hispanicum*), as it is called, is indigenous, it is chiefly used only as a spice. It was introduced as such into England, France, and Italy, and at length was adopted in Germany as a spice to season sauces at the dainty tables of high livers (the pulverised seeds of the still more pungent *Capsicum baccatum*, "or "Cayenne pepper," being often used as a substitute) in order to stimulate the palate to an unnatural appetite, and thus—ruin the health.

In the meantime but little was heard of the medicinal use of this powerful substance. BERGIUS alone (*Mat. Med.*, p. 147) mentions having cured several agues of long standing with two-grain doses of capsicum ; but he did not give it alone, for the old original sin of traditional medicine, *the mixture craze*, induced him to combine it with bay berries, in the proportion of twenty of the latter to three of the former. He does not describe the agues cured by it according to the totality of their symptoms, but only employs the expression "old agues" after the manner of his other old school colleagues, so that the *virtus ab usu* of the mixture prescribed is shrouded in darkness.

On the other hand, the homœopathic physician proceeds much less doubtfully and with much greater certainty in his cures with capsicum, for guided by the peculiar, pure morbid states produced by this powerful medicinal substance in the healthy body (some of which I here record), he only attempts the removal of those natural diseases the sum of whose symptoms is contained in the greatest possible similarity among those of capsicum.

The diseases curable by capsicum are rarely met with in persons of tense fibre.

A very small portion of a drop of the tincture diluted to the trillion-fold degree—each diluting bottle having been only twice succussed—I have found to be quite sufficient for a dose for all homœopathic curative purposes; and as an antidote to diminish the over-strong action of a dose of capsicum in some very sensitive persons, I have found the olfaction of a saturated solution of camphor efficacious.

[HAHNEMANN was aided in this proving by AHNER, HARTUNG, MOSSDORF, and WISLICENUS.

1 From vol. vi, 2nd edit., 1827.

Symptoms are taken from the following old-school sources :
BROWNE, in *Murray's Appar. medic.*, i, 2nd edit.
FORDYCE, in *Murray's Appar. medic.*, i, 2nd edit.
PELARGUS, *Obs.*, tom. ii.
In the *Frag. de Vir.* capsicum has 147 symptoms, in the 1st Edit. 346, in this 2nd Edit. 344.]

CAPSICUM.

Intoxication.

When he wakes up from sleep, his head is so stupid as if he did not know himself.

Cloudiness of the head. [*Btg.*]

In the morning on awaking, dull in the head.

5. During the febrile rigor and coldness at the same time anxiety, dizziness and stupidity in the head, like thoughtlessness and awkwardness, so that she knocks against everything.

Emptiness and stupidity of the head (aft. 12 h.). [*Ar.*]

Dulness and **confusion of the head.** [*Ar.*]

Vertigo, swaying from side to side.

All the senses are more acute.*

10. **When moving the head and when walking, headache, as if the skull would burst.**

Throbbing, beating headache, in one of the temples.

Beating headache in the forehead.

A throbbing, beating headache.

Aching pain in the temples.

15. Aching pain in the temporal region. [*Btg.*]

Pressive pain in the forehead as if it pressed from the occiput forwards out at the forehead, with a cutting from the occiput forwards (immediately).

A continual pressive headache in the forehead above the root of the nose and occasionally some stitches through the ear and over the eye.

A semi-lateral, pressive shooting headache, like a hysterical megrim, which is aggravated by raising the eyes and head, or by bowing the head forwards, and is accompanied by forgetfulness and nausea.

Drawing tearing pain in the left side of the head (aft. 17, 48 h.). [*Ar.*]

20. A shooting headache.

A headache more shooting than tearing, which is worse when at rest, but mitigated by movement.

An outstretching headache, or as if the brain were too full.

A pressing-asunder headache in the forehead.

A drawing headache in the forehead.

25. **Drawing tearing pains in the frontal bone, more on the right side** (aft. 6, 7 h. and 3 d.). [*Ar.*]

Violent deeply-penetrating shooting in the crown. [*Ar.*]

* Reaction of the vital force of the organism, secondary action, curative action,

(Tearing headache.)

On the hairy scalp an eroding itching, as from vermin, which compelled scratching ; after the scratching the roots of the hair and the scalp were as painful as if the hair had been pulled out.

Slight shudder on the hairy part of the head, followed by a burning itching of the integuments of the head, which is diminished by scratching, but then returns with increased violence (aft. 2 h.). [*Htg.*]

30. Unusual redness of the face, without heat, but after half an hour a wretched appearance and pale complexion (aft. 3 h.). [*Htg.*]

Sweat on the forehead. [*Ar.*]

Facial pains, sometimes as pains in the bones, excitable by external touch, sometimes as fine pains penetrating through the nerves, which torment him when going to sleep.

(On the left side of the face pimples, with smarting sensation as from salt.)

In the face red points, and on the forehead a tetter with eroding itching (aft. 2 and 24 h.).

35. Very dilated pupils.

Great dilatation of the pupils. [*Ar.*]

Pressure on the eyes so that he cannot open them wide enough. [*Ar.*]

Eyes projecting out of the head with paleness of face (aft. 16 h.).

An aching pain in the eyes as from a foreign body.

40. In the morning a burning in the eyes, which are red and water.

Fine shooting pain in the eyes.*

Inflammation of the eyes.

In the morning a dimness of vision, as if a foreign substance swam upon the cornea and obscured it, so that by rubbing the eye the transparency can be restored for some instants.

All objects appear black before the eyes.

45. Vision almost quite extinguished, like blindness.

Tearing in the concha of the ear.

An itching pain quite deep in the ear (aft. 16 h.).

An aching pain quite deep in the ear (aft. 1 and 8 h.).

On the petrous bone behind the ear a swelling, painful to the touch.

50. Tearing pain behind the left ear (aft. 6 h.). [*Ar.*]

A pain under the ear.

(An itching mingled with stitches in the nose.)

Contractive twitching pains in the left side of the nose to above the left eye (aft. 5 h.). [*Ar.*]

Burning tensive sensation on the left nostril, as if a pimple would come there. [*Mss.*]

55. **Epistaxis** in the morning in bed, and afterwards frequent blowing of blood from the nose.

Bloody nasal mucus.

Painful pimples under the nostrils.

* From the exhalation.

Burning in the lips. [*Mss.*]

Ulcerated eruption on the lips—not in the angles—which is painful only on moving the part.

60. Swollen lips.

Rough lips.

Chaps on the lips ; fissured lips.

Pains on the left side of the lower jaw, as from a boil or an ulcer, for three-quarters of an hour. [*Ar.*]

Swelling of the gums.

65. Drawing pain in the gums.

A drawing pain in the tooth, which, however, is not increased either by touching the tooth or by eating.

The teeth feel to him as if lengthened and elvated, and as if on edge.

Eruption of pimples on the inside of the cheeks.

On the tip of the tongue, pimples, which when touched cause shooting pain.

70. Flow of saliva.

Twitching tearing pain in the right cervical glands. [*Ar.*]

Pain when swallowing, as in inflammation of the throat, but when not swallowing a drawing pain in the œsophagus.

Pain in the upper part of the œsophagus, when not swallowing, as if the parts were sore and spasmodically drawn together, as in water-brash.

A simple pain in the fauces, only when coughing.

75. In the palate a pain, as if it were pressed or pinched by something hard, at first more when not swallowing, afterwards more whilst swallowing (aft. 1½ h.).

Spasmodic contraction of the œsophagus.

Dryness in the mouth.

On the anterior part of the tongue, a dry feeling, without thirst, in the morning (aft. 8 h.).

Adipsia.

80. **Viscid mucus in the mouth** (aft. 2 h.).

Taste in the mouth as from foul water.

Insipid, qualmish, earthy taste (*e.g.* of butter).

Watery insipid taste in the mouth, then heart-burn.

Heart-burn.

85. Eructation from the stomach only when walking, and at every eructation a stitch in the side ; when sitting no eructations and hence no stitch.

An astringent, sourish taste in the mouth.

Sour taste in the mouth.

Sour taste of soup (aft. 2 h.).

Qualmishness in the stomach (aft. 1 h.).

90. A coldness in the stomach ; a sensation as if cold water were in it—followed by a sensation as if he trembled.

Want of hunger, anorexia.

When he would eat he must force himself to do so ; he has no appetite, although food tasted all right.

After a meal, frequent yawning.

Longing for coffee (aft. 8 h.).

95. Nausea with inclination to vomit, and spitting of saliva after drinking coffee.

Inclination to vomit.

Qualmishness and inclination to vomit in the scrobiculus cordis in the morning and afternoon (aft. 24 h.).

Aching in the scrobiculus cordis, with inclination to vomit.

After a meal, fulness and anxiety in the chest; thereafter sour eructation or heart-burn—finally thin stool.

100. After a meal (at noon), immediately stool with redness of the cheeks (aft. 6 h.).

Immediately after a meal, at noon and evening, a burning over the scrobiculus cordis.

A burning in the stomach up into the mouth, after breakfast.

Deep in the abdomen, a pain in the bowels more burning than shooting—with simultaneous cutting in the umbilical region—when moving, especially when stooping and walking, with ill humour on account of the pain and discontent and tendency to weep about lifeless things (not about persons or moral subjects), and during the crossness a kind of anxiety with perspiration on the face.

An aching tension in the abdomen, especially the epigastric region, between the scrobiculus cordis and navel, which is particularly increased by movement, at the same time with an aching tension in the lower part of the back.

105. Distension of the abdomen two hours after eating; followed by a headache darting towards the occiput, and profuse perspiration.

A tensive pain from the abdomen to the chest, as from distension of the abdomen.

Distension and hardness of the abdomen; she could not bear any tight clothing.

Sensation as if the abdomen was distended almost to bursting, whereby the breathing is impeded to suffocation.

A rumbling in the abdomen going upwards and downwards.

110. Grumbling in the abdomen from flatulence (aft. 1 h.).

Pinching in the epigastrium.

An aching under the short ribs, and in the scrobiculus cordis.

Fine quick stitches in the scrobiculus cordis (aft. some m.). [*Ws.*]

Aching pain in the scrobiculus cordis. [*Ar.*]

115. In the scrobiculus cordis, a pinching, out-boring pain, especially when sitting bent forwards, lasting severely for eight minutes (aft. 1½ h.). [*Ar.*]

Uncommonly strong pulsation of the blood-vessels of the abdomen. [*Htg.*]

A hard pressing almost shooting pain on a small spot in the left hypogastrium (aft. 1 h.).

An aching here and there in the abdomen.

Increased internal heat in the bowels. [*Htg.*]

120. Aching pinching pain in the belly immediately after a meal, like incarcerated flatulence.

Bellyache as from flatulence in the hypogastrium.

The flatulence move about painfully in the abdomen.

Much flatulence. [*Ar.*]

Painless rumbling in the abdomen. [*Htg.*]

125. Along with cutting colic twisting round the navel, diarrhœic evacuations of viscid mucus sometimes mingled with black blood; after every stool thirst, and after every drink shuddering.

A drawing and turning over in the abdomen, without and with diarrhœa.

A flatulent hernia comes forcibly and with pain out at the inguinal ring.

After some flatulent colic in the hypogastrium, small frequent stools which consist of mucus sometimes intermixed with blood, and cause tenesmus.

Slimy diarrhœa with tenesmus.

130. Immediately, diarrhœa; and shortly afterwards, ineffectual urging to stool.

Small stools, consisting of nothing but mucus.

Small stools of bloody mucus.

Tenesmus.

Tenesmus. [BROWNE,[1] in ***Murray, Appar. Medic.*** i, edit. sec., p. 703.]

135. Along with pressive pain in the bowels, he has urging to stool, but he is costive. [*Ar.*]

After drinking he must go to stool, though he is costive, but only mucus is passed. [*Ar.*]

As soon as he has drunk something he feels as if diarrhœa would come on, but every time only a little is passed. [*Ar.*]

Constipation, as if there was too much heat in the abdomen.

Burning pain in the anus (after 3, 4, 8 h.).

140. Burning at the anus. [BROWNE, l. c.]

Itching in the anus (aft. 3, 4, 8 h.).

Smarting, shooting pain in the anus, with the diarrhœic stool.

Blind hæmorrhoids; vascular knots at the anus, which cause severe pain during the evacuation.

Piles at the anus, which sometimes itch.

145. Discharge of blood by the anus for four days.

Strangury, tenesmus of the neck of the bladder; he has urging to frequent, almost ineffectual urination (aft. 4, 8 h.).

Spasmodic contraction, with cutting pain, at the neck of the bladder—not exactly like urging to urinate—sometimes intermitting, sometimes recurring, in the morning in bed; it seems to be somewhat allayed by urinating (aft. 24 h.). [*Ws.*]

The urine is passed only with great difficulty by drops and in spurts (immediately and for a long time).

---

1 General statement.

Frequent urging to urinate, chiefly when sitting, not when walking (aft. 42 h.).

150. **Scalding of urine.**

After urinating a burning, smarting pain in the urethra (aft. 7 d.).

A burning in the mouth of the urethra immediately before, during, and one minute after urinating.

Pain in the urethra, especially in the forenoon.

Immediately after urinating a fine shooting in the orifice of the urethra.

155. When not urinating, pricking as with needles in the fore part of the urethra (aft. 8 h.).

When not urinating, severe stitches in the orifice of the urethra.

When not urinating, a cutting pain in the urethra backwards (aft. 6 h.).

The urethra is painful when touched (aft. 7 d.).

The urine deposits a white sediment.

160. A constant aching and prickling in the glans penis, especially in the morning and evening.

A fine, itching pricking on the glans penis, like gnat bites. [*Ar.*]

In the morning, on awaking, coldness of the scrotum.

Coldness of the scrotum and impotence.

Seminal emission at night.

165. A drawing pain in the spermatic cord and a squeezing pain in the testicle whilst urinating, and for some time afterwards (aft. 48 h.).

Erection in the forenoon, afternoon, and evening.

Stiffness of the penis, in the morning in bed without amorous thoughts.

Violent erection, in the morning on getting up, only to be allayed by cold water.

During amorous toying, an uncontrollable trembling of the whole body (aft. 24 h.).

170. Purulent discharge from the urethra, a kind of gonorrhœa.

Urethral blennorrhœa.* [FORDYCE, in *Murray, App. Med.*, i, edit. sec., p. 704.]

(The gonorrhœa becomes yellow and thick) (aft. 7 d.).

During the menstrual flux, aching in the scrobiculus cordis with inclination to vomit.

* * *

Creeping and tickling in the nose, as in stuffed coryza.

175. Burning formication in the nose, with violent sneezing and flow of mucus† (immediately). [*Ws.*]

Violent, shaking sneezing, with discharge of thin mucus from the nose. (immediately). [*Mss.*]

Stuffed coryza.

Hoarseness.

Feeling of roughness in the throat, for nearly two days. [*Mss.*]

* From wearing on the abdomen next the skin a linen bag filled with the powdered seeds of the Capsicum baccatum.

† From the exhalations.

180. Tickling sensation in the wind-pipe, so that he must sneeze violently several times. [*Ar.*]

Continual stitches in the throat in the region of the epiglottis, which excite dry cough, that, however, does not remove them. [*Mss.*]

Mucus in the upper part of the wind-pipe, which must be expectorated from time to time by hawking and voluntary tussiculation (aft. 3 h.).

Very frequent short cough.

Dry, frequent, short cough.

185. Cough, especially towards evening (from 5 to 9 o'clock).

In the evening, after lying down, a formication and tickling in the larynx, and dry short cough.

Cough, especially after drinking coffee.

Painful cough.

Only when coughing, a pain in the throat, as from a simply painful swelling.

190. Only during the fit of coughing, an aching pain in the throat, as if an abscess were about to burst there.

When coughing headache, as if the skull would burst.

The cough causes inclination to vomit.

Fits of coughing in the afternoon (about 5 o'clock), which cause nausea and vomiting.

With every cough a pressive pain in the ear, as if an abscess would burst there.

195. When coughing a drawing pain in the side of the chest extending up to the throat.

When coughing a deep pressing-in pain on the side of the thigh extending into the knee.

From coughing or sneezing a pain darts through one or other limb.

Whilst coughing and some time afterwards a pressing towards the bladder and some stitches from within outwards in the region of the neck of the bladder. [*Mss.*]

The air from the lungs, when coughing, causes a strange disagreeable taste in the mouth.

200. The cough forces an ill-smelling breath from the lungs.

Pain in the ribs and sternum when fetching a breath.

Pain on the chest, under the right arm, when he touches the place or raises the arm.

A single prick in the left side of the chest, between the third and fourth ribs, as with a blunt needle. [*Ar.*]

Stitches in the left side, at the fifth and sixth ribs (aft. 1 h.). [*Ar.*]

205. Single stitches in the left side of the chest, between the second and third ribs (aft. 5 h.). [*Ar.*]

Shooting in the left side, which takes away his breath (aft. 10 h.) [*Ar.*]

Shooting in the left side of the chest when fetching a breath, between the third and fourth ribs. [*Ar.*]

(Simple pain on a rib, on a small spot, which is worst when touching it, but is not excited either by breathing or by coughing).

When coughing pain like shooting in the side of the chest and in the back.

210. When breathing a shooting pain between the scapullæ and in the region of the stomach, and single stitches in the side of the abdomen, on the ensiform cartilage and in the sternum—pains which do not penetrate, however, but appear to be superficial only.

When breathing, whilst walking, a stitch in the side of the chest; not when sitting.

In the region of the heart several violent stitches, so that he was inclined to cry out.

Anxiety compelling him to breathe deeply.

An involuntary, strong expiratory impulse.

215. He must often draw a single very deep breath, whereby he imagines that he feels alleviation of all his sufferings.

Deep breathing, almost like a sigh.

A pain in the chest when sitting, as if the chest were too full and there was not room enough in it.

Tightness of chest even when at rest, with stiffness of the back, which hurts when stooping forwards, while occasionally a deep sighing inspiration and dry cough occur.

Asthma, feeling of fulness of the chest.

220. **Tightness of chest, which appears to come out of the stomach.**

Easier respiration from day to day.*

Tightness of chest, with redness of face, eructations, and sensation as if the chest were distended.

Tightness of chest when at rest and when moving.

He can only breathe when his body is erect—orthopnœa.

225. **Pain as if the chest were constricted which oppresses the breath, and is increased on very slight movement.**

A pain, like pressure on the chest, on breathing deeply and turning the body.

Tightness of chest when walking.

A throbbing pain in the chest.

An aching pain in the side of the chest on which she lies.

230. In the sacrum a dragging-down pain when standing and moving, with bruised pain.

Pain in the back on stooping.

Drawing pain in the back.

Drawing, aching pain in the back.

Drawing tearing pain in and near the spine. [*Ar.*]

235. Sudden, drawing shooting pain in the middle of the spine. [*Ar.*]

Stiffness in the nape, which is diminished by movement.

* Reaction of the vital force of the organism, secondary action, curative action.

Painful stiffness in the nape, only felt on moving it.

Feeling of weakness over the whole nape, as if it were loaded (aft. 4 h.). [*Htg.*]

A twitching pain in the nape.

240. A pain externally in the neck.

Sweat under the shoulders (aft. 8 h.).

The shoulder-joint pains as if dislocated.

(Drawing, paralytic pain above and below the elbow-joint.)

Drawing, tearing pain, which extends from the right clavicle over the whole of the right arm to the finger tips, for three minutes. [*Ar.*]

245. Shooting in the left elbow-joint, which darted into the hand with flying heat, causing the arm to feel as if asleep. [*Ar.*]

Vibrating pain in the left forearm. [*Ar.*]

Twitching, quivering, painful sensation in the left palm (aft. 8 h.). [*Ar.*]

Contractive pain in the left index finger. [*Ar.*]

Violent, deep stitches in the ball of the left little finger. [*Htg.*]

250. Fine shooting pain in the skin of the wrist.*

Cool sweat in the hands (aft. 3 h.).

A drawing pain in the hip-joint (a pain like stiff-neck), which is aggravated by touching and by bending the body backwards.

From the hip-joint to the feet, a shooting tearing pain, especially on coughing.

In the muscles of the thigh, pain like aching and dislocation.

255. Bruised pain in the right thigh, going off on walking, but returning when at rest. [*Ar.*]

Dislocation-pain in the right thigh ; when he separates the thighs outwards, the pain is severe there, but not otherwise. [*Ar.*]

Convulsive jerking and twitching sometimes of the thigh, sometimes of the forearm. [*Htg.*]

Tearing pain on the inner side of the left thigh. [*Ar.*]

Drawing, shooting, digging pain in the middle of the posterior aspect of the left thigh, going off by movement. [*Ar.*]

260. **Tensive pain in the knee.**

An internal pain compounded of drawing and shooting in the left leg. [*Htg.*]

Stiffness in the calves when walking.

(Bruised pain of the os calcaneum, as if the heel were numbed or bruised by a great leap, sometimes changing into a tearing, in fits) (aft. 2 h.).

Single stitches in the right big toe, ceasing on stamping the foot. [*Ar.*]

265. Shooting out at the tips of the toes.

For many hours, transient drawing pains here and there in the limbs, in the back, in the nape, in the scapulæ, and in the hands, which are excited by moving.

Cracking and grating of the knee and finger-joints.

In all the joints sensation of stiffness and simple pain, worst on

* From the exhalations.

commencing to move, but allayed by continuing to move—together with catarrh of viscid mucus in the wind-pipe.

In the morning, on rising, he feels as if all the joints had been broken on the wheel, a laming stiff pain on commencing to move, especially in the knees and ankle-joints, allayed by continuing to move (aft. 10 h.).

270. When he has lain all the joints are as if stiff, and in the morning on getting out of bed he feels as if all joints were broken on the wheel, the lameness in the knees and ankle-joints especially is much worse after resting than when he is moving.

All the joints are painful as if dislocated, with the sensation as if they were swollen.

Cramp at first in the left arm and then in the whole body; the arms were stiff, she could not straighten them, the feet also were stiff on rising up after sitting, as if asleep and formicating.

Transient aching pains now in one part, now in another.

A crawling here and there in the skin of the body, as if from a fly.

275. Sensation all over the body as if all the parts would go to sleep.*

Formicating sensation in the arms and in the lower extremities, from the foot up to the gullet.

An itching here and there in the skin, but chiefly in the face and on the nose.

(Itching only after touching the part.)

Itching in the hairs of the head and on small parts on the rest of the body, which goes off on scratching gently.

280. Shooting, burning itching all over the body, but chiefly on the chest and face. [*Htg.*]

Corrosive burning on several tender parts (lips, mouth, nose, tip of the nose, alæ nasi, eyelids, &c.).† [*Ws.*]

(Red, round spots on the abdomen and thighs.)

A painless sensation running upwards and downwards in the body, with redness of the cheeks.

Lassitude in the limbs, but more when at rest and when sitting.

285. Weakness and heaviness of the limbs, followed by trembling of the upper extremities and knees; his hands fail him for writing (aft. 7 h.). [*Htg.*]

Great weariness, but not inviting sleep (aft. 2 h.).

Greater weariness in the morning than in the evening.

Trembling weakness in the feet.

Complete prostration of the strength.

290. (Clucking, quick throbbing in some large blood-vessels) (aft. 24 h.). [*Htg.*]

He shuns all movement.

Sleep full of dreams.

Dreams of a sad character of things long passed; on awaking he did not know if it was a reality or not.

Dreams full of obstacles.

* Inhaling sulphur vapour soon relieved this.

† From the exhalations.

295. Sleep interrupted by crying out and starting as if he fell from a height.

During sleep he snores when inspiring by the nose, as if he could not get air through it, and his breath were taken away (aft. 1 h.).

He wakes up several times after midnight.

Complete waking up after midnight and later.

He is wide awake in the night and cannot sleep (aft. 5, 9 h.).

300. The disinclination for everything and the crossness go off by sleep.*

Yawning, almost uninterrupted (aft. $\frac{1}{2}$ h.).

Cool air, and especially a draught, is disagreeable to him ; he cannot bear them (aft. 12 h.).

Gradually diminished temperature of the body.

Coldness on the whole body ; the limbs are cold, without shivering.

305. As the coldness of the body increases† so also does the ill-humour and the contraction of the pupils.

Every time after drinking shivering and rigor.

In the evening, after lying down, uncommon chilliness, followed by coryza (aft. 72 h.).

Evening chilliness.

The feet to up above the ankles are cold and cannot be warmed, along with ordinary temperature of the rest of the body, in the morning (aft. 12 h.). [*Ws.*]

310. He is chilled by letting a little air in under the bed-clothes.

When walking in the open air sensation on the thighs as if they were covered with cold sweat (as when cold air comes in contact with a perspiring part), and yet the thighs did not perspire.

He trembles with chilliness.

In the evening shivering and chilliness in the back, not followed by heat or thirst, but yet by slight perspiration.

(Febrile rigor in the evening, with thirst (without heat, yawning, or stretching), with great exhaustion, short breath, drowsiness, and crossness ; from the smallest movement shivering, without feeling of cold, and without being actually cold, yet it did not feel too warm in a hot room.)

315. The first night chilliness and coldness ; the next night sweat all over.

In the morning sweat all over.

After general heat and perspiration, without thirst, which lasted some hours, shivering at 6 p.m., with shaking and chattering of teeth —at the same time he was thirsty and cold all over, with anxiety, restlessness, want of recollection, and intolerance of noise—similar shivering, rigor, and coldness, with thirst, the following evening about 7 o'clock.

* Reaction of the vital force of the organism, curative action.

† I have seen it increase from capsicum for 11 hours, and it took 12 hours longer to decline and go off entirely.

Heat, and at the same time shivering, with thirst for water.

Heat in the face and redness, with trembling of the limbs (immediately).

320. At noon, after eating, glowing cheeks, with cold hands and feet, without shivering—recurring on two days at the same time.

Red cheeks.

The face is alternately pale and, along with the lobes of the ears, red, with a sensation of burning, but no particular heat is felt with the hand.

(Burning on the hands, feet, and cheeks, which latter are swollen.)

Heat in the hands, but not on the other parts of the body. [*Ar.*]

325. Hot ears, and hot, red tip of the nose, towards evening.

(Internal heat, with cold sweat on the forehead.)

He is silently wrapped up in his own thoughts.

He is indifferent to everything.

Disinclination for work or thinking. [*Htg.*]

330. He is quiet, sullen, and obstinate.

Anxiety and anguish almost to death. [PELARGUS,[1] *Obs.*, tom. ii, p. 206.]

Repugnance and crossness.

Resistance, with howling (aft. 3 h.).

He makes reproaches, and is indignant at the faults of others; he takes trifles ill and finds fault with them.

335. In the midst of joking he takes the slightest trifle in bad part.

He can get angry very easily.

A restless, over-busy disposition.

Disposition to start (aft. 2 h.).

Variable humour; sometimes constantly laughing, and then again weeping.

340. Jocular, given to witticisms.

He is of contented disposition, is jocular and sings, and yet on the slightest cause he is disposed to get angry (aft 4 h.).

Contentedness.*

Staid, easy humour.*

Quiet state of the disposition.* [*Htg.*]

* Curative action, reaction of the organism.

---

1 Poisoning of a girl of 13. It was the observer who feared that death would result.

CARBO ANIMALIS[1]

(*Animal charcoal.*)

(In order to prepare animal charcoal, thick piece of ox-leather is placed among red-hot coals, and allowed to burn until the last flame has completely expired, and then the red-hot piece of leather is quickly placed betwixt two stone plates, so as to extinguish it immediately, otherwise it would continue to smoulder in the air, and thus dissipate the greater portion of its charcoal. A grain of this is triturated with 100 grains of milk-sugar in a porcelain mortar for an hour (every ten minutes being divided between six minutes of trituration and four minutes of scraping); of this product one grain is again triturated in a similar manner with 100 grains of milk-sugar, and of the powder thus made one grain is again triturated for an hour in the same manner with 100 grains of fresh milk-sugar, in order to produce the million-fold potentized attenuation of carbo-animalis.)

Although the animal charcoal presents so much similarity in its effects on the human health to the vegetable charcoal, yet there are so many differences from the latter in it, and so many peculiar symptoms, that I consider it useful to record here what I have observed from it.

Some symptoms were observed by a Russian physician, Dr. Adam; these I have indicated by the letters *Ad.*

A very small portion of a grain of the million-fold ($\frac{I}{I}$) pulverulent attenuation is usually quite sufficient for a dose and acts for at least three weeks in chronic diseases. Camphor proved itself an antidote and alleviating remedy for its too energetic action in highly sensitive persons.

[Besides ADAM, above mentioned, HAHNEMANN got a few symptoms from WEISE in *Rust's Magazin f. d. gesammte Heilk.*, vol. xxii. This medicine makes its first appearance in the 2nd Edit., where its symptoms are 191; in the *Chr. Kr.* there are 728, 214 of these being selected from the 254 symptoms in HARTLAUB and TRINKS'S *R.A.M.L.*, and 23 contributed by WAHLE.]

CARBO ANIMALIS.

Vertigo: it becomes black before her eyes.

Vertigo with nausea, on rising up after stooping.

Vertigo: towards evening (7 o'clock) when she raised up her head all went round in a circle with her; she must always sit in a stooping posture, and when she rose up she staggered to and fro; she felt dull in the head and as if all objects moved; while lying all night long she felt nothing of it—but did so in the morning again on getting up.

Sensation in the head, as on coming out of great cold into a room and going up close to a hot stove—a sensation as if there was something heavy in the forehead, or as if a board was before the head.

1 From vol. vi, 2nd edit., 1827.

5. In the morning, on awaking, headache, as after drinking much wine.

Heaviness of the head. [*Ad.*]

The head, especially **the occiput** (and the left temple) **is heavy** and confused. [*Ad.*]

Rush of blood to the head with confusion of the head.

Aching pain in the occiput. [*Ad.*]

10. Aching pain on a small spot in the occiput.

Headache : aching in both temples.

On the lower part of the temple a pinching pain. [*Ad.*]

Boring pain in the temporal bone extending into the zygomatic process. [*Ad.*]

Boring drawing pains in the head accompanied by tearings ; when the head becomes cold it is worse, especially towards the ear (aft. 7 d.).

15. Shooting in the head, especially in the temple.

Severe tearing in the external parts of the head.

Tearing on the right side of the head.

The left side of the head is painful as if festering.

Anything upon the head pressed him ; his neck-cloth also oppressed him (aft. 18 d.).

20. At night, pain on the head and neck as if both were gone to sleep and dislocated.

Falling out of the hair (aft. 12 d.).

Feeling as if something lay in the forehead above the eyes, so that he cannot look upwards. (aft. 6 h.),

Pressive shooting pain from above downwards above the left eye, the eye-lid, and upper part of the eye-ball. [*Ad.*]

(Shooting in the eyes.)

25. Aching in the eyes in the evening by artificial light.

Aching in the inner canthus (aft. 72 h.).

In the evening the eyes are hurt by the light.

Weakness in the eyes.

In the outer canthus sore burning pain.

30. Disagreeable sensation in the left eye as if something had flown into it, which interferes with vision ; he must always be wiping it ; at the same time the pupil is extremely dilated with great long-sightedness—he could not distinctly recognise any object held near him.

Coppery eruption on the face.* [*Rust's Magaz.*, *f. d. gesammte Heilk.*,[1] vol. xxii, pt. i, p. 198.]

Pimples on the face in quantities without sensation.

Eruption on the cheek like red spots.

Frequently flying heat in the cheeks, with redness.

35. In the afternoon heat of face and head.

* The author prepared his animal charcoal in rather a different manner. He took any kind of flesh freed from fat, added one third by weight of bone to it, and roasted the mixture in an ordinary coffee roaster.

1 Statement from observation (by Weise).

(Smarting of the skin on the cheeks, about the mouth, and on the chin, after shaving). [*Ad.*]

Cramp-pain in the interior of the left ear. [*Ad.*]

Cramp in the ear down towards the gullet on the left side, whereby swallowing was rendered difficult. [*Ad.*]

Drawing in the ear.

40. At night constant ringing in the ears.

Behind the right ear a sort of periosteal swelling, with shooting therein every evening from 5 o'clock onwards.

Swelling in the parotid glands. [*Rust's Magaz.*, l. c.]

Epistaxis (in the morning when sitting).

Nose and mouth swollen.

45. Blisters on the lower lip.

Chapped lips.

Stiffness on the left side of the neck.

The cervical glands are swollen.

The gums are red and swollen and very painful.

50. Pain in the lower gums and looseness of the lower teeth.

Looseness of the teeth and tearing in them, most violent in the evening in bed.

Great looseness of the teeth, so that he cannot chew the softest food without pain (aft. 12 d.).

The upper and lower teeth are loose and too long.

The hollow tooth is dully sensitive and as if projecting ; it is painful when biting and still more in the evening in bed, with much saliva in the mouth.

55. In the teeth a drawing to and fro, also in the front teeth.

Drawing in the teeth, with flying heat in the face.

Vesicles on the tongue which are painful as if burnt.

Blisters in the mouth which cause burning (aft. 21 d.).

(Burning feeling in the throat.)

60. An aching in the throat and dryness on the tongue.

Aching in the throat, only when swallowing.

Internal aching in the gullet down to the stomach.

Bad smell from the mouth.

Bitter taste every morning.

65. Sometimes bitterness in the mouth.

Bitter foul taste in the mouth.

Bitter sour taste in the mouth.

Sour taste in the mouth (aft. 5 d.).

(The appetite quickly goes off while eating.)

70. On commencing to eat, internal chilliness.

After eating a little, with good appetite, soon fulness of the stomach. [*Ad.*]

After eating, aching in the stomach.

After eating, tightness of the chest.

Soon after eating, anxiety and uneasiness in the back, without pain.

75. After eating, palpitation of the heart.

Eructation, with the taste of food that had been long eaten.

Several times eructation. [*Ad.*]

Towards evening qualmishness in the abdomen, with heat rising up (aft. 10 d.).

After much walking, when he comes to sit down, nausea.

80. Aching in the stomach, even when fasting.

Severe aching in the stomach, in the evening, after lying down in bed ; in order to relieve herself she must press her on the gastric region (aft. 16 h.).

On breathing deeply a quick, short, pressive pain in the scrobiculus cordis. [*Ad.*]

In the scrobiculus cordis pain, as after violent coughing (as if bruised) (aft. 6 d.).

Clucking in the stomach. [*Ad.*]

85. **Audible rumbling in the stomach** in the morning on waking. [*Ad.*]

Pressure in the liver, even when lying.

A severe aching pain in the liver, almost like cutting, the region even externally felt as if sore when touched.

A heavy weight in the abdomen like a lump, also when fasting, for several days.

Painful tension in the abdomen, with pain under the ribs, on touching, as if there were a sore there and the parts were festering (aft. 18 d.).

90. Great distension of the abdomen.

The abdomen is always very distended with flatulence.

He is very much troubled with flatulence.

When walking burning in the abdomen.

Cutting in the abdomen, in the forenoon.

95. Pain in the abdomen, as if diarrhœa would come on. [*Ad.*]

Audible rumbling in the abdomen and stomach (immediately). [*Ad.*]

Audible rumbling and grumbling in the large intestine, which then rose to beneath the stomach, and then went down again. [*Ad.*]

After drinking (warm milk), rumbling and grumbling in the right hypogastrium, sometimes above, sometimes below, with ineffectual desire to discharge flatus. [*Ad.*]

(Fermentation in the bowels.)

100. The hernia comes out, and is painful when walking, moving, and touching.

Rumbling in the rectum. [*Ad.*]

Frequent discharge of fetid flatus (while walking, after supper). [*Ad.*]

Frequent pressing on the rectum, but only flatus comes, and then the pressing returns immediately.

Frequent but ineffectual urging to stool in the lower part of the rectum. [*Ad.*]

105. After 24 hours only a scanty stool, hard, and in small pieces.

Before the stool a drawing from the anus through the pudendum (aft. 22 d.).

During the stool tearing from the pudendum internally up into the abdomen (after 22 d.).

(During the evacuation of the stool pains like needle-pricks in the anus.). [*Ad.*]

After the second stool on the same day a great weakness and pain in the bowels, as if they were screwed together.

110. Painful contraction of the anus (aft. 27 d.).

After the stool she had urging to pass urine (which smelt strongly), thereafter she became quite weak and early drowsy, but after lying down she could not sleep; she jumped up again immediately, and after waking she had ringing in the ears as though she should faint; thereafter rigor.

A sticky, odourless moisture passes out of the rectum.

A sticky, odourless moisture exudes in great quantity behind the scrotum from the perinæum.

(He excoriates the nates readily when riding; large blisters appear.)

115. A boil appears on the anus (aft. 16 d.).

Great swelling of the hæmorrhoidal vessels, which are the seat of burning pains when walking.

Tearing transversely across the os pubis and then through the pudendum to the anus (aft. 14 d.).

Pressure on the bladder at night.

Sudden call to urinate. [*Ad.*]

120. The discharge of urine becomes much more copious.

In the morning after waking very profuse discharge of urine (aft. 13 d.).

On slightly pressing, the urine is discharged almost against his will (aft. 16 d.).

Nocturnal seminal emission—for the first time for a long period—with lecherous dreams, without stiffness of penis, and after waking a spasmodic pain along the urethra, especially at its back part. [*Ad.*]

Leucorrhœa (aft. 14 d.).

125. Leucorrhœa which stains the linen yellow (aft. 21 d.).

* * *

Fluent coryza (aft. 10 d.).

Stuffed coryza; he cannot get air through the nose.

Above the nose sensation as at the beginning of a cold in the head—after eating; in the evening this sensation increased. [*Ad.*]

In the wind pipe pain as after much coughing.

130. In the morning, dryness of the throat and coughing therefrom; as soon as mucus is expectorated the cough is gone.

Cough with expectoration.

(Cough which takes away the breath, as if the breath would remain away.)

In the evening, hacking cough, especially in the evening in bed.

In the morning, anxiety on the chest.

135. After a meal, tightness of the chest.

When sitting and writing she gets shooting under the right breast so that she cannot sit quietly on account of it; after rising up it goes off.

In the evening in bed for an hour rattling and wheezing in the chest.

Painful nodes in the breasts. [*Rust's Magazin.* l. c.]

Feeling of coldness in the chest (aft. 7 d.).

140. In the evening, palpitation of the heart without anxiety (aft. 24 d.).

On the coccyx pain, and on touching the part there occurs a burning pain.

In the sacrum a severe stitch.

On breathing deeply, shooting above the sacrum.

Low down in the back, pain.

145. Tension in the nape.

Stiffness in the nape.

Both axillæ secrete very much moisture (aft. 22 d.).

Severe itching in the right axilla.

(A digging down in the arm, as if it worked about in the bone; when she lies on this arm she feels less of it.)

150. Drawing pain in the arms and hands.

The wrist-joint is as if dislocated.

Pain in the wrist-joints, like stiffness, on moving them.

Every day, **the hand goes to sleep**.

The left hand is numb in the morning in bed, this goes off after rising.

155. First the fingers, then the whole hand also, go to sleep.

Tearing in the hands (aft. 10 d.).

The middle joints of the fingers are painful on bending them.

In the proximal joint of the middle finger, a stiffness, on moving.

Itching on a wart on the finger.

160. (In the muscles of the thigh, drawing and tearing.)

When walking some painful stitches in the left hough. [*Ad.*]

At night a painless drawing up the leg.

Jerking drawing on the tibia. [*Ad.*]

Painful tension in the calves, whe walking.

165. For several days, in the morning, cramp in the calves.

One leg bends under him when walking, as from weakness of the joint.

In the morning prickling formication, as if asleep, in the feet.

Inflammatory swelling on the foot which breaks out on one toe.

In the morning the ball of the big toe is swollen; there is much heat in it, and it is painful as if it had been frost-bitten, and as if ulcerated.

170. Great itching of the toes that had once been frost-bitten (aft. 24 d.).

Cramp very often in the toes, by day; on walking on an uneven road they seemed as if they bent under him.

All her limbs are as if numb, especially also the head.

Aching pains in the joints and muscles.

Itching spreads over the whole body, especially in the evening in bed.

175. (At night much pain in the joints) (aft. 20 h.).

At night very vivid dreams. [*Ad.*]

Vivid dreams about scientific subjects; straining of the thinking faculty when dreaming; he composed literary essays in thought and spoke aloud. [*Ad.*]

Sleep full of vivid fancies.

Sleep very restless with frequent waking.

180. Very restless night; about 2.30 a.m. no more sleep on account of internal restlessness.

Sleep very restless; he was very much excited, and could not get to sleep before 2 a.m.

In the morning he can scarcely get warm.

From 9 a.m. until 3 p.m. very cold feet.

In the evening cold hands and cold feet.

185. In the evening **very cold feet,** when she went to bed (aft. 10 h.).

In the evening, in bed, chilly; then sweat during sleep.

At night heat and moisture on the skin (aft. 18 d.).

Profuse night-sweat (aft. 6 d.).

At first indifferent, afterwards increased excitability of the disposition for emotional impressions. [*Ad.*]

190. Takes things in bad part. [*Ad.*]

Extraordinarily gay. [*Ad.*]

CARBO VEGETABILIS.[1]

(Wood-charcoal.)

(The charcoal of any kind of wood, thoroughly heated to redness, manifests a uniformity in its effects on the human health, after adequate disengagement and development (potentization) of its innate medicinal spirit by trituration with a non-medicinal substance (*e.g.* milk-sugar) in the manner I have recorded above when speaking of carbo animalis. I employed the charcoal of birch wood. Some of the provings of others were made with the charcoal of red beech wood.)

From the earliest times physicians have considered charcoal to be non-medicinal and powerless. Empiricism only placed among the ingredients of her highly composite powders for epilepsy, the charcoal of lime-wood, without being able to adduce any evidence of the efficacy of this substance by itself. It is only in recent times, since LOWITZ, of St. Petersburg, discovered the chemical properties of wood charcoal, especially its power of removing from putrid and mouldy substances their bad smell, and of preserving fluids from fœtid odours, that physicians began to employ it externally. They advised rinsing of the mouth with powdered charcoal in cases of fœtor of the breath, the application of the same powder to putrid ulcers, and in both cases the fœtor was immediately removed. Administered internally in the dose of several drachms, it removed the evil odour of the stools in autumnal dysentery.

But this is merely a chemical use of wood-charcoal, for it takes away the foul odour of putrid water when mixed with it in lumps not pulverised, and indeed it does so most effectually in coarse fragments.

This medicinal employment of it was, as I have said, merely a chemical one, and not at all a dynamical employment penetrating into the inner vital sphere. The mouth rinsed out with it only remained free from fœtor for a few hours. The evil smell of the mouth returned every day. The old ulcer was not improved by it and the fœtor, chemically removed from it for the moment, always recurred. The powder ingested in autumnal dysentery removed the fœtor of the stools chemically for but a short time ; the disease remained and the disgusting smell of the stools soon returned.

In such a coarse pulverised state charcoal can exercise almost none other than a chemical action. A considerable quantity of wood charcoal may be swallowed in its ordinary crude condition without producing the slightest alternation of the health.

It is only by prolonged trituration of the charcoal (as of many other

---

1 From vol. vi, 2nd edit., 1827.

dead and apparently powerless substances) with a non-medicinal substance, such as milk-sugar, that its inner concealed, and in the crude state latent and, so to speak, slumbering dynamical medicinal power can be awakened and brought into life. This can be effected by triturating one grain of wood-charcoal for an hour with 100 grains of milk-sugar ; but its power will be developed still more vivaciously and powerfully if one grain of this powder be triturated for the same length of time with 100 grains of milk-sugar, and it will be made far more efficacious (potentized) if one grain of this last powder be again triturated for an hour with another 100 grains of milk-sugar. In this way a million-fold powder-attenuation is produced, a small portion of a grain of which moistened with a drop of water and ingested produces great medicinal effects and derangement of the human health.

The following peculiar, pure effects of wood-charcoal on the human health were caused by the ingestion of a few grains of this million-fold powder-attenuation of wood-charcoal. Its medicinal powers can be developed in a still higher degree by a further trituration with 100 parts of fresh milk-sugar ; but for homœopathic medicinal use a stronger potentization of wood-charcoal than the million-fold attenuation should by no means be employed.

The occasional production in sensitive patients of too energetic action from a small dose of this preparation is soon diminished by smelling several times at a saturated solution of camphor in alcohol, and apparently completely removed by frequent repetitions of the olfaction.

The symptoms marked *(Ad.)* are furnished by the Russian physician, Dr. ADAM ; those marked *(Gff.)* by State-Councillor Baron VON GERSDORFF, of Eisenach, and the few symptoms marked *(Cas.)* by Dr. CASPARI, of Leipzig.

[The records of traditional medicine have contributed no symptoms to this proving. This medicine first appears in the 2nd Edit., where it has 723 symptoms ; in the *Chr. Kr.* there are 1189.]

CARBO VEGETABILIS.

Whirling in the head (aft. 24 h.).

Vertigo on rapidly moving the head (aft. 4 d.).

Whirling all day long.

Vertigo so that he must hold on to something (aft. 15 d.).

5. On waking, vertigo and staggering.

Vertigo when stooping, as if the head wagged to and fro.

Vertigo in bed, after waking from sleep.

In the evening, after sleeping when sitting, he was giddy, with trembling and vibration in the whole body, and on rising from a seat, as if faint, which continued for a quarter of an hour even while lying.

(Pain rising from the stomach into the head, which took away her senses for a short time).

10. Vertigo, only when sitting, as if the head swayed to and fro.

Sudden loss of memory; he could not remember what he had just said to some one nor what the latter had said to him. [*Ad.*]

Slow march of the ideas, which always turn round one subject; at the same time sensation as if the head was too tightly bound (aft. 2 h.). [*Ad.*]

Confusion of head; thinking is difficult for him.

In the morning, immediately after rising, great confusion of the head; he cannot think well, and must collect himself with difficulty as if out of a dream; it went off after lying down again. [*Gff.*]

15. Confusion of the occiput, as after a debauch. [*Ad.*]

Headache; dizzy as after a debauch, which spreads from the occiput to the front, increases towards evening, and involves the whole head, is also aggravated by walking. [*Ad.*]

Confusion of the occiput, more like a tension towards the outside (aft. ½ h.). [*Ad.*]

Stupid feeling in the head after waking from the midday sleep. [*Ad.*]

Sensation in the head as on the occurrence of coryza.

20. Headache involving the whole right side of the head and face (with chilliness, coldness, and trembling of the body and jaws).

Dulness and heaviness before the forehead. [*Gff.*]

A dull headache in the occiput. [*Gff.*]

Heaviness in the head.

Pain in the head as if too full.

25. **Pressure in the occiput,** especially after supper. [*Ad.*]

On and in the occiput, quite low down, violent pressive pain. [*Gff.*]

Constant pressive pain on the crown, during which the hairs are painful when touched. [*Gff.*]

Pain in the crown of the head, with painfulness of the hairs when touched. [*Gff.*]

Aching pain in the upper part of the right side of occiput, with aching in the eyes.

30. **Aching pain in the forehead, especially just above the eyes,** which are painful when moved, all the afternoon. [*Gff.*]

Pressure on the top of the head every afternoon.

Pressive pain above the eyes, extending into the eyes. [*Gff*].

Pressure in both temples and on the top of the head.

Pressure from within outwards in the left temple, lasting several hours. [*Ad.*]

35. A pressure on the top of the head, then drawing all about the head, but chiefly on the left side.

Pressure and drawing in the head, by fits.

Aching pain on a small spot where there had been a wound in former times, on the right side of the forehead (aft. 4 h.). [*Gff.*]

Compressive headache.

A pressure as if something lay on the crown, or as if the integuments of the head were constricted, which spreads thence over the forehead. [*Ad.*]

40. Headache, like a contraction of the integuments of the head, particularly after supper. [*Ad.*]

Headache, as from contraction of integuments of the head.

Contractive pain in the head, especially on movement.

The hat presses on the head like a heavy weight, and when he takes it off the sensation remains, as if the head was bound round with a cloth. [*Ad.*]

Spasmodic tension in the brain.

45. Rush of blood to the head.

Rush of blood to the head, hot forehead, and empty feeling in the head.

For five days severe headaches ; on stooping feeling as if something would come out at the occiput and sinciput.

After a meal pulsating headache in the forehead, and pressure in the occiput, with heat in the head and eructation.

Throbbing headache in the evening in bed, with difficult respiration.

50. After waking from a profound long midday sleep a throbbing in the temples and fulness of the brain. [*Ad.*]

In the afternoon throbbing headache.

Twitching headache.

Very violent headache, throbbing as if gathering in the occiput, from morning till evening (aft. 9 d.).

During a persistent headache a place the size of a hand on the head is quite hot to the touch (aft. 4 d.).

55. In the evening in bed violent pressing and burning headache, especially on the crown and in front to the forehead. [*Gff.*]

In the morning on awaking in bed, in the right half of the head whereon he lay, and in the occiput, a violent headache of a smarting aching character, like what is felt in the nose during abortive sneezing, a pain that was only relieved by raising up the head, but which went off completely on rising from bed. [*Gff.*]

Cutting and squeezing headache above and behind the left ear. [*Gff.*]

Pinching headache in the occiput.

General painfulness of the surface of the brain, with stitches inwards here and there.

60. Shooting upwards in the head towards the temples.

Some stitches in the forehead above the right outer canthus of the eye (aft. 2 h.). [*Ad.*]

Burning shooting on a small spot on the occiput. [*Gff.*]

Painful boring under the left temple.

Drawing pains here and there on the head (aft. 2 h.). [*Gff.*]

65. Drawing headache here and there, especially in the forehead to above the root of the nose. [*Gff.*]

On the right side of the occiput a frequently recurring, short, drawing pain (aft. $2\frac{1}{2}$ h.). [*Gff.*]

Tearing drawing superiorly on the fore part of the head. [*Gff.*]

On the left side of the occiput, on a small spot, a tearing through the head. [*Gff.*]

Drawing and tearing in the left side of the occiput (aft. 6 h.). [*Gff.*]

70. Tearing pain on the left side of the head above the temple (aft. 12 h.). [*Gff.*]

Frequent attacks of tearing pain in the interior of the head, towards the right temple. [*Gff.*]

Tearing in the left half of the head, starting from the left half of the nose. [*Gff.*]

Attacks of dull tearing headache on the crown and in the temples. [*Gff.*]

Tearing on the old scar of a sabre wound on the left side of the top of the head. [*Gff.*]

75. Tearing on the right side of the occiput (aft. 4 h.). [*Gff.*]

Tearing in the left half of the head, and at the same time a rheumatic drawing in the left arm. [*Gff.*]

Tearing in the temples that extends to the molar teeth. [*Gff.*]

Violent tearing on a small spot in the forehead, near the temple. [*Gff.*]

Tearing in the bones of the head for four days (aft. 24 h.).

80. Formication on the integuments of the occiput, as if the hairs moved. [*Ad.*]

The hair of the head falls out very much.

On the forehead, near the hairy scalp, a red pimple, which pains as if sore only when pressed. [*Gff.*]

On the forehead, here and there, eruption of pimples, which are red, smooth, and painless. [*Gff.*]

Itching in the face, especially around the eyes.

85. Itching in the inner canthus of the left eye. [*Gff.*]

Smarting itching sensation, especially in the outer canthus of the right eye. [*Gff.*]

Itching in the left eye and smarting after rubbing, especially in the inner canthus. [*Gff.*]

Smarting in the inner canthus of the left eye. [*Gff.*]

Itching of the right eye, with great dryness of the lid (aft. 14 d.).

90. In the right eye great lachrymation and smarting (aft. 24 h.). [*Gff.*]

Smarting in the right eye with sore feeling, especially in the canthi, and aching in the eye as from a grain of sand. [*Gff.*]

Aching smarting sensation in the outer canthus of the right eye. [*Gff.*]

Aching in the eyes, with confusion of the head (aft. 6½ h.). [*Gff.*]

On the left eye a tearing pressure. [*Gff.*]

95. Painful pressure from above on the right eyeball (aft. ½ h.). [*Gff.*]

On moving in the open air a pressure in the upper lids and in the upper half of both eyeballs. [*Ad.*]

Obtuse pain in the left eye. [*Gff.*]

Swelling of the left eye.

The left eye-lids appear to him to be stuck together, which, however, is not the case.

100. At night she cannot open the eye-lids, though she could not go to sleep.

Inflammation of the right eye.

In the morning the eye-lids are stuck together.

The muscles of the eye are painful when he looks upwards. [*Gff.*]

Drawing in the right eye-lid (aft. 13 d.).

105. Drawing above the right eye through the head.

(During the headache pain in the eye as though it would be torn out.)

Quivering of the eye-lid (aft. 9 d.).

Extreme short-sightedness ; he can only recognise an acquaintance when he comes within a couple of paces (aft. 3 d.).

Black spots before the eyes.

110. Glittering before the eyes, immediately on rising in the morning, for a quarter of an hour. [*Gff.*]

A weight upon the eyes so that he must make a great effort to see anything while reading and writing.

In the afternoon great pallor of the face (aft. 9 d.).

Many pimples on the face and forehead (aft. 3 d.). [*Cas.*]

A white papule on the lower part of the cheek.

115. Swelling of the cheek.

Drawing pain in the cheek for two days (aft. 24 h.).

Pain in the left side of the cheek as if something burned and bored round about in it, in a jerking manner, by fits (aft. 6 d.).

Fine tearing prick on the right cheek (aft. 3 h.). [*Gff.*]

Pain of the bones of the face of the upper and lower jaw.

120. Tearing in the face.

Tearing pain on the left angle of the mouth and thence into the cheek. [*Gff.*]

Tearing by jerks in the right **upper jaw.**

Drawing pain in the right and left **upper** and **lower jaw,** with drawing in the head and confusion in it (aft. 2½ h.). [*Gff.*]

Tearing pain in the depression behind the right ear. [*Gff.*]

125. Violent tearing by jerks in the left zygomatic process, in front of the left ear, in the evening in bed. [*Gff.*]

Single stitches, or tearing jerks in the right internal meatus auditorius. [*Gff.*]

Tearing in the interior of the right ear. [*Gff.*]

Earache in the left ear. [*Gff.*]

A kind of earache in the right ear, in the evening. [*Gff.*]

130. A kind of forcing outwards in both ears (aft. 17 d.).

Violent formicating itching in the interior of the right ear, which recurred after boring in with the finger. [*Gff.*]

Fine pinching in the left ear. [*Cas.*]

Ringing in the ears.

Ringing in the left ear, with whirling **vertigo.**

135. Roaring in the ears.

Great rushing noise before both ears (aft. 36 h.).

Loud speaking is painful to the hearing and very disagreeable. [*Ad.*]

A weight upon the ears like two sand-bags lying at the entrance of the meatus auditorius. [*Ad.*]

A weight in and upon the ears; they feel stopped up to him, but without diminution of the hearing power. (aft. ½ h.). [*Ad.*]

140. Every evening his left ear is hot and red.

Tearing burning pain on the lobe of the left ear. [*Gff.*]

Itching behind the ear.

Great swelling of the parotid gland between the cheek and ear, to the angle of the lower jaw.

Feeling of heaviness of the nose.

145. **Epistaxis, at night**, with ebullition in the blood. (aft. 52 h.).

In the morning, in bed, very severe epistaxis, and immediately thereafter pain in the chest.

Severe epistaxis, that can scarcely be stopped (aft. 48 h.).

(Eruption on the corner of the ala nasi.)

Scabby nose-tip.

150. Swelling of the upper lip and cheek, with twitching pain.

Twitching in the upper lip.

Painful eruption on the upper lip; the red part of the lip is studded with pimples.

Drawing from the right corner of the mouth to the chin.

Spasmodic pain on the lower jaw (aft. 13 d.).

155. Painfulness of the roots of the teeth above and below.

Drawing pain in the hollow tooth.

Drawing and tearing toothache in the upper and lower molars (aft. 4½, 5, 16, 26 h.). [*Gff.*]

Drawing pain in one upper incisor. [*Gff.*]

Gentle drawing in the right molars, mingled with violent jerks. [*Gff.*]

160. Violent drawing jerk in one hollow molar. [*Gff.*]

Tickling, shooting drawing in the first molar on the left side (aft. 26 h.). [*Gff.*]

Squeezing pain in the right lower molars. [*Gff.*]

Pressive toothache in the left upper molars.

Smarting drawing pain in the upper and lower incisors—more in the gums. [*Gff.*]

165. Toothache in the front sound incisors. [*Ad.*]

Gnawing and drawing pain in the hollow tooth, with swelling of the gums.

The gums are painfully sensitive when chewing.

The first upper molar on the left side is often painful as if sore, with drawing pain in it. [*Gff.*]

The gums (by day) **feel sore.**

170. The gum at the hollow tooth is swollen (aft. 21 d.).

The gums are detached from the teeth and sensitive.

Recession of the gums from some of the lower incisors.

A pustule on the gums.

After sucking the gums bloody saliva (aft. 2 d.). [*Cas.*]

175. On drawing with the tongue the teeth and gums bleed profusely. [*Gff.*]

For several days, frequent bleeding of the teeth and gums. [*Gff.*]

The tongue is furred white.

The tongue is covered with brownish-yellow mucus. [*Gff.*]

The tip of the tongue is hot and dry. [*Cas.*]

180. On the left side of the root of the tongue cramp pain (aft. 3 h.). [*Gff.*]

He had a difficulty in speaking, just as if the tongue were difficult to move. [*Ad.*]

Fine tearing pain on the right side of the tongue. [*Gff.*]

Dryness in the mouth, without thirst.

In the morning on awaking very dry mouth.

185. At the back of the palate an aching pain. [*Gff.*]

Burning in the upper part of the fauces.

Frequent burning and smarting in the fauces and palate. [*Gff.*]

Aching pain behind the palate in the fauces.

Smarting sensation posteriorly in the fauces as at the commencement of a coryza, but more smarting. [*Gff.*]

190. Tearing pressure at the back of the fauces and on the left side of the root of the tongue. [*Gff.*]

In the throat and fauces a very violent scraping and formication only relieved for a short time by hawking. [*Gff.*]

Scraping in the throat.

(Feeling of coldness down in the throat).

Painless impediment to swallowing; the saliva swallowed does not go down well and at once, but only gradually. [*Gff.*]

195. The food is not easily swallowed down; the throat feels as if constricted by a spasm, but without pains.

The throat feels swollen internally and as if contracted.

A pressive feeling in the upper part of the gullet, as if it were narrowed or contracted, even when not swallowing. [*Gff.*]

Sore throat, as from swelling on the palate—painful swallowing for four days.

Sore throat; when eating the throat feels excoriated.

200. (Sore throat, uvula inflamed and swollen, and shooting in the throat).

A kind of fulness and pressure down the gullet as far as the stomach—almost like heart-burn.

Eructation (aft. $1\frac{1}{2}$ h.). [*Cas.*]

Frequent almost continual eructation.

Frequent, empty eructation, all day, at least all through the afternoon. [*Gff.*]

205. **Frequent, empty eructation, after short pinching in the abdomen** (aft. $3\frac{1}{2}$, $4\frac{1}{4}$ h.). [*Gff.*]

She has sweet eructations.

Bitter and scraping eructations.

Water-brash.

Salt taste in the mouth all day (aft. 48 h.).

210. (Sour eructation, after taking milk.)

(Sensation as of constant heart-burn ; acidity always rose up into the mouth).

In the forenoon, frequent sensation, as if something hot and acrid rose up in the gullet.

Bitterness in the mouth and eructations.

Bitter taste in the mouth, before and after eating.

215. Little appetite and no taste, as in catarrh.

Little appetite, with heat in the mouth and roughness and dryness on the tip of the tongue (aft. 42 h.). [*Cas.*]

(Anorexia and nausea, also when fasting, but worse after eating, with anxiety, dizziness, darkness before the eyes, and white tongue ; towards evening he must lie down, without sleepiness) (aft. 6, 7 d.).

Absence of hunger ; he could have remained without eating. [*Gff.*]

Little appetite ; she is soon satiated ; she feels pain in the scrobiculus cordis, and as if too empty in the stomach, for half an hour.

220. Anorexia and frequent eructation (with confusion of head).

Towards noon, diminished appetite and nausea (aft. 3 d.).

In the morning, an hour after waking, nausea, and as if qualmish in the stomach.

At night, nausea.

Frequent inclination to vomit, and yet he did not vomit.

225. Constant nausea, without appetite and without stool.

Repugnance to butter.

After eating a painful hiccup in the gullet. [*Ad.*]

After a moderate dinner, repeated hiccup. [*Cas.*]

(After a meal, strong palpitation of the heart.)

230. During and after a meal, pinching in the abdomen. [*Gff.*]

Every afternoon, after a meal, great heaviness in the feet, for eight days.

After eating but little, distension and fulness of the abdomen and rumbling in the bowels. [*Gff.*]

After a moderate breakfast, immediately full and satiated (aft. 68 h.). [*Cas*]

After a meal, headache.

235. A small quantity of wine heats him much. [*Gff.*]

After a moderate breakfast, general perspiration. [*Cas.*]

After a meal, sour taste in the mouth.

Spasm in the stomach and incessant eructation, which was quite sour in the mouth.

An almost burning sensation in the stomach.

240. **A scraping sensation in the stomach up into the throat like heart-burn.**

Throbbing in the scrobiculus cordis.

Anxious pressure in the scrobiculus cordis (aft. 4 d.).

A continued painful pressure in the scrobiculus cordis and epigastrium, as if in the stomach, after 7 o'clock. [*Gff.*]

A pressure as if on something sore in the stomach ; worse on touching.

245. In the evening, pain in the scrobiculus cordis, which was painful even to the touch ; at the same time she had nausea, and she commenced to have loathing when she only thought of eating.

The region of the stomach is very sensitive.

(The stomach is heavy and there is as it were trembling in it.)

(On walking and standing the stomach is as if heavy and hanging down painfully.)

Contractive sensation under the stomach.

250. Contractive pain near the scrobiculus cordis, on the right side, in the morning and afternoon.

Under the scrobiculus cordis, a constrictive pain, which is aggravated by pressure with the finger. [*Ad.*]

Short but violent pain in the right side under the short ribs. [*Gff.*]

Close under the scrobiculus cordis and thence to both sides a very painful, shooting tearing, radiating behind the ribs. [*Gff.*]

Violent shooting in the hepatic region (aft. 48 h.).

255. Continued aching pinching sensation in the epigastrium. [*Gff.*]

Cutting in the abdomen.

Pain in the abdomen as after a chill ; it increases before the discharge of flatus and persists thereafter.

Cutting in the abdomen, only for instants, but very frequently.

Cutting in the abdomen, which darts through the bowels like lightning.

260. In the evening, cutting in the abdomen, like colic.

Pain, as from a sprain, in the abdomen, even when she does something with the hand, whereby the arm is slightly raised ; the same pain also occurs on touching the abdomen.

She dare not lie on the side, for then she has the same pain as is caused by a sprain or over-lifting, chiefly on the left side of the abdomen.

After a meal, sleep, and on awaking, tension in the hepatic region, as if it was too short there.

Constantly distended abdomen. [*Gff.*]

265. Day and night as if overloaded with food, and as if full and pressed in the abdomen, with eructation.

(Great anxiety in the abdomen.)

In the left epigastrium, under the short ribs, going towards the back, a squeezing pain from imprisoned flatulence. [*Gff.*]

Frequent squeezing pain in the abdomen, especially in the right side of the abdomen. [*Gff.*]

Squeezing pressure deep in the abdomen. [*Gff.*]

270. **Squeezing pain in the abdomen**, in the hypogastrium. [*Gff.*]

Sensation as if her abdomen hung heavily down ; she must walk quite bent down (aft. 3 d.).

Aching pain in the hypogastrium (immediately). [*Gff.*]

Aching pain under the short ribs, after breakfast. [*Gff.*]

Dull aching pain in the abdomen, on the right side, on a small spot. [*Gff.*]

275. Pressure in the right inguinal region. [*Gff.*]

Aching pain in the abdomen, with some urging to stool and discharge of hot flatus, which relieves (aft. 26 h.). [*Gff.*]

Aching pain in the anus (after 48 h.). [*Gff.*]

Under the coccyx, aching sore pain. [*Gff.*]

Aching pain in the abdomen, with rumbling and discharge of inodorous, moist, warm flatus, whereupon the bellyache ceases (aft. $\frac{3}{4}$ h.). [*Gff.*]

280. Aching pain on the left side of the abdomen ; there is a movement about in the bowels, with pinching. [*Gff.*]

Pinching pressure, deep in the right hypogastrium, extending towards the hip (aft. $3\frac{1}{2}$ h.). [*Gff.*]

When sitting bent forward, fine pinching in the abdomen. [*Cas.*]

After partaking of a small quantity of harmless food, violent pinching about the umbilical region, which is quickly removed by eructation and the discharge of some flatus. [*Gff.*]

Pinching pain in the right inguinal region (aft. 10 h.). [*Gff.*]

285. Pinching in the abdomen with good stool.

Pinching, obtuse stitches, as from below upwards in the abdomen (aft. $3\frac{1}{2}$ h.). [*Gff.*]

Shooting and pinching pains in the left hypogastrium. [*Gff.*]

Pricking, creeping, running pain deep in the hypogastrium (aft. 28 h.). [*Gff.*]

Shooting pain in the left side of the abdomen (and chest), increased by drawing a breath. [*Gff.*]

290. Tearing stitch in the hypogastrium extending to the navel. [*Gff.*]

Tearing pain in the hypogastrium up to the navel (aft. 48 h.). [*Gff.*]

Burning in the abdomen.

Burning about the umbilical region. [*Gff.*]

Burning pain in the skin, near the navel, frequently recurring (aft. 4 h.). [*Gff.*]

295. Under the navel a sore painful spot. [*Gff.*]

Sore pain in the hypogastrium, also felt when touched (aft. $4\frac{3}{4}$ h.). [*Gff.*]

Imprisoned flatus in the left epigastrium, more towards the back.

Flatulent colic, with discharge of inodorous flatus. [*Gff.*]

Flatulent colic ; the flatulence goes about in the abdomen, and there are single stitches here and there, especially in the left side towards the back. [*Gff.*]

300. He has working about in the bowels (immediately). [*Gff.*]

He has working about in the abdomen deep in the hypogastrium. [*Gff.*]

He has working about in the abdomen, and several discharges of moist flatus take place, sometimes loud, sometimes noiseless. [*Gff.*]

Clucking in the left hypogastrium. [*Gff.*]

Audible rumbling works slowly round about in the bowels (aft. 3½ h.). [*Gff.*]

305. Audible rumbling in the umbilical region. [*Ad.*]

Audible rumbling in the abdomen with some pinching. [*Ad.*]

After the rumbling great discharge of flatus. [*Ad.*]

Audible rumbling in the hypogastrium, with noiseless discharge of almost inodorous (moist, warm, and sometimes hot) flatus. [*Gff.*]

Wind works about in the abdomen, and some inodorous flatus is passed (aft. ½ h.). [*Cas.*]

310. In the morning on awaking enormous discharge of flatus, without smell.

Food that was usually easily digested creates much flatulence and distension of the abdomen.

Flatus of a fœtid smell (aft. 1½ h.). [*Gff.*]

Along with colicky forcing towards the sacrum and thence to the abdomen discharge of very offensive, and latterly, moist flatus (aft. 2 h.). [*Gff.*]

The urging to stool goes off with loud discharge of flatus. [*Gff.*]

315. Discharge of flatus with burning in the anus, and sensation as if a stool were coming. [*Gff.*]

Burning on the right side of the anus (aft. 6 h.). [*Gff.*]

Pappy stool, which causes burning in the rectum.

During the stool, consisting of a few, hard, unconnected masses of fæces, burning in the anus. [*Cas.*]

Drawing pain through the abdomen **transversely across**, before the stool. [*Cas.*]

320. In the evening a couple of violent stitches **in** the anus. [*Cas.*]

During the stool cutting in the anus. [*Cas.*]

The hard stool passes with a cutting pain in **the anus**. [*Gff.*]

During the stool pricking in the rectum as with needles.

Itching at the anus and after rubbing burning therein. [*Gff.*]

325. Itching at the anus, in the morning in bed, increased by scratching, and thereafter burning. [*Cas.*]

Smarting at the anus. [*Gff.*].

Sudden sensation of fulness in the rectum as if for an evacuation, which soon went off. [*Ad.*]

The urging to stool passes off with loud discharge of flatus. [*Gff.*]

Pain in abdomen and sacrum, like a call to stool. [*Gff.*]

330. A kind of hæmorrhoidal colic ; violent urging to stool, formication in the anus, and violent pressure on the bladder and towards the sacrum, spasmodically recurring in fits ; in spite of the great urging it seems that no stool will come ; on the other hand, there occur violent labour-like pains in the hypogastrium to the front and back, with burning in the anus and a sensation as if diarrhœa would ensue ; on trying to have a motion there comes after such a pain, and after much effort, some fæces consisting of soft pieces, whereupon the urging to stool and the pain in the bowels go off immediately. [*Gff.*]

After breakfast call to stool, which though not hard is only passed with much straining. [*Gff.*]

Great urging to stool whereby only a scanty and hard one is passed (aft. 50 h.). [*Gff.*]

Hard stool (aft. 62 h.). [*Gff.*]

Hard stool passed much later than usual, and with much effort (aft. 36 h.). [*Gff.*]

335. Ineffectual urging to stool (aft. 80 h.). [*Gff.*]

The first week during stool there comes first mucus, then followed hard and then soft fæces, afterwards cutting pain in the abdomen.

Stool with discharge of much mucus.

Discharge of much mucus from the rectum, during several days.

The stool is enveloped with yellowish, thread-like mucus, which in the latter portion of the stool is quite bloody. [*Ad.*]

340. Rush of blood to the anus.

With every stool discharge of blood.

Swollen hæmorrhoidal veins (blind hæmorrhoids) which are painful (aft. 2 d.).

The latter portion of the stool is coloured with blood. [*Ad.*]

An acrid biting moisture escapes from the rectum (aft. 24 h.).

345. Acrid stool with furred tongue.

At night a viscid, musty-smelling fluid escapes in considerable qnantity from the anus.

At night, moisture on the perinæum from the anus to the scrotum, with itching and excoriation.

Excoriation on the perinæum; on touching the part it itches painfully.

Excoriation at the anus.

350. Shooting pain in the perinæum, near the anus (aft. $2\frac{1}{2}$ h.). [*Gff.*]

After stool repeated pain in the abdomen towards the sacrum and bladder, almost as after taking rhubarb. [*Gff.*]

After the stool forcing pain in the abdomen. [*Gff.*]

After the stool squeezing pain in the abdomen. [*Gff.*]

In the morning, after a hard scanty stool, a pinching shooting in the left hypogastrium and incomplete call to stool, like a pressure on the rectum, all day (aft. 4 d.). [*Gff.*]

355. After the stool complete emptiness in the abdomen, particularly observable when walking. [*Cas.*]

The urine is reddish and turbid. [*Gff.*]

The urine is dark coloured.

Red, dark urine, with roughness of the larynx. [*Gff.*]

Dark red urine, as if it were mixed with blood (aft. 2 d.).

360. Reddish, turbid urine.

Red sediment in the urine.

Urine of very pungent odour.

After drinking but little, copious discharge of urine (aft. 6 h.). [*Gff.*]

The urine is much more scanty (aft. 48 h.). [*Gff.*]

365. He must rise several times during the night to make water, and the quantity of urine passed is increased; he has at the same time pressure on the bladder.

Frequently during the day pressing on bladder, but yet she could retain the urine.

When urinating there is often tearing in the urethra ; the last drops consist of mucus and pass with pain.

In the morning, after urinating, tearing and drawing in the urethra. [*Gff.*]

On the prepuce itching and excoriation.

370. On the prepuce a great itching, and on its inner surface a vesicle and an excoriated spot.

Formication in the testicles and scrotum.

Itching near the scrotum on the upper part of the thigh ; the part exudes moisture (aft. 24 h.).

Swelling of the scrotum which is hard to the touch.

A seminal emission that effects the nerves violently and painfully, and is followed by an extremely violent burning in the anterior part of the urethra, and when urinating, a severe cutting and burning, which lasts long and is renewed by slight external pressure. [*Gff.*]

375. Persistent erection of the penis, at night, without lascivious feeling or ideas. [*Gff.*]

Complete want of sexual desire in the morning, which is not excitable even by sensual thoughts (aft. 24 h.). [*Gff.*]

Great excoriation on the female pudendum anteriorly, in the evening.

Burning on the female pudendum.

A sore pain on the female pudendum, with discharge of much leucorrhœa for two days, thereafter occurrence of the menses, which had not appeared for several months previously ; they flow for three days but are quite black ; thereafter very little leucorrhœa without soreness.

380. Menses five days too soon (aft. 21 d.).

Just before the occurrence of the menses, pain in the abdomen, like spasms, from morning till evening.

During the menses, very violent headache, which drew her eyes quite together.

Cutting in the hypogastrium, during the menses.

Severe itching of a tetter, before the occurrence of the menses.

385. In the morning, on rising, much very thin leuccorrhœa, and then no more all day.

Discharge of white mucus from the vagina (aft. 4 d.).

* * * *

Stoppage of the left nostril for an hour. [*Gff.*]

The left nostril is stopped (aft. 1½ d.). [*Cas.*]

Sneezing followed by stoppage of the left nostril. [*Gff.*]

390. **Stuffed coryza.**

Frequent sneezing with constant and violent tickling and formication in the nose, and catarrhal roughness in the nose and upper part of the chest, at night in bed. [*Gff.*]

Very frequent sneezing without coryza. [*Gff.*]

Sneezing with watering of the left eye, which causes smarting in the inner canthus. [*Gff.*]

Violent sneezing followed by severe smarting pain above and in the nose and watering of the eyes as if severe coryza were about to burst forth; this pain in the nose also came on when blowing it. [*Gff.*]

395. Formication in the right nostril, discharge of nasal mucus, then violent sneezing, watering of the right eye; coryza. [*Gff.*]

Incomplete abortive irritation to sneeze, returning at one time more at another less strongly. [*Gff.*]

Sneezing which occasions stitches in the abdomen. [*Gff.*]

Sneezing, which is followed by burning on a large portion of the right side of the abdomen. [*Gff.*]

In the root of the nose feeling of a commencing coryza. [*Ad.*]

400. Pressing pain in the root of the nose and nasal bones, as in a severe coryza, but he could get air through the nose. [*Ad.*]

Ineffectual irritation to sneeze with formication in the left half of the nose; it then became moist, and after blowing the nose the right nostril remained stopped up; at the same time some feeling of coryza—a formication and smarting on the left side of the palate (aft. 5 h.). [*Gff.*]

Fluent coryza with sneezing (almost immediately). [*Gff.*]

For several days, at night and in the morning on awaking, irritation like coryza which (with the exception of occasional sneezing) went off during the day. [*Gff.*]

Severe fluent coryza.

405. Coryza and catarrh (aft. 7 d.).

Hoarse, in the evening (aft. 12 d.).

Catarrh, owing to which he could scarcely speak loud (aft. 8 d.).

In the evening, suddenly great hoarseness, so that he could scarcely utter a sound, with great tightness of the chest, so that when walking in the open air he had scarcely any breath (aft. 6 d.).

Roughness and hoarseness of the larynx; she could not speak loud without great exertion.

410. Great roughness of the larynx; the voice is deep and rough, and when he exerts it it fails him, but without pain in the throat on swallowing. [*Gff.*]

Roughness on the chest and frequent irritation to cough. [*Gff.*]

In the evening and morning, scraping in the throat, which excites her to dry cough.

Scrapy in the throat, with some cough, during which the left eye especially waters (aft. $3\frac{1}{2}$ h.). [*Gff.*]

Formication in the upper part of the wind-pipe, as if something adhered there, exciting cough (aft. 3 h.). [*Gff.*]

415. Itching in the larynx exciting cough (with viscid, salt expectoration), in the evening on going to sleep, and in the morning an hour after rising. [*Cas.*]

Irritation to cough, as from sulphur fumes, with choking.

Frequent short hacking cough (aft. $3\frac{3}{4}$ h.). [*Gff.*]

Irritation to cough at the back of the throat, with short cough, **frequently recurring.** [*Gff.*]

Great formication in the throat removed for a short time by hawking, with great flow of saliva. [*Gff.*]

420. Constant rough feeling in the throat, with formication and frequent semi-voluntary, rough cough, which causes pain in the upper part of the chest. [*Gff.*]

After formication and irritation in the throat, some deep coughs, whereupon the chest pains as if pressed in. [*Gff.*]

(When coughing, pain on the chest as if raw.)

During the cough-irritation, in the evening, a chilliness and a drawing in the cheeks.

Cough, in the evening in bed.

425. Spasmodic cough, daily, in three or four fits.

(In the evening, cough, which causes vomiting and retching).

Along with tightness of chest and burning on the chest, a fatiguing cough.

Expectoration of mucus from the larynx by hawking or short cough.

Expectoration of masses of green mucus.

430. **Tearing, pressive pain on (in) the left side of the chest** (aft. 26 h.). [*Gff.*]

In the morning, in bed, tearing from the chest towards the back (in the arms and left ear), with internal heat, especially in the head.

Drawing (rheumatic) pain on the right short ribs. [*Gff.*]

Tearing in the right side of the chest. [*Gff.*]

Rheumatic pain from the left short ribs to the hip. [*Gff.*]

435. Aching rheumatic pain in the right side on the short ribs, for a quarter of an hour. [*Gff.*]

Painful drawing in the chest, shoulders, and arms, more on the left side, with hot sensation and rush of blood to the head, during which she feels cold.

Obtuse pain first in the left, then in the right, side of the chest, more perceptible on expiring than on inspiring. [*Gff.*]

Obtuse pain on the right side of the chest (aft. 6 h.). [*Gff.*]

Obtuse stitch in the left side of the chest towards the short ribs [*Gff.*]

440. Obtuse shooting, oppressive pain in the region of the heart, which goes off with audible rumbling in the left side, as from incarcerated and now liberated flatulence (aft. $3\frac{1}{4}$ h.). [*Gff.*]

Shooting pain in the right side of the chest (and of the abdomen) increased by drawing a breath. [*Gff.*]

On going to sleep, some very painful stitches through the chest, which impeded respiration. [*Gff.*]

On drawing a deep breath a deep stitch in the right side of the chest. [*Gff.*]

Violent, obtuse stitches, as if darting outwards, deep in the lower part of the right side of the chest. [*Gff.*]

445. Severe stitches under the left breast (without chill or heat) ; on

account of them she could not sleep or walk ; even when sitting they continued.

Pains more of a burning than a shooting character in the region of the heart.

Severe burning in the chest, as from red-hot coals (almost uninterruptedly).

Burning pain near the scrobiculus cordis and on the left side of the chest.

Burning and rush of blood in the chest.

450. She always felt as if the blood rose into her chest, and at the same time she was cold in her body.

Rush of blood to the chest in the morning on awaking, and furred tongue.

Palpitation of the heart, chiefly when sitting.

Frequent palpitation of the heart, some quick beats.

In the evening, on going to sleep, palpitation of the heart and intermitting pulse (aft. 16 d.).

455. Excessively violent palpitation of the heart for several days.

Spasmodic oppression and contraction of the chest for three or four minutes.

Pain in the chest as from displaced flatulence.

Tightness of the chest and **short** breathing, as from flatulence pressing upwards (aft. 48 h.). [*Gff.*]

Feeling of oppression in the chest, which goes off immediately after eructation.

460. In the morning, after rising from bed, chest and shoulders as if pressed together.

(Pain on dilating the chest).

In the evening, when lying in bed, difficult respiration and throbbing in the head.

(The breath is quite cold ; also coldness in the throat, mouth, and teeth.)

Difficult respiration, chiefly when sitting.

465. Frequent attacks of constriction of the chest, which stops the breathing for instants.

Frequent oppressive aching on the chest. [*Gff.*]

Pressure on the left side of the chest. [*Gff.*]

Pressive pain superiorly in the right side of the chest, through into the right scapula. [*Gff.*]

On the sternum, just above the scrobiculus cordis, a dull pain on a small spot, excited by stooping forwards and also by touching. [*Gff.*]

470. **Feeling of weakness and fatigue of the chest.**

On awaking he feels the chest as if fatigued.

Itching internally in the chest.

Pricking itching in the region of the coccyx, in the evening in bed. [*Cas.*]

In the sacrum, sensation of coldness, numbness, and tension.

475. Tensive pain and stiffness in the sacrum.

(Severe sacral pain ; she cannot sit, she feels like a plug in the back, she must put a pillow below her.)

Tearing pressure in the sacrum. [*Gff.*]

Aching, tearing pain in the left side through to the back, near the left hip. [*Gff.*]

Violent external burning on the right hip. [*Gff.*]

480. Tearing low down in the back, near the sacrum. [*Gff.*]

Heaviness in the back and oppression on the chest.

Drawing in the back, chiefly when sitting.

Pressive pain near the lowest part of the back (aft. 3 h.).

Squeezing pressive pain near the lowest part of the spine.

485. Pain in the side of the back, as if bruised.

Jerking of the muscles in the left side of the back. [*Gff.*]

Burning on the upper part of the left side of the back.

(Shooting betwixt the scapulæ, taking away the breath, at night.)

After the (accustomed) washing with water by no means cold, rheumatic pains at the upper part of the left scapula (aft. 26 h.). [*Cas.*]

490. Rheumatic sensation in the whole of the left scapula when writing (aft. 6 h.). [*Cas.*]

On bending back the left arm, violent tearing in the left scapula. [*Gff.*]

Burning sensation on the right scapula. [*Gff.*]

Burning on the right shoulder. [*Gff.*]

Burning on the shoulder-joint (aft. 3 h.). [*Gff.*]

495. Drawing pain in the left shoulder-joint. [*Gff.*]

Drawing pain in the shoulder.

Rheumatic drawing in the right shoulder. [*Gff.*]

Violent tearing pain in the right shoulder-joint, especially on moving, with drawing in the shafts of the arm-bones. [*Gff.*]

Paralytic tearing in the right shoulder-joint, frequently recurring.

500. Paralytic weakness of the right shoulder and right arm (aft. $\frac{1}{4}$ h.) [*Cas.*]

Shooting in the right shoulder by day and night.

Tearing in the posterior cervical muscles. [*Gff.*]

Aching, tearing pain in the cervical muscles. [*Gff.*]

In the muscles on the neck (right side) violent aching pain. [*Gff.*]

505. Pressive pain on the neck (aft. 6 d.).

Pricking itching on the neck and nape, and red spots there (aft. 38 h.). [*Cas.*]

An aching drawing pain under the right axilla, felt especially when moving. [*Gff.*]

Burning pain in the right axilla. [*Gff.*]

Itching, moisture, and excoriation in the axillæ.

510. Bruised pain of the right arm.

Drawing in the right arm.

Cramp in the arms.

On the inner side of the left upper arm, dull drawing (aft. 4 h.). [*Cas.*]

The upper arm is particularly heavy. [*Cas.*]

515. Drawing pain, with burning, on the upper arm (aft. 48 h.). [*Gff.*]

Burning superiorly on the upper arm, first on the left then on the right (aft. 5 h.). [*Gff.*]

Tearing in the left upper arm (aft. 4 h.). [*Gff.*]

A large boil on the upper arm, surrounded by many itching pimples (aft. 7 d.).

Burning on the right elbow. [*Gff.*]

520. Drawing pain in the shaft of the ulna towards the wrist (aft. 20 m.). [*Cas.*]

Drawing tearing pain in the upper side of the left forearm, near the elbow, where also the part is likewise painful when the shalf of the bone is pressed (aft. 3½ h.). [*Gff.*]

Burning itching on the forearm near the elbow. [*Gff.*]

Tearing drawing from the left elbow to the hand (aft. 48 h.). [*Gff.*]

Paralytic pain in the wrist on moving it.

525. Arms and hands go to sleep, especially at night, so that she does not know where to put them in bed ; also by day they go to sleep.

Tendency of the hands to become numb.

In the morning, when washing the hands she feels as if they would go to sleep.

Icy cold hands (aft. 48 h.). [*Gff.*]

On making certain movements, sensation in the left wrist-joint as if the tendons were too short.

530. Sensation in the hands as if the muscular power were weakened, felt especially when writing (aft. 6 h.). [*Gff.*]

Writing is performed slowly and with difficulty (aft. 1½ h.), [*Cas.*]

Tearing in the right or left wrist. [*Gff.*]

On the hands an itching fine eruption.

Bruised pain on the back of the left hand. [*Gff.*]

535. Drawing in the right metacarpal bones (aft. ¾ h.). [*Cas.*]

Great itching in the palms, at night.

Tearing in the inside of the left hand from the root of the little finger inwards. [*Gff.*]

Violent tearing in the proximal joint of the left index (aft. 28 h.). [*Gff.*]

Tearing pain in the fingers of the right hand (aft. 6 h.). [*Gff.*]

540. Fine **tearing in the fourth** and fifth **fingers of the right hand.** [*Gff.*]

Fine tearing in the middle-joint of the right index. [*Gff.*]

Fine burning tearing in the tip of the right thumb. [*Gff.*]

Tearing in the tip and beneath the nail of the left fourth finger (aft. 48 h.). [*Gff.*]

Tearing in the joints of the fourth and fifth fingers. [*Gff.*]

545. Tearing beneath the thumb-nail. [*Gff.*]

Tearing in the right little finger, increased by movement. [*Gff.*]

A drawing in the right index forwards towards the tip.

In the inner side of the middle-joint of the left index, when at rest, a boring pain, but on flexing it a fine pricking as from a splinter, for six hours. [*Ad.*]

Boring pain in the proximal joint of the middle-finger and in the proximal joint of the thumb, when at rest. [*Ad.*]

550. A slow throbbing pain in the distal phalanx of the thumb. [*Ad.*]

Pulsation on the back of the thumb for some minutes and recurring. [*Cas.*]

Throbbing pain in the metacarpal bone of the middle-finger. [*Ad.*]

Tearing shooting in the middle-joints of the fingers.

Stitch in the proximal joint of the middle-finger (aft. $\frac{3}{4}$ h.). [*Cas.*]

555. Pricking as from a splinter in the distal phalanx of the fourth finger. [*Cas.*]

Shooting in a finger, on rising from a seat.

Shooting in the ball of the thumb proceeding from the wrist-joint.

Fine pricks in the skin of the right index, renewed on flexing the arm (aft. 2 h.). [*Cas.*]

Chilling burning in the proximal joint of the right middle and ring fingers. [*Gff.*]

560. Violent itching on the outer side of the left thumb. [*Gff.*]

Tearing in the right hip. [*Gff.*]

Tearing aching pain below and near the left hip towards the back and sacrum, frequently repeated (aft. 2 h.). [*Gff.*]

Severe, **paralytic drawing pain proceeding from the abdomen down into the left lower extremity.** [*Gff.*]

Jerking of the muscles in the superior posterior part of the left thigh, in the morning in bed. [*Gff.*]

565. Obtuse stitch in the upper part of the thigh. [*Gff.*]

Burning on the thigh at night in bed.

Burning sensation on the outer side of the thigh superiorly.

In the left thigh, rheumatic drawing, in the evening in bed, alleviated by lying on that thigh. [*Gff.*]

Tearing pain in the middle of the thigh, frequently recurring. [*Gff.*]

570. At the lower and outer part of the left thigh, cramp-pain when walking, especially when raising the thigh and going up-stairs ; the part is also painful to the touch (aft. 35 h.). [*Cas.*]

When walking, numbness of the thighs.

Stiffness in the thighs above the knees, in the morning on rising.

Stiffness and drawing in the left thigh, as if paralysed and dislocated (the first 4 d.).

Feeling of restlessness in the right thigh and leg, which causes him to be constantly changing his position in his chair. [*Cas.*]

575. Pain in both lower extremities, especially in the legs, when sitting and lying ; he knows not where to put them.

Tearing in the right thigh and leg. [*Gff.*]

Tearing in the left thigh and leg (aft. 29 h.). [*Gff.*]

Heaviness in the lower extremities (aft. 5 d.).

In the lower extremities, numbness and insensibility.

580. Drawing pain in the knees when standing.

In the knees and ankle-joints, tenseness (aft. 5 d.).

Paralytic pain in the knee when sitting and rising from a seat, and at night when lying, on turning round, or extending the **knee.**

On slightly knocking on the knee, great pain in the **bone.**

On going upstairs, pain in the knees.

585. Weakness and unsteady feeling in the knees when walking and standing. [*Gff.*]

Weakness and stiffness in the knee.

Great burning in the right knee. [*Gff.*]

After rising from a seat, shooting in the patella, as if the knee were swollen.

In both knees aching tearing, and also in the legs.

590. Drawing sensation in the lower extremities, especially from the knee down the leg. [*Gff.*]

Tearing in the right leg. [*Gff.*]

Tearing in the leg from the calf down to the inner ankle. [*Gff.*]

Drawing and gnawing in both legs ; he cannot let them lie quiet, and must stretch them out or draw them up, for half an hour, in the afternoon.

Paralytic sensation in the left leg.

595. At the lower part of the calf a swollen spot that is painful when touched.

On the calves, itching wheals.

Severe cramp in the leg, especially in the sole of the foot, when walking in the open air.

Severe cramp, at night in bed in the whole leg, especially in the sole of the foot.

Cramp in the sole of the right foot, in the evening, after lying down ; the toes are drawn crooked.

600. Tearing in the bone above the left inner ankle (aft. 4 h.). [*Gff.*]

Drawing in the feet, chiefly when sitting.

Tearing pain under the big toe of the right foot, increased by walking. [*Gff.*]

Tearing in the middle toe of the right foot. [*Gff.*]

Severe tearing under the nails of the toes, from the evening into the night ; it extended into the soles of the feet (the first 4 d.).

605. Pain in the right big toe under the nail. [*Gff.*]

On treading pain in the metatarsal bones, as if they were lacerated.

Restlessness in the left foot ; she must move it to and fro.

Burning in the soles of the feet, after standing.

Great sweat of the feet (aft. 9 d.).

610. (During the pains, great anxiety and heat.)

(After the pains great exhaustion.)

Bruised pain in all the limbs (aft. 24 h.).

In the morning, after waking, in bed, great bruised feeling in the joints, relieved by stretching out the limbs, gradually going off after rising. [*Gff.*]

Every limb of the body is painful, so also is the back (with much headache and great weakness).

615. The limbs go to sleep.

The limbs on which he is lying are apt to go to sleep.

Formication all over the body.

In the morning in bed, a shooting under the left ribs, which radiates into the abdomen, the scrobiculus cordis, and the left and right side of the chest, showed itself as aching in the larynx, was aggravated by expiration, and when it went off was renewed by pressure on the abdomen. [*Gff.*]

Itching pricks on the side on which he is lying, in the evening in bed.

620. Itching like flea-bites on several parts of the body. [*Cas.*]

Itching and shooting on several parts of the body. [*Cas.*]

Nettle-rash for some weeks (aft. 4 d.).

Itching and **burning on various parts of the body**, on the back, chest, navel, thighs, &c. [*Gff.*]

Burning on various parts of the body, at night in bed.

625. Here and there, on the back and in the sides, as also in the right side of the abdomen, a burning sensation on the skin, as from a mustard plaster (aft. 12 h.). [*Gff.*]

Stiffness in the knees and hip-joints, in the morning on awaking.

Tension in the knees and left hand as if they had been fatigued by too great exercise.

Drawing pain in the limbs.

Drawing and tearing pains on various parts of the body. [*Gff.*]

630. Drawing in the back and feet, only when sitting.

Drawing in the wrist, elbow and shoulder-joints, which goes off by moving.*

Tearing in various parts of the body, at night in bed.

Rheumatic sensation in the whole body, with coldness of the hands and feet. [*Gff.*]

In the morning, on awaking, tearing sensation in the left shoulder, then in the right hand, then in the right upper jaw in the incisor teeth. [*Gff.*]

635. Frequent, tearing pains here and there, *e. g.* in the left half of the face, then as if in the left side of the occiput, in the left thigh, and left shoulder, at the same time great pressure in the arms and lower extremities. [*Gff.*]

(A healed ulcer again breaks out, and discharges, instead of pus, lymph mixed with blood ; the part is hard and painful when touched.)

The pus of the ulcer becomes fœtid like asafœtida.

The sore of the issue excretes a corrosive moisture.

After sitting for a long time he feels, on rising from his seat, heaviness and stiffness in the limbs, which is relieved by walking a little.

640. Indisposed for bodily exertion. [*Cas.*]

Want of energy in the muscular movements (aft. 1 h.). [*Cas.*]

Exhaustion. [*Ad.*]

---

*Especially by exposure to the morning wind.

Exhaustion in the morning in bed (aft. 48 h.). [*Gff.*]

Great feeling of fatigue, in the morning in bed, especially in the joints, which goes off after rising from bed. [*Gff.*]

645. In the morning, weak, lazy, trembling in the limbs and readily perspiring (aft. 2 d.). [*Cas.*]

Trembling in the body, with faintness.

In the morning feeling of great exhaustion, with trembling in the limbs and round about the stomach, as after drinking wine in excess (aft. 24 h.). [*Gff.*]

Attacks of sudden faint weakness.

Very frequent, but only momentary attacks of fainting, causing him to sink down, also accompanied by vertigo—followed by cutting in the abdomen and griping in the bowels as if diarrhœa would ensue—but yet only an ordinary stool was passed (aft. 24 h.).

650. Exhaustion after a short slow walk in the open air. [*Gff.*]

Whilst walking in the open air sudden fatigue came on, which, however, soon went off (aft. 3 d.).

Weakness, especially in the lower extremities. [*Gff.*]

In the forenoon, weakness, as from stupefaction.

Exhaustion in the evening.

655. In the evening, laziness, drowsiness, indisposed for exertion.

Yawning. [*Ad.*]

Much stretching and yawning (aft. 2 h.). [*Gff.*]

Drowsiness and frequent yawning. [*Gff.*]

Drowsiness in the forenoon, when sitting (and when reading), **which goes off on moving.** [*Ad.*]

660. After the midday meal, inclination to sleep, without being able to sleep.

After a meal uninterrupted sleep for hours which is beset with anxious dreams. [*Ad.*]

After a meal over-powered by sleepiness.

Very early in the evening inclined for sleep.

Great sleepiness in the evening.

665. When he gets into bed, in the evening, he is attacked by anxiety so that he can scarcely keep lying (aft. 19 d.).

Late of falling to sleep—not till 1 a. m.

At night though his eyes are heavy with sleep he cannot get to sleep.

She cannot get to sleep at night, but yet cannot open the eyes.

In the evening very cold feet and hands.

670. In the evening, before going to sleep, a severe internal shivering, without chilliness, and at the same time much eructation.

She frequently wakes up at night with coldness of the lower extremities and knees.

In the evening, after lying down in bed, his eyes were painful.

At night heaviness in the lower limbs and back, like fatigue.

In the evening before going to sleep, a drawing sensation in both lower limbs.

675. At night, in bed, the corns ache.

At night he cannot lie quiet except with both lower extremities drawn up to the abdomen.

At night he wakes up several times on account of pulsation in the head and anxiety as if about to have a fit of apoplexy ; some instants after awaking he was composed and felt that it was an illusion, and then the beating in his head went off ; when he attempted to await in slumber what would happen to him, the lower extremities and knees were drawn up to the upper part of his body and the back became bent—both involuntarily—and he felt that if he put off awaking longer he would have fainted.

In the evening, after going to sleep, in bed, he wakes up several times, with a feeling of rush of blood to the head, with hair on end, anxiety accompanied with shivering, and a feeling over the body as if some one stroked him with the hand, and as if ants were running over the skin, at every movement in bed—at the same time the hearing is so sensitive and so extremely acute that the slightest noise echoed in his ear.

In the evening, during sleep, deception of the hearing ; he thought he heard some one approach his bed, this woke him up with anxiety.

680. At night, he started at a noise, with shudder in the back.

Much connected talking in dreams, whereby he woke up and remembered what he had dreamt.

Nights very full of dreams (aft. 16 h.). [*Gff.*]

At night, **vivid**, but unremembered dreams. [*Gff.*]

Frightful dreams.

685. Extremely anxious dreams. [*Gff.*]

Restless sleep, anxious dreams, and at night a pressure under the stomach.

Restless sleep, frequent waking, and in the morning in bed, headache, with burning here and there on the body. [*Gff.*]

Restless sleep with many dreams until after 3 a.m., when he awoke with violent squeezing and forcing-down pains in the abdomen, which pressed particularly on the sacrum and somewhat on the bladder also, with rumbling in the bowels. [*Gff.*]

Very restless sleep full of anxious dreams, until 1 a.m. [*Gff.*]

690. Restless sleep, without refreshment ; in the morning he was in perspiration.

Feverish coldness in the evening ; he did not feel the heat of the stove (aft. 48 h.).

Anxiety in the form of fever, the hands become cold and he trembles.

In the evening, great anxiety and sensation of heat, though she was cold all over to the touch.

(Weak, depressed pulse.)

695. Frequent chilliness, especially at night, chilliness and coldness.

In the evening weariness and febrile rigor, and before going to sleep flying heat (aft. 10 d.)

Chilliness and heat towards evening (aft. 12 d.).

All day long, much heat, but always attended by cold feet.

At night, heat in bed.

700. She could not sleep at night owing to heat in the blood.
Warm perspiration in the morning (aft. 29 h.). [*Cas.*]
Sour smelling sweat (aft. 8 d.).
Out of humour (after a meal). [*Ad.*]
Indifferent, unsympathetic. [*Ad.*]

705. Music, which he is fond of, he does not care for all day. [*Ad.*]
Anxious, as if oppressed, for several days.
Very oppressed and full.
In the evening, restlessness.
In the evening, anxiety increasing for several hours, with much heat in the face.

710. Great irritability.
Excessive irritation, as if she were too much hurried, or had too much to do.
Irritability, sensitiveness. [*Ad.*]
Ill-humoured, very sensitive (aft. $4\frac{1}{4}$ h.). [*Gff.*]
Peevish, impatient and desperate, so much so that he would like to shoot himself.

715. Peevish, irritable disposition, with confusion of the head. [*Gff.*]
Irritable, violent temper.
Involuntary angry outbursts (aft. 36 h.).
Sensitive, lachrymose disposition.
Sensitive, easily irritated humour, which, however, on cause given is apt to change into silly gaiety, that, on laughing, is attended by relaxation of the muscles of the arms and hands especially. [*Gff.*]

720. Excessively cheerful, but apt to be easily put out of humour. [*Ad.*]

CHAMOMILLA.[1]

(*Camomile.*)

(This juice of the whole plant, *Matricaria chamomilla*, freshly expressed, and mixed with equal parts of alcohol.)

It will be seen from the following symptoms of camomile, though they are far from being exhaustive, that this plant must evidently be reckoned among the medicines of many uses (polychrests). Hence in their domestic practice the common people have employed it in all kinds of maladies, especially those of an acute character. On this account physicians in their ludicrous pride have not deigned to regard it as a medicine, but, giving it the contemptuous name of "domestic remedy," they permitted their patients to use it by handfuls in infusion as a tea or as a clyster along with the medicines they prescribed,* just as if camomile, being but a vulgar domestic remedy, was of no account. In like manner they allowed their patients to apply bagfuls of the warmed flowers in any quantity they pleased to painful parts, whilst they themselves directed quite different medicines to be taken internally. Obstetric practitioners permitted the midwives and mothers to mix camomile tea in almost all the drinks and food of children at the breast and wet-nurses, as though it were a purely wholesome, non-injurious, or at least a perfectly unimportant and indifferent matter.

To such an extent did the blindness of physicians go with respect to a plant which belongs to the category of powerful medicines, whose exact power and importance it was their duty to ascertain, in order not only to learn how to make a rational and wholesome employment of it, but also to prevent its misuse by the common people, and to teach them in what particular cases camomile could only be employed beneficially, and in what cases its use was to be avoided.

But hitherto physicians have neglected their duty in all these respects ; on the contrary, they vied with the common people in the thoughtless recommendation or permission to use this powerful

* In order to avoid the degradation of admitting into their elegant prescriptions a vulgar folk's-remedy like the ordinary camomile, when it was desired to give a medicine of this sort, they preferred to order the dearer and more aristocratic *Chamomilla romana off*, without considering that this, being quite a different plant, belonging, indeed, to a totally different genus of plants (*Anthemis nobilis*, L.), must possess different properties and actions. But what does a man who *only wants a name* in his prescriptions care about the peculiar actions of medicines ?

1 From vol. iii, 2nd edit., 1825.

medicinal plant in all cases of disease, *without any distinction*, in any quantity or dose the patients chose.

But it does not require much sense to perceive that no medicine in the world can be useful in all diseases, and that every one possesses an accurately defined curative sphere of action, beyond which every powerful medicinal substance, like camomile,* must act in a thoroughly injurious manner, and so much the more injuriously the greater its powers are. Hence the physician who does not desire to act like a charlatan ought to be able to tell beforehand, not only the cases in which camomile must be beneficial, but also those in which its use must be injurious. Finally, he should be able also to determine the exact dose, which shall be neither too large nor too small for the disease. By the administration of the appropriate dose the cure of the disease by this plant may be anticipated with the greatest certainty.

Did we not know by thousands of other instances in what a melancholy state, in what incomprehensible blindness, so-called practical medicine has groped through so many centuries, and how it has done every thing to emulate the common herd in their folly, it would only be necessary to direct the attention of an unprejudiced person to the proceedings of physicians in regard to this powerful medicinal plant, camomile.

For as it is impossible that any one medicine, be it ever so useful, can be serviceable and curative in one tenth part of the enormous number of different morbid states that exist in nature, so neither can camomile.

But let us suppose the impossible case, that camomile is curative in a tenth of all known diseases, must it not, if employed as hitherto, in almost all cases of disease without distinction, do harm in the other nine tenths? Is it wise to purchase a single benefit† by a ninefold injury? "What! injury?" retorts the ordinary practitioner; "I never saw any injury from camomile." Yes, as long as you are ignorant of the morbid symptoms and ailments that camomile as a powerful medicine is capable of developing *per se* and in a peculiar manner in the healthy human body, you cannot recognise the ailments due to its employment in diseases, as the injurious effects of camomile; and in your ignorance you often attribute them to the course of the disease itself, to the malignity of the disease, and thus you deceive yourself and the poor tortured patient.

Look in this mirror, look at the following camomile symptoms, and when you are practising your ordinary slipshod treatment with an unlimited simultaneous employment of camomile, behold the serious

* Every medicine that is capable of curing serious ailments must naturally be a powerful medicine.

† It would be sufficiently stupid if one should purchase all the tickets of a class-lottery in order to obtain the several prizes in it, without considering that he thereby incurs a palpable loss of ten per cent. But what could possibly be more foolish than, supposing there was a lottery which obviously brought a loss of nine tenths to its subscribers, for a person to buy up all the tickets and so incur a certain loss of nine whilst he could only win one? And yet the ordinary practitioner who employs camomile in every case is far more foolish; he does a much greater proportion of injury, only with this difference, that the injury does not touch himself, but only his wretched patient.

hurtful symptoms and ailments caused by camomile, consider how much discomfort and torture you inflict on your patients by the abuse of this powerful plant in unsuitable cases and in excessive doses.*

See from this list of symptoms, incomplete though it be, how often, where the disease would frequently have passed away by itself, you have prolonged, doubled, multiplied the sufferings of the patient by exciting an accumulation of the peculiar camomile ailments by your senseless continued abuse of this drug ! As long as you really did not know, did not suspect the peculiar sufferings camomile is capable of occasioning, you sinned out of pure ignorance ; but now that you have here displayed before you a list of the pure pathogenetic effects of camomile, you may well begin to be ashamed of your sin in inflicting so much suffering on your patients, who come to you in order to obtain from you an alleviation of their sufferings, a cure and relief of their diseases, by your every-day employment or unlimited permission to take it in cases for which it is unsuitable, and moreover, in such enormous doses.

From the symptoms and ailments which camomile excites *per se* in the healthy human being (and the same is the case with all dynamically acting medicines) we see what are the natural morbid states it can and must cure rapidly, certainly, and permanently. I need not point out these to him who knows how to employ it homœopathically.

In the cases for which this plant is suitable, indicated by the correspondence of the symptoms of the disease with the peculiar camomile symptoms, it effects a perfect cure in very small doses, *when the patient is protected from all other foreign medicinal influences*, as he ought to be in every rational mode of treatment. I have found a single drop of the quadrillion-fold attenuation of the juice of the plant, prepared as above directed, not only sufficient, but sometimes (when the patient was very sensitive) rather too strong. Any one who has a fancy to compare these doses with the ordinary ones of a couple of ounces of camomile flowers in infusion, the drug being also given at the same time in clysters and fomentations, as it often is in the ordinary stupid routine practice, may do so. Well-attested truth is on *my* side.

Chamomilla has not a long duration of action. but in large doses its action extends over some, occasionally many days.

The injurious effects of its employment in excessive doses and in unsuitable cases are soon removed, according to the symptoms, sometimes by *raw coffee*, sometimes by *ignatia*, sometimes by *pulsatilla* ; but if they consist of tearing and shooting pains relieved by moving the affected part, by *aconite*. *Coffee*, when it is not used by the patient as his daily beverage, also removes many of the sufferings caused by camomile, and, on the other hand, camomile is often a powerful antidote to the hurtful effects of coffee, when the symptoms do not rather

*Often, when, in the ordinary *hap-hazard* practice, camomile may have been administered in an appropriate case (for it must occasionally happen that a polychrest medicine, which is given in all sorts of cases, will by chance meet with a case of disease for which it is suited), it does harm, owing to the excessive quantity in which it is taken. It removes the symptoms of the malady to which it is homoeopathic, but inflicts in addition many useless sufferings, by producing some of its other severe symptoms which are not developed by a small dose, and thus it does harm in even the most appropriate cases by the unnecessarily strong dose.

point to *nux vomica.* But when the injurious effects of coffee are continually renewed by its daily use as a beverage, camomile can no more relieve the coffee-drinker of his morbid symptoms than wiping up can avail while the rain continues to fall.

Camomile in the smallest dose seems to diminish in a remarkable manner over-sensitiveness to pain or the too acute sufferings of the organs of the emotions from excessive pain. Hence it alleviates many of the affections caused by coffee-drinking and by courses of treatment with narcotic palliatives. On this account it is unsuited for persons who bear pain calmly and patiently. I attach great importance to this observation.

Of late I have seldom been able to employ camomile as a curative agent. When in new patients the symptoms indicated the employment of camomile I have usually found that they were not original symptoms of disease, but as the history showed, symptoms resulting from the abuse of camomile, so that I had only to give antidotes for the ailments occasioned by the latter in order to cure the disease that had been artificially produced thereby.

[The only one of his disciples who assisted HAHNEMANN in this proving was STAPF.

The old-school authorities are very few.

CULLEN, *Mat. Med.*, is quoted for one symptom : "diarrhœa."

LIND, MONRO, PRINGLE, and ROSENSTEIN (no reference being given to their works) are cited for another : "vomiting."

SENAC, *De Recondita Febrium Intermit. et Remitt. Natura*, supplies a third : "pungent heat." All the other symptoms were observed by HAHNEMANN himself.

The *Frag. de Vir.* had 275 symptoms, the 1st Edit. 481, and this 2nd Edit. 493.]

CHAMOMILLA.

(Vertigo on stooping forwards.)

Giddy when sitting upright, not when lying. [*Stf.**]

Vertigo, especially when talking (aft. 16 h.).

Vertigo after a meal.

5. Soon after a meal, when walking, vertigo as if he would fall, just as if the head were top-heavy.

Vertigo after drinking coffee.

Vertigo in the morning.

Drunken, staggering vertigo in the morning on rising from bed.

Vertigo with dizziness.†

10. Vertigo in the evening, as if he could not recollect himself properly.

(Vertigo and dimness of vision after lying down, with flying heat in the face.)

Syncopal vertigo.

Slight attacks of syncopal vertigo (aft. ¼ h.).

*In a girl of 19, from some cupfuls of strong camomile tea. [Apparently all Stapf's symptoms were observed in this subject.]

† See also the following symptoms of dizziness, also 245.

Obtuseness of the senses, diminished power of collecting himself (aft. 4, 5, 6 h.).

15. **Joyless obtuseness of the senses with drowsiness, but without being able to sleep.**

Stupidity in the head. [*Stf.*]

He does not rightly understand a question, and answers wrongly, with low-toned voice, as if he was delirious (aft. 6 h.).

He is easily fatigued by thinking.

He understands and comprehends nothing properly, just as if he were prevented doing so by a sort of dulness of hearing, or a waking dream (aft. 1½ h.).

20. A state of distraction ; he sits as if absorbed in thought.

His thoughts leave him.

When writing and speaking he leaves out whole words.

He stammers, he makes mistakes in speaking (aft. 4 h.).

Unobservant, inattentive ; external things make no impression on him ; he is indifferent to everything (aft. 2 h.).

25. Dull aching headache when sitting and thinking.

Heaviness in the head.

Heaviness in the head. [*Stf.*]

Headache compounded of heaviness and bruised feeling (aft. 3 h.).

Headache felt even when asleep.

30. Headache, in the morning in bed, while the eyes are still shut, in a half waking state, which goes off when quite awake and after getting up.

On awaking from sleep, pain in the head, as if it would burst (aft. 13 h.).

Repeated attacks of tearing pain in the forehead.

(When sitting up or turning in bed, tearing pains in the forehead, with the sensation as if a lump fell forward. [*Stf.*]

Very violent tearing headache at midnight, which, however, only wakes him up for instants on account of the very profound sleep.

35. **Semilateral drawing headache** (aft. 3, 4 h.).

Tearing headache on one side in the temple.

Shooting tearing pain in the forehead, which extends to the chest.

Pain in the bone on both sides of the forehead (aft. 3 h.).

Tearing and shooting **outwards at the temples.**

40. Single stitches in one-half of the brain, especially the right (aft. 11 h.).

Single severe stitches in the brain.

Severe stitches in one-half of the head, as after a chill.

Fine shooting headache.

Headache like needle-pricks, as if the eyes would fall out of the head.

45. **Transient attacks of throbbing in one-half of the brain.**

Throbbing headache (aft. 14 h.).

Single beats in the head (aft. ¼ h.).

Twitching headache in the forehead, especially after a meal.

A cracking and grating in the left half of the brain.

50. The left temple is swollen, and painful when touched (aft. 6 h.).

The forehead wrinkled above the nose. [*Stf.*]

Her head waggles to and fro. [*Stf.*]

Puffiness of the face and hands.*

An eroding itching on the skin of the forehead.

55. When the consciousness has returned and the drowsiness is past the pupils become more dilated (aft. 7 h.).

Pupils very contracted, or rather having a tendency to contract † (aft. several h.).

Contracted pupils (the first 4 h.).

A great dryness (of the Meibomian glands) on the border of the upper and lower eyelids (aft. 1 h.).

Feeling of soreness in the outer canthi of the eyes, and sore excoriated lips (aft. 36 h.).

60. The canthi in the morning full of matter.

The eye is swollen in the morning, and sealed up with mucus.

After sleeping the eyelids are gummed together.

Painless extravasation of blood in the white of the inner angle of the right eye (aft. 14 h.).

Aching in the eyes; the eyes are inflamed and full of mucus in the morning.

65. An aching pain under the upper eyelid on moving the eye and on shaking the head.

Severe stitches in the eyes.

Sensation as if fire and heat came out of the eyes‡ (immediately).

Glittering before the eyes (immediately).

Glittering before the eyes; she did not see where she was. [*Stf.*]

70. Obscuration of the sight on one side, when he fixes his look on a white object.

Eyes dull and weak in the morning, more rarely in the evening; with the candle a ray of light seems to extend from the eyes to the candle flame.

Dimness of vision, with chilliness.

It became black before his eyes. [*Stf.*]

Red miliary rash on the cheeks.

75. Tearing in the ears, earache.

(Tearing in the lobe of the right ear.)

Single coarse stitches in the ear, especially when stooping, with taking things ill and vexation about trifles.

Some stitches on the neck near the ear.

When stooping obtuse pressure in the internal ear, as from a blow.

80. Sensation as if the ears were stopped up, and as if a bird were rustling and scratching in them.

In the evening he has dulness before the ears.§

* 52, 53,—see 91, 104, 105.
† See 411.
‡ See 412.
§ See 410.

Roaring in the ears as from rushing water.

Ringing in the ears (aft. 1, 3, 4 h.).

Epistaxis.

85. Ulcerated nostrils ; sore nose.

The lips become cracked and desquamate (aft. 16 h).

The lower lip parts in the middle in a crack (from the 3rd to the 10th h.).

Scabby ulceration on the border of the lip (from 1 to 4 h.).

Swelling of the gums.

90. Looseness of the teeth.

Toothache, with swelling of the cheek.*

After midnight (3 a.m.), wakened by toothache (a gnawing pain as if the nerve were scraped), which ceased about 7 a.m., so that only occasional stitch-like jerks remained.

In the teeth of the upper jaw a stirring up and formication.

Stirring-up drawing toothache in the jaw.

95. Drawing pain in the teeth.

Toothache as from a chill from exposure to the open air while perspiring profusely.

Toothache on taking something warm into the mouth.

(Toothache renewed in the warm room.)

Toothache particularly severe after warm drinks, especially after coffee.

100. After eating and drinking, especially warm things (but also from cold things), the toothache comes on either immediately or after a minute.

Drawing pain in the teeth after eating and drinking.

Toothache after eating and drinking, although neither was either warm or cold (later).

On opening the jaws, pain as if the masseter muscles ached as from cramp, which pain at the same time extends into the teeth.

Toothache recurring intermittently in fits, with swelling of the cheek and accumulation of saliva ; the pain darts hither and thither, and extends even to the eyes, and is aggravated by drinking cold water.

105. Tearing toothache in the jaw towards the ear, with swelling of the cheek.

In the lower jaw, towards the front, drawing toothache (aft. ½ h.).

Drawing toothache, he knows not in which tooth exactly, which goes off while eating, and rages particularly at night, during which the teeth feel too long.†

* See 104 and 105, also 50 and 53. The toothache which camomile can cause (see 89 to 108) corresponds very closely to that so frequently prevailing in recent times (generally resulting from drinking coffee) and hence this will be homoeopathically and specifically cured by small doses of camomile.

† The camomile-pains have this peculiarity as a rule, that they are most severe in the night, and then often drive the victim almost to despair, not unfrequently with incessant thirst, heat, and redness of one cheek ; sometimes also hot sweat in the head even in the hair. The pains of camomile seem generally intolerable, and not to be endured (see 457). All these characteristic symptoms of camomile point to the similar cases of disease capable of being cured homoeopathically by it.

Single stitches in the jaw into the internal ear.
Spasmodic drawing pain in the palate towards the fauces.
110. **On and under the tongue vesicles with shooting pain.**
A severe smarting at the back of the tongue and on the palate (aft. 1 h.).
Red tongue. [*Stf.*]
Simple pain at the back of the throat, which is increased on moving the neck and on swallowing.
Sore throat, as from a plug in the throat, on swallowing (aft. 4 h.).
115. Sore throat, with swelling of the parotid gland.
(Throbbing pain in the submaxillary glands (aft. 4 h.).
Throbbing at the back of the throat (aft. ¼ h.).
Ptyalism.
Teeth covered with mucus.
120. Slimy taste (aft. 2 and 12 h.).
Sour taste (aft. 3 and 18 h.).
Bread tastes sour.
Everything he takes tastes like old rancid fat (aft. 2 h.)
What he hawks up tastes putrid.
125. (At night he has a putrid taste in the mouth.)
He has a putrid smell from the mouth after dinner, like fœtid breath (aft. 3 h.).
In the morning bitter taste in the mouth (aft. 24 h.).
Want of appetite.
Anorexia, but on eating his appetite returns.
130. He has no appetite and he relishes nothing ; the food will not go down.
No desire for food ; nothing tastes good.
He shudders when food is placed before him ; he has repugnance to it.
Want of appetite, as if he loathed the food, though it tastes all right.
No hunger and no appetite.
135. (He dislikes soup.)
Beer smells ill.
He dislikes coffee.
After his early coffee nausea, as if he would vomit, with suffocative attacks.
In the morning, after drinking coffee, heat all over and perspiration, with vomiting of bitter mucus ; afterwards bitter taste in the mouth, weakness in the head, and inclination to vomit.
140. Great appetite for coffee.* (aft. 7 h.).
(Appetite for raw sour crout.)
Unnatural hunger, in the evening (aft. 3 h.).
During supper the food seems to go no further than the pit of the throat and to stick there, with sensation of fulness, sickness, and eructation.
Empty eructation (aft. ¼ h.).
145. Sour eructation.

* 140 seems to be alternating action with

The pains present are aggravated by eructation.
Frequently a single hiccup (aft. 1 h.).
During the meal fulness, and after the meal nausea.
After a meal, fulness of satiety in the stomach even till the next day ; inclination to vomit.
150. After breakfast inclination to vomit, all the morning.
After a meal the abdomen becomes distended.
Nausea after meal.
After a meal fulness, anxiety, and tearing pain in the back, which then goes into the abdomen.
In the morning dryness in the mouth, then distension of the abdomen, and the stool is incompletely evacuated.
155. Nausea, with inclination to vomit, as if about to faint.
Qualmishness and faint-like nausea.
The qualmishness (faint-like nausea) in the scrobiculus cordis goes off by eating.
Nausea, inclining to vomit, with collection of saliva in the mouth.
In the morning nausea, inclining to vomit.
160. Vomiting. [LIND.—MONRO.—PRINGLE.—ROSENSTEIN.]
(Vomiting without previous eructation.)
(Sour vomiting ; she also smells sour from the mouth.)
The food is returned by eructation, it is belched up (aft. 5 h.).
Vomiting of food, which is first excited by fulness of the abdomen, but afterwards by intolerable nausea.
165. **After eating** and drinking **heat** and sweat **on the face** (aft. 14 h.).
After a meal aching in the hypochondria and stomach.
He cries out anxiously about a pain in the scrobiculus cordis, as if it were pressed down, and he sweats profusely during it.*
Painful flatulent distension of the epigastric region in the morning.
In the hypochondria the flatulence pushes upwards (later).
170. Pressure on the stomach, as if a stone pressed downwards.
Pressive pain in the stomach and under the short ribs that tightens the breath, especially after drinking coffe (aft. 1 h.).
Pressive pain above the navel.
Flatulent colic ; flatulence presses now here now there with great force, as if it would bore through the abdominal muscles, with loud rumbling and grumbling ; it presses especially on the inguinal rings ; when the colic subsides very little flatus is passed, and then scarcely any is felt in the abdomen (aft. 3 h.).
Flatulent colic (aft. 1 and several h.).
175. Colic returning from time to time ; the flatulence accumulates in the hypochondria, and stitches dart through the chest (aft. 8 h.).
Continued tensive pain beneath the ribs, with a tension about the brain (and dry catarrh in the chest) (aft. 1 h.).
Clucking in the side down into the abdomen.
Bruised pain of the hypogastric muscles (aft. 9 h.).
Hard distended abdomen.
180. Compressive pain in the abdomen (immediatel).

* See 247, 249, 457.

Intolerable pain in the abdomen in the morning at sunrise.

Extraordinary pain in the abdomen, owing to which he did not know how to rest.

Sensation as if the whole abdomen were hollow, and at the same time a perpetual movement in the bowels (with blue rings round the eyes), and when the attack comes on in the evening it is for a short time combined with anxiety (aft. 24 h.).

Colic, more cutting than pinching.

185. Colic, more cutting than shooting, with collection of saliva in the mouth.

Drawing pain in the abdomen.

Single attacks of violent pinching in the abdomen ; each of these pains lasts for full a minute (aft. 12 h.).

Pinching, tearing colic in the umbilical region and further down on both sides, with a pain in the sacrum as if it was broken.

Constant tearing colic, as if rolled up in a ball, in the side of the abdomen.

190. Pain in the abdomen, as if caused by costiveness of the motion, the evacuation of which is delayed.*

Sufferings in the abdomen, as from constipation (aft. 4 h.).

Constipation.

Constipation from inaction of the rectum, so that the excrements can only be pressed out by the efforts of the abdominal muscles (aft. 1, 4 h.).

In the midst of sharp pinching pain in the abdomen, bright coloured fæces are passed (aft. 12, 24 h.).

195. (Undigested excrements.)

(Hot, diarrhœic stool, smelling like rotten eggs.)

Diarrhœa. [CULLEN, *Arzneimittell.*, Tom. ii, p. 94.]

Painless, diarrhœic, green, watery stools, composed of fæces and mucus.

Watery diarrhœa, with (and without) cutting in the abdomen.

200. Nocturnal diarrhœa, with pains in the abdomen, so that he must crouch together.

Excrements covered with mucus, and with mucus in the intervals between the lumps of fæces.

Only white slimy diarrhœa with bellyache (aft. 1, 3 h.).

Shooting pain in the rectum after every stool.

A forcing towards the inguinal ring, as if that part were now too weak to resist, as if a hernia would come (aft. 3 h.).

205. Tendency to blind piles.

Fluent piles.

Blind piles.

Itching pain in the anus (aft. ½ h.).

(The discharge of urine is held back by pains in the belly.)

210. Shooting pain in the neck of the bladder, when not urinating.

* 190, 191, 192, 193. All the constipation symptoms are secondary action, *i.e.* reaction of the organism against the efforts of the camomile to produce diarrhoea in its primary action.

Burning in the neck of the bladder when urinating.

Smarting pain in the urethra while urinating.

Anxiety whilst urinating, without any mechanical obstacle.

Weakened power of the bladder ; the urine passes in a sluggish stream (aft. 20 h.).

215. Anxiety with ineffectual urging to urinate, though there is not much urine in the bladder.

Involuntary discharge of urine (aft. 3, 4 h.).

Itching of the scrotum (aft. 6 h.).

Sexual desire (later).

Nocturnal seminal emission.

220. In the morning in bed, erection of the penis.

Excoriation on the border of the prepuce.

On the border of the prepuce, itching pricking pain (aft. 3 h.).

Sore burning in the vagina

Yellow, smarting leucorrhœa.

225. Acrid, smarting, watery discharge from the vagina after dinner.

Forcing towards the womb, like labour pains, with very frequent urging to urinate.

Cutting pain in the abdomen and drawing in the thighs before the menses.

Amid severe pains as if going to get a child, and like labour pains in the womb, frequent discharge of clotted blood, with tearing pains in the blood-vessels of the legs.

Drawing from the anterior part of the sacrum, grasping and griping in the womb, and then large pieces of blood are always passed.

230. Metrorrhagia.

Metrorrhagia, even in old persons.

(On the advent of the menses, cross, intolerant, and disposed to quarrel sooner than give in.

Suppression of the menses, with swelling of the scrobiculus cordis and a pain as if it would be pressed down, with swollen abdomen, labour-like pains, and anasarca.

* * *

Stoppage of the nose, as from stuffed coryza (aft. 1 h.).

235. Catarrhal stoppage of the nose, with flow of mucus from the nose.

Coryza lasting five to eight days (aft. 2 h.)

Whistling, wheezing, rattling in the wind-pipe when breathing.

Hoarseness from viscid mucus sticking in the larynx, which can only be brought away by violent hawking (aft. 8 h.).

Catarrhal hoarseness in the wind-pipe, with dryness of the eyelids (aft. 1 to 8 h.).

240. Hoarseness and cough on account of rattling mucus in the upper part of the wind-pipe, and where the mucus is detached by coughing the part is painful (aft. 2 h.).

A burning in the larynx.

Short, croaking respiration. [*Stf.*]

Fetches short deep breath, with great elevation of the chest. [*Stf.*]

A burning pain under the sternum up into the mouth.

245. A burning in the chest with stupidity of the head,* as if he did not know where he was, with anxiety.

The chest internally is painful, as if bruised (aft. 24 h.).

An aching pain under the sternum, which does not interfere with breathing, and is not increased either by breathing or by the touch (aft. 12 h.).

A pressive pain under the sternum that tightens the breath (aft. 10 h.).

It lies heavy on his stomach, pain in the pit of the stomach as if it were pressed down.†

250. Quick stitches at the heart when moving, which oppress the breathing. [*Stf.*].

A drawing pain, or sensation as if the right side of the chest were repeatedly drawn inwards (aft. 12, 16 h.).

Contraction of the chest.

Oppression of the chest.

Tensive pain over the chest on inspiring.

255. Across the upper part of the chest a squeezing pain (in the evening) (aft. 5 h.).

Oppression of the chest, as from flatulence which is dammed up in the epigastrium, with pressive pain ; at the same time stomachache, as at the commencement of heart-burn ; afterwards a burning in the spinal column.

Constriction of the upper part of the chest, which then also is painful on coughing (aft. 4 h.).

Suffocative tightness of the chest (the larynx feels constricted) in the region of the pit of the throat, with constant irritation to cough (aft. $\frac{1}{4}$ h.).

About midnight a fit of coughing, whereby something seems to rise up in the throat, as if she would suffocate.

260. **Almost uninterrupted tickling irritation to cough under the upper part of the sternum, but it does not always result in coughing.**

Dry cough on account of an itching irritation and constant tickle in the part of the trachea behind the pit of the throat (aft. 4 h.).

A severe dry cough in sleep (aft. 11 h.).

Dry cough four or five times daily.

(The child gets angry and then has cough.)

265. Before midnight, stitches radiating from the abdomen into the chest, with constant thirst, without heat.

(Rather obtuse) **stitches, which dart from the abdomen into the**

* See 9, 10, 14, 15, 17, 18, 19 to 26, 298.

† The word here translated stomach is "Herz," respecting which Hahnemann says in a note, "Common people mean by this usually the pit of the stomach ; see also 167," where "Herz" is also the word used. This being so the symptom ought properly to be laced beside 167.

middle of the chest, as from flatulence (aft. 2, 4 h.).

After every start, waking or sleeping, stitches from the abdomen up into the chest.

Stitches **in** the side of the chest, under the ribs and scapulæ, on breathing (aft. 4 h.).

Pricking in the chest like needle-pricks.

270. At times **single severe stitches in the chest** (aft. 2, 4 h.).

Stitches **right** through the chest at every breath.

Stitches **from** the middle of the chest towards the right side, after every expiration (aft. 1½ h.).

Scirrhous hardness of the mammary glands.

A hard lump under the nipple, painful when touched, and also sometimes with drawing tearing pains *per se.*

275. In the region of the clavicle and neck tearing pain (aft. 2 h.).

(Tensive stiffness of the cervical muscles.)

Drawing pain in the scapulæ, chest and hands, as from a chill (aft. 15, 16 h.).

Fine shooting pains in the back.

Tearing in the back.

280. **Drawing pain in the back**, for an hour (aft. 1 h.).

Contractive sensation in the spine.

Drawing tearing pain in the back.

Pain in the sacrum, especially at night.

Sacrum as if bruised.

285. (A kind of irregular labour-pains) from the sacrum into the thighs, a drawing paralytic pain (aft. 1, 2 h.).

After sitting a stiff pain in the loins (aft. 16 h.).

At night, intolerable pain in the loins and hip-joint, when he lies on the opposite side.

From midnight onwards an uninterrupted fine, painful aching in the articular ligaments and the periosteum of the arm, from the shoulder to the fingers, which resembles a drawing or tearing (almost as bad when not moving as when moving) ; late at night it is at its worst, especially when lying on the back, and it is easiest when lying on the painful arm (aft. 8 h.).

A crawling tearing in the shafts of the arm-bones to the fingers, as if the arm were numb or asleep, or had no feeling.

290. **A stiffness of the arm, as if it would go to sleep, on grasping anything with the hand.**

The arms go to sleep immediately, when she grasps anything strongly ; she must immediately let it go.

The left arm goes to sleep without having lain on it. [*Stf.*]

Drawing paralytic pain in the elbows and hands.

Late in the evening a drawing pain in the interior of the arm, from the elbow to the tips of the fingers (aft. 1 h.).

295. Drawing pain in the wrist-joint.

Pain of the thumb and index finger, as from a sprain, or as from too great exertion, or as if they were broken, felt when moving them.

Burning pain in the hand, in the afternoon (aft. 72 h.).

The hands are cold ; she feels a paralytic stiffness in them, and cloudiness of the head ; she is sensitive to the open air as if she would easily take cold.

Coldness of the hands, with cold sweat on the palms, the rest of the body being sufficiently warm (aft. 2. h.).

300. The fingers become cold and have a tendency to go to sleep, when sitting (aft. 1 h.).

In the morning the fingers go to sleep (aft. 12 h.).

Tearing pain in the thighs and legs.

In the hip-joint pain as if dislocated, on treading after sitting (in the evening) (aft. 5 h.).

Lame stiffness with weakness in the thigh like a paralytic stroke.

305. In the thigh an indescribable pain, on attempting to rise after sitting, and when lying on stretching out the leg.

Transient bruised pain in the thighs (aft. $\frac{1}{4}$ h.).

Creaking and cracking in the knee on moving it (aft. 3 h.).

Tension in the knee. [*Stf.*]

Late in the evening, drawing pain from the knee through the leg.

310. In the knee a drawing tearing pain down into the ankles.

Sensation in the legs as if they would go to sleep.

He must stretch out the legs from time to time in order to get rest.

At night in bed, on stretching out and pressing the feet against something he gets cramp in the calves, which is relieved by flexing the knees (aft. 8 h.).

Cramp in the calves (aft. 10 h.).

315. Especial tendency to cramp in the calves.

Tensive cramp-like pain in the calves on moving the feet (aft. 8 h.).

Tension in the legs up the calves. [*Stf.*]

She must draw the legs up on account of pain in the calves and knees ; when she stretches herself out they go to sleep. [*Stf.*]

Nocturnal paralytic powerlessness of the feet ; they have no strength, he cannot tread, and when he stands up he sinks down to the ground, with drawing pain in the leg and stiffness and numbness of the soles of the feet.

320. Feet are as if paralysed.*

Tearing pain in the feet ; he dare not cover them with the bed clothes.

In the night the soles of the feet burn, and he puts his feet out of bed.

In the feet a burning and itching as if they had been frost-bitten (aft. 3 h.).

Rapid swelling of one foot and of the sole.

325. In the interior of the heel an itching pain (aft. 3 h.).

Itching on the sole of the foot.

* The paralytic sensation of camomile in any part is never without accompanying drawing or tearing pain, and the drawing or tearing of camomile is almost always accompanied by paralytic or numb sensation in the part. See 285, 293 (288, 289), 320, 347 (357, 364).

Spasmodic contraction of the toes with tearing pain in the limbs.

Feeling as if the toes would bend and go to sleep, while sitting, especially the big toes (aft. 1 h.).

Great dread of the wind.

330. The hands and feet easily become benumbed in the cold, as if they would be frost-bitten (aft. 5 h.).

Pain compounded of itching and pricking, now in one part now in another, in a small spot ; after scratching the pain increases (aft. 4 h.).

A slightly elevated cutaneous eruption in the nape, which causes a smarting sensation that compels scratching.

Pustule-like pimples here and there in the face, which are not painful and only itch when touched.

Red miliary eruption on the cheeks and forehead, without heat.

335. Small red spots on the skin, which are covered with miliary papules.

Thick eruption of red **papules**, which are crowded together on a red spot on the skin, which itches and smarts somewhat, particularly at night, on the lumbar vertebræ and the side of the abdomen ; from time to time, especially in the evening, there occurs a shudder round about.

The skin becomes œdematous, unhealthy, and every injury takes on a bad character and tends to suppurate.

An existing ulcer becomes painful (aft. $\frac{3}{4}$ h.).

In the ulcer there occurs twitching and shooting pain.

340. **In the ulcer there occurs at night a burning and smarting pain, with creeping in it and painful over-sensitiveness to the touch,**

(Round the ulcer on the foot there occurs redness, swelling, and bruised pain.)

There arise around the ulcer papules covered with a scab and going on to suppuration with itching (the border round the base of the ulcer is very red).

Cracking in the joints, especially of the lower limbs, and pains in them, as if bruised, and yet no proper feeling of fatigue (aft. 8 h.).

Simple pain of all the joints on moving, as if they were stiff and would break (aft. 6 h.).

345. All the joints are painful, as if bruised and beaten ; there is no power in the hands and feet, but without proper feeling of fatigue.

All his limbs are painful.

Pain in the periosteum of the limbs with paralytic weakness.

Tearing pain in the limbs, which can only be allayed by perpetually turning about in bed.

Attack of tearing pains in the evening.

350. Single, rare, drawing tearing jerks in the shafts of the bones of the limbs, or in the tendons.

Convulsive, single twitches of the limbs when on the point of falling asleep.

Twitching in the limbs and eyelids.

Single twitchings of the limbs and head in the morning sleep.

Infantile convulsions: alternately first one then the other leg is moved up and down; the child grabs at and tries to get something with its hands, and draws the mouth to and fro, with staring eyes.

355. The child lies as if unconscious, completely devoid of sense, its face is frequently transformed, the eyes distorted, the facial muscles drawn awry; it has rattling in the chest, with much cough; it yawns and stretches much.

General stiffness for a short time.

In the parts whence the pain has departed sensation of paralysis.

Weariness, especially of the feet (aft. 10 h.).

Weakness; she wants to be always seated (aft. 5 h.).

360. Dreads all work.

Greater weakness when resting than when moving; he is strong enough when moving.

The greatest weakness in the morning, which does not allow him to rise from his bed.

After breakfast he feels at first very well, but after a few minutes a faint-like sinking of the strength (aft. 8 h.).

When the pain begins there immediately occurs weakness, so that he feels like to sink down; he must lie down.

365. The child insists on lying down, it will not allow itself to be carried (aft. 2 h.).

The child will not put its foot to the ground nor walk; it weeps piteously (aft. 4 h.).

The greatest weariness and weakness, which borders on fainting (aft. 4 h.).

Fainting fits.

Sinking feeling about the heart.

370. **Fainting fits** that return sooner or later (aft. ½, 3, 4, 5 h.).

A kind of faint: he becomes sick, and has a sinking feeling about the heart; the legs become suddenly as if paralysed, and he has pains in all the limbs as if they had been beaten.

Heaviness of the limbs, yawning and drowsiness all day.

Frequent very violent yawning, without sleepiness, with gay activity (aft. 1 h.).

Frequent, interrupted (ineffectual attempts at) yawning (aft. ¼ h.).

375. By day, drowsiness and laziness.

Drowsiness when eating.

Uncommon sleepiness (aft. ¾ to 1½ h.).

When seated by day he feels like to go to sleep, but when he lies down he cannot sleep, but remains awake.

In the morning, in bed, half-open, downward-directed eyes, pupils somewhat dilated, stupefied drowsiness. [*Stf.*]

380. Nocturnal sleeplessness, accompanied by attacks of anxiety; very vivid visions and fantastic pictures hover before him (aft. 1 to 4 h.).

In the drowsy state of awaking he imagines one about him to be quite another (stouter) person.

At night it seems to him as though he heard the voices of absent persons.

He chatters unintelligibly in his sleep, directing this or that obstacle to be removed.

At night, when awake and sitting up in bed, he talks nonsense.

385. Sleep full of fantastic dreams.

Vivid, distinct dreams, as if a story were being acted before him while awake.

In his dream he carries on conversations with lively memory and thoughtfulness.

Moaning in sleep.

Weeping and howling in sleep.

390. Quarrelsome, vexatious dreams.

His sleep seems to him to be more fatiguing and tiresome ; his expression in sleep is gloomy, cross and sad.

At night in sleep he starts with affright.

Starting up, crying out, tossing about and talking in sleep (aft. 6 h.).

He tosses about anxiously at night in bed, is full of fantasies.

395. He cannot stay in bed.

He has the greatest anxiety in bed, but not when he is out of bed ; at the same time the pupils dilate and contract rapidly.

|The nocturnal pains can be allayed by warm compresses.
|(Sitting up in bed alleviates the nocturnal pains.)

Snoring inspiration in sleep.

400. In sleep snoring inspiration which is shorter than the expiration, with mouth somewhat opened, and hot clammy sweat on the forehead. (aft. 3 h.).

Groaning in sleep, with hot clammy frontal sweat.

Waking stupefied slumber, or rather inability to open the eyes ; slumber without sleep, rapid expiration and tearing pain in the forehead, with inclination to vomit. (aft. 1½ h.).

Shivering on single parts, which are not cold, with drowsiness (aft. 2½ h.).

He has shivering on certain parts, in the face (aft. ½ h.), **on the arms** (aft. 2 h.), **with or without external coldness.**

405. He is cold, and at the same time the rigor usually courses from the back to the abdomen (aft. 1 and 4 h.).

When he uncovers himself, he shivers.

Chilliness (immediately) ; none of his articles of clothing are warm enough for him.

He shivers at cold air (aft. 2 h.).

In the evening on lying down, coldness, a kind of dulness of hearing, in which the sound appears to come from a distance, nausea, restlessness, tossing about in bed, a kind of stupefaction of the head and diminished sensibility of the skin, so that the skin when scratched feels numb.

410. Icy coldness of the cheeks, hands and feet, with burning heat of the forehead, neck and chest ; then again heat and redness on the right cheek, during which the hands and feet become again properly

warm, with contracted and not dilatable pupils ; thereafter snoring sleep (aft. 1 to 3 h.).

Coldness of the whole body, with burning heat of the face, which flames out at the eyes.

Cold limbs, with burning heat of the face, burning heat in the eyes, and burning breath (aft. 5 h.).

(Violent internal chill, without coldness of the external parts, excepting the feet which are cold, with thirst ; then great heat with sweat ; when he then stretches his arms out of bed, chill, and when he covers them again with the bed-clothes, perspiration ; at the same time tearing in the forehead).

(After a meal chill all over, followed by heat in the cheeks.)

415. Shivering over the posterior aspect of the body, the arms, the thighs and the back, which recurs in fits, without external coldness, rather with internal dry heat, and external heat, especially of the forehead and face.

Chill only over the anterior aspect of the body ((aft. $\frac{1}{4}$ h.).

(Fever : during the chill he is compelled to lie down, thirst during the chill, no thirst during the heat ; sweat after the heat ; during the perspiration only, shooting pain in the left half of the brain ; the following morning bitter taste in the mouth.)

In the afternoon (about 4 o'clock) chill (during which he says things he did not wish to say), with nausea in the abdomen, until 11 p.m. ; in addition to this throbbing shooting pain in the forehead, aggravated by lying down.

(Fever : rigor in the afternoon, he cannot get warm, with flow of saliva from the mouth, bruised pain in the back and side, and aching stupid pain in the forehead, then at night extreme heat with violent thirst and sleeplessness.)

420. In the evening chilliness ; at night much sweat and thirst.

Immediately after throwing off the clothes violent chill. [*Stf.*]

In the evening burning in the cheeks, with transient rigor.

Repeated attacks of redness in one cheek, without shivering or internal heat (aft. 4 and 12 h.).

Internal heat with shivering.

425. External heat with shivering.

Continual alternation of heat and cold in various parts ; the hands are at one time cold, at another warm—sometimes the forearm, sometimes the upper arm at one time cold at another warm—sometimes the forehead cold while the cheeks are hot, &c. [*Stf.*]

Before midnight, when he tries to go to sleep lying on his back, immediately heat attended by general perspiration (aft. 6 h.).

At night the lips were dry and stuck together, without thirst.

Along with febrile heat and redness of cheeks, thirst.

430. Glowing heat in the cheeks with thirst.

Hot face with redness of cheeks. [*Stf.*]

Along with febrile heat and redness of cheeks he tosses about in bed and talks nonsense, with open eyes.

Feeling of external heat, without actual external heat (aft. 1 and 3 h.).

Feeling of heat, without external heat and without thirst.

435. The lightly covered parts are burning hot, the uncovered parts almost cold. [*Stf.*]

Excites a pungent heat. [SENAC, [1] *De recondita febrium interm. et remitt. natura*, p. 188.]

At night terrible feeling of heat, with burning unquenchable thirst, dry tongue, stupefaction. [*Stf.*]

At night great heat with sleeplessness (aft. 24 h.). [*Stf.*]

General heat, in the forenoon from 9 till 12 o'clock; then profuse perspiration. [*Stf.*]

440. His tongue is dry, with thirst for water, anorexia, flying heat, perspiration on face and palpitation of the heart followed by unnatural hunger.

Violent thirst for water. [*Stf.*]

Unquenchable thirst and dryness of the tongue (aft. 5 h.).

Evening thirst and waking at night with pain.

On account of feeling of external heat he cannot bear the bed clothes.

445. (General morning sweat with smarting sensation in the skin.)

Nocturnal general perspiration (from 10 p.m. till 2 a.m.), without sleep.

Profuse sweat of the covered parts. [*Stf.*]

Perspiration on the face, neck, and hands (aft. 6 h.).

Perspiration, especially on the head under the temples.

450. Frequent transient perspirations on the face and palms.

Involuntary groaning during the heat of the face.

Repeated attacks of anxiety by day.

Anxiety as if he must go to stool and evacuate his bowels.

Trembling anxiety, with palpitation of the heart (aft. 1 h.).

455. Rush of blood to the heart (immediately).

Extreme restlessness, anxious agonised tossing about, with tearing pains in the abdomen (aft. 1 h.), followed by obtuseness of the senses and then intolerable headache.

Hypochondrial anxiety.

He feels a sinking in the precordium; he is beside himself with anxiety, moans and sweats profusely therewith.

Weeping and howling.

460. (Attacks lasting some minutes, every two or three hours): the child makes itself stiff and bends backwards, stamps with its feet on the nurse's arm, cries in an uncontrollable way, and throws everything away.

Lachrymose restlessness; the child wants this thing and the other, and when given anything he refuses it or knocks it away from him (aft. 4 h.).

---

1 When used in agues. Original not accessible, but Caldwell's translation (Philadelphia, 1805) gives the quality of heat as "pungent," by which word Hahnemann's "beissend" may also be rendered.

With weeping and ill-humour, she complains of sleeplessness on account of bruised pain in all the limbs. [*Stf.*]

The child can only be quieted by carrying it in the arms.

Lamentable howling of the child when refused what it wanted (aft. 3 h.).

465. Very anxious ; nothing she does seems to her to be right ; she is irresolute ; at the same time transient heat in the face and cold sweat on the palms of the hands.

Trembling apprehensiveness.

He has a tendency to start (aft. 24 h.).

She starts at the least trifle.

Howling on account of a slight, even an imaginary insult, which, indeed, occurred long ago.

470. Cannot cease talking about old vexatious things.

Suspicion that he may have been insulted.

His hypochondriacal whims and his crossness at the smallest trifles appear to him to proceed from stupidity and heaviness of the head and constipation.

Moroseness after dinner.

Moroseness for two hours.

475. Sulky moroseness ; everything others do is displeasing to him ; no one does anything to please him.

He vexes himself inwardly about every trifle.

He is always morose and disposed to crossness.

Crossness about everything, with tightness of the chest.

He cannot stand being talked to or interrupted in his conversation, especially after rising up from sleep, with sluggish pupils that dilate and contract with difficulty* (aft. 10 h.).

480. She cannot bear music.

Excessively sensitive to all smells.

Irritated disposition.

Sullen, disposed to quarrel (aft. 12 h.).

The disposition is inclined to anger, quarrelsomeness and disputation (aft. 2 h.).

485. Quarrelsome crossness ; she seeks for everything vexatious (aft. 3 h.)

Groaning and moaning from low spirits (aft. 5 h.).

He is silent and does not speak when he is not obliged to answer questions (aft. 6 h.).

She sits stiffly on a chair like a statue, and seems to take no notice of anything about her (aft. 24 h.). [*Stf.*]

Speaks unwillingly, in disjointed phrases, curtly. [*Stf.*]

490. (She has scruples of conscience about everything.)

* (See 77.) The sometimes dangerous illness resembling acute bilious fever, that often comes on immediately after a violent vexation causing anger, with heat of face, unquenchable thirst, taste of bile, nausea, anxiety, restlessness, &c., has such great homoeopathic analogy with the symptoms of camomile, that camomile cannot fail to remove the whole malady rapidly and specifically, which is done as if by a miracle by one drop of the above-mentioned diluted juice.

Serious reservedness ; calm submission to his profoundly felt fate (later).

Very reserved ; one cannot get a word out of her. [*Stf.*]

Fixed ideas (later).[1]

---

1 The number of symptoms, 493, does not correspond with the numeration in the original, 461 + 33 = 494. This is owing to a mistake in the reckoning of his own symptoms by Hahnemann. The symptom he has marked 395 is actually 394, and the whole subsequent numeration is vitiated by the error. In place of his tale of symptoms being 461 it is actually only 460.

CHELIDONIUM.[1]

(Celandine.)

(The expressed juice of the root of Chelidonium majus, mixed with equal parts of alcohol.)

The ancients imagined that the yellow colour of the juice of the plant was an indication (signature) of its utility in bilious diseases. The moderns from this extended its employment to hepatic diseases, and though there were cases where the utility of this plant in maladies of that region of the abdomen was obvious, yet the diseases of this organ differ so much among one another, both in their origin and in the attendant derangements of the rest of the organism ; moreover, the cases in which it is said to have done good have been so imperfectly described by physicians, that it is impossible from their data to tell beforehand the cases of disease in which it must certainly be of use ; and yet this is indispensably necessary in the treatment of diseases of mankind which are of such serious importance. Hence, a recommendation of this sort *(ab usu in morbis)* is of but a general, undefined, and dubious character, especially since this plant was so seldom given simply and singly by physicians, but almost always in combination with heterogeneous, powerful substances (dandelion, fumitory, water-cresses), and along with the simultaneous employment of the so-called bitters, which vary so much in their effects.

The importance of human health does not admit of any such uncertain directions for the employment of medicines. It would be criminal frivolity to rest contented with such guesswork at the beside of the sick. Only that which the drugs themselves unequivocally reveal of their peculiar powers in their effects on the healthy human body—that is to say, only their pure symptoms—can teach us loudly and clearly when they can be advantageously used with certainty ; and this is when they are administered in morbid states very similar to those they are able to produce on the healthy body.

From the following symptoms of celandine, which it is to be hoped will be completed by other upright, accurate observers, a much more extensive prospect of the real curative powers of this plant is opened up than has hitherto been dreamt of. It is, however, only the physician who is conversant with the homœopathic doctrine who will be able to make this advantageous employment of it. The routine practitioner may content himself with the uncertain indications for the employment of celandine to be found in his benighted materia medica.

1 From vol. iv, 2nd edit., 1825.

[HAHNEMANN was assisted in this proving by BECHER, GROSS, HARTMANN, HERMANN, LANGHAMMER, MEYER, TEUTHORN, and WALTHER.

The old-school authorities quoted are :

Horn's Archiv, Bd. xi.

WENDT, in *Hufel. Journ.*, xvi.

The 1st Edit, gives 151 symptoms, this 2nd Edit. only 5 more.]

CHELIDONIUM.

(His senses left him.)

Cloudiness (aft. 10 m.). [*Gss.*]

Contractive headache.

Dull headache, with beating synchronous with the pulse on the right temple, as if the vessels were too full of blood (aft. 2 h.). [*Trn.*]

5. Headache, aching pressing from within outwards, especially towards the forehead, which is very much aggravated by open air, coughing, blowing the nose and stooping but is absent while eating, lasting all day. [*Htn.*]

A forcing in the cerebrum, as if it had not room in the skull, and would be forced through the ear, wherein is heard a noise like a distant water weir. [*Wth.*]

Disagreeable sensation in the left temple as if the blood stagnated there all at once, followed by an obtuse shooting pain in the same place (aft. ½ h.). [*Wth.*]

Aching pain in the right temporal region, during which the right nostril was stopped up (aft. 6 h.). [*Myr.*]

Pressive tearing headache betwixt the eye-brows, which tended to press the eyelids to, went off after eating and returned three quarters of an hour later (aft. ½ h.). [*Bch.*]

10. Tearing pain in the right side of the occiput, with long severe stitches towards the front (aft. 15½ h.). [*Htn.*]

Violent tearing stitches in the left frontal eminence (aft. 3½ h.). [*Htn.*]

Obtuse shooting extending across the whole forehead. [*Lr.*]

Sensation of transient drawing under the frontal bone (aft. ¼ h.). [*Gss.*]

Formications in the frontal eminences in intermittent, short intervals. [*Gss.*]

15. Shooting, aching headache in the vertex, by fits, especially on walking rapidly.

Slow, drawing, pressive-like stitch from the left side of the occiput towards the forehead (aft. ½ h.). [*Htn.*]

Pinching stitches in the right side of the occiput (aft. 1½ h.). [*Htn.*.]

Pinching stitches on the left side of the occiput, as if externally, but neither increased nor diminished by pressing on it (aft. 7 h.). [*Htn.*]

(In the eyeballs a tickling itching.)

20. Stupefying pressure on the right orbit as if from without inwards, [*Gss.*]

Contraction of the pupils (immediately). [*Bch.*]

Contraction of the pupils immediately after taking the medicine, but after an hour they dilated to their ordinary size. [*Trn.*]

Pressive pain over the left eye that seemed to press down the upper lid (aft. ¾ h.). [*Htn.*]

Pressure on the right upper eyelid. [*Hrr.*]

25. A pimple on the left upper tarsal cartilage containing pus, with aching pain in it on touching it and on shutting the eyes. [*Hrr.*]

A dazzling spot appeared before the eye, and when he looked into it the eye watered.

Tension and drawing in the left zygoma, only when lying (aft. 9 h.). [*Gss.*]

Pale face. [*Trn.*]

Pain as from a contusion in the left ear lobe, and immediately afterwards burning in the right lobe as from a live coal (aft. 13 h.). [*Myr.*]

30. **A long-lasting stitch in the right external ear that gradually disappears** (aft. 3 h.). [*Htn.*]

When walking, ringing in the left ear (aft. 9 h.). [*Lr.*]

Ringing before the ears, like whistling (aft. ½ h.). [*Myr.*]

Roaring before the ears, like a strong wind (aft. 1½ h.). [*Myr.*]

Intolerable sensation in both ears, as if wind rushed out of them, so that he must often introduce the finger in order to remove this sensation (aft. ½, 3, 4 h.). [*Wth.*]

35. In both ears a noise like distant **thundering of cannon.** [*Wth.*]

Intermitting tearing pressure in the right internal meatus auditorius (aft. 2 h.). [*Hrr.*]

Tearing pain in the right internal meatus auditorius (aft. ¾ h.). [*Hrr.*]

Tearing in the inner ear; by boring in the finger in order to relieve it, ringing came on in addition. [*Myr.*]

Toothache in the left upper jaw. [*Lr.*]

40. In the tip of the nose a trembling and quivering.

A digging tearing in the Antrum Highmorianum (aft. 3 h.).

The teeth of the left lower jaw have a dull pain when touched, and are loose (aft. 3 to 21 h.). [*Bch.*]

Great tension on and in the throat, above the larynx, as if it were constricted, whereby, however only the gullet was narrowed (aft. ½ h.). [*Gss.*]

Sensation as if the larynx were pressed upon the œsophagus from without, whereby not the breathing but the swallowing was rendered difficult (aft. 5 m.). [*Gss.*]

45. **A choking in the throat, as if too large a morsel had been too hastily swallowed.** [*Gss.*]

Tongue covered with a white fur. [*Wth.*]

Slimy tongue. [*Gss.*]

Disgusting flat taste in the mouth, as after drinking elder-flower tea, but the food tastes quite right. [*Gss.*]

Bitter taste in the mouth, whilst food and drink tasted all right (aft. 2 h.). [*Myr.*]

50. Diminution of the appetite. [*Bch.*]

Diminution of the thirst.

Much thirst for milk, followed by comfortable feeling through the whole body ; though he took a good deal of it, he did not suffer any inconvenience, whereas formerly a great deal of flatulence was produced (aft. 36½ h.). [*Bch.*]

Frequent eructation of air. [*Trn.*]

Empty eructation. [*Gss.*]

55. Inclination to vomit. [*Horn's Archiv*, vol. xi,[1] ii.]

Nausea with inclination to vomit (from external use).

Great nausea with increased temperature of the body (aft. ¼ h.). [*Wth.*].

Hiccup (aft. 1½ h. and oftener). [*Lr.*]

Pinching aching pain in and under the scrobiculus cordis, increased by touch (aft. 3 h.). [*Bch.*]

60. Cramp-like throbbing in the scrobiculus cordis, which caused anxious breathing (aft. 5 h.). [*Htn.*]

Burning on the left side under the ribs on a level with the scrobiculus cordis. [*Gss.*]

Pain in the stomach. [*Horn's Archiv*, l. c.]

A tension over the epigastric region.

Constant gurgling and rumbling in the abdomen. [*Gss.*]

65. Pain in the abdomen.

Pain in the abdomen. [*Horn's Archiv*, l. c.]

Painful pressure just above the navel. [*Gss.*]

Dull pinching in the umbilical region, followed by discharge of flatus (aft. 1 h.). [*Htn.*]

Spasmodic retraction of the navel accompanied by transient nausea (aft. 6½ h.). [*Bch.*]

70. Burning pain in the abdomen, just under the short ribs of the left side (ast. 14 h.). [*Gss.*]

Continued cutting in the bowels, immediately after eating, the food, however, was relished. [*Gss.*]

Pinching pain in the left inguinal region (aft. 9 h.). [*Htn.*]

Flatus is passed in large quantities.

Constipation : the stool is passed in small, hard lumps, like sheep's dung (for two successive days). [*Trn.*]

75. Diarrhœa. [*Horn's Archiv*, l. c.]

Every night three diarrhœic stools.

Mucous diarrhœa.

Urging to urinate, all day long, with scanty discharge of urine (aft. 2 h.). [*Lr.*]

He must urinate during the day ten to twelve times, and at night two or three times, and each time copiously (aft. 24 h.).

---

1 Not accessible.

80. Just before passing urine, a burning. [*Myr.*]

Reddish urine (from the external application).

Burning in the urethra, immediately before the urine comes away.

A shooting and cutting in the urethra when urinating, and during bodily exercise.

Urethral blenorrhœa.[1] [WENDT, in *Hufel. Journ.*, xvi, iii.]

* * *

85. Stuffed coryza (aft. 2 h.). [*Lr.*]

Pain in the chest. [*Horn's Archiv.*, l. c.]

Tightness of the chest.

Oppression of the chest and respiration. [*Gss.*]

Oppression of the thoracic cavity during expiration. [*Gss.*]

90. Tearing pressure in the left axilla and further forwards towards the nipple (aft. 30 h.). [*Hrr.*]

Sharp shooting near the vertebræ in the middle of the back. [*Gss.*]

Obtuse stitches, in rapid succession, in the left lumbar region more towards the back (aft. 10 m.). [*Gss.*]

Tearing pressure on the lowest lumbar vertebræ, extending forwards to the neighbourhood of the os ilii ; it feels as if the vertebræ were broken away from one another, only when bending forwards and on again bending backwards, for several days, felt also when walking (aft. 86 h.). [*Hrr.*]

Pinching spasmodic pain on the inner border of the right scapula, that prevented him moving the arm (aft. 1 h.). [*Htn.*]

95. (When sitting) shooting in the left axilla (aft. 2 h.). [*Lr.*]

Tearing in the muscles of the right upper arm (aft. 28 h.). [*Hrr.*]

Paralytic pressure on the left upper arm (aft. 2 d.). [*Hrr.*]

A kind of paralysis in the muscles of the upper arm, on moving it. [*Gss.*]

Cramp-like pain in the left elbow-joint, which a bent position of the arm made still more painful (aft. 4½ h.). [*Htn.*]

100. A drawing in the left forearm and thence into the palm of the hand, in which there was a quivering movement.

Relaxation of the muscles of the right forearm, so that they can only be brought into movement with difficulty, and every movement and grasping anything caused pain (aft. 26 h.). [*Htn.*]

The left wrist-joint was as if stiff in the evening.

In the right wrist-joint an impediment to movement and stiffness, only perceptible on moving.

Squeezing tearing pain in the back of the right hand (aft. 1½ h.). [*Htn.*]

105. Tearing shooting pain in the right metacarpal bones, which is much increased by pressing on them (aft. 26 h.). [*Htn.*]

---

1. This is the return of a suppressed gonorrhoea, occurring while Chelidonium was being taken for the swollen testicle which had resulted.

Fine tearing in the metacarpal bone and carpal bone of the right thumb (aft. 7 h.). [*Hrr.*]

Paralytic tearing in the metacarpal bones and the proximal joints of the thumb and index finger of the left hand. [*Hrr.*]

The distal phalanx of the fingers of the right hand became yellow, cold, and as if dead, the nails blue (aft. 1 h.). [*Myr.*]

Fine tearing in the tips of the fingers of the right hand. [*Hrr.*]

110. Frequently recurring tearing in the distal phalanx of the little finger of the right hand, independent of moving or touching (aft. 3¼ h.). [*Htn.*]

Burning itching in the left-hip-joint on its anterior aspect (aft. 10 m.). [*Gss.*]

A pain above the left hip, as if something were swollen and bulged out there.

From the hip-bone to the toes of the right foot, a paralytic drawing pain, which remained the same when walking, sitting, and lying, and suddenly disappeared (aft. 39¼ h.). [*Bch.*]

Some red papules with white apices on both thighs, with smarting eroding itching.

115. Gone-to-sleep feeling of the anterior surface of the thigh, with fine stitches and sore pain (from external application).

A kind of paralysis and loss of power in the left thigh and knee when treading. [*Gss.*]

The knees bend under him when standing and walking (aft. 12. h.). [*Htn.*]

Hard pressure two fingers' breadth under the right patella [*Hrr.*]

Hard pressure, two fingers' breadth under the left patella, more towards the inner side. [*Hrr.*]

120. Shooting in the right hough (when sitting) (aft. 2 h.). [*Lr.*]

Down-drawing pain in the left calf. [*Lr.*]

Some burning painful spots, with stitches in their centre, above the tendo Achillis; the pain is increased by scratching. [*Trn.*]

Some stiffness in the ankle-joint, as if sprained.

Aching pain in the right ankle-joint, when sitting (aft. 1½ h.). [*Myr.*]

125. Clucking pain in the dorsum of the left foot (aft. 9 h.). [*Myr.*]

Cramp in the sole of the right foot, which together with the toes was bent downwards; the toes were as if dead and insensible; the cramp was relieved by compressing the calf with the hand, but was aggravated by attempting to tread (aft. 12 h.). [*Bch.*]

Single transient needle-pricks alternately on various parts, sometimes on one hand or one arm, sometimes on one foot, on the knee, on the abdomen, &c. [*Gss.*]

(Apoplectic insensibility and numb sensation of the whole body, with trembling, but with unaltered pulse.)

Fatigue and laziness of the limbs; it is impossible for him to move a limb quickly, he is disinclined to move and avoids doing so ; at the same time, yawning and drowsiness (aft. 15 h.). [*Htn.*]

130. After a meal very great laziness and disinclination for work, with drowsiness. [*Htn.*]

In the morning on awaking, such great weariness, that he can with difficulty make up his mind to get up. [*Wth.*]

Great laziness and drowsiness without yawning (aft. 9 h.). [*Gss.*]

Great discomfort : he feels not at all well, without knowing what is actually the matter with him ; he must lie down but could not sleep, and everything was intolerable to him. [*Gss.*]

Desire to lie down, without being sleepy or able to sleep. [*Gss.*]

135. After a meal, desire to lie down, without actually being able to sleep ; he started up several times in this slumber, and when he got up, the headache was worse. [*Htn.*]

Sleep with dreams about the occupations of the day. [*Lr.*]

Restless sleep full of dreams. [*Myr.*]

Restless sleep, without particular dreams. [*Bch.*]

Very restless sleep with quick waking and with profuse sweat, which occurred during sleep and continued till the morning, even when awake. [*Htn.*]

140. Morning sweat. [*Myr.*]

Sweat during the morning sleep. [*Wth.*]

Diminished temperature.

While lying in bed in the evening, he is seized with a violent rigor, that lasted about an hour, with external warmth all over the body, and yet with goose-skin, followed by sweat which lasted all night (aft. 38 h.). [*Htn.*]

Every time he goes out into the open air rigor, without coldness (in summer), which did not leave off until he again came into the room (for 2 d.). [*Htn.*]

145. Sometimes he had a feeling of warmth all over the body at once, sometimes a feeling of coldness ; he had often an alternation of this sort in single limbs (aft. 18 h.). [*Bch.*]

Shivering through the whole body, with unaltered temperature thereof, without thirst, (aft. 3 h.). [*Lr.*]

Shivering all over the body, with unaltered temperature thereof. [*Gss.*]

Strong, not rapid pulse (when sitting) (aft. $\frac{3}{4}$ h.). [*Lr.*]

Cold hands (aft. $2\frac{3}{4}$ h.). [*Lr.*]

150. Rigor (with cold hands) over the whole body. [*Myr.*]

Rigor with nausea, without eructation (aft. $\frac{1}{4}$ h.). *Myr.*

Shivering in the hands, which are warmer than usual (aft. $\frac{1}{4}$ h.). [*Gss.*]

The right leg, up to the knee, is icy cold, with feeling of coldness in it, whilst the other leg and all the rest of the body are normally warm and the blood-vessels of the hand and arms are swollen (aft. $3\frac{1}{2}$ h.). [*Htn.*]

Extraordinarily depressed, full of gloomy thoughts about the present and future, causing him to weep; he could get no rest in any place. [*Myr.*]

155. Sad to weeping, and depressed about the present and future. [*Wth.*]

Cheerful disposition.* [*Lr.*]

* Curative secondary action.

CHINA.[1]

(*Cinchona Bark.*)

(The alcoholic tincture of the *thin tubular* as well as the *royal bark, Cinchona officinalis.*)

Excepting opium I know no medicine that has been more and oftener misused in diseases, and employed to the injury of mankind, than cinchona bark. It was regarded not only as perfectly innocuous, but as a wholesome and universally beneficial medicine in almost all morbid states, particularly where debility was observed, and was often prescribed in large doses several times a day for many weeks, and even months, together.

In so acting the ordinary physicians were guided by an utterly false principle, and they confirmed the reproach I have already frequently made against them to the more sensible portion of the public, that they have hitherto sought in traditional opinions, in guesses prompted by false lights, in theoretical maxims and chance ideas what they could and should find only by impartial observation, clear experience, and pure experiment, in a pure science of experience such as medicine from its very nature must only be.

Setting aside all guess-work and all traditional unproved opinions, I adopted the latter method, and I found, as with the other medicines, so especially with cinchona bark, by testing its dynamical powers on the healthy human being, that as certainly as it is extremely curative in some cases of disease, so surely can it also develop the most morbid symptoms of a special kind in the healthy human body; symptoms often of great intensity and long duration, as shown by the following true observations and experiments.

Thereby, first of all, the prevailing delusion as to the harmlessness, the child-like mildness and the all-wholesome character of cinchona bark is refuted.*

* As long ago as the year 1790 (see W. CULLEN's *Materia Medica*, Leipzig, bei Schwickert, ii, p. 109, note) I made the first pure trial with cinchona bark upon myself, in reference to its power of exciting intermittent fever. With this first trial broke upon me the dawn that has since brightened into the most brilliant day of the medical art; that it is only in virtue of their power to make the healthy human being ill that medicines can cure morbid states, and, indeed, only such morbid states as are composed of symptoms which the drug to be selected for them can itself produce in similarity on the healthy. This is a truth so incontrovertible, so absolutely without exception, that all the venom poured out on it by the members of the medical guild, blinded by their thousand-years old prejudices, is powerless to extinguish it; as powerless as were the vituperations launched against HARVEY's immortal discovery of the greater circulation in the human body by RIOLAN and his crew to destroy the truth revealed by HARVEY.

---

1 From vol. iii, 2nd edit., 1825.

But equally evident is it, from thesymptoms of disease produced by cinchona bark in healthy observers recorded below, that the numerous unhappy results of the treatment by this bark occurring in the practice of ordinary physicians, and the frequently incurable aggravations of disease developed where bark in long continued and large doses was the main remedy in their prescriptions were owing solely to the noxious character of this drug when employed in *unsuitable cases*, and in too frequent and too large doses. This noxious character is demonstrated by the medicinal symptoms recorded below, which physicians till now were not aware of, and which they made no effort to ascertain. On the contrary, they innocently ascribed these aggravations to the natural course of the disease itself.

But I refrain from blaming these physicians, whose judgment is biassed by the prejudices of their schools, on this account, (their conscience will doubtless reproach them for it) I will content myself with expressing my own convictions in a few remarks.

1. Cinchona bark is one of the most powerful vegetable medicines. When it is accurately indicated as a remedy, and when the patient is seriously and intensely affected by a disease that china is capable of removing, I find that one drop of a diluted tincture of cinchona bark, which contains a quadrillionth (1/1000000,000000,000000,000000,th) of a grain of china-power, is a strong (often a too strong) dose,* which can accomplish and cure all alone all that china is capable of doing in the case before us ; generally without it being necessary to repeat this dose in order to effect a cure ; a second dose being rarely, very rarely, required. In the case neither of this nor of any other medicine did a preconceived opinion or an eccentric fancy lead me to this minuteness of dose. No, multiplied experience and faithful observation led me to reduce the dose to such an extent. Led by experience and observations I clearly saw that larger doses, even where they did good, acted much more powerfully than was needed for the cure. Hence the smaller doses ; and, as I repeatedly observed from these the same effects though in a less degree, I gave still smaller, and the very smallest doses. These proved sufficient to effect a complete cure, and they did not display the violence of larger doses, which tends to delay the cure.

These opponents of an inextinguishable truth fought with the same despicable weapons as do to-day the adversaries of the homoeopathic medical doctrine. *Like their modern congeners they also refrained from repeating his experiments in a true, careful manner*, (for fear lest they might be confuted by facts), and confined themselves to abuse, appealing to the great antiquity of their error (for GALEN's predecessors and GALEN himself had arbitrarily decided that the arteries contained only spiritual air, and that the source of the blood was not in the heart but in the liver), and they cried out : *Malo cum Galeno errare, quam cum Harveyo esse circulator !* This blindness, this obstinate appeal to the extreme antiquity of their delusion (it was only after thirty years and more that HARVEY had the satisfaction of seeing his true doctrine universally adopted), was in those days not more stupid than the blindness of to-day, and the present aimless rancour against homoeopathy which exposes the pernicious rubbish talked about ancient and modern arbitrary maxims and unjustifiable practices, and teaches that it is only by the responses given by nature when questioned that we can with sure prescience change diseases into health rapidly, gently, and permanently.

* Compare this with the large doses of this drug given in ordinary practice !

2. A very small dose of china acts for but a short time, hardly a couple of days, but a large dose, such as is employed in the practice of every day, often acts for several weeks if it be not got rid of by vomiting or diarrhœa, and thus ejected from the organism. From this we may judge how excellent the ordinary practice is of giving every day several and moreover large doses of bark!

3. If the homœopathic law be right—as it incontestably is right without any exception, and is derived from a pure observation of nature—that medicines can easily, rapidly, and permanently cure cases of disease only when the latter are made up of symptoms similar to the medicinal symptoms observed from the administration of the former to healthy persons; then we find, on a consideration of the symptoms of china, that this medicine is adapted for but *few* diseases, but that where it is accurately indicated, owing to the immense power of its action, one single very small dose will often effect a marvellous cure.

I say *cure*, and by this I mean a "recovery undisturbed by after-sufferings." Or have practitioners of the ordinary stamp another, to me unknown, idea of what constitutes a *cure*? Will they, for instance, call cures the suppression by this drug of agues for which bark is unsuited? I know full well that almost all periodic diseases, and almost all agues, even such as are not suited for china, must be suppressed and lose their periodic character by this powerful drug, administered as it usually is in enormous and oft-repeated doses; but are the poor sufferers thereby really cured? Has not their previous disease only undergone a transformation into another and worse disease, though it may no longer manifest itself in intermittent attacks recurring periodically; but has become a continued and, we may say, a more insidious disease by this very powerful and, in this case, unsuitable medicine? True, they can no longer complain that the paroxysm of their original disease reappears on certain days and at certain hours; but note the earthy complexion of their puffy faces, the dulness of their eyes! See how oppressed is their breathing, how hard and distended is their epigastrium, how tensely swollen their loins, how miserable their appetite, how perverted their taste, how oppressed and painful their stomachs by all food, how undigested and abnormal their fæcal evacuations, how anxious, dreamful, and unrefreshing their sleep! Look how weary, how joyless, how dejected, how irritably sensitive or stupid they are as they drag themselves about, tormented by a much greater number of ailments than afflicted them in their ague! And how long does not such a china-cachexy often last, in comparison with which death itself were often preferable!

Is this health? It is not ague, that I readily admit; but confess—and no one can deny it—it is certainly not health. It is rather another, but a worse, disease than ague. It is the china-disease, which must be more severe than the ague otherwise it could not overcome and suppress (suspend) the latter.

Should the organism, as it sometimes will, recover from this china-disease after many weeks, then the ague, which has till now remained suspended by the superior force of the dissimilar china-disease, returns in an aggravated form, because the organism has been so much deteriorated by the improper treatment.

If the attack be now renewed in a still more energetic manner with cinchona bark, and continued for a longer time in order, as it is said, to ward off the fits, there then occurs a chronic china-cachexy, a faint picture of which will be found in the symptoms recorded below.

Such are most of the bark treatments of our physicians, because they know not what are the cases for which bark is suited. They are suppressions of the original affection by the production of a stronger china-disease, which is mistaken for a manifestation of the obstinacy of the original disease, the development of new symptoms being attributed to its peculiar malignity ; because it is not known that these ailments are due to china, because it is not recognised what they are, namely, artificially induced china-disease.

The following symptoms caused solely by bark acting on the healthy body, will open the eyes of physicians on this subject, those of them at least who have not yet acquired the faculty of silencing their consciences, and in whose bosoms a warm heart for the welfare of their fellow creatures still beats.

Most intolerable and unjustifiable, however, is the monstrous abuse made by the dominant school of medicine, which plumes itself on being the only rational school, of this powerful drug in all kinds of *debility*.

There is no disease which is attended by weakness (as almost every one is naturally), or which physicians by their unsuitable allopathic medicinal mixtures have reduced to exhaustion of the vital powers—where they did not consider it necessary to give this bark in large doses in order to *strengthen* as they call it ; no patient prostrated, ruined and enfeebled by improper drugs to a condition of complicated cachexy whom they have not endeavoured to set up and restore to a healthy condition by tonic potions of infusion, decoction, extract, electuary of china, or by the same drug in powder. He is stuffed and tortured with it for weeks and months under the pretence that it will do him good. Of the consequence of such treatment I would prefer to say nothing. If the death-rolls could speak, they would most eloquently speak the praises of this abuse of bark ; and so also would the crowds of the living victims of asthmatic, dropsical, and icteric diseases, and those other unfortunates who remain affected with neuralgic or spasmodic maladies, or with malignant growths, abdominal sufferings or lingering fever, if they but knew what mischief had been done to them.

I would appeal to the common sense of these practitioners and ask them how, without being guilty of the most unpardonable slipshod practice, they can venture to administer bark in all those infinitely various diseases, which of themselves, as also especially in consequence of the traditional medical treatment, must necessarily be attended by weakness ? How can they ever imagine that they can strengthen a sick person whilst he is still suffering from his disease, the source of his weakness ? Have they ever seen a patient rapidly cured of his disease by *appropriate* remedies who failed to recover his strength in the very process of the removal of his disease ? If, however, as is natural, it is only by the cure of the disease that the weakness of the patient can cease and give place to strength and activity, and if, on the other hand, there can be no question of a removal of the weakness as long as its source is not dried up, that is to say, as long as the disease on which it depends is not cured, what a perverse treatment must not that be, which seeks to make strong and active by the administration of china (and wine) a patient at whose vitals the disease is still gnawing! These practitioners cannot *cure* diseases, but they attempt to *strengthen* these uncured patients with cinchona-bark. How can such a stupid idea ever enter their heads? If bark is to make all sick persons strong, active and cheerful, it must needs be the universal panacea which shall at once deliver all patients from all their maladies, from all morbid sensations and abnormal functions, that is to say, make them in all their ailments in every respect well and free from disease! For so long as the plague of disease deranges the whole man, consumes his forces and robs him of every feeling of well-being, it is a childish, foolish, self-contradictory undertaking to attempt to give such an uncured person strength and activity.

That cinchona-bark is no panacea for all diseases, we are taught by the sad experience of the ordinary practice; but its symptoms show that it can be an appropriate, real remedy for only a *few* cases of disease.

It is no doubt true that *by the first doses* of bark the strength of the patient, be he ever so ill, is increased for a few hours; he is able to raise himself up in bed all alone, as if by a miracle; he wants to get out of bed and put on his clothes; all at once he speaks in a stronger more resolute manner, venturing to walk alone, and grows animated, eagerly desires to eat this or that,—but a careful accurate observer easily sees that this excitation is only an unnatural tension (see below the note to § 895). A few hours pass and the patient sinks back, sinks deeper down into his disease, and the fatal result is often accelerated.

Do not these gentlemen perceive that no one can become well (truly strong and active) as long as his disease lasts?

No! the always suspicious semblance of strength communicated to the patient for a few hours by bark is invariably attended by the saddest results, and this will ever be so, except in those *rare* cases where cinchona-bark is at the same time the right remedy for the disease on which the weakness depends. In such cases the patient's weakness ceases immediately with the disease. But, as I have said, such cases are rare, for cinchona-bark is the *true remedy* (which relieves rapidly, permanently, and *without after-ailments*) for but *few* diseases. In all the many other cases bark, as a medicine and so-called tonic, must to harm, and the more so the stronger its medicinal power (injuring when given improperly) is. For all medicines, *without exception*, can do no good when unsuitable for the case of disease, and must inflict so much the more injury the greater their medicinal strength (and the larger the doses in which they are given).

Hence, physicians should first learn the peculiar power of action of cinchona-bark, and exactly what particular alterations in the health of human beings it is capable of causing, before they presume to undertake the cure of diseases, and consequently the morbid weakness, with this powerful medicinal agent. They should first know the symptoms of china before attempting to determine for what collection of morbid symptoms, that is, for what case of disease it may be curative; it can be curative for none but those whose symptoms are to be found in similarity among the symptoms of china. He who fails to do this will always commit mistakes, and do infinitely more harm than good to the patient.

When china has been selected according to conscientious homœopathic conviction (but not as hitherto, according to theoretical views, deceptive names of diseases, or the misleading authority of equally blind predecessors), and is consequently the truly appropriate remedy of the case of disease to be treated, in such a case, and for that very reason, it is also the true strengthening remedy. It strengthens inasmuch as it removes the disease, for *it is only the organism free from disease that restores the defective strength*; strength cannot be materially poured into it by a decoction of china (or by wine).

There are no doubt cases where the disease itself consists of weakness, and in such cases bark is at once the most appropriate curative and strengthening remedy. Such a case is that where the sufferings of the patient are solely or chiefly owing to *weakness from loss of humours*, from great loss of blood (also from repeated venesections), great loss of milk in nursing women, loss of saliva, frequent seminal losses, profuse suppurations (profuse sweats), and weakening by frequent purgatives, where almost all the other ailments of the patient are wont to correspond in similarity with the china symptoms (see notes to 837 and 860). If, then, there is here no other disease in the background to produce dynamically or to keep up the loss of humours, then for the cure of this peculiar weakness (from loss of humours), which has here become the disease, one or two doses as small as those above mentioned,* together

* Here as elsewhere I insist on the sufficiency and efficacy of such small doses. And yet the vulgar herd can never understand me, for they know nothing of the pure treatment with one single simple medicinal substance to the exclusion of all other sorts of medicinal irritants, and their thoughts are enchained in the mazes of their old routine. Even when the ordinary physicians now and then *constrain* themselves to give in some (acute) disease one single medicine, they never have the heart to refrain from using at the same time several other things possessing medicinal power, which, however, they regard as of no consequence, and to which they apply the trivial name of *domestic remedies*. They must always use simultaneously either a poultice of so-called aromatic or solvent herbs applied to the most painful part (just as though these could have no effect on the patient through his olfactory nerves, nor act as a heterogeneous medicine through the skin!), or they must rub in some medicinal ointment, or give a medicated vapour-bath, or a medicinal gargle, or apply a blister or a sinapism, or prescribe several half, whole or foot-baths, or order clysters of valerian, camomile, &c. (just as though all these were a mere nothing and did not act on the human system as heterogeneous powerful medicine through the skin, the mouth, the rectum, the colon, &c.!), or they must administer simultaneously a tea of mint camomile, elder-flower, so-called pectoral herbs, &c. (just as though a handful of such herbs or flowers infused in boiling water counted for nothing!). In such an onslaught with heterogeneous drugs, which, although ignorance looks upon them as innocuous domestic remedies, are to all intents and purposes medicines, and some of them very *powerful* medicines; in this accessory quackery, I say, even a large dose of medicine of another kind can, of a truth, never display its peculiar action, and such an uncommonly small dose as homoeopathy requires is completely powerless; it will be instantaneously overpowered and annihilated. *No! in the language of rational men that*

with appropriate treatment in other respects, by nourishing diet, open air, cheerful surroundings, &c., are as efficacious to effect recovery as larger and repeated doses are to cause secondary and injurious effects, as is the case with every nimium, every excess even of the best thing in the world.

This suitableness of cinchona-bark in diseases of debility from loss of humours led physicians of the ordinary sort, as it were instinctively, to a mode of treatment of many diseases which has been, and still continues to be, the most prevalent of all modes of treatment—*the weakening treatment by means of squandering the humours* (under pretence of loosening the morbid matter and expelling it from the body) by means of frequently repeated so-called solvents (that is, drugs of various kinds that purge the bowels), by means of exciting an increased flow of urine and copious perspirations (by many tepid and warm drinks and

alone can be called giving a single medicine in a disease, when, excepting this one, all other medicinal influences are excluded from the patient and carefully kept away from him. But he who will do this must know what things brought in contact with the human body act medicinally on it. So long as he does not know this it must be ascribed to his ignorance that he considers as nothing, as not at all medicinal, such things as herb-teas and clysters, poultices and baths of herbs and salts, and the other things just mentioned, and continues to use them thoughtlessly under the name of domestic remedies during the employment of medicine internally. Still more heedlessly in this respect is the treatment of chronic maladies conducted ; for, in addition to what the patient takes from medicine chests and bottles, and the external applications and so-called domestic remedies that are usually administered to the patient, lots of superfluous hurtful things are allowed, and even prescribed, which are also regarded as indifferent matters in spite of the disturbing effects they may exercise on the patient's health, and of the confusion they may cause in the treatment. Besides the internal and external use of medicines the patient is allowed, for example, to take (for breakfast) mulled beer, vanilla chocolate, also (even several times a day) strong coffee or black and green tea, not unfrequently—to strengthen the stomach (?)—claret-cup, liqueurs containing strong spices, seasonings of all sorts in the food, and especially in sauces (made of soy, cayenne pepper, mustard, &c.)—these things are supposed merely to increase the appetite and promote digestion, but to possess no hurtful medicinal quality !—moreover, quantities of uncooked herbs cut small and sprinkled over the soup—which are regarded as supremely wholesome, but are really medicinal—also various sorts of wine—one of the main reliances of ordinary practice—must not be forgotten. Besides all these there are tooth-powders, tooth-tinctures, and tooth-washes —also composed of medicinal ingredients, and yet considered innocuous because forsooth they are not swallowed ; just as though medicines only taken into the mouth or their exhalations drawn into the nose did not as surely act on the whole organism through its living sensitive fibres as when they are swallowed ! And then the various kinds of perfumes and washes (musk, ambergris, peppermint drops, oil of bergamot and cedar, neroli, eau-de-Cologne, eau-de-luce, lavender water, &c.), besides perfumed sachets, smelling bottles, scented soaps, powders and pomades, pot-pourri, and any other noxious *articles de luxe* the patient may desire. In such an ocean of medicinal influences the otherwise adequate homœopathic dose of medicine would be drowned and extinguished. But is such a medley of medicinal luxury necessary and useful for the life and well-being or compatible with the recovery of the patient ? It is injurious, yes, extremely injurious ; and yet, perhaps, it has been invented by physicians themselves for the upper classes in order to please, to stimulate and to keep them ill. But even though physicians may not directly recommend it, it is sufficiently sad that they do not know the medicinal noxiousness of all this luxury, and that they do not prohibit it to their chronic patients. This hotch-potch of noxious influences, due partly to the luxurious habits of the patient himself, partly to the simultaneous use of domestic remedies ordered or permitted by the doctor, is so much the rule, so universally prevalent, that the ordinary practitioner cannot think of

quantities of tepid and warm-bath), by means of blood-letting by venesection and leeches, by means of salivation, by means of drawing off imaginary impure humours by open blisters, issues, setons, &c. If such a treatment, especially that by mild purgatives the use of which is so general, be long enough continued, then, by means of irritation of the intestinal canal, not only is the greater disease of the abdomen that keeps in suspense the acute disease, so long kept up until the natural termination of the acute disease is reached, but also a disease of debility from loss of humours is induced, for which, then, after months of treatment, when the strength and humours are much exhausted, cinchona-bark will assuredly restore the health in the only remaining malady (the artificially produced disease of debility from loss of humours). But none perceived by what a circuitous round-about way such a cure was effected. Thus, *inter alia*, the spring tertian fevers, and most other diseases of an acute character, having of themselves a

treatment without such a simultaneous medical confusion, and hence, under these circumstances, he is unable to promise any decided effect from the internal administration of a single medicinal substance in a disease, even when it is given in a large dose, far less from a very small dose of medicine homoeopathically employed! CONRADI was acquainted with no other treatment than such as is constructed amid such a confused medley of medicinal influences, as is evident when he says (*Grunariss der Pathologie und Therapie*, Marburg, 1801, p. 335), that the action ascribed by me to such small doses is beyond all belief. Here, not to dwell upon the trifling circumstance that the determination of the action of medicinal doses is hardly a *matter of belief*, but rather of *experience*, he seems no more than other ordinary practitioners to have either the slightest conception or the slightest experience of the action of a small dose of appropriate medicine *in a patient completely excluded from the simultaneous irritation of all other kinds of medicinal substances*, otherwise he would have spoken in a different manner. A pure treatment with a single homoeopathic medicine, all counter-acting medicinal contaminations being removed (for it is only of such I speak and only such I teach), never is seen or dreamt of in routine practice. But the difference is enormous and incredible.

So the glutton just risen from his luxurious meal of highly-spiced food is incapable of perceiving the taste of a grain of sugar placed upon his over-stimulated tongue; whereas a person contented with simple fare will, when fasting in the morning, experience an intense sweet taste from a much smaller quantity of the same sugar. Similarly amid the multifarious noises in the most crowded part of a large town we can often not comprehend the loudly spoken words of a friend at the distance of five or six paces, whereas in the dead of night, when all the sounds of day are hushed and perfect stillness prevails, the undisturbed ear distinctly perceives the softest tone of a distant flute, because this gentle sound is now the only one present, and therefore it exercises its full action on the undisturbed organ of hearing.

So certain is it, that when all accessory medicinal influences are withheld from the patient (as should be done in all *rational* treatment), even the very minute doses of a simple medicinal substance, especially of one chosen according to similarity of symptoms, can and must exercise its adequate and complete action, as a thousand-fold experience will teach any one whom prejudice does not deter from repeating the experiment accurately.

Quite small doses of medicine are all the less likely to fail to exercise their peculiar action, inasmuch as their very smallness cannot excite the organism to revolutionary evacuations (what is morbid in the organism is altered by the small dose), whereas a large dose, by the antagonism it excites in the system, will often be rapidly expelled and bodily ejected and washed away by vomiting, purging, diuresis, perspiration, &c.

Will the ordinary physicians at last understand that the small and smallest doses of homoeopathically selected medicines can only effect great results in a *pure* genuine treatment, but are quite unsuitable in routine treatment?

duration of only a few weeks, are spun out into (rational ?) treatments of many months' duration ; and the ignorant patient is happy in having escaped with his life, *whereas a real cure of the original disease ought only to have occupied a few days.*

Hence the everlastingly repeated warnings in so-called practical works, not to administer cinchona-bark in agues, until all the (imaginary) impurities and morbid matters have been energetically and repeatedly evacuated upwards and downwards, or, according to the euphemistic expressions of the moderns (though the same thing is meant), until the solvent treatment (*i.e.* laxatives and purgatives to produce many liquid stools) has been employed to a sufficient extent and long enough ; in reality, until the artificially produced abdominal disease has lasted longer than the normal duration of the ague, and so the disease of debility from loss of humours which alone remains can be transformed into health by cinchona-bark, as of course it will be.

This is what was and is still called methodical and rational treatment, in many, many cases of disease.

With equal justice might we rob widows and orphans in order to establish an asylum for the poor.

* * *

As cinchona-bark in its primary action is a powerful laxative (see the symptoms, 497 *et seq.*) it will be found to be very efficacious as a remedy in some cases of diarrhœa when the other symptoms of china are not inappropriate to the rest of the morbid symptoms.

So also in those cases where we have to do with so-called moist gangrene in the external parts, we shall generally notice in the remainder of the patient's ailments, morbid symptoms similar to the symptoms peculiar to cinchona-bark ; hence it is so useful in such cases.

The too easy and too frequent morbid excitation to seminal discharges of the genitals, caused sometimes by slight irritation in the hypogastrium, is very permanently removed by the smallest dose of bark (in conformity with its peculiar symptoms of this character).

Those attacks of pain which can be excited by merely touching (or slightly moving) the part, and which then gradually increase to the most frightful degree are, to judge by the patient's expressions, very similar to those caused by china. I have sometimes permanently removed them by a single small dose of the diluted tincture, even when the attacks had been frequently repeated. The malady was homœopathically (see note to 685), as it were, charmed away, and health substituted for it. No other known remedy in the world could have done this, as none other is capable of causing a similar symptom in its primary action.

Bark will hardly ever be found curative when there are not present disturbances of the night's rest similar to those the medicine causes in the healthy (which will be found recorded below).

There are some, though but few, suppurations of the lungs (especially accompanied by stitches in the chest, almost always only aggravated or excited by external pressure), that may be cured by bark. But in these cases the other symptoms and ailments of the patient must be found in similarity among the symptoms of china. In such cases only a few, sometimes but a couple of doses of the above minuteness, at long intervals, suffice for the cure.

So also there are a few icteric diseases, of such a character that they resemble the symptoms of china ; when this is the case the disease is removed as if by magic by one, or at most two, small doses, and perfect health takes its place.

An intermittent fever must be very similar to that which china can cause in the healthy, if that medicine is to be the suitable, true *remedy* for it, and then a single dose of the above indicated minuteness relieves —but this it does best when given immediately after the termination of the paroxysm, before the operations of nature are accumulated in the body for the next fit. The usual method of suppressing an ague not curable by cinchona bark, by means of large doses of this powerful substance, is to give it shortly before the paroxysm ; it is then most certain to produce this act of violence, but its consequences are very injurious.

Cinchona-bark can only permanently cure a patient affected with intermittent fever in marshy districts of his disease resembling the symptoms of china, when the patient is able to be removed from the atmosphere that causes the fever during his treatment, and until his forces are completely restored. For if he remain in such an atmosphere he is constantly liable to the reproduction of his disease from the same source ; and the remedy, even though frequently repeated, is unable to do any further good ; just as the morbid state induced by over-indulgence in coffee is rapidly relieved by its appropriate remedy, but while the hurtful beverage is continued to be taken, it will recur from time to time.

* * *

But how could physicians act so stupidly as to think of *substituting* other things for cinchona bark, which in its dynamic action on the human health, and in its power to derange that health in a peculiar manner, differs so immensely from every other medicinal substance in the world ?* How could they dream of finding a *surrogate* for china, that is to say, a medicinal substance of identical and precisely the same medicinal power among other extremely different substances ? Is not every kind of animal, every species of plant, and every mineral something peculiar, as entity never to be confounded, not even in external appearance, with any other ? Could any one be so short-sighted as from their external appearance to mistake a cinchona tree for a willow tree, an ash or a horse-chestnut ? And if we find these plants differ so much in their external characters, though nature cannot offer so much difference to a single sense—that of vision—as she can, and actually does, to all the senses of the practised observer in the dynamic action of these various plants on the health of the living healthy human organism, shall no attention be paid to these latter, the multiform peculiar symptoms which each single one of these plants elicits in a manner so different from those of the second and third, and whereon alone depends the specific medicinal power of each medicinal plant with which only we are concerned in curing disease ? Shall we fail to perceive

* See the peculiar symptoms it causes, recorded below.

their high significance, shall we fail to recognise them as the highest criterion of the differences of drugs among one another? Or shall we consider all things that have a bitter and astringent taste as identical in medicinal effects, as a kind of cinchona-bark,* and thus constitute the coarse sense of taste in man (which can scarcely judge of similarity of taste, but never of identity of medicinal power) the supreme and sole judge for determining the medicinal significance of the various plants? I should think it were impossible to act in a more short-sighted and foolish manner in matters of such extreme importance for the welfare of humanity!

I grant that all the medicinal substances that have been proposed as substitutes for cinchona bark, from the lofty ash down to camomile and the lichen on the wall, as also from arsenic down to James's powder and sal-ammoniac, I grant, I say, that every one of those medicinal substances I have named, and others I have not named, has of itself cured particular cases of ague (their reputation proves they have done this now and then). But from the very circumstance that observers state of one or other that it was efficacious even *when cinchona bark did no good or was hurtful*, they prove clearly that the ague which the one medicine cured was of a different kind from that the other cured! For had it been an ague suited for china, this medicine must have removed it, and none other could have been of use. Or else there must be foolishly attributed to the china in this case a peculiar malignity and spitefulness, making it refuse to be helpful, or to the other vaunted medicine, which was efficacious, a peculiar amiability and obligingness, causing it to do as the doctor wished! It would almost appear as if some such foolish notion was entertained!

No! the truth of the matter, which has not been perceived, is as follows: It is not in the bitterness, the astringent taste, and the so-called aroma of the cinchona bark, but in its whole intimate nature, that resides the invisible dynamical working spirit, that can never be exhibited in a material separated condition (just as little as can that of other medicinal substances), whereby it differentiates itself from all other medicines in the derangements of the human health it causes. See the observations recorded below.

Every one of the medicinal substances recommended in agues has its own peculiar action on the human health, differing from the medicinal power of every other drug, in conformity with eternal immutable laws of nature. Every particular medicinal substance, by the will of the Creator, differs from every other one in its externals (appearance, taste, and smell), and even much more so in its internal dynamic properties, in order that we may be enabled by means of these differences to fulfil all possible curative intentions in the innumerable and various cases of disease. Is it to be supposed that the all-good and omnipotent Creator of the infinite varieties of nature could, would, or should have done less?

Now, if every one of the vaunted ague remedies, whilst leaving other

* As W. CULLEN amongst others does (see *Abh. uber die Materia Medica*, ii, p 110, Leipz., 1790).

agues uncured, has really cured some cases—which I will not deny as far as regards those cases where the observers have given the remedy *by itself*—and if every single one of these remedies has effected its cure, not as a matter of especial favour towards the doctor who prescribed it, but, as it is more rational to suppose, owing to a peculiar power bestowed on it in conformity with eternal laws of nature, then it must necessarily be that the case in which this remedy, and not another, did good, was a peculiar form of agüe, adapted for this medicine only, and different from that other ague which could only be cured by some other remedy. And so all agues, each of which requires a different medicine for its cure, must be agues absolutely dissimilar to one another.

Again, when two agues betray their difference, not only by symptoms palpably different from one another, but also, as I have said, by this, that the one can only be cured by one remedy and the other by another remedy, it plainly follows from this, that these two remedies must differ from one another in their nature and action,* and cannot be identical, consequently cannot be considered as the same thing, and therefore cannot reasonably be substituted for one another; in other words, the one ought not to be represented as a surrogate for the other.

Or have those gentlemen, who do not see this, some mode of thinking peculiar to themselves and unknown to me, some logic of their own that stands in direct contradiction to that of the rest of mankind?

Infinite nature is much more multiform in her dynamic endowment of medicinal substances than the compilers of medicinal virtues, called teachers of Materia Medica, have any idea of, and immeasurably more multiform in the production of innumerable deviations in human health (diseases) than the bungling pathologist enamoured of his natty classification is aware of, who, by his couple of dozen, not even correctly† designated, forms of disease, seems only to give expression to the wish that dear nature might be so good as to limit the host of diseases to a small number, so that his brother therapeutist and practitioner—his head stuffed full of traditional prescriptions—may the more easily deal with the little collection.

* * *

That the ordinary physicians, by mingling iron in the same prescription with bark, often dish up for the patient a repulsive-looking and unsavoury ink, may be overlooked, but they must be told that a compound results from this mixture that possesses neither the virtues of cinchona bark nor those of iron.

The truth of this assertion is manifest from the fact that when cinchona bark has done harm iron is often its antidote and the remedy for its injurious action, as cinchona bark is for that of iron, when indicated by the symptoms caused by the unsuitable medicine.

* Otherwise the one medicine must have been able to cure just as well that ague which yielded to the other medicine, if the action of both was the same.

† What physician, except HIPPOCRATES, has ever described the pure course of any disease where no medicine has been given from the beginning to the end? Consequently, do not the recorded histories of diseases contain the symptoms of the diseases mixed up with those of the domestic remedies and drugs given during their course?

Still iron can only remove some of the untoward symptoms, those, namely, which it can produce in similarity in healthy persons.

After long-continued treatments with large doses of china many symptoms often remain for which other medicines are required; for we frequently meet with china-cachexias of such a severe character that it is only with great difficulty that the patient can be freed from them and rescued from death. In these cases, *Ipecacuanha* in small doses, more frequently *Arnica*, and in some few *Belladonna*, is of use, the indication for the antidote being determined by the symptoms of the china-disease. Veratrum is useful when coldness of the body and cold sweats have been caused by bark, if the other symptoms of this drug correspond homœopathically.

[HAHNEMANN was assisted in this proving by ANTON, BAEHR, BECHER, CLAUSS, FRANZ, GROSS, HARNISCH, HARTMANN, HARTUNG, HERRMANN, HORNBURG, CH. LEHMANN, J. G. LEHMANN, MICHLER, MEYER, STAPF, TEUTHORN, WAGNER, WALTHER, WISLICENUS.

The following old-school authorities are quoted:

ALPINI, *Hist. Febr. epid.*

BAGLIVI, *Praxis*, Lib .ii. BAKER, in *Medical Transactions*, vol. iii. Lond., 1785. BAUER, J. Fr., in *Acta Nat. Cur.*, iii. BERGER, JOH. GOTTFR., *Diss. de Chinchina ab iniquis judiciis vindicata.* Viteb., 1711. *Breslauer Samml.*, 1728.

CARTHEUSER, J. F., *Diss. de Febre intermitt. epid.* Francof ad V., 1749. CLEGHORN, *Diseases of Minorca.* CRUGER, DAN., in *Misc. Nat. Cur.*, Dec. iii, ann. 3.

ETTMULLER, B. M., *Diss. de usu et abusu præcepit.*

FISCHER, C. E., in *Hufel. Journal f. pr. A.*, iv. FORMEY, *Med. Ephem.*, i, 2. FOTHERGILL, *Essays*, tom. ii. FRIBORG, *Diss. de usu cort. Peruv.*, 1773.

GESNER, J. A. PH., *Sammlung. v. Beob.*, i. Nordlingen, 1789. GREDING, in *Ludw. Advers.*, tom. i.

HILDENBRAND, J, V. VON, in *Hufel. Journ.*, xiii.

JUNCKER et FRITZE, *Diss. de usu cort. peruv. discreto.* Halæ, 1756.

KOKER, JOH. DE (work not given). KREYSIG, *Diss. Obs. de Febr. Quart.* Viteb., 1797.

LIMPRECHT, J. A., in *Acta Nat. Cur.*, ii.

MAY, W., in *Lond. Med. Journ.*, 1788. MORTON, *Opera*, ii. MURRAY, *Apparat. Medicam.*, 2nd edit., i.

PELARGUS, *Obs.*, ii. PERCIVAL, *Essays*, vol. i.

QUARIN, *Method. Med. Febr.*

RAULIN, J., *Observat. de Med.* Paris, 1754. RICHARD, *Recueil d' Observ. de Med.*, ii. ROMBERG, J. W., *Misc. Nat. Cur.*, Dec. iii, Ann. 9, 10. ROSCHIN, in *Annalen der Heilkunde*, 1811, Feb.

SCHLEGEL, in *Hufel. Journ.*, vii. STAHL, J. E., *Diss. Problem. de Febribus*, —*Obs. Clin.* SYDENHAM, *Opusc. Lips.*, 1695.

THOMPSON, AL., in *Med. Inqu. and Observ.*, iv, No. 24. THOMSON, THOM., *Med. Rathpfleg.* Leipzig, 1779.

In the *Frag. de Vir.* China has 221 symptoms, in the 1st Edit. 1082, and in this 2nd Edit. 1143.]

CHINA.

Vertigo. [J. F. CARTHEUSER,[1] *Diss. de Febre intermitt. epid.* Francof. ad V., 1749.]

First vertigo and giddy nausea, then general feeling of heat.*

Vertigo in the occiput, when sitting. [*Fz.*]

Vertigo ; the head tends to sink backwards, worse when moving and walking, diminished by lying down (aft. a few m.). [*Hrr.*]

5. Constant vertigo, the head tends to sink backwards, in every position, but worse when walking and moving the head (aft. 6 h.). [*Hrr.*]

Stupidity. [CARTHEUSER, l. c.]

He is long in collecting his thoughts, is much disinclined for movement, and more disposed to sit and to lie.

Confusion of the head. [C. E. FISCHER,[2] in *Hufel Journal*, iv, pp. 652, 653, 657.]

Confusion of the head, like vertigo from dancing and as in catarrh.†

10. Confusion and emptiness in the head and laziness of the body as from watching at night and sleeplessness‡ (aft. 1 h.).

Confusion of the head, like a catarrh§ (aft. 9 d.). [*Ws.*]

Confusion of the head in the forehead. [*Hbg.*]

Confusion of the head, as after a debauch, with aching in the temples. [*Hbg.*]

A cloudiness spread all over the head, for half an hour (aft. ¾ h.). [*Htg.*]

15. Stupefaction of the head, with aching in the forehead (aft. ¼ h.).

A dull feeling in the lower part of the head behind, as from awaking from sleep. [*Bch.*]

Heaviness of the head (at noon vertigo rises up into the head, without pain).‖

Heaviness of the head.¶ [J. E. STAHL,[3] in various works, particularly in his *Diss. Problem. de Febribus.*]

Heaviness in the head, which tends to sink backwards, when sitting. [*Hrr.*]

20. Headache, like heaviness and heat in it, worst when turning the eyes, at the same time with twitching pains in the temples.

In the morning, on awaking from sleep, dull, stupefying headache.

* Comp. with 1, 3, 4, 5.
† Comp. with 11 and 49.
‡ 10, 15, 21, comp. with 6, 8, 11, 12, 13, 14, 16 and 23.
§ See 9 and 49.
‖ 17, 20, comp. with 18, 19, 22.
¶ 18, 19, 22, see 17, 20.

---

1 Results of suppression of intermittents by china.
2 Effects of china in agues.
3 As 1.

In the morning, on awaking from sleep, heaviness of the head and weariness in all the limbs. [*Lhm.*]

In the morning quite dazed in the head, as after a debauch, with dryness in the mouth. [*Fz.*]

Headache in the frontal region. [*Fz.—Gss.*]

25. Aching shooting pain in the forehead and temple of one side (aft. 4 h.).

Headache in the temples. [*Hbg.*]

Headache, exhaustion, then some coldness. [*Fz.*]

Aching pain in the occiput* (aft. 3 h.). [*Myr.*]

Pressure on the left temple. [*Hrr.*]

30. Compression in the temples (aft. 5 h.). [*Fz.*]

In the evening, aching pain in the temple. [*Fz.*]

Headache from afternoon till evening, an aching in the middle of the forehead.

Aching pain in the right side of the forehead. [*Gss.*]

Aching pain in the forehead ; on bending backwards it came with increased intensity in both temples ; when sitting it remained confined to the forehead. [*Bch.*]

35. Aching pain when walking, first over the forehead, then in the temples† (aft. 6 h.).

Headache, first an aching in the forehead, which then spreads all over the head. [*Bch.*]

Headache as if the brain was compressed from both sides and pressed out at the forehead, very much increased by walking in the open air.

Violent aching pains deep in the brain, and like constriction, especially in the right side of the forehead and in the occiput, very much increased by walking.‡ [*An.*]

Aching pain, especially in the occiput. [*An.*]

40. **Aching, pressing headache, which is aggravated by open air** (aft. 9 h.). [*Htn.*]

Hard pressure in the occiput, as if the cerebellum were pressed out (aft. $5\frac{1}{2}$ h.). [*Myr.*]

Painful aching and pressing in the head, towards the forehead, as if all were too heavy and would be pressed out, relieved by pressing strongly on it with the hand (aft. 8 h.). [*Htn.*]

Aching pressing headache in the side towards which he leans. [*Htn.*]

A kind of aching, as if oppressed in the head, with frontal sweat (aft. $\frac{1}{2}$ h.). [*Wr.*]

45. An aching, like fulness, in the head just over the eyes (aft. 2 h.). [*Wr.*]

The brain feels as if pressed by excess of blood.§

Headache over the orbits, which comes on in the forenoon hours, is increased by walking, but is removed by the mid-day meal (aft. 18 h.).

* 28, 29, 30, 31, 33, 34, 36, see 35 and 39.

† Comp. with 28, 29, 30, 31, 33, 34, 36, 39.

‡ See 37, 40—46, 48, 50, 51, 53—63, 65—67, 69, 70.

§ 37, 46, comp. with 38 and 40—45, 48 and 70.

Headache as if the brain were kneaded together, with too great excitement of the mind, restlessness, inordinate and too rapid attentiveness and over-strainedness of the imagination. [*Fz.*]

Headache in the temples like stuffed coryza.*

50. **Pressive tearing in the temporal region as if it would press out the bone.**† [*Hrr.*]

Tearing pain in the left temple. [*Lr.*]

Headache now in one part then in another part of the brain.

Tearing on several spots in the head, aggravated by walking and by moving the head. [*Hrr.*]

Tearing headache from the right occipital bone to the right frontal protuberance. [*Hrr.*]

55. Drawing headache from the occiput to the forehead, as if the whole forehead were contracted, which ended in the temples like a beating ; it was alleviated by walking, increased by sitting and standing, and ceased by pressing on it with the hand. [*Trn.*]

Drawing headache in the occiput, when sitting. [*Fz.*]

Drawing pain in the head behind the ears to the mastoid process. [*Htg.*]

Drawing pain in the left side of the occiput, that goes off on bending back the head. [*Fz.*]

Drawing pain in the forehead. [*Hbg.*]

60. When he places his hand on his forehead there occurs there a to-and-fro drawing pain. [*Fz.*]

Violent twitching tearing on several spots in the head, which is increased by movement and by walking, diminished when lying (aft. 1 h.) [*Hrr.*]

Twitching tearing on the frontal protuberances. [*Gss.*]

Twitching tearing in the right temporal region, for three days. [*Hrr.*]

Twitching headache in the temple to the upper jaw.‡

65. Twitching from both parietal bones of the head along the neck.§ [*Hbg.*]

Headache, like a twitching towards the forehead, increasing in severity till evening, when it went off. [*Ln.*]

Digging headache in the left side of the forehead, when he sits doing nothing, or occupies himself with something for which he has no inclination. [*Gss.*]

Headache, first spasmodic in the vertex, then on the side of the head as if bruised, increased by the slightest movement.

Headache, a digging in the left side of the head, when sitting (aft. $9\frac{1}{4}$ h.) [*Htn.*]

70. Headache so painful, as if the skull would burst asunder ; the brain beats in an undulating manner against the skull. [*Trn.*]

* Comp. with 9 and 11.

† Tearing (drawing) pressure, and pressive tearing (drawing), seems to be a chief character of pain with china, see also, 686, 687, 739, 746, 779, 780.

‡ Comp. with 65, 66, also partly with 61, 62, 63.

§ 63, 65, see 64.

Violent hammering in the head towards the temples. [*Ln.*]

Headache in the left parietal bone, like beating. [*Hbg.*]

An uninterrupted, dull, cutting pain from both temples and occiput up into the orbits, more acute and severe when moving and when stooping. [*Lhm.*]

Shooting headache, especially in the left frontal region (aft. 1½ h.). [*Htg.*]

75. Shooting betwist forehead and temple on the left side ; on touching the temple he felt a strong throbbing of the artery, and the shooting went off hy this touching.*

Betwist forehead and vertex burning, severe stitches. [*Htg.*]

Continued shooting sensation in the right temple. [*Wth.*]

Shooting headache in the forehead (when sitting). [*Lr.*]

Fine shooting in the temple. [*Fz.*]

80. Shooting headache between the right temple and forehead, with strong pulsation of the temporal artery† (aft. ½ h.). [*An.*]

Single stitches, which darted from the internal ear upwards through the brain. [*Trn.*]

Shooting tearing on several parts in the head, increased by moving the head. [*Hrr.*]

Headache when walking in the wind, compounded of bruised and sore pain.

Headache, as if the brain were sore, which is increased by the slightest touching of the head or any part of it, but especially by strained attention and profound reflection, indeed, even by speaking.

85. The integuments of the whole head are so sensitive to touch that all thereon is painful, and the roots of the hair in especial seem to suffer (aft. 36 h.). [*Gss.*]

Painful drawing on the right side of the occiput. [*Fz.*]

Drawing pain in the occipital joint when touched, so that he must bend the head backwards. [*Fz.*]

Painful drawing in the occipital bone. [*Fz.*]

Contractive pain on the left side of the occiput in the skin. [*Gss.*]

90. **Contractive, external pain on the left side of the occiput ; it feels as if the skin were drawn together on one point ; not increased by touching.** [*Hrr.*]

Pain as if the skin on the upper part of the head was grasped by a whole hand. [*Gss.*]

A pain drawing together in a circle on the middle of the head superiorly (aft. ½ h.). [*Hrr.*]

Sweat among the hair of the head.

Profuse sweat among the hair of the head when walking in the open air.

95. Sharp stitches on the left side of the hairy scalp. [*Fz.*]

Shooting itching in the hairy scalp (aft. 1 h.). [*Fz.*]

(A crawling in the skin of the forehead.)

Shooting aching externally on the left frontal protuberance, accompanied by vertigo and some nausea in the throat. [*Hrr.*]

* Comp. especially with 80, also with 74, 76, 77, 78.

† See 75.

Shooting aching on the right from protuberance, more violent when touched (aft. 10 m.). [*Hrr.*]

100. Frequent alteration of the colour of the face.

Paleness of the face.*

Bad, earthy complexion.

Pinched, pale face.

Hippocratic face (pointed nose, hollow eyes with blue rings), indifference, insensibility; he wants to know nothing about those around him, nothing about things that he most liked (aft. 1 h.).

105. Pinched sharpened features, pale, unhealthy-looking complexion, as after debauches.† [*Stf.*]

Redness of the cheeks and of the ear-lobes.

Puffy, red face. [FISCHER, l. c.]

Heat of the face. [J. RAULIN,[1] *Observed. de Med*, Paris, 1754, pp. 243, 248.]

On coming from the open air into the not warm room, there occurred burning heat in the face. [*Stf.*]

110. Alternate heat and redness in the face. [STAHL, l. c.]

Momentary contraction of the skin of the forehead, as if the skin in the middle of the forehead were drawn together on one point (aft. ½ h.). [*Ws.*]

Burning pain on the forehead and hot frontal perspiration. [*Lhm.*]

Aching over the face, especially near the nose and cheeks, together with a contraction of the eyelids, as if the upper and lower lids were drawn towards one another (aft. 3 h.). [*Ws.*]

Shooting pressure on the forehead, above the nose and on the cheeks (aft. 32 h.). [*Fz.*]

115. A pecking pain in the zygomatic process and in a right molar tooth. [*Htg.*]

Fine stitches in the right malar bone, which go off by pressure. [*Htn.*]

A boil on the cheek.

Soft pressure going upwards over the root of the nose and on the eye-brow, which goes off on touching, with tension of the skin of the left ala nasi. [*Fz.*]

Aching in both eye-brows, more externally, aggrevated by moving the frontal muscles (aft. 3 h.). [*Myr.*]

120. Pain above the left orbit.

Tearing on the outer canthus of the left eye. [*Lr.*]

Fine itching pain above the orbits. [*Hbg.*]

Itching on the left eye-lid. [*Fz.*]

A tickling sensation on the eye-lids (aft. 5 h.). [*Htg.*]

125. Violent pain in the eye-lids. [*Css.*]

Dry feeling betwixt the eye-lids and eye-ball, causing rubbing pain

* 101 to 104, comp. with 105.

† See 101 to 104.

---

1 Not accessible.

on moving the eye-lids, without alteration in the appearance of the eye. [*Htg.*]

Eye gum in the outer canthus (after sleep).

Aching pain in the outer canthi. [*Fz.*]

Smarting first in one, then in the other eye, accompanied by watering of them.

130. Aching smarting pain in the eyes as from salt, she must always rub them* (aft. ½ h.).

Painless pressure in the eyes, such as is apt to occur from fatigue and want of sleep (aft. 10½, 12 h.). [*Htn.*]

On awaking, at night, the right eye felt as if it were swimming in water (aft. 19 h.). [*Stf.*]

In the eyes a sensation, as in general weakness, as if they were much sunk, which they are not (aft. ¼ h.). [*Fz.*]

A quivering, winking, trembling in both eyes (aft. 2¼ h.). [*Ln.*]

135. Twitching to and fro of the left lower eye-lid (aft. 6 h.). [*Ws.*]

Lachrymation of the eyes, with creeping pains in them on the inner surface of the eye-lids. [*Bch.*]

The eyes are somewhat red, with aching burning pain in them, and much heat (in the afternoon) (aft. 6 h.). [*Stf.*]

Contracted pupils.

Contracted pupils (immediately and aft. 3½ h.). [*Bch.*]

140. Contracted pupils (aft. ¾ h.). [*Htn.*]

Very contracted pupils (aft. 1 h.). [*Stf.*]

Pupils mobile, but more disposed to contraction than dilation (aft. 20 h.).

Dilated pupils (aft. 1½ h.). [*Htn.*]

Very dilated pupils (aft. ¼ h.). [*Htn.*]

145. Extreme dilatation and almost immobility of pupils, with weakness of vision, so that he cannot see distant things distinctly (myopia), with high complexion and liveliness (aft. 6 h.). [*Fz.*]

Black points fly before the sight† (aft. 4 h.).

Darkness before the eyes.‡ [*Lhm.*]

Dimness of vision. [CARTHEUSER, l. c.]

Amaurosis. [*Breslauer Samml.*,[1] 1728, p. 1066.]

150. A ticking noise in the ear, as from a distant watch.

First a beating sensation in the ear, then a loud ringing.§

Ringing in the ears.

Frequent ringing in the right ear, and at the same time a tickling crawling in it, as if an insect had crept in.‖ [*Bch.*]

Ringing in the ears with headache in the temples. [*Fz.*]

155. Ringing in the ears with headache in the temples. [*Lr.*]

Roaring in the ears.¶

* From the exhalation, compare with 137.

† Comp. with 147—149.

‡ 147—149, see 146.

§ 151, 152, comp. with 153—155.

‖ 153—155, comp. with 151, 152.

¶ Comp. with 157.

1. Results of suppression of intermittents by china.

Roaring in the ears.* [*Css.*]

Something seems to come before the hearing internally (as from deafness)† (aft. 1 h.).

Hardness of hearing.‡ [MORTON,[1] *Opera*, ii, pp. 76, 81.]

160. Tearing in the lobes of the ears.§

Heat of the external ear.

A tickling in the ear. [*Hbg.*]

Vesicles behind the ears.

Eruption in the concha.

165. **Tearing on the cartilage of the ear and in the external meatus auditorius.**|| [*Hrr.*]

(Aching pain in the internal ear, like ear-ache) (aft. 3 h.).

Pain in the left ear only when touched (aft. 6 d.). [*Ws.*]

Aching pain in the root of the nose (after the heat of the cheek has gone) that spreads on to the side of the nose (aft. 5 h.).

Tearing pain on the back of the nose.

170. Smarting deep in the left nostril, every inspiration causing a sudden stitch-like pain; on compressing the nose the smarting becomes worse, and then it also itches externally on the back of the nose, in the evening (aft. ½ h.). [*Fz.*]

Fine needle-pricks on the cartilage of the septum narium. [*Hrr.*]

Redness and heat only on the nose (aft. 12 h.).

(He fancies he smells a corpse-like odour.)

Epistaxis, in the morning between 6 and 7 o'clock, after rising from bed, for several successive days. [*Htg.*]

175. Frequent profuse epistaxis. [RAULIN, l. c.]

Epistaxis after blowing the nose strongly. [*Ws.*]

On the upper lip, on the right side near the commissure of the mouth, sore feeling as after much wiping in coryza.¶ [*Fz.*]

On the lower lip, near left commissure of the mouth, pain as if an eroding ulcer were there. [*Fz.*]

The inner surface of the lower lip pains as if sore and excoriated.**

180. Eruption on the lips and tongue; small ulcers which itch and burn much. [SCHLEGEL,[2] *Hufel. Journ.* vii, iv, p. 161.]

(Puckered, wrinkled epidermis of the lips) (aft. 5 h.).

The lower lip cracks in the middle (on sneezing).

(Chapped lips.)

Dry lips, without thirst (aft. 7 h.). [*Fz.*]

185. Blackish lips. [DAN. CRUGER,[3] in *Misc. Nat. Cur.*, Dec. iii, Ann. 3.]

Speechlessness. [RICHARD,[3] *Recueil d'Observ. de Med.*, ii, p. 517.]

* Comp. with 156

† Comp. with 159.

‡ See 158.

§ Comp. with 165.

|| See 160.

¶ 177, 178, see 179.

** Comp. with 177, 178.

1 Observed effects of overdosing.

2 Effects of china in agues. This eruption is said to be critical.

3 Results of suppression of intermittents by china.

Slight rigor, followed by speechlessness. [A. THOMPSON,[1] in *Med. Inq. and Observ.* iv, No. 24.]

At night (before 12 o'clock) tearing pressure in the right upper and lower jaw.*

On the upper jaw a cutting, burning pain (when standing) (aft. 7 h.). [*Fz*]

190. Twitching, obtuse stitches in the right lower jaw.† [*Wth.*]

Tearing on the left lower jaw. [*Hrr.*]

Swelling of the gums and lips. [FORMEY,[2] *Med. Ephem.*, i, 2.]

Drawing toothache readily occurs in the open air and when exposed to a draught of air.

Toothache ; stuffed coryza and watering eyes.

195. Toothache, a shooting outwards in the front teeth.‡

Toothache with looseness of the teeth (aft. 3 h.).

Loose teeth only painful when chewing.

On biting the teeth together aching pain in the crowns of the right molars. [*Fz.*]

Toothache, like an aching drawing in the left lower jaw.§ [*Fz.*]

200. **Twitching tearing in the upper back molars of the left side** (aft. 5 h.). [*Htn.*]

Digging in the upper molars, diminished momentarily by biting the teeth together and pressing on them (aft. 40 h.). [*Htn.*]

(During the accustomed tobacco-smoking) tearing toothache extending upwards and backwards in the upper jaw followed by a sort of fainting fit. [*Fz.*]

Aching, drawing pain in the left upper row of molars, with sensation as if the gums or the inside of the cheek were swollen (aft. 1 h.). [*Fz.*]

In the morning, drawing, aching toothache in one upper molar, with sensation of numbness in it (aft. 24 h.). [*Fz.*]

205. The lower incisors are painful, as if they had been knocked.

In the morning, drawing pain in the incisor teeth.‖ [*Fz.*]

Small, fine stitches, with tearing in the right upper molars, neither diminished nor increased by touching or drawing in cold air¶ (aft. 2½ h.). [*Htn.*]

Throbbing toothache.**

Pecking pain in one of the upper molars.†† [*Htg.*]

210. Sore-throat.[3] [STAHL, l. c.]

In the pit of the throat, sensation as if it would be painful on

* Comp. with 199, 203, 204, partly also with 191, 198, 200, 202, 206.
† See 195, 207.
‡ Comp. with 190 and 207.
§ See 188, 203, 204.
‖ For 204 and 206 Rhus toxicodendron seems to be an antidote.
¶ See 190, 495.
** Comp. with 209.
†† See 208.

1 Results of suppression of intermittents by china. This symptom, with S. 448, 574, 602, 676, 698, occurred in a hysterical subject instead of a paroxysms of ague.
2 Not accessible.
3 In original "angina faucium."

swallowing, like a sore-throat (and yet it does not hurt when he swallows).

Painful deglutition, swollen submaxillary glands, which are painful, especially when he swallows.

A shooting on the right side in the throat only when he swollows.

Throat internally as if swollen; shooting pain on the left side of the tongue only when swallowing; there is only aching pain at this spot when speaking and breathing.

215. Shooting in the throat from a slight draught of air, when not swallowing.

In the evening, after lying down, shooting in the throat, not when swallowing. but when breathing.

Contractive sensation in the throat.* [*Hbg.*]

(A choking and contraction in the gullet without impediment to breathing.)

Deglutition difficult, as if caused by narrowing of the throat. [*An.*]

220. On bending back the head, tension in the gullet, which, however, does not prevent deglutition. [*Fz.*]

Scratching on the palate, also when not swallowing (aft. 8 d.). [*Ws.*]

Tobacco-smoke seems to him unusually acrid and stinging at the back of the palate (aft. 24 h.). [*Fz.*]

Tiresome rough feeling in the throat. [*Stf.*]

Painless swelling of the velum palati and uvula† (aft. 3 h.).

225. **Painful swelling on the side of the tongue posteriorly.**

It smarts on the middle of the tongue as if the part was excoriated or burnt.

A vesicle under the tongue, which is painful when the tongue is moved.

Fine stitches in the tip of the tongue.‡

Sensation on the tongue as if it were dry and covered with mucus§ (aft. 1 h.).

230. Smarting on the tip of the tongue as from pepper, then accumulation of saliva at this part. [*Fz.*]

Burning stitches on the tongue.‖ [*Hrr.*]

Here and there in the parotid gland flying shooting pains.

Simply painful submaxillary glands (under the angle of the lower jaw), especially on touching and on moving the neck.

A choking or squeezing aching in one of the right submaxillary glands *per se*, but more when moving the neck or touching it.

235. Contractive sensation in the salivary glands; ptyalism. [*Fz.*]

Much saliva in the mouth with nausea (aft. 2 h.). [*Ln.*]

* 217, 219, see 224, 225.

† 224, 225, comp 217, 219.

‡ Comp. 231.

§ Comp. 239 to 241.

‖ See 228.

Collection of saliva, combined with nausea. [*Hbg.*]

After an agreeable surprise much bright blood came rapidly into the mouth (aft. 24 h.). [*Stf.*]

Dryness in the mouth.* [STAHL, *Obs. Clin.*, pp. 144, 171.]

240. Dryness in the mouth with thirst. [*Hbg.*]

Great feeling of dryness in the throat, with cool breath (aft. 1 h.). [*Ln.*]

(Yellowish tongue, not covered with dirty fur).

Thickly furred tongue, especially in the afternoon (aft. 7 h.). [*Htg.*]

In the morning very white furred tongue.

245. Tongue covered with a thick, dirty white crust (aft. ¼ h.). [*Gss.*]

Yellow furred tongue, [FISCHER, l. c.—*Bch.*]

Yellowish furred tongue. [*Bch.*]

Clean tongue, with bitter taste. [SCHLEGEL, l. c.]

The mouth is slimy, and the taste watery and insipid.

250. Slimy taste in the mouth, which makes butter nauseous.

After drinking, flat, qualmish taste in the mouth.

Bitter taste of food, especially of flour-cakes† (aft. 6 h.).

Though he has no bitter taste *per se* in the mouth, yet all he eats tastes bitter ; after swallowing the food there was no longer bitterness in the mouth.

Constant bitter taste in the mouth.‡

255. In the morning, bitter taste in the mouth.

Bitter taste§ [FISCHER, l. c.]

Bitterness of the mouth. [QUARIN,[1] *Method Med. Feb.*, p. 23.]

Bitter taste in the mouth ; tobacco tastes bitter when smoking. [*Fz.*]

Bitter taste in the throat, causing him to swallow his saliva constantly (immediately) [*Htn.*]

260. A nasty, sometimes bitter taste in the mouth, especially in the morning ; the food did not taste nice, but not bitter. [*Hrr.*]

Bitter taste in the mouth on drinking coffee. [*Css.*]

Beer tastes bitter and goes to his head.

Bread when chewed tastes well, but is bitter when swallowed. [*Fz.*]

Bitter salt taste of roll and butter, with dryness in the palate and thirst ; when not eating there is no abnormal taste in the mouth, only dryness and thirst. [*Bch.*]

265. Salt taste in the mouth.||

All food tasted uncommonly salt, afterwards bitter. [*Myr.*].

Sourness in the mouth.¶ [*Fz.*]

* 239 to 211, see 229.

† 252, 253, 262, comp. with 261, partly also with 258, 263, 266.

‡ 254, 255, comp. with 256 to 260.

§ 256 to 260, see 254, 255.

|| Comp. with 660, partly also with 264 and 271.

¶ See 268, 272, 275.

---

[1] Physical effects of powder.

Frequently a sour taste in the mouth as if his stomach was deranged by fruit.

Black bread tastes sour* (aft. 3 h.).

270. Coffee tastes sourish.

A sweetish salt taste in the mouth (aft. 3 h.). [*Stf.*]

First sweetish then sour taste in the mouth, much saliva. [*Fz.*]

Sweetish taste in the mouth. [*Wth.*]

Tobacco when smoked tastes sweetish. [*Wth.*]

275. A sensation in the mouth causing collection of saliva, as if he had smelt strong vinegar.†

Nasty taste in the mouth as after cheese. [*Hsch.*]

Sensation as of a putrid exhalation out of the mouth.

Towards morning a nauseous, putrid smell out of the mouth, which goes off as soon as she eats something.

Mucus in the mouth in the morning after walking and after some prolonged exertion, which he thinks must smell ill to those about him ; he thinks he smells badly out of the throat.

280. He has no taste in consequence of smoking tobacco. [*Hbg.*]

Tobacco has no taste when he smokes.‡ [*An.*]

He cannot bear his (accustomed) tobacco smoking, it affects his nerves.§

He feels always as if he had eaten, drunk, and smoked to satiety, and yet he has a proper, good taste of all those things‖ (aft. some hours).

Aversion from coffee, though food tastes right.

285. Aversion from beer.

Aversion from water and inclination for beer.

Great longing for wine.

Supper has little taste.¶ [*Hbg.*]

Supper is relished, but he is immediately satiated, and hence can eat but little.

290. **No desire for food, but the taste is all right.**

Anorexia. [J. W. ROMBERG.[1] *Mis. Nat. Cur.*, Dec. iii, Ann. 9, 10, Obs. 109.]

Little appetite. [*Hrr.*]

Indifference to food and drink ; it is only when he begins to eat that some appetite and relish for food comes (aft. 6 h.).

No desire for food or drink.**

295. Want of appetite as from slight nausea.†† [*Htg.*]

The midday meal is not at all relished.‡‡

* 269, 270, comp. with 316, partly also with 315.
† 268, 275, comp. with 267, 272.
‡ See 282.
‖ 283, 290, comp. with 297.
§ Comp. with 281, partly also with 274, 280.
¶ See 296.
** Comp. partly with 299, 300.
†† See 298.
‡‡ Comp. with 288, partly also with 210.

1 Effects of china in agues.

Little appetite at noon from feeling of satiety.* [*Bch.*]

Extreme aversion from and loathing of not disagreeable food, even when it is not present and he only hears it mentioned, with dread of work, constant day-drowsiness, and yellowness of the eye-balls† (aft. 8 h.).

Little thirst. ‡ [*An.*]

300. No thirst when eating. [*Bch.*]

Canine hunger, with insipid taste in the mouth.

She is hungry, but does not relish her food.

Hunger and yet want of appetite ; the food which tasted right was disagreeable to him in his mouth. [*An.*]

Hunger at an unusual time in the afternoon. [*Htn.*]

305. Longing appetite ; he has longings, but he knows not for what.§

He has appetite for many things, but knows not rightly for what.

Longing often for unknown things.

In the morning (8 o'clock) great hunger and appetite, he knows not for what.‖ [*Lhm.*]

Great desire for sour cherries. [*Bch.*]

310. A kind of ravenous hunger, with nausea and inclination to vomit (aft. 2 h.).

Feeling of emptiness in the fauces and œsophagus (aft. 11 h.). [*Ws.*]

First a burning, then an agreeable warming sensation from the upper part of the chest to the stomach. [*Htg.*]

Scraping sensation in the fauces, especially on the border of the larynx, as after rancid eructation or heart-burn.

Eructation¶ (immediately). [*Htn.*]

315. After bread and butter bitter, sourish eructation.** [*Lhm.*]

After partaking of milk incomplete, sourish eructation†† (aft. $1\frac{1}{2}$ h.). [*Fz.*]

Tasteless eructation after eating. [*Stf.*]

A nasty slime often rises up.

After a meal bitter eructation‡‡ (aft. 2 h.).

320. Eructation with the taste of the food he had eaten.

Empty eructation of nothing but air§§ (aft. 2 h.).

A sighing kind of movement with eructation, intermediate between sighing and eructation (aft. $\frac{3}{4}$ h.).

Eructation, as if caused by loathing, and pain in abdomen (aft. $\frac{3}{4}$ h.) [*Wr.*]

An eructation, as from inclination to vomit (aft. 1 h.). [*Wr.*]

325. Whilst eating and drinking shooting in the side and back, and constant inclination to vomit (aft. 5 h.).

Whilst eating drawing twitching pain in the side of the abdomen (aft. 2 h.).

* See 283, 290.
† Comp. with 295.
‡ See 294.
§ 305, 306, 307, comp. with 308.
‖ See 305, 306, 307.
¶ 314, 317, see 321.
** See 319.
†† See 269, 270.
‡‡ Comp. with 315.
§§ Comp. with 314, 317.

After a meal, nausea in the region of the pit of the throat. [*Hrr.*]

Want of appetite and nausea, he has always an inclination to vomit without being able to do so (forenoon and afternoon).

After eating fulness, and yet good appetite before the meal*.

330. After eating, distension of the abdomen, like fulness.

After eating a motion of the bowels.

After eating drowsiness.†

After the midday meal great desire to lie down and sleep.

After eating exhaustion, so that he would like to lie down and sleep.

335. After eating the loathing, the flying heat and ebullition of blood go off.

Nausea [BAKER,[1] *Med. Transact.* iii, p. 162.—QUARIN, l. c.]

Nausea with good appetite. [SCHLEGEL, l. c., p. 161.]

He feels as if some food remained up in his throat (aft. 3 h.). [*Stf.*]

After a meal he remains for a long time as full as when he had just eaten ; the food seems to stick high up.

340. Inclination to vomit. [*Mch.*]

Nausea without vomiting. [*Lhm.*]

Inclination to vomit and vomiting.

Vomiting [MORTON, l. c.—BAKER, l. c.—FRIBORG,[2] *Diss. de usu cort. Peruv.*, 1773.]

Continued vomiting. [J. FR. BAUER,[3] *Acta Nat. Cur.* iii, obs. 70.]

345. Half an hour after the midday meal pressing aching headache that lasted till bed-time. [*Wr.*]

After a moderate meal followed by walk, while sitting sick anxiety in the stomach, as from over-loading and derangement of the stomach, and yet at the same time hunger.‡ [*Fz.*]

Weariness and laziness after dinner.§ [*Htn.*]

Exhaustion and drowsiness after supper (aft. 12 h.). [*Htn.*]

After a meal a hard pressing pain in both sides below the navel.‖ [*Bch.*]

350. After a moderate supper, eaten with appetite, immediately colic, that is : distended abdomen and here and there sharp aching pains mixed with pinching in all the bowels.¶

Stomachache, spasm of stomach.**

* 329, 330, 339, comp. with 338.
† 332, 333, 334, comp. with 347, 348.
‡ See 364, 366, 367, 368, 369.
§ 347, 348, see 332, 333.
‖ See 350.
¶ Comp. with 349.
** Comp. with 352—355 and 359, 360, 362, 363, 365.

---

1 Effects of Cinchona rubra. This symptom in both from the powder.
2 Physical effects of the powder.
3 Results of suppression of intermittents by china.

Pressure in the stomach.* [ROSCHIN,[1] *Annalen der Heilkunde* 1811, Febr.]

In the morning in bed, when lying on the side a pressure in the stomach (as if it were constricted), which went off on lying on the back. [*Stf.*]

In the stomach a pressure as from fullness. [*Hbg.*]

355. In the stomach violent aching, which went off while eating.† [*Stf.*]

After eating any food, however little, immediately a hard long-continued pressure in the stomach.‡ [*Hrr.*]

After every meal hard pressure in the stomach.§

With a good appetite, after eating (vegetables), at first stomachache, then accumulation of flatulence, then vomiting.

Weight and pressure in the stomach.‖ [PERCIVAL,[2] *Essays*, vol. i.]

360. Heavy pressure in the stomach. [KREYSIG,[3] *Diss. Obs. de Febr. Quart.*, Viteb., 1797, p. 17.]

After aching in the stomach, a burning rises half way up in the chest.

Oppresses the stomach. [BAKER, l. c.]

Feeling of fulness in the stomach. [*An.*]

The food partaken of at supper remains undigested in the stomach.¶

365. Feeling of heaviness in the stomach. [QUARIN, l. c.]

Milk readily deranges the stomach.

By taking rather too much food, even of the most innocent kind, the stomach is immediately deranged, and an insipid taste in the mouth, a fulness in the abdomen, crossness and headache come on.

Indigestion. [FRIBORG, l. c.]

Feeling of emptiness and qualmishness in the stomach.

370. Feeling of coldness in the stomach.

After every mouthful of drink feeling of internal coldness in the epigastrium, which is renewed at every breath (aft. 4 h.).

Pain in the region of the stomach, like aching, which is alleviated every time he rises from his seat, recurs on sitting down and lasts two hours (aft. $\frac{3}{4}$ h.). [*Wr.*]

Tearing aching under the last true ribs, at the left side of the ensiform cartilage. [*Gss.*]

Sore sensation with pressure (or pain as if a wound were pressed on) in the region of the scrobiculus cordis (several mornings). [*Gss.*]

* 352 to 355, see 351.

† Alternating action with 356.

‡ See 357, 358.

§ 357, 358, comp. with 356, and, on the other hand, the alternating action 355.

‖ 359, 360, 362, 363, 365, see 351.

¶ 364, 366, 367, partly also 369, comp. with 346 and 368.

---

1 Not accessible.

2 Physical effects of powder.

3 Not accessible.

375. A violent aching under the scrobiculus cordis, as if all were excoriated there, the same in all positions, also when touched ; soon after this a violent diarrhœa, whereby the pain in the scrobiculus cordis was not relieved (aft. 7 h.). [*Myr.*]

Stomachache, which takes away the breath. [STAHL, l. c.]

A squeezing together in the scrobiculus cordis, which impedes inspiration (aft. ½ h.). [*Htn.*]

Sufferings under the short ribs. [STAHL, l. c.]

Hypochondrial sufferings. [STAHL, l. c.]

380. Anxiety in the region of the scrobiculus cordis, especially after a meal. [STAHL, l. c.]

Anxiety in the region of the scrobiculus cordis. [CARTHEUSER, l. c.]

Pain in the abdomen, aching, pinching (shooting), under the scrobiculus cordis, as if diarrhœa would ensue, but no stool comes, in the evening* (aft. 36 h.). [*Fz.*]

Twitching shooting in the stomache (aft. 3 h.). [*Wth.*]

Under the last rib tearing drawing, when standing. [*Fz.*]

385. Under the last rib contractive pain and as if bruised, only when walking† (aft. 24 h.). [*Fz.*]

Flying stitches here and there in the stomach and abdomen.‡

After every drink a stitch in the precordial region.§

After every mouthful of drink shivering or chilliness with goose-skin (aft. 6 h.).

After drinking griping as from a purgative.

390. Sharp stitches in the scrobiculus cordis.‖ [*Hrr.*]

Sharp stitches in front under the last ribs, without relation to expiration or inspiration.¶ [*Gss.*]

Shooting pain in the scrobiculus cordis to the sternum. [*Lhm.*]

Shooting aching in several spots of the epigastrium, in the morning in bed (for four successive days). [*Hrr.*]

After moderate eating, at noon and in the evening, a pinching aching somewhat above the navel in the epigastrium, which becomes intolerable on walking, and is only allayed by perfect rest.

395. In the umbilical region severe cutting, with cold sweat on the forehead for a quarter of an hour (aft. a few minutes). [*Wr.*]

Pains in the abdomen in the umbilical region, combined with shivering.

In the region of the spleen cutting aching, as if the spleen were indurated. [*Fz.*]

Sharp stitches in the left side of the epigastrium, just beneath the ribs, from within outwards, increased by inspiring (aft. 7 h.). [*Hrr.*]

When walking, even slowly, shooting in the spleen. [*Fz.*]

400. Pinching stitches in the left epigastric region (aft. 1½ h.). [*Htn.*]

* 382, 383, but especially 390 to 392, comp. with 386, 459.

† See 433, 455, also 446 to 453.

‡ Comp. with 391, 398, 399, 402, 403, and 464 to 469.

§ Comp. with 638.

‖ See 649.

¶ See 386, 398, 399, 402, 403, and 464 to 469.

Obstruction of the spleen. [MURARY,[1] *Apparat Medicam.*, edit., sec., i, pp. 856, 857.]

Continued stitches under the right ribs in the hepatic region, neither diminished nor increased by inspiration or expiration (aft. 4 h.). [*Htn.*]

Violent stitches from within outwards in the hepatic region, only during expiration (aft. 5 h.) [*Htn.*]

Several attacks of intermittent aching in the hepatic region. when standing, which goes off on bending the body forwards ; on touching the region is painful as if gathering (aft. 5 d.). [*Fz.*]

405. Swelling of the liver. [KREYSIG, l. c., p. 27.]

Obstruction of the liver. [MURRAY, l. c.]

Induration in the abdomen. [STAHL, l. c.]

Indurations[2] of the intestines. [JOH. GOTTER. BERGER, *Diss. de Chinchina ab iniquis judiciis vindicata*, Viteb., 1711.]

The epigastrium feels tightened. [*Hrr.*]

410. Fulness of the abdomen.* [KREYSIG, l. c.]

Obstinate and anguishing tension of the abdomen. [STAHL, l. c.]

Flatulent distension. [FISCHER, l. c.]

Painful distension of the abdomen, and especially of the hypogastrium.†

415. In the morning distension of the abdomen, without flatulence.

At noon before eating and soon after eating, cutting in the abdomen, as in incarceration of flatulence.

Fermentation in the abdomen from eating fruit (cherries).

Flatulence and frequent discharge of flatus.‡ [*Hbg.*]

Tympanitis,§ [STAHL, l. c.—THOM. THOMSON,[3] *Med. Rathpflege*, Leipzig, 1779, p. 117.]

420. Distension of the abdomen as from drinking much, and partaking of flatulent food. [*Hbg.*]

Distension of the abdomen, pain in the abdomen and diarrhœa. [KREYSIG, l. c., p. 25.]

Attacks of hardness, distension, and pains of the abdomen.[4] [AL. THOMPSON, in *Med. Inq. and Observ.*, iv, No. 24.]

Tiresome, tight distension of the abdomen. [*Stf.*]

Swelling of the abdomen. [CARTHEUSER, l. c.]

425. Ascites, encysted dropsy. [STAHL, l. c.]

Rumbling in the abdomen (aft. 1 h.). [*Stf.*]

Rumbling in the epigastrium (aft. 2 h.). [*Wth.*]

* 410 to 413, see 414, 415.

† 414, 415, comp. with 410 to 413, and 419 to 424.

‡ See 492.

§ 419 to 423, see 414, 415.

---

1 Supposed ill-effects of china, mentioned only to reject them.

2 In the original, "angustia et firmitas." All other effects of china referred to this writer are mentioned by him only to reject them.

3 Results of suppression of intermittents by China.

4 This with S. 740 and 882, occurred instead of the ague paroxysm, five days after beginning China.

Rattling in the left side of the abdomen, backwards and downwards, as if in the descending colon. [*Fz.*]

Grumbling in the hypogastrium. [*Lr.*]

430. Cruel, intolerable colicky pains. [J. FR. BAUER, l. c.]

Colics. [STAHL, l. c.]

Flatulent colic (aft. 2 h.).

Flatulent colic deep in the hypogastrium ; the lowest bowels are as if constricted, and the flatulence vainly attempts to force its way out with aching and tensive pains, and even under the short ribs it causes tension and anxiety.

Pain in the abdomen with nausea. [W. MAY,[1] in *Lond. Med. Journ.*, 1788.]

435. Pain in the abdomen, and at the same time great thirst (aft. 1 h.). [*Bch.*]

Scorbutic colic. [CRUGER, l. c.]

Indescribable pains in the abdomen. [J. A. LIMPRECHT,[2] *Acta Nat. Cur.*, ii, Obs. 129.]

Ulcers in the abdomen. [STAHL, l. c.]

Inflammation in the abdomen. [STAHL, l. c.]

440. Heat in the umbilical region. [*Hbg.*]

Aching in the umbilical region. [*Hbg.*]

During the aching in the abdomen some chilliness. [*Wr.*]

Hard pressure in the left side of the hypogastrium (aft. 3 m.). [*Gss.*]

Aching pain in the region of the cæcum (when sitting). [*An.*]

445. In the evening severe aching pain in the abdomen, as if diarrhœa would come on, when sitting, which was dissipated by walking and standing. [*Fz.*]

Contractive pain in the abdomen, in the evening when sitting, which goes off on raising himself up, but still more on standing and wallking.* [*Fz.*]

On the right side, below the navel, a contractive aching, as if an induration were there, when sitting. [*Fz.*]

Contraction of the abdomen and of the sides with heavings and fallings of the scapulæ.[3] [AL. THOMPSON, l. c.]

Pain in the abdomen, like pinching and drawing, mostly when sitting. [*Fz.*]

450. Sensation of contraction of intestinal canal, and grumbling in the hypogastrium. [*Hrr.*]

Cramp pain in the groin coming in jerks, when standing. [*Fz.*]

pinching and colic-like constriction of the bowels above the navel, when he rises up after stooping. [*Fz.*]

Pinching together, as if it were externally, under the right side of the navel, when sitting, in the evening (aft. 13 h.). [*Fz.*]

Violent pinching in the epigastrium (he must crouch together to

* 446, to 453, See 385, 433 and 455.

1 Physical effects of powder.
2 Effects of China in agues.
3 See note to S. 187.

relieve himself) (aft. 1 h.), alternating with inclination to vomit and urging to stool, with rigor all over; after the pinching aching in the epigastrium. [*Wth.*]

455. Spasmodic pain in the abdomen, compounded of aching and constriction (aft. 24 h.).

Aching and heaviness in the abdomen.

Pinching, aching pain in the abdomen when walking, towards evening. [*Fz.*]

Pinching in the abdomen with increased hunger and exhaustion (aft. 3 h.).

Pinching, shooting pains in the abdomen* (aft. 1½ h.)

460. Violent pinching in the abdomen, which went off on rising up from his seat. [*Wr.*]

In the abdomen above the pubes pinching going here and there, as if a diarrhœa would occur, with small discharges of flatus, while sitting (aft. 27 h.). [*Fz.*]

Beating in the right side of the abdomen. [*Hbg.*]

Extremely violent aching shooting on the left side below the navel, on walking quickly and afterwards (aft. 2 h.). [*Gss.*]

Obtuse shooting pain in the region of the right kidney, worse on bending the body† (aft. 24 h.). [*Hrr.*]

465. Obtuse shooting on the left side of the abdomen, round about the navel, and at the same under the right nipple towards the interior (aft. 1 h.). [*Hrr.*]

Obtuse shooting above the navel on the right, worse when touched. [*Hrr.*]

Obtuse shooting in the left hypogastrium, in the region of the kidney. [*Hrr.*]

Obtuse stitches in the lumbar regions. [*Hrr.*]

When sitting, during inspiration, stitches darting downwards in the abdomen. [*Fz.*]

470. Cutting in the abdomen, in frequent fits, in the umbilical region.‡ [*An.*]

When walking, drawing pain in the right side of the abdomen. [*Fz.*]

Great discharge of flatus, together with a drawing in the abdomen during a hard stool, which is evacuated with difficulty§ (aft. 48 h.). [*Ws.*]

When flatus is about to be discharged, the abdomen is pinched together with violent pains.||

In the evening, between 6 and 10 o'clock, great grumbling and rolling about of much flatulence in the abdomen, with aching sensation, whereupon very fœtid flatus is discharged. [*Bhr.*]

475. Tearing in the navel. [*Gss.*]

* Comp. with 382, 400.
† 464—469, see 386, 391.
‡ See 491, 549.
§ See 495, 496, also 481 and 516.
|| See 461, 490, 491.

Extremely violent tearing on the right side near the navel, towards the groin, in the whole inguinal region, diminished by bending back. [*Gss.*]

In the abdomen, under the navel, tearing and rumbling. [*Hbg.*]

Pain in the abdominal muscles, as if bruised (aft. 1 h.).

In the inguinal ring excoriation-pain, and sensation as if a hernia would come out through the sore ring (aft. 4 h.).

480. Aching tearing pain on the left, near the pubes. [*Hrr.*]

Increased peristaltic movement in the hypogastrium, associated with aching. [*Hbg.*]

Aching in both sides of the abdomen, as if a stool ought to come but cannot.

(With urging and straining to stool, nothing but flatus comes away.)

Call to stool. [*Hrr.*]

485. During the day a soft stool. [*Bhr.*]

Stool thinner than usual* (aft. 24 h.). [*Bch.*]

Looseness of the bowels. [MORTON, l. c.]

Lumpy, yellow, soft stool, in the morning. [*Fz.*]

Bilious stools. [ALPINI,[1] *Hist. Febr. Epid.*, p. 93.]

490. Pain in the bowels before a discharge of flatus.

Before a discharge of flatus, cutting pains dart in all directions through the abdomen† (aft. 1 h.).

Accumulation of and then great discharge of flatus ‡ (aft. ½ h.).

Discharge of extremely fœtid flatus (aft. 10 h.).

Much horribly fœtid flatus is discharged. [*Stf.*]

495. Bellyache before the stool.§

Stool with bellyache.

Three times soft stool with smarting burning pain in the anus, and with bellyache before and after each stool.||

Looseness of the bowels, like diarrhœa.

Frequent, diarrhœic, blackish stools.[2] [QUARIN, l. c.]

500. Severe purging. [SYDENHAM,[3] *Opuscula*, Lips. 1695, p. 382.]

Diarrhœa of undigested fæces, like a kind of lientery.

Diarrhœa : it is as if the excrement contained undigested food ; it comes away in separate pieces (aft. 12 h.), and when it is passed, there still remains desire to go to stool, but no more passes.¶ [*Hrr.*]

He must press out the motion with the greatest effort, although it is not hard, but pappy, and is followed by ineffectual urging to stool, with pain.** [*Fz.*]

* 486, 487, see 497—502.
† Comp. with 470, and 549.
‡ Comp. with 418,
§ 495—497, comp. with 472, 481.
|| 497, 498, 501, Comp. with 486, 487, 499, 500, 502.
¶ See 501.
** 503, 507, 509, see 504, 505.

---

1 General statement from observation.
2 From the extract ; the stools looking (says the author) like the extract itself.
3 Observed effects of China. This symptom not found.

Costiveness and accumulation of the fæces in the bowels, with heat of head and dizziness.*

505. The stool comes after long urging only, with great pressing, and then it causes much pain.

Stoppage of the evacuations. [MURRAY, l. c.]

All day long constipation, and in the evening costive stool.† [*Trn.*]

Constipation. [QUARIN,—BAUER,—FISCHER, l. c.]

Constipation: long-continued accumulation of hard fæces in the rectum.[1] [FOTHERGILL, *Essays*, tom. ii, p. 92.]

510. Hæmorrhoidal bleeding. [ALPINI, l. c.]

Sensation in the anus during the stool, as from an acrid matter.

A burning and burning itching at the orifice of the anus (immediately).

Diarrhœa with burning pain in the anus.

Stitches in the anus during an evacuation mixed with blood‡ (aft. 5 h.).

515. Penetrating stitches in the anus and rectum, not during evacuation (aft. 5 d.).

Sharp stitches in the lower part of the rectum, especially in the sphincter ani; also during and after the stool, shooting drawing for three days§ [*Hrr.*]

After the stool a crawling in the rectum, as from thread-worms.

Crawling in the rectum, as from thread-worms, and evacuation of many of them.

A crawling in the anus.

520. A constant burning pain in the rectum after the midday sleep (aft. 4 d.).

An aching in the rectum (aft. 2, 6 h.).

Tearings and tearing jerks in the rectum while lying in bed (aft. 10 h.).

Contractive pain in the rectum, especially when sitting (aft. 72 h.).

Fine stitches in the inguinal flexure, on the pubes, almost only when walking. [*Fz.*]

525. In the inguinal flexure, especially on the tendon (of the psoas muscle), an aching drawing, when sitting. [*Fz.*]

Shooting pain in the perinæum, especially acute when sitting down.

The urine is not passed more frequently, but is paler, and yet deposits a cloud (aft. 3 h.). [*Fz.*]

In the evening, when passing urine, a burning smarting in the anterior part of the urethra.||

A throbbing in the region of the bulb of the urethra (aft. 6 h.).

* 504, 505, comp. with 503, 507 to 509. The costiveness of china is secondary action or reaction of the organism to the great tendency of this medicine to excite diarrhœa in its primary action.

† 507, 509. see note to 504, 505.

‡ 514. 515, 526, comp. with 516.

§ See 514, 515, 526.

|| Comp. with 539 and 540.

---

1 No such symptom to be found.

530. While urinating a shooting in the urethra.

Painful sensitiveness in the urethra, especially when the penis is erect, also observable while sitting and standing up.

After frequent and almost ineffectual urging to urinate, a pressing in the bladder.

The first twelve hours scanty secretion of urine, but thereafter more copious.

The urine flows in a weak stream and slowly, and there is very frequent call to urinate.

535. Very frequent urination (aft. 24 h.).

Frequent and such urgent call to urinate that the urine is involuntarily pressed out.

Burning pain in the orifice of the urethra during and after urination (aft. 3 h.).

A continual burning in the orifice of the urethra.

Increased discharge of urine, with burning at the orifice of the urethra* (aft. 2 h.). [*Ws.*]

540. Continual burning at the orifice of the urethra, with a feeling of excoriation at the seam of the prepuce, both especially painful from the friction of the clothes† (aft. 2 h.). [*Ws.*]

A twitching pain betwixt glans and prepuce when walking.

Pressing pain in the glans before urinating.

Itching on the glans penis, which makes him rub it, in the evening in bed.

A pain as of fine needle-pricks on the frenum of the glans ; on touching it the pain became more severe, namely, shooting and tensive ; nothing was to be seen externally.

545. Excites urination. [ALPINI, l. c.]

Whitish cloudy urine with white sediment.‡

Scanty, yellowish-green urine. [FISCHER, l. c.]

Pale yellow urine, which, the following morning, deposits a dirty yellow, rather loose sediment. [*Bhr.*]

Pressing and cutting in the bowels during and after the discharge of a white cloudy urine.§

550. White stool and dark urine|| (aft. 48 h.).

Dark coloured urine with brick-red sediment¶ (aft. 24 h.). [*Trn.*]

Scanty urine with brick-red sediment, and red-spotted, hard prominent swelling of the foot.**

Spasmodic contractive pain from the rectum through the urethra to the glans penis, and through the testicles, in the evening.

A crawling running and itching in the anus and urethra, with a burning in the glans penis.

555. Increased sexual desire.

Frequent erections of the penis (aft. 6 h.).

Nocturnal seminal emissions.††

* 539, 540, see 528.

† Comp. with 754, 819.

‡ Comp. with 527.

§ See 470 and 491.

|| Comp. with 856, 857.

¶ See 552.

** Comp. with 551.

†† Comp. with 558.

Great seminal discharge, about 3 a.m.* [*Bch.*]

Swelling of the spermatic cord and testicle, especially of the epididymis, painful to the touch.

560. Drawing pain in the testicles.

A kind of tearing pain in the left testicle and the left side of the prepuce, in the evening in bed.

An itching crawling in the scrotum, in the evening in bed, compelling him to rub it.†

Shooting itching in the scrotum. [*Fz.*]

Hanging down of the scrotum (aft. 1 h.).

565. Increase of the menses that are present, to the extent of metrorrhagia ; the discharge passes in black clots‡ (aft. 1 h.).

Suppression of the menses.§ [RAULIN, l. c.]

*   *   *

Sneezing (aft. $\frac{1}{4}$, 2, 3 h.).

Sneezing with coryza (aft. 1, 2 h.).

Several times violent, dry sneezing (aft. 7 h.). [*Stf.*]

570. Watery discharge from the nostril, which, nevertheless, is stopped up (aft. 13 h.). [*Fz.*]

Coryza, with sensitiveness of the nose and some papules on the border of the nostrils and the septum nasi painful to the touch (aft. 9 d.). [*Ws.*]

Coryza, so that there is running from the nose for two hours. [*Fz.*]

Symptoms of a stuffed coryza. [*An.*]

Noisy breathing through the nose.[1] [AL. THOMPSON, l. c.]

575. **Something is adherent in the throat (the larynx), so that the tones of the voice and of singing become deeper and deficient in clearness** ‖ (aft. 2 h.).

A whistling and wheezing in the wind-pipe when breathing (aft. 2 h.).

Tightness on the chest (at night) ; whistling, rattling, snoring, and wheezing in the wind-pipe, and yet the viscid mucus does not excite coughing (aft. 5 h.).

In the larynx stitches and feeling of roughness.¶ [*An.*]

Sensation of accumulation of mucus in the larynx. [*An.*]

580. Mucus adheres in the larynx, which he continually hawks up, and which makes the voice hollow and hoarse. [*Stf.*]

Hoarse rough voice. [*An.*]

A kind of suffocative attack, as if the larynx were full

* See 557.

† Comp. with 563.

‡ 565 seems to be the primary action of china, and 566 the secondary action or reaction of the organism ; for excitement of the circulation and hæmorrhages from the nose 174 to 176, from the mouth 238, and from the lung 586, are its not infrequent primary effects.

§ See 565.

‖ 575, 576, 577, comp. with 578 to 581.

¶ 578 to 581, see 575 to 577.

1 See note to S. 187. "Geräusch" in original is 'sibilus."

of mucus, especially towards evening, and (at night) on awaking from sleep* (aft. 8 h.).

Violent cough immediately after eating (aft. 4 h.).

In the evening tickling causing cough, which he could suppress.

585. Cough excited by laughing.

(Coughing up of bloody mucus)†

At night about 2 and about 4 a.m. suffocative cough lasting half a quarter of an hour (a kind of whooping-cough) ; she screams out from it, but not before she has coughed several times.‡

He wakes up after midnight with a cough ; at each cough-impulse he feels a sharp shooting in both sides of the chest, and yet he could cough in the lying position.

Pain in the trachea and sternum when coughing.

590. From the cough, pressive pain in the chest and excoriation feeling in the larynx.§

(During the chill of an ague) troublesome cough with stitches in the side. [FISCHER, l. c.]

Continual irritation to hacking cough, in the morning after rising, as from sulphur fumes, whereby nothing is expectorated, for several mornings. [*Gss.*]

Suspicious cough‖ [JUNCKER et FRITZE,[1] *Diss. de usu cort. peruv. discreto,* Halæ, 1756, p. 26.]

In the wind-pipe under the larynx, a kind of drawing, followed by cough with one impulse. [*Fz.*]

595. Tightness of the chest.¶ [BAGLIVI,[2] *Praxis,* lib. ii, § 2, 3.—AL. THOMPSON, l. c.]

Tightness of the chest. [CARTHEUSER, l. c.]

Oppression on the chest. [*Fz.*]

Inclination to breathe deeply before the mid-day meal.

In the evening a feeling of oppression and uneasiness in the chest ; he feels compelled to breathe deeply and then must expire in a sighing manner, whereby the oppression is diminished for the moment, with weak, scarcely perceptible pulse and anxious impatient humour. [*Bhr.*]

600. **Great oppression of the chest in the region of the scrobiculus cordis, as if something was digging around therein** (aft. 4 h.) [*Gss.*]

Tightness of the chest with difficult, sometimes rattling, expiration (chiefly when walking) and roughness of the chest (aft. 4 h.). [*Htn.*]

Impeded respiration, for half an hour.[3] [AL. THOMPSON, l. c.].

Heavy, difficult, painful inspiration, and rapid expiration.

* 582, 603, comp. with 595 to 597, 599 to 602, 604 to 606.
† Comp. with 593.
‡ 587, 588, 589, comp, with 591, 653.
§ 590, 610, 613, 621, comp. with 611, 612, 614, 615, 617, 620, 622.
‖ Comp. with 586.
¶ 595 to 597, 599 to 602, 604 to 606, comp. with 582, 603.

1 From China given for gangrene of foot, with alkermes and syrup of Canella.
2 Results of suppression of intermittents by China,
3 See note to S. 187.

Suffocative asthma.[1] [AL. THOMPSON, l. c.]

605. Fatal oppression of the chest.* [JOH. DE KOKER, l. c.]

An agreeable fulness in the chest, as from satiety, with (sweet) pleasant taste of the saliva (aft. 1 h.). [*Fz.*]

Tensive pain, especially in the external pectoral muscles (in the morning).

Some twitching and subsultus here and there in the pectoral muscles. [*An.*]

(A creeping in one side of the chest as if something were running about in it.)

610. A sharp aching combined with creeping in one side of the chest.)

Pressure on the chest.† [*Fz.*]

Aching pain in the chest. [*Css.*]

Pressure on the whole anterior part of the chest, at night when he lay on the back.

Pressure on the left side near the ensiform cartilage. [*Hrr.*]

615. External pressure on the middle of the sternum when the upper part of the body is bent forward, also when standing, which is removed by pressing upon it (aft. 26 h.). [*Fz.*]

Pressure outwards in the region of the lowest ribs (aft. 24 h.). [*Ws.*]

Great pressure in the sternum after a meal ; worst when he sat in a stooping position and had his arms elevated.

On inspiring severe stitches under the last ribs, that take away his breath.

Under the right last rib a small spot, which causes a shooting pain both by the slightest pressure and when walking

620. When sitting in a stooping attitude, pressure externally on the sternum, which causes anxiety and does not allow the breath to be drawn in enough, going off when raising himself up (aft. 6 h.). [*Fz.*]

In the side of the chest a pressive pain that impedes respiration.

Hard pressive pain in the right side of the chest, in the region of the fourth and fifth ribs.‡ [*Fz.*]

On the right side of the chest drawing aching when sitting, which is relieved when standing and walking. [*Fz.*]

Pain in the side, as if bruised or as if from a blow.

625. Drawing pain behind the sternum. [*Hrr.*]

In the whole chest a burning inward-pressure.

Inferiorly over the chest aching drawing pain when sitting, which causes anxiety ; it goes off when standing and walking. [*Fz.*]

On the right side of the chest, in the middle, on a not large spot, a contractive pain so that he must almost involuntarily suddenly jerk out and expel the breath. [*Fz.*]

* When the cinchona-bark was administered in the cold stage of ague.

† See 590, 610, 613, 621.

‡ See 590, 610, 621.

1 In the original, simply "asthma."

Over the chest, when sitting in a stooping attitude, an intermitting cutting aching, which goes off on raising himself up, but still more completely when standing and walking. [*Fz.*]

630. Aching, fine shooting on the left side of chest (aft. 8½ h.). [*Htn.*]

Stitch in the side. [RICHARD, l. c.]

Shooting in the chest, in the morning. [*Hsch.*]

Shooting in the left side of the chest. [*Lhm.*]

Shooting in the side, at night, but during the day only when moving or touching it (aft. 13 d.).

635. Shooting in the chest on walking quickly, which went off when at rest. [*Lr.*]

Some violent stitches in the chest, immediately above the precordial region, when he was not moving, especially when reading (aft. 3½, 16, 18 h.). [*Ln.*]

Stitches in the side when sitting and reading. [*Ln.*]

Some stitches from the sternum through to the back soon after drinking* (aft. 8 h.).

Sharp stitches in the thoracic cavity, from within outwards, in the region of the sixth and seventh true ribs, without relation to expiration or inspiration (aft. ¾ h.). [*Hrr.*]

640. **Regularly recurring obtuse stitches, from within outwards, in the thoracic cavity, when at rest and when moving, and without relation to respiration** (aft. 1 h.). [*Ws.*]

In the right side of the chest, in the region of the fourth rib under the arm, a shooting, as if it were in the pleura, almost like a persistent stitch, which goes off by pressing on it and by stooping down (aft. 6 h.), [*Fz.*]

Sharp stitches between the seventh and eighth left ribs. [*Hrr.*.]

Pain in the bone in the joints of the ribs, as if bruised, on inspiration.

Sharp stitches near the right nipple, from within outwards (aft. 10 h.). [*Hrr.*]

645. **Sharp stitches, from within outwards, on the sternum where the ribs join on to it on both sides, without reference to expiration or inspiration** (aft. 2 d.). [*Hrr.*]

Sharp shooting pain on the left, near the ensiform cartilage and in the scrobiculus cordis, only when expiring (aft. 60 h.). [*Hrr.*]

Shooting in the left side of the chest (during expiration) when sitting (aft. 2 h.). [*Lr.*]

A tickling shooting in the left side of the chest towards the region of the heart. [*Htg.*]

When drawing in the breath severe stitches in the scrobiculus cordis† (aft. 3 h.).

650. Obtuse stitches on the chest, which compel him to expire. [*Fz.*]

Obtuse shooting on the cartilages of the third and fourth left false ribs, without relation to inspiration or expiration. [*Hrr.*]

* Comp. with 387.

† Comp. with 390, 392.

Stitches in the side with great heat, strong, hard pulse, and staring eyes. [J. A. PH. GESNER,[1] *Sammlung v. Beob.*, i, p. 244, Nordlingen, 1789.]

Fever like a kind of false pleurisy.* [GREDING,[2] in *Ludw. Advers.*, tom. i, p. 90.]

A boil on the pectoral muscles.

655. (Throbbing in the sternum, in the evening and morning.)

Palpitation of the heart.†

Palpitation of the heart and rush of blood to the face, which became hot and red, and at the same time coldness of the hands (aft. 1 h.). [*Bch.*]

Violent beating of the heart, with depressed pulse and coldness of the skin. [*Wth.*]

Strong beating of the heart combined with an anxious feeling. [*Htg.*]

660. Pain as from dislocation in the scapula (aft. 24 h.).

Tearing in the region of the left scapula, on inspiration. [*Gss.*]

Drawing tearing pain in the left scapula (aft. 9 h.). [*Htn.*]

Contractive pain between the scapulæ, when standing (aft. 3 h.). [*Fz.*]

Needle-pricks over the right scapula and in the left side of the chest (aft. ¼ h.). [*Ws.*]

665. Pain in the back on the slightest movement, as if bruised (aft. 3 h.).

Throbbing, shooting pain in the back.‡

Small stitches on the middle of the spine§ (aft. 5 h.). [*Htn.*]

Shooting in the left side of the back (when sitting.) [*Lr.*]

Intolerable pain in the sacrum, as from cramp, or as if beaten and crushed, which on the slightest movement forces out a sudden cry.‖

670. A crawling itching on the coccyx, which goes off for a short time only by rubbing (aft. 1 h.)

Twitching tearing on the left side in the sacrum. [*Gss.*]

Severe shooting, drawing pains in the middle of the sacrum towards the lumbar vertebræ. [*Htg.*]

Twitching over the sacrum (aft. ½ h.). [*Wth.*]

Painful jerks on the sacrum¶ (aft. 21 h.). [*Ws.*]

675. (Stretching) pain in the sacrum, as from a heavy weight, or as after long stooping (aft. 23 h.). [*Htn.*]

The neck drawn obliquely on one side.[3] [AL. THOMPSON, l. c.]

Several stitches in the nape (which leave behind a kind of stiffness therein.** [*Htg.*]

* 591, 653, comp. with 587 to 589.
† Comp. with 657 to 659.
‡ Comp. with 667, 668.
§ 667, 668, see 666.
‖ Comp. with 674.
¶ See 669.
** See 680, 682, 683.

1 Not accessible.

2 In an epileptic, taking Hyoscyamus. After an intermediate dose of China, he had "diarrhœa, dolores rheumatici, *febrisque pleuritiden spuriam æmulans.*"

3 In original, simply "contractions of the neck." See note to S. 187.

Slow drawing stitches in the anterior cervical muscles, when at rest. [*Bhr.*]

(Anteriorly on the neck red miliary eruption, without itching.

680. Movement of the nape is painful*

Pain in the nape towards the neck, on turning the head as if he had swollen cervical glands (though he has none) ; on touching the pain is still more severe, as if bruised (after a walk).

Drawing pain on the right side of the neck inferiorly, at the commencement of the nape, when standing, which goes off when stooping.† [*Fz.*]

Drawing pains in the nape. [*An.*]

On the slightest movement sweat on the nape and back.

685. **Paralytic twitching tearing on the top of the shoulder, which is acutely painful when touched, and when the pain is gone it can be excited anew by touching ; even the pressure of the coat on the shoulder excites it.**‡ [*Hrr.*]

Tearing pressure in the left axilla and on the anterior and inner border of the scapula. [*Hrr.*]

Intermittent pressive drawing pain on the border of the right axilla towards the front (aft. 3 d.). [*Hrr.*]

Paralytic twitching tearing, which proceeds from the head of the humerus, and extends (in the muscles and bones) to the phalanges of the fingers, where it becomes less painful ; at the same time the whole arm is weaker ; the pain is increased by touching (aft. 3 h.). [*Hrr.*]

A weakness in the arms, observable when he tightly closes the hands.§

690. Shooting pains in the upper arm which however went off immediately on moving it (aft. $\frac{3}{4}$ h.). [*Wr.*]

Twitching tearing in the humerus towards the upper and inner part (aft. 2 h.). [*Hrr.*]

Tearing, first in the left, then in the right upper arm (aft. $\frac{1}{2}$ h.). [*Lr.*]

Paralytic pain on the right upper arm, which begins at the head of the humerus, and becomes lost in the hand as a fine and feeble tearing, during which the whole body, and especially the forehead, is warm (aft. 8 h.) [*Hrr.*]

Tearing and drawing in the arm when she stands at the window.

695. **Paralytic twitching tearing in the long bones of the upper extremities, more violent when touched** (aft. 1 h.). [*Hrr.*]

* Comp. with 677, 682, 683.

† 682, 683, see 677 and 680.

‡ It is peculiarly characteristic of China that its pains are aggravated not only by movement, and especially by touching the part (see 466, 619, 634, 688, 695, 696, 701, 704, 713, 761, 776, 830), but also that they are renewed when not present by merely touching the part, as in this symptom and 749, 772, and then often attain a frightful intensity, hence this medicine is often the only remedy in cases of this description.

§ Compare partly with 688 and 693, 695, 696.

Paralytic tearing in the upper extremities, which spreads into all their parts, increased more by touching than by movement. [*Hrr.*]

A tension in the arms and hands (aft. 2 h.).

Stretching out the arms with bent fingers.[1] [THOMPSON, l. c.]

A tearing darting through the left elbow-joint, frequently recurring.

700. On the elbow-joint, sensation, as if blood were extravasated in the skin. [*Htg.*]

Painful drawing in the coronoid process of the left elbow (in the bend of the elbow), worse when touched. [*Hrr.*]

Tearing pain in the left elbow-joint, worse on movement (aft. 2 h.). [*Hrr.*]

Shooting in the left elbow-joint. [*Fz.*]

Tearing in the shafts of both ulnæ, worse when touched.* [*Hrr.*]

705. From the elbow to the fingers drawing pain in the bones, in the evening† (aft. 24 h.).

Tearing extending hither and thither, at one time in the right forearm (which went off by rubbing), at another in the left (aft. 4 h.). [*Myr.*]

Drawing pain on the bones of the forearm, as from scraping on the periosteum with a blunt knife. [*Fz.*]

The forearm goes to sleep when flexed (*e. g.* when writing), with a fine shooting in the tips of the fingers.‡

Sharp drawing shooting across the left wrist (in the evening) (aft. 13, 14 h.). [*Fz.*]

710. In the hollow of the hand, across the roots of the fingers, drawing pain. [*Fz.*]

The hand is painful (cramp-like drawing) on grasping. [*Fz.*]

Trembling of the hands when writing (aft. 1 h.). [*Lr.*]

Twitching tearing in the metacarpal bones and fingers, aggravated by touching § [*Gss.*]

Twitching tearing in the wrist and metacarpal bones. [*Hrr.*]

715. Tearing where the metacarpal bones join the wrist (aft. 5 h.). [*Hrr.*]

Obtuse shooting on the metacarpal bone of the right index. [*Hrr.*]

On moving the left hand a drawing pain over the back of the hand, which is swollen.

Tearing in the bones of the distal phalanges of the fingers of the right hand, especially severe in the joints, without relation to movement (aft. ½ h.). [*Hrr.*]

A drawing upwards in the left thumb, index, and middle finger.

720. Fine shooting tearing in the distal joint of the right thumb.‖ [*Hrr.*]

* 704, 707, see 705.

† Comp. with 704, 706, 707.

‡ Comp. with 731, 828.

§ 713, 714, see 722.

‖ Shooting tearing and shooting drawing (which sometimes passes into twitching

1 See note to S. 187.

Twitching tearing on the metacarpal bone of the right little finger.* [*Gss.*]

Twitching pain in the left little finger.†

Knuckle of the middle finger swollen; he cannot move it on account of stiffness and pain.

Twitching tearing in the phalanges of the fingers (aft. 24 h.). [*Gss.*]

725. The hands are sometimes warm, sometimes cold.

One hand is icy cold, the other warm.

Blue nails. [CRUGER, l. c.]

Superiorly in the flesh of the right nates, on the coccyx, aching increasing in a pulsating manner, while sitting, which goes off on standing up. [*Fz.*]

Tearing drawing in the left nates when sitting.‡ [*Fz.*]

730. Drawing in the nates, and at the same time in the knees, when standing, which leaves off when seated.[1]

The lower extremities go to sleep when seated.§

Pain, like shooting and burning, in various parts of the lower extremities at the same time. [*Gss.*]

Exhaustion and relaxation, as from a long journey on foot, in the thighs and legs. [*Hbg.*]

Weakness and unsteadiness in the hip- and knee-joints, for two successive mornings, as if he had made a long journey on foot the previous day; on prolonged movement the feeling goes out of the joints, and gives place to a bruised pain, the first day in the thighs, but the second day more in the legs. [*Bhr.*]

735. Exhaustion in the lower extremities when walking, all day long (aft. 2 h.). [*Wr.*]

Exhaustion in the thighs.‖

Painful drawing in the long bones of the lower extremities¶ (aft. 2 d.). [*Hrr.*]

Spasmodic (stitch-like) drawing in the thighs and legs (aft. ½ h.). [*Wth.*]

In the inguinal and knee-joints aching drawing when sitting, which goes off on walking and standing. [*Fz.*]

740. Pain in the hip-joint, in the knees and feet, as if they were dislocated or cut to pieces.[2] [AL. THOMPSON, l. c.]

Drawing pain on the thigh bones, as if the periosteum were scraped with a blunt knife. [*Fz.*]

tearing, seems also to be one of the characteristic pains of china, see also 709, 738, 798, 799, 800.

* 721, see 722.

† Comp. with 713, 714, 721, 724.

‡ 729, 730, see 748.

§ See 828.

‖ Comp. with 733.

¶ See 748.

---

1 This symptom, though unaccompanied by the name of any authority, is not among Hahnemann's own observations.

2 See note to S. 422.

Slow, painful drawing in the inside of the left thigh, which seems to be only in the skin. [*Fz.*]

Pain of the posterior muscles of the thigh, as if they were beaten when sitting.

In the anterior muscles of both thighs tension when walking.

745. (A burning anteriorly on the upper parts of the thighs.)

Spasmodic drawing in the right thigh from the hough upwards (with sensation of pressure), just as if it would draw up the leg, in the evening when sitting, which goes off by standing and walking. [*Fz.*]

In the middle of the left thigh a twitching (aft. 5 h.). [*Wth.*]

A tearing by jerks in the thigh.

Twitching tearing on the right and left thighs forwards and outwards, excited only by touch, not by movement. [*Hrr.*]

750. **Twitching tearing on the anterior aspect of the left thigh** (aft. 2 h.). [*Gss.*]

Tearing in the thigh bones, from above downwards, when at rest and when moving, in fits, for several days (aft. 72 h.). [*Ws.*]

Tearing, that extends from the knee-joint to the thigh, accompanied by a weakness which renders walking and standing difficult. [*Hrr.*]

In the shaft of the thigh-bone a painful, aching drawing downwards, chiefly when sitting, in the afternoon. [*Fz.*]

Painful sensitiveness of the skin on the thighs, from the friction of the clothes, as if the skin were rough and covered with papules (aft. 8 d.). [*Ws.*]

755. In the left thigh, when standing, a sensation as if there were a hardened node in the flesh, with drawing pain in it* (aft. 2 h.). [*Fz.*]

Hard swelling of the thighs, which sometimes goes down over the knees to the beginning of the feet, becomes thinner below, is reddish, and is painful when touched.†

Stitch darting upwards in the right thigh posteriorly, when standing. [*Fz.*]

When he rises from a seat, burning and formication, as of having gone to sleep, in the thigh on which he was sitting, especially in the hough, particularly observable when standing. [*Fz.*]

Cramp-like, paralytic pain in the right thigh and knee-joint on rising up from a seat, when he has sat for a considerable time, and when walking (aft 5½ h.). [*Htn.*]

760. Twitching tearing internally in the patella. [*Gss.*]

Paralytic tearing in the right knee-joint, which spreads now towards the thigh and now towards the leg, with weakness of the part, and aggravation more by touch than by movement. [*Hrr.*]

In the right knee, on rising up from a seat and when walking, a sharp drawing pain, which went off again when sitting (in the afternoon). [*Stf.*]

* See 771.

† Comp. with 785, 792, 793.

Shooting in the left knee-joint. [*Fz.*]

Slight trembling of the knees on rising up after sitting, which went off whilst walking. [*Bch.*]

765. Knuckling together of the knees, especially on going upstairs. [*An.*]

When walking the knees give way and knuckle together. [*Fz.*]

Coldness and chilliness of the knees (aft. ½ h.).

In the knees twitching pain.*

Hot swelling of the right knee with drawing tearing pains, from which he awakes at midnight.

770. Pain in the knee on the slightest motion, as if bruised† (aft. 3 h.).

(Pain in the knee on bending it, preventing sleep, with nodes‡ [lumps in the skin there].)

A pain on the side of the patella when touched (aft. 2 h.).

On the tendons of the flexor muscles in the hough jerking drawing, synchronous with the pulse.§ [*Fz.*]

Sensation in the leg as if a garter were too tightly tied about it, and as if it would go to sleep and become benumbed.

775. An internal uneasiness in the legs compelled him to bend them and draw them up.‖ [*Fz.*]

Bruised pain of the bones of the leg when treading, and still worse on touching; when she touched them the whole foot shivered and was chilly, as if she had immersed it in cold water.

Drawing pain in the right tibia inferiorly, near the heel, and then in the whole foot (when sitting). [*Lr.*]

Pain in the lower half of both legs, as if the periosteum were bruised and swollen, only when standing; on touching it sore pain as if on an excoriated bruised spot.

On extending the left leg, when sitting, an aching drawing pain superiorly on the inside of the shaft of the tibia below the patella, which goes off on flexing the leg. [*Fz.*]

780. Aching drawing on the tibia, in the evening, when sitting, which goes off when standing and walking. [*Fz.*]

When walking shooting in the tibiæ, which went off when at rest (aft. 5 and more h.). [*Lr.*]

Painful cramp in the left calf, at night, on extending and flexing the foot, which prevents sleep (aft. 16 h.).

When walking in the open air, single, sharp, rapidly recurring stitches in the upper part of the calf. [*Fz.*]

Tearing in the calf. [*Lr.*]

785. Hard, dark red swelling on the calf, which went on to suppuration.¶ [PELARGUS,[1] *Obs.* ii, i, p. 72.]

* Comp. with 760, and partly with 773.
† Comp. with 759.
‡ Comp. with 755.
§ See 768.
‖ See 837 to 840.
¶ See 756, 792, 793.

1 Results of suppression of intermittents by china.

Over the tendo Achillis a severe burning tension. [*Htg.*]
Weariness of the feet, as if they were bruised (aft. 4 h.).
Paralysis of the feet. [CRUGER, l. c.]
Violent shooting burning on the dorsum of the foot close to the tibia (when sitting). [*Gss.*]

790. Coldness of the feet, in the evening.
Shooting in the left foot. [*Lr.*]
Swelling of the feet. [STAHL, l. c.]
Painful swelling of the feet. [FISCHER, l. c.]
Very soft swelling of the soles of the feet.

795. Contractive pinching pain on the outer side of the right foot, on the side of the sole (aft. 6 h.). [*Htn.*]
Violent itching on the right sole when walking and sitting, relieved for a short time by scratching. [*Hrr.*]
Pricking formication from the big toe up to the dorsum of the foot, as if the part had been frost-bitten, in the evening when sitting, which goes off when walking and standing.* [*Fz.*]
Shooting drawing in the heel (aft. 48 h.). [*Gss.*]
Shooting tearing in the sole of the foot in the region of the heel, while sitting and walking. [*Hrr.*]

800. Very violent tearing shooting in the soles, when sitting and walking. [*Fz.*]
Drawing pain in the metatarsal bones of the right foot. [*Hrr.*]
When standing, drawing with sore pain on the dorsum of the foot, which goes off when sitting. [*Fz.*]
Cramp-like drawing in the inner side of the left foot when sitting. [*Fz.*]
Twitching tearing in the bones of the foot and metatarsus. [*Hrr.*]

805. **Twitching tearing in the metatarsal bones and toes.** [*Gss.*]
Twitching tearing, increased only when touched, not by movement, in the metatarsal bones and phalanges of the toes, especially in the joints (aft. 31 h.). [*Hrr.*]
Twitching tearing where the metatarsal bones unite with the bones of the tarsus (aft. 25 h.). [*Hrr.*]
Boring stitches in the tips of the toes.†
Shooting now in the tibiæ, now in the back, now in the chest, when sitting (aft. 14 h.). [*Lr.*]

810. Excessive, almost painful sensitiveness of the skin of the whole body, even of the palms of the hands‡ (aft. 10 h.).
In the wound a digging pain.
In the ulcer boring pain.

* Although the china pains and sufferings are most frequently (next to touch, see 685) aggravated and increased by movement of the part, yet there is a not altogether rare alternating action, where they are diminished and allayed by movement, as here and 682, 728, 739, 746, 775, 779, 780, and also where they are especially produced when at rest, 729, 743, 753, 837, 838, 839.

† Comp. with 791.

‡ Comp. with 540, 754.

In the wound (the ulcer) a shooting itching pain for two hours* (aft. some h.).

(In the ulcer shooting throbbing pain, even when at rest.)

815. The ulcer becomes painfully sensitive, and there occurs a boring pain in it.

In the ulcer throbbing pain on moving the part, but not when at rest.

(In the ulcer there appears fœtid-smelling ichor ; there is burning and aching in it ; he dares not let the foot hang down ; the foot is painful when standing.)

Itching, particularly in the evening, on the arms, loins, and chest ; after scratching papules appear.

Smarting itching almost confined to the parts on which he lies in bed ; scratching allays it for instants only ; but if he lies on the unaffected side, so that the itching parts come uppermost, the itching soon goes off (aft. 8, 9 h.).

820. Smarting itching almost confined to the parts whereon he does not lie (in the midday sleep), and which are turned uppermost (aft. 26 h.).

Itching of the skin ; after scratching blisters appear, as from nettle-stings.

Itching of the skin : on scratching blood exudes.

In the warmth and at night in bed a burning itching in the hough and on the inner side of the arms, with an eruption of small vesicles, which contain water, but disappear in the cold air.

Fine shooting on various parts of the skin. [*Fz.*]

825. (Shooting in a cicatrized wound on the left foot.†) [*Fz.*]

In the skin, especially of the abdomen, on some parts a tugging as if a hair were pulled. [*Fz.*]

Spasmodic twitching in various muscular parts. [*An.*]

The limbs on which he lies go to sleep.‡

Stiffness and numbness of the limbs.

830. **Twitching tearing§ on various parts of the limbs, especially of the hands and feet, aggravated by touching.** [*Gss.*]

Bone pains in the joints of the ribs, of the limbs, of the shoulders and scapulæ, as if they were beaten, when he stirs or moves in the very least.‖

In the bones he feels like a drawing. [*Fz.*]

Stretching, extremely acute drawing pain in almost all the bones, now in one; now in another, which at first went off for a few moments on lying down, but then recurred all the more violently (aft. 14 h.). [*Bch.*]

Gout. [MURRAY, l. c.]

835. Rheumatic pains. [GREDING,—RAULIN, l. c.]

Pains in the limbs, especially in the joints.¶ [FISCHER, l. c.]

* 813, 814, comp. with 825. † See 813, 814. ‡ See 708, 731.

§ The chief pain produced by china seems to be *twitching tearing.*—HERRMANN.

‖ 831 is alternating action with 837, 838, and 840.

¶ See 831, 837—840.

Pain of the joints when sitting and lying; the limbs will not allow him to lie quietly in one position, as after excessive fatigue from a long journey, or as after great debility caused by excessive blood-letting or too frequent seminal emissions; the limbs must be laid now here, now there, and be sometimes flexed and at another time extended.*

Pain of all the joints as if beaten, in the morning slumber; the longer they are left lying still the more painful are they;—hence it is necessary to turn the limbs frequently, because the pains are diminished by movement; on awaking completely they go off.

Pain in all the joints, as from a great weight pressing on them, in the morning in bed, which goes off on getting up.

840. While sitting, pain in all the joints, as from a heavy weight pressing on him; the longer he sits the more weary he becomes.

On rising from (the noon) sleep all the joints feel stiff.

On rising from sleep in the morning and from the midday sleep, a paralytic stiffness of all the limbs, that causes dejection of mind.

Cracking in the joints.

Everywhere he is in pain, the joints, the bones, and the periosteum, as if he had sprained himself, and like a drawing and tearing, especially in the spinal column, in the sacrum, in the knee and thighs.

845. Tensive pains. [B. M. ETTMULLER,[1] *Diss. de usu et abusu præcipit.*, cap. 3, § 5.]

Oppression of all parts of the body, as if his clothes were too tight (after a walk in the open air).

Wandering rheumatism, sometimes in one part, sometimes in another, without swelling or fever, alternating with pains in the interior of the body.† [SYDENHAM, *Opusc.*, p. 351.]

* 837 to 840 comp. with 775. The weakness here described, as if proceeding from a great loss of humours, is in conjunction with the phenomena indicated under 860, 862, 863, 865, 889, and 893, together with the symptoms of the disposition of china (1095, 1096, 1103. 1107 to 1110, 1113, 1125, 1126. 1131), the symptoms of deranged digestive organs (229, 242, 249 to 255, 265, 269, 277 to 279, 283, 289, 290, 293, 294, 296, 298, 301, 302, 305 to 307, 310, 318 to 321, 829, 330, 339), the suffering after food (332, 333, 350, 351, 357, 358, 364, 366, 367, 369 to 371, 387, 394, 414, 416), the too-easily excited perspiration, especially in the back on movement and during sleep (684, 1058, 1060, 1061, 1064), and the confusion of the head (6, 8, 11 to 16, 18, 19, 21 to 23), exactly that for which china is the only suitable remedy, and which almost without exception occurs in persons who have experienced a very considerable loss of strength by hæmorrhages and frequent blood-letting, by prolonged escape of milk from the breasts and unduly prolonged suckling, by excesses in venery and onanism, or frequent involuntary seminal emissions, by profuse morbid sweats or taking sudorifics in excess, by diarrhœas, or frequently repeated purgatives. In morbid debility of other kinds, when the disease itself is not suitable for this remedy, the administration of china is always followed by injurious, often fatal consequences, although even in such unsuitable cases a stimulation of the strength is produced by it in the first few hours; but the unnatural, over strained character of this is easily perceived, and but too often a premature death is the consequence of this over-stimulation, and if in such cases its use is long continued, the patient falls into a cachectic condition hard to cure, and which is the result of the physician's maleficent art.

† From the long-continued employment.

1 Results of suppression of intermittents by china.

A burning, mingled with some formication and itching, in various parts of the body, by day. [*Gss.*]

Consumption. [MURRAY,—BAGLIVI, l. c.]

850. Cachexiæ. [MURRAY,—BERGER, l. c.]

Lingering fevers. [BAGLIVI, l. c.—STAHL, *Obs.*, *Clin.*]

Dropsy. [MURRAY,—BAGLIVI,—BERGER,—RICHARD,—RAULIN,—ROMBERG,—STAHL,—THOMPSON, l. c.]

Anasarca. [STAHL, l. c.]

Swelling of the limbs.* [CARTHEUSER, l. c.]

855. Erysipelatous swelling of the whole body. [FORMEY, l. c.]

Yellow colour of the skin. [FISCHER, l. c.]

Jaundice. [BERGER,—STAHL,—THOMPSON,—RICHARD, l. c.]

He feels ill all over ; he is not at all well.

The sensitiveness of the whole nervous system is, as it were, morbidly increased, strained and irritated.

860. Excessive sensitiveness of all the nerves, with a morbid feeling of general weakness.†

Internal feeling, as of an illness about to come on.

Over-irritation, with pusillanimity and intolerance of all noises.

Languishing condition of mind and body, with over-sensitiveness.‡

Ailments from a slight draught of air.

865. Too great delicacy and over-sensitiveness of the nervous system ; all impressions of sight, smell, hearing, and taste are too strong for him, they offend his inner sensibility and affect his disposition.

The former pains are as if kept back and forcibly suppressed, and at the same time a great heaviness in the whole body.

Weariness.

Trembling powerlessness of the limbs, with dilated pupils.§

Inclination to lie down.

870. Exhaustion. [GESNER, l. c.]

Exhaustion in the limbs. [STAHL, *Obs.*]

Chronic weakness.[1] [THOMPTON, l. c.]

Sinking of the forces. [ROMBERG, l. c.]

Sunken forces. [CLEGHORN,[2] *Diseases of Minorca*, pp. 191, 213.]

875. Feeling of exhaustion, especially when he rises from a seat ; he would like to sit down again, and unless he strains his muscles he sinks back on his chair, whereupon an agreeable feeling of rest ensues (aft. 3, 4 h.). [*Bhr.*]

He had a difficulty in walking, and felt soon exhausted, as from a feeling of weight and paralysis in the thighs. [*Stf.*]

* 854, 855, see 756, 785, 792, 793, 794.

† 860, comp. with the symptoms mentioned in the note to 837. Here is described the peculiar weakness which china especially excites in a high degree, and it is especially this form that is permanently relieved by china, when at the same time the other symptoms resemble those produced by it. This particular kind of weakness is especially characteristic of those exhausted by loss of humours.

‡ Comp. with 888.

§ Comp. with 890.

1 Not found.

2 Effects of china in agues.

Heavy feeling of the body. [RAULIN, l. c.]

Heaviness in all the limbs, especially in the thighs, as if lead hung upon them.* [*An.*]

Laziness. [*Wth.*]

880. When he tried to keep himself erect for some minutes there ensued stiffness, paleness and loss of consciousness. [GESNER, l. c.]

Unconsciousness and exhaustion at the same time. [*Lhm.*]

Slight attacks of[1] apoplexy and unconsciousness. [THOMPSON, l. c.]

Exhaustion and relaxation of the whole body. [*Hrr.*]

Severe fainting fit.† [BAKRR, in *Medical Transactions*, vol. iii, Lond., 1785.]

885. Syncopes. [MORTON,—MURRAY,—CRUGER,—GESNER, l. c.]

Syncope—death.‡ [DE KOKER, l. c.]

Asphyxia, apparent death. [CRUGER, l. c.]

Exhaustion and relaxation of body and mind (aft. 1 h.). [*Hrr.*]

Exhaustion : he can scarcely hold up his head, and falls asleep. [*Fz.*]

890. Flaccidity in all the limbs and trembling in the hands.§ [*Lhm.*]

Relaxation of the whole body, felt also when seated, but far more **when walking.** [*An.*]

Sometimes weakness, sometimes feeling of excessive strength in the joints.‖ [*Fz.*]

He feels quite weak and faint in the open air, and as if sinking away about the stomach and chest, although he has plenty of strength for walking. [*Fz.*]

Extraordinary facility of all movements, as if he had no body¶ (aft. 2 to 3 h.). [*Fz.*]

895. Liveliness, but with staring eyes, all the evening.** [*Hsch.*]

Comfortable feeling, in the evening. [*Lhm.*]

Trembling in all the limbs, felt not seen, combined with feeling of coolness. [*Hbg.*]

Twitchings. [GESNER, l. c.]

She cannot sleep all night ; she is occupied with nothing but disagreeable thoughts, one after the other.

900. He cannot fall asleep on account of many ideas and reflections, each of which only engages him for a short time, but is always supplanted by another ; hence almost all night long no sleep comes

* Comp. with 733, 736.

† In a powerful man, to whom a drachm of best red cinchona-bark had been given in one dose ; the fainting fit was so severe that he could not be roused from it until an emetic was given to him.

‡ SYDENHAM also (*Opera*, Lips., 1695, p. 379) mentions two men having died in his time from cinchona-bark taken a few hours before the attack of ague.

§ See 868.

‖ Alternating action in a healthy person.

¶ Alternating action after previous feeling of weakness caused by cinchona-bark.

** A kind of unnatural excitement, as in the so-called strengthening treatment of ordinary practitioners, when they are unable to remove from the patient his disease, and yet will hypocritically procure for him strength and liveliness for a few hours.

---

1 Should be "as of," See note to S. 422.

to his eyes; towards morning he becomes quite warm all over yet cannot bear throwing off the bed-clothes, without thirst (aft. 30 h.).

Sleeplessness after midnight; but sleepy though he is, his thoughts remain wide awake, he shuts his eyes and often changes his position in bed.

He fell asleep late; on account of many thoughts he could not go to sleep, he did not sleep soundly, and on rising he was in a very exhausted state.

Sleeplessness until midnight, with aching pain over the whole head.* [*Bch.*]

When about to fall asleep he is awakened by horrible fancies.†

905. He starts up when about to go sleep.

Before midnight till 2 a.m. unusual wakefulness. [*Lhm.*]

Drowsiness, with palpitation of the heart.

Incessant yawning, without sleepiness.‡

Drowsiness by day.§

910. The eyelids will close from weariness and sleepiness (aft. ½ h.).

Constant day-drowsiness; he falls asleep unexpectedly.

When sitting invincible drowsiness.

As soon as she sits down, by day, she immediately nods and slumbers; but if she lies down, she becomes wide awake from the least noise.

Sleepiness and soon thereafter again wakefulness. [*Hbg.*]

915. Drowsy lassitude. [STAHL, l. c.]

Drowsiness all day, with stretching of the limbs and yawning. [*An.*]

He wakes in the morning two hours earlier than usual. [*Bhr.*]

He starts up at night in sleep.

Sleeps only from 3 till 5 a. m. [*Lhm.*]

920. Very deep sleep, like that of an intoxicated person, without once waking; in the morning his head is quite dazed, as if he had not slept enough, and he gets aching in the temples on shaking the head ‖ [*Fz.*]

Snoring and whining in sleep, in children.¶

Snoring inspiration and expiration in sleep.

Snoring inspiration (through the nose) **in sleep** (aft. 3 h.).

In sleep there occurs at one time snoring inspiration, at another **blowing (puffing) expiration.**

925. In sleep one eye is open, the other half shut, with eye-balls turned backwards like a dying person (aft. 1 h.).

In sleep he lies on the back, with head bent back, the arms

* 903, 906, 919, comp. with 889, 899, 900. The aching pain in the head at night seems to be characteristic of china; comp. with 920, 936, 951. Also the pressure in the umbilical region, in the evening in bed, 932, is allied with it.

† 904, 905, 933, 938, 946. Restless sleep at night, with anxious, frightful dreams, after which on waking consciousness is not quite perfect, or the anxiety they cause continues (934, 935), are quite peculiar to china, see 936, 937, 939 to 947.

‡ 908, and 955, 958, are alternating action with 916.

§ 909 to 913, comp. with 915, 916.

‖ Comp. with 951.

¶ Comp. with 938.

stretched out above the head, with slow expiration and strong quick pulse.

Restlessness, sleeplessness. [RAULIN, l. c.]

Restless sleep, with tossing about, without waking. [*Htg.*]

Restless sleep. [CLEGHORN, l. c.]

930. Restless sleep ; he could not fall asleep ; when he got to sleep he soon woke up again, with perspiration on the hair of the head and on the forehead, and chilliness over the back. [*Wr.*]

Restless sleep, and after waking in the night, slight sweat all over. [*Hbg.*]

In the evening in bed a pinching pressure in the umbilical region. [*Fz.*]

At night a frightful dream (aft. 8 h.).

Heavy dreams in the night sleep, which make him anxious after waking.

935. Anxious dream : he has to go perpendicularly down into an abyss, whereupon he wakes, but retains the dangerous place so vividly in his imagination (especially when he shuts his eyes) that he remains for a long time in great fear about it and cannot calm himself.

All night long alternately headache and dreams, from which he starts up in affright.* [*Lhm.*]

At night restless sleep, from which he started up from time to time, and then every time remained for some instants without being able to collect himself. [*Myr.*]

Restless sleep full of dreams and crying out.

In the evening, on going to sleep, confused dream-pictures, from which he wakes up again (aft. 16 h.). [*Ws.*]

940. At night, on awaking out of frightful dreams, anxiety. [*Hrr.*]

At night fearful, startling dreams of falling from a height, with waking up full of restlessness and inability to collect himself for some instants. [*Wth.*]

Fearful dreams of misfortunes, from which he wakes up, but without being able to come to himself. [*Gss.*]

Anxious dreams at night, from which he awoke in a half-conscious state, and for some time continued afraid. [*Wth.*]

A sleep disturbed by confused and disconnected dreams, with repeated awakings ; he woke up but could not quite recollect himself. [*Bch.*]

945. **Confused, nonsensical dreams after midnight, mingled with semi-conscious waking.** [*Hrr.*]

When he wakes at night, he cannot recollect himself.

Confused, absurd dreams, by which he is often woke up from sleep. [*Hrr.*]

At night restless sleep, with vexatious dreams and tossing about, from which he wakes up every time. [*Fz.*]

Voluptuous dreams with pollutions. [*Hbg.*]

950. As soon as she closes her eyes to go to sleep, she dreams about nasty things.

At night, in sleep, he tosses about hither and thither, throws off

* 936, 937, 939 to 945, 947 see note to S. 904.

the clothes, and has all kinds of vexatious dreams about things that have occurred long ago ; in the morning he cannot get quite awake on account of emptiness and confusion of the head ; in the morning he is as if broken on the wheel and not at all refreshed by sleep. [*Fz.*]

On awaking at night he feels giddy, so that he could not trust himself to sit upright.

In the morning on awaking, anxious ideas and thoughts.

Towards morning heat in the head and oppression of the chest.

955. Inclination to yawn. [*Ws.*]

Yawning.

Stretching.

Yawning and stretching of the limbs. [*Htn.*]

Dread of the open air.

960. In the open air great shuddering, with rigor and goose-skin. [*Wth.*]

He gets shuddering and chilliness in the open air which is not cold. this goes off immediately in the room. [*Fz.*]

In the open air of moderate coldness, trembling of the limbs from chilliness, and shudder passing over the thighs. [*Fz.*]

Though the room is cold he does not feel chilly (aft. 9 h.). [*Fz.*]

Cold hands and chilliness externally all over the body, as if he had cold water poured over him, in the open air, where it went on to chattering of the teeth ; in the room this went off, but the hands remained cold. [*Trn.*]

965. Coldness of the hands and feet, even in the warm room. [*Fz.*]

Cold hands (aft. $\frac{1}{4}$ h.).

Sensation of icy coldness in the left hand which, however, is not colder externally to the touch than the right*

Coldness of the hands, feet, and nose.

Coldness of the hands. [*Lr.*]

970. Cold feet in the evening (aft. 4 h.). [*Mch.*]

A cold feeling of the left leg from the knee to the foot. [*Hbg.*]

A shudder of the same kind over both elbows and knees. [*Fz.*]

Icy cold feet with warmth of the rest of the body (aft. 1 h.). [*Hbg.*]

Sensation of coldness on the lower extremities, whilst the face and chest are still warm (aft. 1 h.). [*Hrr.*]

975. The right hand is warm (while writing), the left cold.† [*Hbg.*]

The right hand is perceptibly colder than the left. [*Wth.*]

In the morning cold hands and feet, and rigor over the thighs, which increases when walking (aft. 28 h.). [*Fz.*]

Shivering (aft. $\frac{1}{4}$ h.). [*An.*]

A slight shiver all over the body. [*Htg.*]

980. Flying chill, especially over the back (immediately). [*Wr.*]

A slight shivering in the back (aft. 3 h.). [*Stf.*]

Along with chilliness of the body, yawning.

* Alternating action with 975, 976.

† 975, 976, alternating action with 967.

Chilliness of the whole body, with very cold feet (aft. 2 h.). [*Fz.*]

He is cold all over.*

985. **Rigor all over the body, without thirst.** [*Lr.*]

Chilliness all over the body, with cold hands (aft. ½ h.). [*Myr.*]

Chilliness in the whole body, without external coldness. [*Lhm.*]

Chilliness in the whole body, more internally (aft. 3½ h.). [*Myr.*]

Palpitation of the heart, followed immediately by chilliness† (aft. 20 m.).

990. Chilliness on the body, as if a cold wind blew on him, especially when walking, seldom with shivering, which only comes on when he sits down, over the arms, loins, and thighs (aft. 8 h.). [*Fz.*]

Shuddering all over the body, with goose-skin (aft. 1 h.). [*Htn.*]

Shuddering and rigor all over the body. [*Wth.*]

(In the evening, on lying down, severe rigor.)

Rigor internally and externally in the whole body, sometimes more in the marrow of the bones of the feet, which are colder than the hands (aft. ½ h.). [*Gss.*]

995. Internal coldness, periodically with shuddering and rigor all over the body (immediately). [*Wth.*]

Internal chill, without externally perceptible coldness‡ (aft. 4 h.). [*Ws.*]

Internal feeling of coldness, chiefly in the arms and hands. [*Bch.*]

Rigor on the chest and arms when walking in the open air.

Chill over ther arms, with sickness about the stomach, then cold limbs, with shuddering and recurring nausea.

1000. Chilliness, without coldness of the body, without thirst§ (in the interval betwixt heat and chill, 1½ h.). [*Hrr.*]

In the morning rigor for half an hour, without thirst, and without subsequent heat.

(During the febrile chill, thirst.‖

* Alternating action with 996, 997, 1000.

† The china-fever often commences with an accessory symptom, with palpitation of the heart, 989, or with sneezing, 1083, or great anxiety, 1016, 1093, or nausea, 999, 1017, or great thirst, 1048, or ravenous hunger, 1053, 1054, or aching pain in the hypogastrium, 1014, or headache, 1015.

‡ 996, 1000, alternating action with 984.

§ On the second and third day after taking the drug, in the febrile attacks the interval betwixt chill and heat became always greater—HERRMANN.

‖ This, as also 1046, seems not to have been properly observed, for in every other observation I found that in the china-fever there is no thirst during the chill or rigor, 985, 1000, 1001, 1003 to 1005, 1007, 1008, 1040; on the contrary, the thirst only came after the chill or rigor, as we learn from the observations 1009 to 1011, or which comes to the same thing, immediately before the heat, as in 1048. So also the thirst during the china-fever is not met with even during the fully-developed febrile heat, see 1036, 1038, 1042, 1043, 1054, 1055, 1056, 1093, except some burning of the lips, see 1053, or dryness of them, see 1037 and 1055; which dryness is indicated by the expression—"Sensation of *some* thirst during the heat," 1020, for "Thirst during the flying heat," 1047, does not refer to fully-developed febrile heat. The thirst is rather only *after* the heat in the china-fever, 1018, 1049, 1052, or, which is the same thing, during the perspiration, 1064. But the febrile heat accompanied by stitches all over the body seems to be exceptional, 1074, 1075.

Along with internal chill, external rigor and shivering, during which at first the left hand and left foot are colder, afterwards both hands and feet are equally cold, without thirst (aft. ½—1 h.). [*Wth.*]

Shivering all over the body, but less violent on the limbs, without thirst ; the body is not cold, only the hands (aft. ½ h.). [*Hrr.*]

1005. Shivering all over the body, without thirst (aft. 2½ h.). [*Hrr.*]

Shivering and chill when he comes from the open air into the warm room* (aft. 5 h.).

Rigor all over the body, with icy cold hands, without thirst [aft. 1—3 h.). [*Htn.*]

Rigor and internal coldness, for several hours, without thirst (aft. ½, 1 h.). [*Wth.*]

After the shivering through the skin, thirst.

1010. After the chill thirst, not followed by heat. [*Trn.*]

All day long, from time to time, febrile chill over the whole body, especially on the forehead, which is bedewed with cold sweat ; a quarter of an hour after the first chill, great thirst (aft. 1 h.). [*Bch.*]

Febrile chill (aft. ¾ h.), alternately coming and going off, at the same time weakness of the knees and tibiæ when walking and standing, less when sitting. [*Bch.*]

In the morning (about 5 o'clock) severe febrile shivering, with weakness of the feet (aft. 12 h.). [*Css.*]

During the febrile chill, aching pain in the hypogastrium (aft. ½ h.). [*Bch.*]

1015. Shivering throughout the body, without external coldness, then dull, cutting headache extending into the orbits. [*Lhm.*]

Shuddering and rigor through the whole body, with cold hands and oppression of the mind (aft. 1 h.). [*Wth.*]

In the morning and forenoon shivering, with cold hands, feeling of nausea, and quick pulse. [*Fz.*]

In the evening (about 5 o'clock) coldness and shivering when walking in the open air, going off in the room (aft. 10 h.) ; an hour afterwards great heat, especially in the face, which is increased by movement and when walking ; an hour after the disappearance of the heat, thirst comes on. [*Fz.*]

Two attacks of chilliness at different times before the febrile heat. [FISCHER, l. c.]

1020. Heat alternating with chill ; from half an hour to an hour after the chill the heat comes on ; some thirst for cold water in the heat. [*Hrr.*]

While walking in the open air, shivering on the back, then heat in the back, with breaking out of perspiration, followed immediately by renewed sensation of coldness and shivering. [*Wr.*]

Quick and hard pulse, with flying heat alternating with chilliness in the back, which is covered with cold sweat, as is also the forehead (aft. a few m.), without thirst in the chill and heat, for five hours. [*Wr.*]

All the afternoon chilliness alternating with heat, at the same

* A rare alternating action in comparison with the much more frequent 960 to 964, 998, 1018.

time weakness in the lower extremities; all much worse when walking in the open air. [*Wr.*]

Heat in the head, with distended blood-vessels on the hands* (aft. 4 h.).

1025. **The blood mounts to the head, the forehead is hot and the limbs are cold.**†

During the feeling of heat, intermingled with alternating redness of face, lasting all day, febrile attacks of chill and perspiration, with but little thirst. [*An.*]

All over the body sometimes warmth, sometimes coldness (aft. ½—1 h.). [*Wth.*]

Redness and heat in the cheek and lobe of the ear, with chill over the arms and abdomen (aft. 1 h.).

Redness and heat in the cheek and ear-lobe of one side or the other, and before this goes off, chill all over the body, at last on the lower extremities (aft. 4 h.).

1030. Heat in the face, and after some hours shivering and chilliness, with coldness of the whole body.

In the evening, cold hands with hot cheeks. [*Fz.*]

During the heat he can scarcely uncover the hands without suffering.

Warmth and redness in the face, whilst the rest of the body was cold; at the same time a disagreeable cold feeling (chill) on the warm forehead. [*Bch.*]

Very great internal heat in the whole face, the trunk and the thighs, with cold sweat on the forehead, cold cheeks and cold feet (aft. 10½ h.). [*Htn.*]

1035. Warmth in the face with chilliness of the rest of the body, and shortly afterwards coldness of the forehead, with warm feeling of the rest of the body. [*Hbg.*]

Very great feeling of heat on the whole body, with red cheeks, heat on the trunk and arms, moderately warm thighs, legs, and feet, with damp forehead, without thirst. [*Htn.*]

During the heat, immediately after midnight, no thirst, only dry lips.

Feeling of heat and redness of the cheeks, without externally perceptible warmth in them, without thirst, with cold feet (aft. 9 h.). [*Fz.*]

After previous increased warmth in the not warm room, whilst walking in the open air, feeling of coldness about the ankles, and coldness of the rest of the body, in the forenoon before a meal. [*Fz.*]

1040. He eats his dinner with relish and great appetite, and an hour

* In the china-fever the blood-vessels are generally distended, even during heat in the head alone, as here, or during considerably increased temperature of the body, 1042, or during mere feeling of heat without externally perceptible heat, 1041, and so also during actual external heat, 1056.

† 1024, 1025. In the china-fever rush of blood to the head is very frequent, generally with redness and heat of face, 1030, 1055, often with chilliness of the rest of the body, 1028, 1029, 1035, also with external coldness, 1031, 1033, or only internal feeling of heat on the face, with cheeks cold to the touch, and cold sweat on the forehead, 1034.

afterwards there occurs chilliness, without thirst, then feeling of heat. [*Fz.*]

Sensation of heat throughout the body, with distended veins and cold feet ; on the rest of the body also there is no perceptible external increase of temperature.

Temperature of the whole body somewhat elevated and distended blood-vessels, but without thirst, with readily dilated pupils (aft. 8, 12 h.).

Heat all over the body without thirst (aft. 3 h.).

Heat and feeling of heat on the body ; at first the limbs are at the same time still cold, and he has also a feeling of coldness in them (aft. ½ h.), with slight thirst for cold water. [*Hrr.*]

1045. **Dry heat**, all day long. [*An.*]

Unquenchable thirst during the chill and heat of an ague. [J. V. VON HILDENBRAND[1] in *Hufel. Journal,* xiii, i. p. 142.]

Feeling of flying heat, with thirst for cold drinks. [*Gss.*]

Very great thirst, for an hour (aft. 9½ h.), and thereafter a burning heat all over the body, with throbbing in all the blood-vessels, without sweat, and without thirst, with violently burning ears and burning in the forehead, but only normally warm cheeks, hands, and feet, notwithstanding which all these three parts seem to his inward feeling to be too hot (aft. 10½ h.). [*Htn.*]

In the evening, an hour after the heat, dry palate and thirst. [*Fz.*]

1050. After the febrile heat, during the sweat on the back and forehead, thirst. [*Wr.*]

Fever with anorexia. [FISCHER, 1 c.]

In the evening, an hour after the heat, thirst and hunger, then, after eating, there ensued coldness and rumbling in the abdomen. [*Fz.*]

Heat of the body and redness and heat of face, for three hours, with great hunger ; the lips burn when he brings them together ; in the skin about the lips, also, there is burning shooting pain (afternoon). [*Fz.*]

Heat of the whole body (in the afternoon from 5 to 7 o'clock), which on walking in the open air increases, and sweat breaks out on the forehead, with great hunger preceding and lasting into the commencement of the heat, returning also after the fever ; when walking he feels in the abdomen as if hot water ran down it (heat running all over the abdomen and down the thighs), with red cheeks, without thirst (aft. 12 h.). [*Fz.*]

1055. Warmth in the face and redness of the cheeks, with dry, sticky lips, without thirst, in the afternoon about 3 o'clock. [*Fz.*]

Heat on the whole body with swollen blood-vessels on the arms and hands, without perspiration and without thirst (aft. 4½ h.). [*Htn.*]

Irregular, acute fever, with profuse sweat. [STAHL, l. c.]

He perspires incessantly at night, even under light bed-clothes.

On covering himself up with the bed-clothes he immediately sweats

---

1 Effects of china in agues.

profusely all over ; disagreeable as this is to him, he is at the same time so drowsy that he cannot collect himself nor get up.

1060. Sweat during sleep.

Sweat during sleep in the morning.

Greasy sweat in the morning.

In the morning, as soon as he gets up, sweat came on his face.

After awaking (about 3 a. m.), sweat of the body with thirst, but no sweat on the feet, and on the head only where the cheek lies on the pillow.

1065. Profuse sweat. [MORTON, l. c.]

Debilitating sweat at the end of the febrile heat. [SCHLEGEL, l. c.]

General profuse sweat. [ALPINI, l. c.]

In the morning, after the night sweat, the skin is not sensitive to the open air, nor apt to be chilled ; he can throw off the clothes without injury.

Profuse sweat all over the body when walking in the open air.

1070. Cold sweat on the face with thirst.

Cold sweat all over the body (aft. $\frac{1}{2}$ h.).

The whole body is very warm, especially the face and chest (aft. $\frac{1}{2}$ h.). [*Hrr.*]

Heat through the whole body, internally and externally, as from drinking wine, with redness of the face. [*Wth.*]

Heat all over, and fine needle-pricks in the skin of the whole body, particularly on the neck, at the same time great thirst for cold water (aft. 22 h.). [*Hrr.*]

1075. **Over the whole body a transient feeling of heat and actual heat, and on some parts of the skin fine weak needle-pricks, with thirst for cold water** (aft. 1 h.). [*Hrr.*]

Great thirst for cold water, and yet chilliness and heat, especially in the morning immediately after waking. [*Hrr.*]

More thirst every morning than after noon. [*Hrr.*]

Towards evening some heat, quite without chilliness, with quicker pulse (aft. 12 h.). [*Bch.*]

Quick irregular pulse-beats (aft. 6 h.). [*Bch.*]

1080. Pulse much slower and weaker (in the first h.).* [DE KOKER, l. c.]

Slow weak pulse (aft. $1\frac{1}{2}$ h.). [*Htn.*]

Slow weaker pulse, which gradually becomes quicker and stronger (aft. $\frac{1}{2}$ h.). [*Htn.*]

The febrile attack commences with sneezing.

(Fever returning earlier†.) [SCHLEGEL, l. c.]

1085. (Decrease of the febrile chill, and increase of the febrile heat.) [SCHLEGEL, l. c.]

(Increased febrile heat.)† [FISCHER, l. c.]

(Talking nonsense during the febrile heat. [SCHLEGEL, l. c.]

(Talking nonsense.)† [CLEGHORN, l. c.]

(Delirium.)† [GESNER, l. c.]

* From a half-ounce dose.

† From its employment in agues.

1090. Anxiety, anguish. [CLEGHORN,—QUARIN,—ROSCHIN, l. c.]
Extraordinary anguish. [STAHL, l. c.]
Great anxiety—death.* [DE KOKER, l. c.]
Intolerable anxiety (about 8 p.m. and 2 a.m.); he jumps out of bed and wants to make away with himself, and yet he fears to go near an open window or to approach a knife—with corporeal heat, without thirst.
Quite besides himself, and in despair he tosses about in bed.†

1095. **Too anxious caution.**
An over-anxious concern about trifles (aft. 1½ h.).
Dejection. [GESNER, l. c.]
Gloominess, hopelessness.‡ [*Gss.*]
Inconsolableness.§

1100. **Discouragement.** [*An.*]
Want of the (usual) cherful humour; he prefers to be alone. [*Htn.*]
Piteous, subdued whining and crying out.
She falls from time to time into a lachrymose humour, without external cause, from some self-made, trivial whim, *e.g.* from some imaginary want, such as that she cannot eat enough, &c. (aft. 20 h.)
In the midst of cheerful humour, sudden, short-lasting crying out and tossing about, without visible or appreciable cause.

1105. What formerly appeared to him in a bright genial light, seems now to be lustreless, unworthy, and shallow. [*Stf.*]
Morose, disposed to quarrel.‖ [*Trn.*]
He is cross, angry, and easily moved to anger¶ (aft. 4 h.).
Ill-humour, going on to the most violent anger, so that he could have stabbed some one.
Cross when cause is given, otherwise stupid, perplexed, embarrassed.

1110. Extremely disposed to be vexed, and to take every occasion to get cross; afterwards quarrelsome and disposed to vex others, and to make reproaches and give annoyance to others (aft. 2 h.).
He is inwardly very cross. [*An.*]
Discontented and sensitive, disposed to quarrel. [*Wth.*]
Discontented; he thinks himself unfortunate, and fancies he is opposed and tormented by everybody (aft. 5 h.).
Disobedience.

1115. Indisposed to think, alternately gay and gloomy for three hours (aft. 2 h.). [*Wth.*]
Distaste for mental and serious occupations. [*Bch.*]
No desire for work; he is idle.
Serious humour. [*Htg.*]

* From cinchona-bark taken during the chill of ague.
† Comp. with 1091, 1092.
‡ 1098, 1100, see 1094.
§ Comp. with 1098, 1100.
‖ 1106, 1112, see 1107, 1108, 1110.
¶ 1107, 1108, 1110, comp. with 1106, 1112.

Humour gloomy, no wish to live.

1120. Contempt for everything* (aft. 1 h.).
Indifference to all external impressions, and disinclination to speak.† [*Bch.*]
Tranquillity of mind.‡ [*Lr.*]
Ill-humour, but neither sad nor quarrelsome, yet not at all disposed for rapid thinking.§
Quiet ill-humour, and not disposed to speak (the first day). [*Hrr.*]

1125. Complaining ill-humour.
Sighing ill-humour.‖
Ill-humoured, laconic, disposed to reverie. [*Stf.*]
He is silent and will not answer.
Obstinate silence ; he will not answer at all.

1130. Caresses increase his ill-humour.
Ill-humoured irresolution ; she can never come to the point, and is disobliging at the same time.
Dislike to mental work and drowsiness. [*Hrr.*]
Dislike to bodily and mental exertion. [*An.*]
Liking for work, reading, writing, and thinking ; particularly well-disposed and industrious.¶

1135. He makes a number of grand plans for the future.** [*Htn.*]
He makes many plans, and thinks over their accomplishment ; many ideas force themselves upon him at once. [*Hrr.*]
He has many ideas, undertakes to carry out all sorts of things, builds castles in the air (aft. some h.). [*Wth.*]
He has a number of plans in his head which he greatly desires to carry into execution, in the evening. [*Gss.*]
A quantity of scheming ideas.††

1140. **Slow flow of ideas.**
Periodical cessation of thoughts. [*Lhm.*]
He is lost in thought (as if the flow of ideas stood still) (aft. 3 h.).
He cannot keep his ideas in order, and commits mistakes in writing and speaking, inasmuch as he puts words first that should come afterwards ; the talking of others distracts him much (aft. 2 h.).

* Comp. with 1121.
† See 1120.
‡ Curative action, apparently.
§ Comp. with 1115, 1116, 1132, 1140, to 1142.
‖ 1126, 1128, 1129, comp. with 1124, 1127.
¶ Curative action.
** 1135 to 1138, see 1139, 1143.
†† 1139, 1143, together with 1135 to 1138 are alternating actions with 7, 1140, 1141 and 1142.

CICUTA VIROSA.[1]

(Long-leaved Water Hemlock.)

(The freshly expressed juice from the root gathered when the plant is commencing to flower, mixed with equal parts of alcohol.

The following symptoms can only be regarded as a commencement of a thorough proving of the peculiar effects of this powerful plant in altering the human health.

Further and more complete provings will show that it is useful in rare cases where no other remedy is homœopathically suited, and particularly in chronic cases, for I have seen its effects last for three weeks, even when given in small doses.

Traditional medicine has never made any internal use of cicuta virosa; for when cicuta was prescribed, as it was very often some years ago, it was actually conium maculatum that was meant by that name.

The juice of cicuta was used only for external application in preparing the cicuta plaster on LINNÆUS's recommendation, particularly by the *Danish Pharmacopœia* (Empl. de cicuta, *Pharm. Dan.*). It was applied for the purpose of allaying gouty pains.

The juice of the fresh root (for it has little action when dried) is so powerful that ordinary practitioners did not dare* to give it internally in their accustomed big doses, and consequently had to do without it and its curative power altogether.

Homœopathy alone knows how to employ with advantage this powerfully remedial juice in the decillion-fold dilution (30th dilution).

[In this proving HAHNEMANN had the assistance of his son FRIEDRICH HAHNEMANN, HORNBURG, and LANGHAMMER.

The only authorities of traditional medicine quoted are :

ALLEN, *Synopsis.*

Bresl. samml., 1727.

WEPFER, *De cicuta aquat.*

The number of symptoms is the same in both Editions.]

CICUTA VIROSA.

In the morning after rising from bed, confusion of the head.

Stupid and dazed (after 10 m.). [*Fr. H—n.*]

Stupid in the head, with rigor; at the same time the neck felt stiff and the muscles too short. [*Fr. H—n.*]

* "Nec ulli auctor essem, ut interno usui dicaret," says MURRAY (*Apparat. Medicam.*, tom. i, 2nd edit., p. 402).

1 From vol. vi, 2nd edit., 1826.

Absence of thought, difficulty of recollecting himself, deprivation of the senses. [WEPFER, *De cicuta aquat.*,[1] and ALLEN *Synopsis.*[2]]

5. Intoxication, staggering. [WEPFER, l. c.]

When walking, vertigo, as though he would fall forward to the left (aft. 72 h.). [*Lr.*]

On stooping he feels as if he would fall head-foremost (aft. 80 h.). [*Lr.*]

Vertigo, staggering.[3] [WEPFER, l. c.]

Staggering and swaying when walking (aft. 82 h.). [*Lr.*]

10. When sitting, standing, and walking, he is as if intoxicated (aft. 5 m.). [*Fr. H—n.*]

All objects appear to him to move round in a circle, especially when he is seated—for many hours (aft. 2 h.). [*Fr. H—n.*]

Objects seem to him to move hither and thither, from one side to the other, although they all retain their right shape (aft. 10 m.). [*Fr. H—n.*]

She thinks she must place or seat herself more firmly, because she sees nothing steady or firm about her, and she consequently thinks that she herself is unsteady; everything dazzles her (aft. 15 m.). [*Fr. H—n.*]

She imagines she is swaying to one side or another, or that the objects around her are moving to and fro; it seems to her that nothing is standing still, but that everything swings backwards and forwards like a pendulum. [*Fr. H—n.*]

15. When she has to stand still, she wishes she could lay hold of something, because the objects seem at one time to come near her and then again to recede from her. [*Fr. H—n.*]

Staggering, so that she thinks she must fall (aft. 6 h.). [*Fr. H—n.*]

Vertigo; he fell to the ground. [WEPFER, and ALLEN, l. c.]

He is always inclined to fall to the ground. [WEPFER, l. c.]

He fell to the ground without saying a word. [WEPFER, l. c.]

20. He falls to the ground and rolls about. [WEPFER, l. c.]

A hammering pain in the forehead, from noon till evening (aft. 2 h.). [*Fr. H—n.*]

Anxiety in the head. [*Fr. H—n.*]

Stupefied and heavy in the head (aft. 74 h.). [*Lr.*]

Heaviness in the head when sitting. [*Hbg.*]

25. In the morning on waking, headache, just as if the brain were loose and shook when walking; when he set himself to think what sort of pain it was exactly, it was gone.

Headache pressing together from both sides. [*Hbg.*]

Aching in the left frontal bone. [*Hbg.*]

---

1 Two boys and six girls are largely of it. (Quite half of the symptoms referred by Hahnemann to this authority are not to be found, after the most diligent search, in his pages.)

2 Poisoning of four children.

3 Not found.

Pressive, stupefying headache externally on the forehead, more when at rest (aft. 1, 36 h.). [*Lr.*]

Semilateral headache, like an aching more externally.

30. Severe headache in the occiput like dull pressure, accompanied by some coryza (aft. 48 h.).

(After sickness in the abdomen, violent headache lasting two days; shooting, which extended from the nose and right eye to the occiput) (aft. 15 d.).

(After the headache, dazedness for two days.)

The headache went off on sitting upright.

The headache is relieved by discharge of flatus.

35. Creeping in the forehead as from ants (aft. 2 m.) [*Fr. H—n.*]

Shooting pain in the frontal bone. [*Hbg.*]

Stitches extending along the eyebrow (aft. 12 h.). [*Lr.*]

Great eruption on the hairy scalp and face. [*Fr. H—n.*]

Exanthematous elevations, the size of a lentil, all over the face (and on both hands), which caused a burning pain when they first appeared, then became confluent, of a dark red colour, lasting nine days, when desquamation ensued, which lasted three weeks.* [*Fr. H—n.*]

40. Redness of the face.[1] [WEPFER, l. c.]

Face (and neck) swollen.[2] [WEPFER, l. c.]

Eyes protruded from the head[2] [WEPFER, l. c.]

Staring look.[2] [WEPFFR, l. c.]

He keeps staring at one and the same spot, whereby everything appears to him like black stuff (aft. 6 h.). [*Fr. H—n.*]

45. Staring (aft. ¼ h.); she looks fixedly at one and the same place, and cannot help doing so, much as she would like to; at the same time she has not full command of her senses, and must be very strongly excited in order to answer correctly; if she compels herself forcibly, by turning away her head, to cease having her eyes directed on the object, she loses consciousness, and all becomes dark before her eyes. [*Fr. H—n.*]

Even though she keeps her look steadily fixed on an object, she sees nothing distinctly; everything runs together, as when one has looked too long on one and the same object, when the sight becomes blurred. [*Fr. H—n.*]

If she looks long at the same spot, she grows sleepy, and she feels as if the head were pressed down, though nothing of the sort is noticed, and she then, her eyes being open and staring, is unable to tell the letters of a book. [*Fr. H—n.*]

As often as she is spoken to, and thereby forced out of her unconscious staring, and wakened up by shouting to her, so often does

* I have cured chronic, suppurating, confluent eruptions in the face having only burning pain by means of one or two doses of a small part of a drop of the juice, but I did not venture to give the second dose in less than three to four weeks; when the first dose did not suffice.

1. With S. 206.
2. Not found.

she always relapse again into it, and in this state her pulse is only 50 in the minute. [*Fr. H—n.*]

If she is allowed to sit still for a considerable time her head sinks down gradually, whilst the eyes continue to stare at the same point, so that as thus the head sinks very low, the pupils become almost hidden under the upper eyelids; she then gets an inward shock, which brings her quickly to her senses for a short time; she then falls again into a similar state of unconsciousness, out of which she is from time to time awakened by an internal shivering, which she says is a febrile rigor. [*Fr. H—n.*]

50. Sometimes everything appeared double and of a black colour, sometimes she was affected with dulness of hearing. [*Fr. H—n.*]

First (aft. 2½ h.) **contracted, then** (aft. 8, 9 h.) **very dilated, pupils** [*Lr.*]

At first extremely contracted, soon afterwards extremely dilated, pupils. [*Hbg.*]

Aching in the inner canthus of the right eye, so that he must shut and press to the eyes in order to get relief. [*Hbg.*]

A quivering under the lower eyelid in the orbicularis muscle.

55. Heat and burning round about the eyes.

Sore pain behind the left ear. [*Hbg.*]

Sore sensation behind the left ear, as after a knock or blow. [*Hbg.*]

Pain behind the right ear, such as would remain after a knock or blow. [*Hbg.*]

Great eruption on the ears. [*Fr. H—n.*]

60. Exanthematous pimples below and in front of the ears, their apices filled with pus and painful like a boil. [*Fr. H—n.*]

When swallowing something bursts in the right ear. [*Fr. H—n.*]

Roaring before both ears, worse in the room than in the open air. [*Fr. H—n.*]

Loud ringing in the left ear. [*Hbg.*]

She does not hear well unless one speaks loudly in her ear and attracts her attention. [*Fr. H—n.*]

65. Discharge of blood from the ears. [WEPFER, l. c.]

Yellow discharge from the nose.

The right ala nasi is painful as if excoriated, as from a knock or blow. [*Hbg.*]

A burning itching vesicle on the left side of the upper lip at the edge of the red. [*Hbg.*]

A kind of cramp in the cervical muscles: when he looks round, he cannot immediately turn the head back again; the cervical muscles do not yield, and if he should effect his object by force it would give him great pain.

70. Tension in the cervical muscles. [*Hbg.*]

On bending the head backwards a sore tension in the left cervical muscles. [*Hbg.*]

Drawing pains in the left side of the neck (aft. 6 h.). [*Hbg.*]

Swollen neck.[1] [WEPFER, l. c.]

---

1 Not found.

Bending back of the head (a kind of opisthotonos). [WEPFER, l. c.]

75. Twitching and jerking of the head. [*Fr. H—n.*]

Lock-jaw. [WEPFER,—ALLEN, l. c.]

Teeth firmly closed, lock-jaw. [WEPFER, l. c.]

Grinding of teeth. [WEPFER, l. c.]

Mouth full of foam.[1] [WEPFER, l. c.]

80. Foam before the mouth.[2] [WEPFER, l. c.]

Toothache in the nerves of the lower row of teeth. [*Hbg.*]

A whitish sore place on the border of the tongue, very painful when touched. [*Fr. H—n.*]

On speaking several words he can bring out the first five or six words without hindrance, but with the remainder, in pronouncing the words he gets a small jerk backwards of the head observable by others, and at the same time the arms twitch somewhat, so that he must, as it were, draw back and swallow the syllable about to be spoken, almost like what frequently occurs in hiccup. [*Fr. H—n.*]

Dumbness. [ALLEN, l. c.]

85. **Inability to swallow.** [WEPFER, l. c.]

The throat appears to be grown together internally, and externally it pains as if bruised on being moved or grasped, getting worse for several hours, with eructation from noon till evening. [*Fr. H—n.*]

Dry feeling in the mouth. [*Fr. H—n.*]

Constant hunger and desire for food, even when he has just been eating. [*Fr. H—n.*]

Great thirst (during the convulsions).[2] [WEPFER, l. c.]

90. He had a great longing for coals and swallowed them.[2] [WEPFER, l. c.]

Hiccup [WEPFER, l. c., and *Breslauer Samml.*, 1727, p. 313,[3] and *Hbg.*]

Loud hiccup.[2] [WEPFER, l. c.]

When she was stooping (in the open air) a very bitter yellow fluid was belched up, as by eructation, from the stomach into the mouth, and thereafter she had burning in the œsophagus all the forenoon. [*Fr. H—n.*]

A sensation up from the stomach like water-brash ; he felt qualmish and hot all over, and a quantity of saliva that had risen up from his stomach flowed out of his mouth (aft. 9 to 13 h.). [*Lr.*]

95. Nausea (aft. ½ h.). [*Hbg.*]

Nausea while eating. [*Fr. H—n.*]

In the morning nausea, with shooting tearing headache. [*Fr. H—n.*]

Nausea and shooting in the forehead, all day. [*Fr. H—n.*]

Vomiting. [ALLEN, l. c.]

100. Vomiting without relaxation of the lock-jaw. [WEPFER, l. c.]

Want of appetite on account of dry feeling in the mouth ; food has no wrong taste, but not its full flavour.

At noon, appetite for food, but the appetite went away at the first mouthful.

---

1 Post mortem. 2 Not found.

3 Poisoning of three children by root.

Breakfast is not relished; he felt a stuffy sensation in the abdomen, as if he had already eaten too much.

Immediately after eating cutting in the hypogastrium.

105. Immediately after eating an aching in the scrobiculus cordis, which compels him to draw a deep breath, at the same time tendency to eructation.

Immediately after eating bellyache and drowsiness.

In the morning sick feeling in the abdomen and when this passed off, in the afternoon, headache, a shooting on the right side of the head, which extended from the right eye and the nose—in both of which it was at its worst—to the occiput, for three days, whereon the nose became unstopped, and yellow mucus was discharged (aft. 9 d.).

Vomiting of blood. [*Breslauer Samml.*, l. c.]

Burning scraping sensation from the inside of the throat to the gastric region. [*Hbg.*]

110. **Burning pressure in the stomach.** [*Hbg.*]

Scraping scratching sensation in the stomach. [*Hbg.*]

Tightness in the scrobiculus cordis and anxiety, for eight days, he wishes always to go out in order to cool himself.

A blow in the region of the scrobiculus cordis as with a finger which makes him start, and then only he collects himself and comes to his senses. [*Fr. H—n.*]

Throbbing in the scrobiculus cordis, which is swollen as large as a fist. [Wepeer, l. c.]

115. Great throbbing in the scrobiculus cordis. [Wepfer, l. c.]

Shooting[1] pain in the scrobiculus cordis. [Wepfer, l. c.]

Anxiety about the scrobiculus cordis.[2] [Wepfer, l. c.]

Heat in the abdomen (and chest). [*Hbg.*]

Great accumulation of flatulence, with constant anxiety and crossness.

120. Grumbling and rumbling in the abdomen. [*Hbg.*]

Much flatus is discharged. [*Hbg.*]

Constipation. [Wepfer, l. c.]

Diarrhœa. [Allen, l. c.]

In the right groin a sensation as if an ulcer would break out (while sitting). [*Hbg.*]

125. Itching internally in the rectum, just above the anus; after rubbing there is burning pain, a pain that caused a shudder through him every time it came—after walking, when standing still, and when at stool.

Retention of urine.[3] [Wepfer, l. c.]

At night difficulty of urinating.[2] [Wepfer, l. c.]

Involuntary discharge of urine.[2] [Wepfer, l. c.]

Frequent call to urinate. [*Lr.*]

130. Very frequent urination. [*Fr. H—n.*]

Violent ejection of the urine. [Wepfer, l. c.]

---

1 The author adds "and burning."

2 Not found.

3 With S. 122.

Sore drawing pain under the penis as far as the glans, which compels him to urinate (aft. 12 h.). [*Hbg.*]

Three emissions of semen in the night. [*Hbg.*]

Emission of semen, without voluptuous dreams. [*Lr.*]

135. The menses come later. [*Fr. H—n.*]

* * *

Stoppage of the nose, and at the same time copious secretion of mucus from it.

Very frequent sneezing, without coryza (aft. 29 h.). [*Lr.*]

Aching under the larynx when sitting (aft. 4 h.). [*Hbg.*]

Sensation in the chest and in the throat, as if something that pressed asunder were sticking there, as big as a fist, which hindered respiration, and felt as if it would burst the throat—worse when sitting than when walking. [*Fr. H—n.*]

140. Tightness on the chest, so that she can hardly draw her breath all day long (immediately). [*Fr. H—n.*]

Want of breath all day long (immediately). [*Fr. H—n.*]

On inspiring and expiring some needle-pricks under the last false ribs of the left side, which went off when standing and walking (aft. 3 h.) [*Lr.*]

Hoarseness[1] [WEPFER, l. c.]

Cough, with much expectoration, especially by day. [*Fr. H—n.*]

145. Burning round the nipple (aft. 3 h.). [*Fr. H—n.*]

Itching combined with sensation of heat in the right side of the chest. [*Hbg.*]

Heat in chest (and abdomen). [*Hbg.*]

At the inferior entremity of the sternum an ache, as after a blow, and as if excoriated, when walking. [*Hbg.*]

General heat, and particularly **heat in the chest**, for three quarters of an hour, increased by (accustomed) tobacco-smoking. [*Hbg.*]

150. A tugging at the chest near the scrobiculus cordis (aft. 1 h.). [*Hbg.*]

Tearing twitching in the coccyx. [*Hbg.*]

A blow in the dorsal vertebræ. [*Hbg.*]

Tetanus, bending the back backwards (opisthotonos). [WEPFER, l. c.]

Back bent like a bow. [WEPFER, l. c.]

155. Painful tension above the right scapula. [*Hbg.*]

Painful sensation on the inner surface of the scapulæ. [*Hbg.*]

Sensation as if there were an ulcer on the right scapula. [*Hbg.*]

A red vesicle on the right scapula, that was very painful when touched. [*Hbg.*]

Sore pain, as from a blow, in the right shoulder-joint. [*Hbg.*]

160. Painful sensation under the right arm. [*Hbg.*]

Twitching in the left shoulder (aft. 20 m.). [*Fr. H—n.*]

Sensation of cracking in the shoulder-joint, which is not audible. [*Fr. H—n.*]

---

1. Not found.

Tearing pain in the whole of the left arm aown to the fingers. [*Fr. H—n.*]

On raising it the arm feels very heavy, and at the same time there are such violent shoots in the shoulder that she cannot bring the arm on to the head without screaming loudly ; she dare not even move the fingers. [*Fr. H—n.*]

165. Sensation in the left arm as if he had no power in it, with a shooting tearing pain on raising it. [*Fr. H—n.*]

Powerlessness of the whole arm and fingers. [*Hbg.*]

Twitching in the left arm, so that the whole body is jerked (aft. 4 m.). [*Fr. H—n.*]

Frequent involuntary twitching and jerking in the arms and fingers (lower extremities and head). [*Fr. H—n.*]

(On the inside of the left elbow-joint, a swelling, as if a boil would come there ; on raising the arm it was painful there, as when one presses on an ulcer.)

170. Stitch-like tearing in the muscles of the right forearm when writing, which went off when the body was perfectly inactive (aft. $1\frac{1}{4}$ h.). [*Lr.*]

Sore pain, as from a knock or blow, in the left forearm. [*Hbg.*]

Distended blood-vessels on the hands. [*Hbg.*]

Feeling of cracking in the wrist, which is not audible. [*Fr. H—n.*]

Exanthematous elevations, the size of a lentil, on both hands, even on the balls of the thumbs, which on their appearance cause a burning pain ; they then become confluent, of a dark colour, and last nine days. [*Fr. H—n.*]

175. Twitching together of several fingers and of the thumb of the right hand. [*Fr. H—n.*]

Dying away (gone-to-sleep feeling, numbness, coldness) of the fingers. [*Fr. H—n.*]

In the right pelvic region, on the border of the os-ilii, a kind of sore, drawing, pulsating pain, as after a violent blow. [*Hbg.*]

Burning shooting in the left hip-bone. [*Hbg.*]

Frequent involuntary twitching of the lower extremities. [*Fr. H—n.*]

180. Painful tense and stiff feeling in the muscles of the lower extremities, so that he cannot walk at all, for three hours (aft. 1 h.). [*Fr. H—n.*]

Tearing pain in the thighs and heaviness of them when walking. [*Fr. H—n.*]

Pain, like tearing in the thighs, immediately after rising from a seat, and pain, as if bruised, in the knees ; on walking the pain in the thighs increases, like a deep-seated stiffness. [*Fr. H—n.*]

Burning itching on the right thigh, so that he must scratch, whereupon it went off. [*Hbg.*]

Creeping close beneath the skin of the thighs and legs, and especially of the soles of the feet, as if the limbs would go to sleep, only when sitting. [*Fr. H—n.*]

185. Perceptible trembling of one thigh. [*Fr. H—n.*]

Very violent trembling of the left leg. [*Fr. H—n.*]

When walking she does not tread properly on the soles of the feet; they tip over towards the inside. [*Fr. H—n.*]

Tearing round the ankles of the left foot. [*Hbg.*]

Frequent needle-pricks in the heel, when sitting. [*Hbg.*]

190. Tingling and "pins and needles" in the left sole. [*Hbg.*]

Drawing twitching pains in the toes. [*Hbg.*]

Trembling in the upper and lower extremities. [*Hbg.*]

Burning itching all over.

Itching all over the body, so that he must scratch. [*Fr. H—n.*]

195. Spasmodic stiffness of all the body, with coldness thereof. [*Bresl. Samml.*, 1727, p. 314.]

(About noon, anxiety, perspiration in the face, and trembling of the hands; about his heart [in the middle of the chest] he feels as though he would faint.)

Whilst lying in bed a peculiar sensation, as if his whole body were swollen, and at the same time (while awake) frequent starting, as though he were falling out of bed (aft. 15 h.). [*Lr.*]

Catalepsy; the limbs hang down loosely, as in a corpse, without breathing.[1] [WEPFER, l. c.]

The most violent (tonic) spasms, so that neither can the flexed fingers be stretched out, nor the limbs be either flexed or extended.[1] [WEPFER, l. c.]

200. Tossing of the limbs to and fro. [WEPFER, l. c.]

He threw the limbs now on one side now on the other. [WEPFER, l. c.]

Epileptic convulsions in three children, one of whom recovered. [*Breslauer Samml.*, l. c., p. 313.]

Spasmodic distortions of the limbs which threw him a distance of two feet.[1] [WEPFER, l. c.]

General convulsious. [WEPFER, l. c.]

205. Very violent convulsions. [WEPFER,—ALLEN, l. c.]

Epilepsy. [WEPFER,—ALLEN, l. c.]

Frightful **epilepsy**, recurring first at shorter, then at longer intervals, the limbs, head, and upper part of the body are moved in a wonderful manner, with closed jaws. [WEPFER, l. c.]

Epileptic fits with wonderful distortions of the limbs, upper part of the body, and head, with bluish complexion, and, for some instants, interrupted respiration, with foam before the mouth; and after the convulsions, when the breathing was free, he was unconscious and lay as if dead, gave no sign of sensation when called to or pinched.*[1] [WEPFER, l. c.]

She lies like a corpse, with closed jaws. [WEPFER, l. c.]

* In a young man of twenty, whose death took place in two hours, the body remained warm for a whole day without any blue discoloration or swelling; the limbs were stiff, the lungs full of blue and yellow spots, the blood red and fluid, the heart empty of blood, the œsophagus internally bluish and dry.

---

1 Not found.

210. Immobility.[1] [WEPEER, l. c.]

They all lay prostrated with weakness, without consciousness and immovable, like blocks or corpses.[1] [WEPFER, l. c.]

Frequent yawning. [*Hbg.*]

Frequent yawning, as if he had not slept enough (aft. $1\frac{3}{4}$ h.). [*Lr.*]

Drowsiness, so that his eyes always closed. [*Hbg.*]

215. **At night, vivid dreams about events that had occurred during the day.**

Vivid but unremembered dreams. [*Lr.*]

Many confused dreams with much restlessness. [*Hbg.*]

Sleeplessness, all night (immediately). [*Fr. H—n.*]

Sleeplessness ; he woke up every quarter of an hour with a painful feeling of weight in the head. [*Fr. H—n.*]

220. Every morning he has not slept enough, is not satiated with sleep. [*Fr. H—n.*]

Frequent waking up out of sleep, in which he perspired all over, but from which he felt strengthened. [*Lr.*]

They all wish to come near the warm stove.[1] [WEPFER, l. c.]

She has a feeling of coldness running down her thighs, then coldness in the arms—the coldness seems to come chiefly out of the chest—then comes on a greater inclination to stare fixedly at one point. [*Fr. H—n.*]

Uncommonly strong heat in all parts of the body from beginning to end of the action of the drug. [*Hbg.*]

225. Perspiration on the abdomen at night.

He became indifferent to everything, and began to doubt whether this was really the condition in which he was.

He confounded the present with the past.

He thought with anxiety of the future and was always sad.

Anxiety ; he was violently affected by sad stories.[1] [WEPFER, l. c.]

230. **Moaning, whining and howling.** [WEPFER,—ALLEN, l. c.]

Excitement, with concern for the future, he represented to himself as dangerous everything that would happen to him.

When others were gay he was sad.

Sadness for several days.[1] [WEPFER, l. c.]

Great liability to be startled ; every time a door is opened, or a word spoken, even not loudly, he starts and feels stitches in the (left) side of the head. [*Fr. H—n.*]

235. He did not think he was living in the ordinary conditions ; everything appeared to him strange and almost frightful ; it was as if he woke up out of an acute fever and saw all sorts of figures, and yet he did not feel corporeally ill.

Mania ; after unusual sleep, heat of the body ; she leapt out of

---

1 Not found.

bed, danced, laughed, and did all sorts of foolish things, drank a great deal of wine, jumped about constantly, clapped her hands, and at the same time was very red in the face—all night long. [*Bresl. Samml.*, l. c, p.[1] 58.]

Depreciation and contempt of mankind ; he fled from his fellow-creatures, was in the highest degree disgusted with their follies, and his disposition seemed to change into misanthropy ; he withdrew into solitude. [*Lr.*]

Want of trust in people and anthrophoby ; he fled from them, remained solitary, and thought seriously about their errors and about himself. [*Lr.*]

Suspicious.

240. He felt like a child of seven or eight years old, objects were very dear and attractive to him, as toys are to a child.

Tranquillity of mind ; he was extremely satisfied with his position and with himself, and very cheerful.* [*Lr.*]

* Curative secondary action.

---

1 In an adult woman.

CINA.[1]

(*Semen cinæ, Semen santonici, contra.*)

(The tincture obtained by macerating, for a week, without heat, one part of the unpowdered buds with twenty parts of spirits of wine ; twenty drops of this represent one grain of the drug.)

Even the best generally consists only of small oblong, light yellowish-green buds, mixed with a few stalks, from a shrub-like plant, *Artemisia contra.* The finest comes to us from Aleppo. It has also been improperly called zedoary seed, Semen zedoariæ, merely because its odour has a great resemblance to that of the zedoary root.

For centuries no other use has been made of this very important vegetable substance, except for the expulsion of lumbrici in children, in doses of 10, 20, 30, 60, and more grains. I pass over the not unfrequently dangerous, or even fatal, effects of such doses, nor will I dwell on the fact that a few lumbrici are not to be considered as an important disease in otherwise healthy children, and are common in childhood (where psora is still latent), and generally unattended by morbid symptoms. On the other hand, this much is true, that when they are present in large numbers, the cause of this is always some morbid condition of the body, namely, the evolution of psora, and unless this be cured, though large numbers of the lumbrici may be expelled by cina, they are soon reproduced. Hence, by such forcible expulsion of the worms not only is nothing gained, but such improper treatment, if persisted in, often ends in the death of the tortured children.

This vegetable substance has much more valuable curative properties, which may be easily inferred from the subjoined characteristic morbid symptoms produced by it in the healthy.

Experience of what it can do, for instance, in whooping-cough, and in certain intermittent fevers accompanied by vomiting and ravenous hunger will excite astonishment. I will not dwell on the other morbid states for which it is adapted, as the initiated homœopathic physician will be able to discover these by himself.

Formerly I used to employ the tincture potentised to the trillion-fold dilution, but I have found that when raised to the decillion-fold development of potency, it displays its medicinal powers still more perfectly. One, tow, or three smallest globules moistened with this serve for a dose.

[In this proving HAHNEMANN was assisted by AHNER, GROSS, LANGHAMMER, RUCKERT, jun., STAPF.

---

1 From vol. i, 3rd edit., 1830.

The medical writers quoted are :
ANDRY, *De Generations Vermium.*
BERGIUS, *Mat. Med.*
PELARGUS, *Observ.*, tom. i, ii.
In the 1st edition of the *R.A.M.L.* cina had 48 symptoms, in the 2nd edition 287, the 3rd, as we see, has 301.]

CINA.

On rising from bed blackness before the eyes, dizziness in the head, faintness ; he staggers to and fro ; on lying down he is immediately better.

Violent headache. [PELARGUS,[1] *Observat.*, tom. i, pp. 8. 31, 275.]

Headache, with a feeling of general discomfort. [*L. Rkt.*]

On the middle of the vertex intermittent pressure, as from a heavy weight, as if the brain were pressed down ; pressing upon it increases and renews the pain. [*Gss.*]

5. A pain, pressing from above downwards, externally on the forehead, as if a weight gradually sank down there (aft. ¾ h.). [*Lr.*]

All day long some headache, a tearing aching, spreading even into the zygoma.

Aching pain in the head all day, in the evening also in the forehead. [*L. Rkt.*]

When walking in the open air stupefying, internal headache, especially in the sinciput, afterwards also in the occiput (aft. 3 h.). [*Lr.*]

On waking from sleep an out-pressing pain in the right parietal bone, and the right side of the forehead.

10. (While sitting) pressive stupefying pain externally on the forehead and temples, which at length involved the whole head (aft. 36 h.). [*Lr.*]

Pressure on the frontal bone, and at the same time internally a fluctation like the beating of waves. [*Gss.*]

Headache, as if the whole head were screwed in, with numbness. [*Gss.*]

Pain, as if the upper part of the frontal bone were strongly pressed together from both sides. [*Gss.*]

Immediately after a meal and later, a dull drawing pain in the interior of the head, increased by reading and mental work [*L. Rkt.*]

15. The headache is increased by reading and thinking, relieved by stooping. [*Gss.*]

Cramp-like drawing in the temples, increased by pressing on them. [*Gss.*]

Stretching tearing pain in the right temple. [*L. Rkt.*]

On the left side of the sinciput drawing aching. [*Gss.*]

---

1 Observation of effects of over-dosing. The symptom occurred in a child, with S. 242 and 291.

Aching pain, like fine tearing, in the temporal region, that went off on moving the head (aft. 11 h.). [*Lr.*]

20 Confusing drawing from the left frontal protuberance towards the root of the nose. [*Gss.*]

In the left frontal protuberance a paralytic tearing with stupefaction of the head ; immediately afterwards in the right frontal protuberance. [*Gss.*]

Drawing tearing pain on the whole left side of the head. [*Ar.*]

A small spot on the right parietal bone feels numb and as if asleep. [*Gss.*]

Obtuse stitches in the brain, especially in the left side of thecrown (aft. $1\frac{1}{2}$ h.). [*L. Rkt.*]

25. In the frontal bone over the right temple severe obtuse stitches deep into the brain, which threaten to stupefy him. [*Gss.*]

When the headache goes off there occurs an aching pain in the abdomen, and when this goes off the headache returns.

Over the upper orbital border a slow obtuse stitch extending deep into the brain. [*Gss.*]

Palpitation of the muscle of the eyebrow, a kind of convulsion. [*Gss*]

Dull headache, affecting the eyes, in the morning. [*L. Rkt.*]

30. Obtuse pain in the eyes while reading, and during mental labour. [*L. Rkt.*]

Pressing ache in the interior of the eye, generally with dilatation of the pupils. [*L. Rkt.*]

Dilated pupils (aft. $\frac{1}{2}$ h.). [*Lr.*]

Contracted pupils (aft. $3\frac{1}{2}$ h.). [*Lr.*]

Great contraction of the pupils (aft. 1 h.). [*L. Rkt.*]

35. In the evening when he wishes to see accurately (read) by candle-light, he sees everything as through a veil ; on wiping the eyes he sees better for a short time. [*Gss.*]

On reading a book there comes a dimness before the eyes, so that he can only read again after rubbing the eyes strongly with the finger. [*Ar.*]

(In the morning) fatigue in the eyes ; the upper lids were so weak he could scarcely open them, lasting all the forenoon. [*Ar.*]

Burning pain in the outer canthus of the eye, mingled with itching, and on the border of the upper lid (aft. 2 h.).

(Burning in the eyelids, especially in the inner canthus, in the evening, by candle-light.) [*Gss.*]

40. In the evening, by candle-light, dryness of the eyelids and an aching feeling in them, as if sand had got into them. [*Gss.*]

Feeling of dryness in the interior of the eye, and drawing aching pain, when he only exerts the eyes a little in reading. [*L. Rkt.*]

Formication in the eyelids, so that he must rub them. [*Gss.*]

Tickling itching in the right inner canthus, compelling him to rub (aft. 1 h.). [*Lr.*]

Tickling itching on the left outer canthus, compelling him to rub (aft. 36 h.). [*Lr.*]

45. (In the morning, after rising, the inner canthi are stuck together, as with matter.) [*Gss.*]

He looks ill about the eyes and pale in the face. [*Gss.*]

On the lower border of the orbit an obtuse pressure ; by pressing on it it increases, and may be excited anew. [*Gss.*]

Pain as if both zygomatic arches were seized and compressed by pincers ; the pain is aggravated by external pressure. [*Gss.*]

Cramp-like twitching in the zygoma, a pain which, even after it is gone, can be excited anew by pressing strongly on it, only it then comes as a continued cramp-like or paralytic pain. [*Gss.*]

50. Periodical, stretching tearing pain in the zygomatic arches, going from one place to another, aggravated by pressure. [*L. Rkt.*]

In the external ear, cramp-like twitching, like ear-ache. [*Gss.*]

Under the mastoid process, obtuse shooting, like a pinching pressure ; on pressing on it, as from a blow or knock. [*Gss.*]

White and bluish round the mouth. [PELARGUS, l.c., tom. ii, p. 458.]

Puffy, bluish face. [*Stf.*]

55. The child often bores so long in his nose that blood comes from it.

On the cheek a boil, with hardness round about it.

Aching pain in the submaxillary glands.

Obtuse shooting pain in the right ramus of the lower maxilla, aggravated by pressure. [*L. Rkt.*]

Single fine pricks as with needles on the left lower maxilla, aggravated by pressing on it with the hand. [*Ar.*]

60. Twitching pain in the left side of the lower jaw. [*Ar.*]

Toothache as if from excoriation.

The inspired air and cold drinks cause pain in the tooth.

The child leans the head on one side.

Paralytic feeling in the nape. [*L. Rkt.*]

65. Boring stitches in the right cervical muscles, synchronous with the pulse, which go off on moving the neck (aft. 11 h.). [*Lr.*]

Dryness and roughness of the interior of the mouth, especially of the palate, with sick qualmishness (aft. $3\frac{1}{2}$ h.). [*Lr.*]

Cannot swallow.

Inability to swallow ; liquids roll about in the mouth for a long time. [*Stf.*]

Great hunger shortly after a meal. [*Gss.*]

70. Thirst.

In the morning when fasting, empty eructation. [*Gss.*]

After a meal, eructation with the taste of the food. [*Gss.*]

Not long after a meal, belching of a bitter-sour fluid up into the mouth. [*Gss.*]

Qualmish feeling in the scrobiculus cordis with a shudder running over him (immediately). [*Gss.*]

75. (Several lumbrici come up through the child's mouth.) [*Stf.*]

Sickness, with empty feeling in the head. [*Ar.*]

Frequent hiccup (aft. $1\frac{1}{4}$ h.). [*Lr.*]

(At night, a continued pressure in the stomach.)

Transversely across the epigastrium, in the region of the scrobiculus cordis, a pinching or cramp-like pressure, after a meal. [*Gss.*]

80. In the scrobiculus cordis, a pain that hinders respiration (aft. 4 h.). [*Lr.*]

A digging, wriggling pain in the epigastric region (scrobiculus cordis), as if bruised. [*Gss.*]

Obtuse shooting, on the left below the scrobiculus cordis, aggravated by pressure, and relieved by deep breathing. [*Gss.*]

Boring pain above the navel, going off by pressure. [*Lr.*]

Continued pinching in the abdomen. [PELARGUS, l. c., t. i.]

85. Intermitting needle-pricks in the left side of the abdomen, like colic, when sitting (aft. 10 h.). [*Lr.*]

Sudden, deep, sharp, intermitting stitches internally, on the left near the navel, especially on inspiring, and always at the same time stitches on the internal side of the scapula, towards evening (aft. 12 h.). [*L. Rkt.*]

Cutting pinching in the abdomen, that does not cease until he has been to stool (aft. 48 h.). [*Lr.*]

Violent pain in the navel and in the umbilical region, as if the navel were forcibly pressed in, or as if he had been struck there, at first for a short time, afterwards for a longer time, when it was aggravated by breathing. [*Ar.*]

About the navel a painful twisting, also pain when pressing on the navel. [*Gss.*]

90. After a meal an aching pain in the navel, also when pressing on it. [*Gss.*]

Cutting in the small intestines, in the morning. [*Gss.*]

Disagreeable warm feeling in the abdomen, that at last changed into pinching (aft. 4 h.). [*Lr.*]

Labour-like, frequently-recurring pains in the abdomen, as if the catamenia were about to come on (aft. 2 h.).

In the abdomen, immediately above the pubes, a pulsation, as if he felt the pulse beat in the interior. [*Gss.*]

95. Flatus explodes with little noise and goes quietly about in the bowels. [*Gss.*]

During discharge of flatus single stitches in the lower part of the rectum. [*Ar.*]

Feeling of emptiness in the abdomen, with silent discharge of flatus (aft 1 h.). [*Lr.*]

(A voluptuous itching on the anterior part of the anus, which compels him to scratch) (aft. 4 h.). [*Lr.*]

Frequent urging to pass water, with copious discharge of urine, all day (aft. 3 h.). [*Lr.*]

100. Turbid urine (immediately).

Urine that soon becomes turbid.

Uterine hæmorrhage as long as she (a girl of ten years) takes cina seeds. [BERGIUS,[1] *Mater. Med.*, p. 709.]

* * *

1 Observation.

In the left nostril, deep in, a not disagreeable, hot, burning sensation, as if blood would come, or as if brandy had been sniffed up. [*Gss.*]

In the left nostril on the septum narium a burning pain, as if a scab had been scratched off; aggravated by external touch. [*Gss.*]

105. Violent sneezing (aft. $\frac{1}{8}$ h.). [*L. Rkt.—Lr.*]

Sneezing so violent that it rushed into the head and pressed out at the temples; the headache pressing out through the temples remained some time afterwards. [*Gss.*]

Sneezing so violent that it seems as if it would burst the thorax on both sides; afterwards he still feels a pain, especially in the right side. [*Gss.*]

Fluent coryza (aft. $\frac{3}{4}$ h.). [*Lr.*]

A kind of coryza; in the morning he must frequently blow his nose, the nose is always full of loose mucus (aft. a few days). [*Gss.*]

110. Discharge of purulent matter from the nose.[1] [PELARGUS, l. c., t. i.]

In the evening the nose is stuffed, after having had fluent coryza in the forenoon. [*Gss.*]

Mucus in the larynx, which he expels by voluntary tussiculation and hacking cough (aft. 6 h.). [*Lr.*]

On walking in the open air short, rattling respiration, as if he had much mucus in the chest, without being obliged to cough (aft. 6 h.). [*Lr.*]

Difficult, loud breathing (aft. $\frac{1}{2}$ h.).

115. Very short, rattling respiration.

Very short breathing, sometimes with interruptions, so that some respiration are awanting.

The child is very short breathed, with loud rattling in the chest. [*Stf.*]

On inspiring a loud whistling whooping in the wind-pipe, not audible during expiration (aft. 12 h.). [*Lr.*]

In the morning after getting up, mucus adheres to the larynx, so that he must often hawk, after which, however, it is soon formed again. [*Gss.*]

120. In the morning he must always hack, and scrape, and clear the throat on account of mucus, which is constantly produced at the back of the throat and in the larynx. [*Gss.*]

In the morning great dryness at the back of the throat (trachea); a feeling of catarrh. [*Gss.*]

Inclination to cough is caused by deep breathing. [*Gss.*]

Tickling irritation to cough, rather deep in the wind-pipe, and if he does actually cough there occurs expectoration of whitish phlegm (aft. 24 h.). [*Lr.*]

Tickling irritation to cough in the region of the trachea, under the sternum, with expectoration of white mucus (aft. 16 h.). [*Lr.*]

125. Before the cough the child suddenly rises up, stares about; the whole body is somewhat stiff; she is unconscious, just as if going to have an epileptic fit, and then the cough comes.

---

1 With S. 2, 242, 291.

After the cough the child whines, Au, Au ! a gurgling-down sound is heard ; she is anxious, gasps for breath, and becomes at the same time quite pale in the face—in fits of two minutes' duration.

Attacks of violent coughing from time to time.

Hoarse hacking cough consisting of few impulses, with long pauses before the exciting irritation recurs ; in the evening. [*Gss.*]

In the morning, after rising, hoarse hacking cough, the exciting irritation to which (as if from feather dust) occurs after a long pause on inspiring. [*Gss.*]

130. In the morning, after rising, hollow cough ; violent succussions against the upper part of the wind-pipe, whereby mucus is detached, though with difficulty (after several days). [*Gss.*]

In the morning, in order to get rid of the mucus accumulated during the night, he must cough so violently that tears come into the eyes. [*Gss.*]

During the morning cough, the upper part of the chest (under the top of the sternum) is painful, and when he detaches something with difficulty this part continues to have raw and burning pain for a long time, as if something were torn away. [*Gss.*]

Squeezing on the chest during inspiration. [*Gss.*]

Tightness of the chest when standing (lasting half an hour) with anxiety, during which he perspires profusely on the chest. [*Ar.*]

135. **A kind of oppression of the chest ; the sternum seems to press on the lungs and the breathing is somewhat impeded.** [*L. Rkt.*]

In the left half of the chest, cramp-like contraction. [*Gss.*]

Pain anteriorly under the sternum only *per se.* [*Gss.*]

When running, a squeezing pain on the sternum. [*Gss.*]

Sudden oppressive pain in the left side of the chest. [*Ar.*]

140. Under the sternum cramp-like digging pain, as if the thorax would burst asunder. [*Ar.*]

On the clavicle, a fine squeezing, like the pressure of a blunt point. [*Gss.*]

An out-pressing pain sometimes in the left side of the chest, sometimes in the sacrum, the latter as from prolonged stooping, especially during expiration (aft. 4 h.). [*Lr.*]

Painful digging superiorly under the sternum. [*Gss.*]

In the left side of the chest, pinching pains, increased by every inspiration (aft. 30 h.). [*Ar.*]

145. Pinching pain in the left side of the chest, between the second and third ribs. [*Ar.*]

Pinching, shooting pain in the left side of the chest (lasting a quarter of an hour. [*Ar.*]

From time to time single stitches in the chest. [*L. Rkt.*]

Prickling burning, intermitting, fine stitches in the side, on one of the true ribs. [*Gss.*]

Obtuse stitches near the sternum on one of the costal cartilages, increased by pressing on it and by expiration, diminished by inspiration. [*Gss.*]

150. Near the sternum underneath the left clavicle on deep inspiration, two obtuse, penetrating stitches, in rapid succession ; during expiration he feels nothing, on pressing on it it is very painful. [*Gss.*]

In the right side of the chest, between the sixth and eighth ribs, twitching shooting pains, not affected by pressing or by inspiration or expiration. [*Ar.*]

Sudden twitching stitch in the left side of the chest, between the fifth and sixth ribs. [*Ar.*]

In the middle of the right side under the ribs, a boring shooting pain, that goes off on pressing thereon. [*Ar.*]

Bruised pain in the sacrum, not increased by movement (aft. 35 h.). [*Ar.*]

155. Tearing in the left hip and buttock.

Paralytic drawing in the loins. [*Gss.*]

After a meal, sensation as if the lumbar region just above the hips were constricted by a tight ligature. [*Gss.*]

In the loins, a weary pain as if he had stood long. [*Gss.*]

Pain of the loins and spine when he bends to the side or backwards, as if he had over-fatigued himself. [*Gss.*]

160. Tearing twitching pain in the middle of the spine. [*Ar.*]

Shooting pain in the middle of the spine, that went off on moving the body, but returned when at rest. [*Ar.*]

In the evening in bed, when lying on the side, the spine is painful, as if broken. [*Gss*].

When lying on the back in bed, the spine is painful as if broken. [*Gss.*]

Drawing tearing pain downwards throughout the whole spine (aft. 29 h.). [*Ar.*]

165. Tearing shooting pain in the upper part of the spine towards the right scapula. [*Ar.*]

Shooting pain on the outer border of the right scapula. [*Ar.*]

In the scapulæ pain when he moves them. [*Gss.*]

A squeezing on the top of the shoulder. [*Gss.*]

Needle-prick on the top of the left shoulder. [*Ar.*]

170. Shooting pain on the top of the left shoulder, which does not go off by pressure or by moving the arm (aft. 32 h.). [*Ar.*]

Single stitches anteriorly in the left shoulder. [*L. Rkt.*]

Paralytic drawing down through the right arm, especially when he lets it hang down, or when he lays it down anywhere, particularly on a hard place. [*Gss.*]

Paralytic pain in the arm, so that he must let it sink down. [*Gss.*]

Paralytic sensation in the whole of the right arm ; it felt as if stiff in the joints, so that he could not move it (aft. 29 h.). [*Ar.*]

175. Stretching tearing pain in the arms, with paralytic pain ; on touching it, bruised pain, as after great muscular exertion. [*L. Rkt.*]

Paralytic drawing through the upper arm from above down to the middle, so that he hardly dare move it ; on pressing on the affected part it is painful, as if he had received a knock or blow there. [*Gss.*]

Boring cramp-like pain in the left upper arm, not removed by pressure (aft. 25 h). [*Ar.*]

Drawing tearing pain in the right upper arm, going off by pressing on it, but immediately returning (aft. 27 h.) [*Ar.*]

Violent squeezing pain in the right upper arm, that went off on moving it, but returned when at rest. [*Ar.*]

180. On the upper arm, above the elbow joint, pain as from a knock or blow. [*Gss.*]

Paralytic pain in the bend of the elbow towards the outside, like a twitching, in fits. [*Gss.*]

Tearing pain in the right elbow-joint, when at rest, not affected by movement (aft. 27 h.). [*Ar.*]

In the left forearm, a drawing digging pain from the wrist to the elbow-joint (aft. $1\frac{3}{4}$ h.). [*Ar.*]

In the whole right forearm, a drawing tearing pain, that did not go off by movement (aft. 7 h.). [*Ar.*]

185. Cramp-like aching pain in the muscles of the forearm, especially when bending it. [*L. Rkt.*]

Paralytic twitching from above downwards on the under surface of the forearm, but especially violent in the place where it commences. [*Gss.*]

In the morning, after rising, when he extends the arm forcibly, cramp-like pain in the forearms, especially from the elbow downwards; if he bends the hands to and fro whilst keeping the arms extended, the same pain comes in the wrist-joints. [*Gss.*]

Contractive tearing, like cramp, in the inferior muscles of the left forearm, close to the wrist, quickly going off on movement (aft. 17 h.). [*Lr.*]

Drawing pain in the wrist-joints (aft. 12, 24 h.).

190. Wrist-joint as if dislocated.

Pinching, boring pain in the right wrist (aft. 3 h.). [*Ar.*]

Intermittent, cramp-like contraction of the hand. [*Gss.*]

Twitching tearing pain in the palm of the left hand, increased by extending the hand. [*Ar.*]

Single stitches in the left hand, towards the little finger. [*Ar.*]

195. **Single, small, twitching stitches, sometimes in the right, sometimes in the left hand** (aft. 33 h.). [*Ar.*]

On the back of the left hand an itching, that compels scratching, whereby it is removed (aft. $6\frac{1}{2}$ h.). [*Ar.*]

Itching tickling externally on the border of the right hand near the thumb and index, compelling him to scratch (aft. 35 h.). [*Lr.*]

Fine stitches on the upper end of the metacarpal bone of the ring finger ; on pressing on it it pains as if bruised. [*Gss.*]

Spasmodic contraction, with cramp-like pain, of the middle finger of the right hand ; it was bent inwards. [*Ar.*]

200. Quick inward twitching of the fingers of the right hand. [*Ar.*]

Cramp-like twitching in the fingers. [*Gss.*]

Drawing in the fingers (aft. 48 h.).

Cramp-like pain in the muscles of the outside of the left little finger, going off on moving it (aft. 12 h.). [*Lr.*]

On the proximal joint of the middle finger, burning pain. [*Gss.*]

205. Paralytic drawing in the ring finger, when at rest and when moving it. [*Gss.*]

In the proximal joint of the thumb a formication, almost as if asleep. [*Gss.*]

Formication in the tip of the thumb, as if asleep ; it is as if numb. [*Gss.*]

In the ball of the thumb pains as after a severe blow, when he presses on it, and also when he moves the metacarpal bone of the thumb towards the palm. [*Gss.*]

An out-boring pain below the glutæi muscles, when sitting, going off by pressing on them and by movement, but soon returning when at rest. [*Ar.*]

210. When sitting the nates are painful, as if tired by prolonged sitting. [*Gss.*]

When walking, pain in the great trochanter, as if he had fallen on it. [*Gss.*]

A shudder runs over the thighs. [*Gss.*]

Whilst standing, cramp-like pain in the anterior muscles of the left thigh (aft. $\frac{1}{2}$ h.). [*Lr.*]

Drawing tearing pain on the anterior part of the right thigh, going off by active movement. [*Ar.*]

215. **Paralytic pain in the left thigh, not far from the knee.** [*L. Rkt.*]

The child stretches out the legs spasmodically. [*Stf.*]

The left leg of the child is in constant spasmodic motion ; at last it remains much averted from the body, lying motionless. [*Stf.*]

Now and then single, obtuse stitches in the knees. [*L. Rkt.*]

Single needle pricks on the patella (aft. 10 h.). [*Lr.*]

220. On the knee a hot flush, with a not disagreeable sensation, as if a hot body, *e. g.* a live coal, were brought near the knee. [*Gss.*]

Paralytic twitching on the front of the leg, betwixt the tibia and fibula. [*Gss.*]

While walking in the open air, cramp-like pain sometimes in the muscles of the right, sometimes in those of the left leg, quickly going off on standing and sitting (aft. 30 h.). [*Lr.*]

Under the left knee, on the tibia, a digging pain (aft. $8\frac{1}{2}$ h.). [*Lr.*]

In the left tibia, close under the knee, intermittent pricks as with a fork. [*Ar.*]

225. In the middle of the left calf tearing pains (while sitting). [*Ar.*]

Twitching tearing in the interior of the foot. [*L. Rkt.*]

Stitches in the ball of the right foot. [*L. Rkt.*]

Cutting pain in all the toes of the left foot, as if they were being detached, not relieved by movement (aft. 2 h.). [*Ar.*]

Tearing shooting pain in the left heel (while sitting). [*Ar.*]

230. Here and there on the trunk, but especially on the abdomen, very painful stitches ; when sitting (aft. 8 h.). [*Ar.*]

Obtuse stitches here and there on the body (aft. several d.). [*L. Rkt.*]

Here and there on the body, sometimes on the limbs, arms, feet,

toes, sometimes in the side, or on the back, sometimes on the nasal bone, but especially on the posterior crista ilii (on the hip), obtuse stitches, sometimes like a squeezing, sometimes like aching, sometimes like knocks or jerks, sometimes like an itching ; on pressing on the part it pains as if sore or bruised. [*Gss.*]

Burning fine pricks here and there, removed by scratching. [*Gss.*]

Prickling, itching, formicating sensation on several parts of the body, that soon goes off on slightly scratching. [*Gss.*]

235. Severe itching here and there in the skin, at night.

In the evening eruption of red itching pimples which soon go off.

Transparent miliary rash. [PELARGUS, l. c., t. i and t. ii.]

(Whilst sitting) cramp-like contractive stitches sometimes in the muscles of the right, sometimes in those of the left thigh, sometimes in the muscles of the left, sometimes in those of the right upper arm, and sometimes up along the sacrum like pains in the back, which however go off when walking in the open air (aft. 27 h.). [*Lr.*]

Whilst sitting, cramp-like tearing, sometimes in the muscles of the right, sometimes in those of the left leg. sometimes in the muscles of the left, sometimes in those of the right forearm, which went off when walking in the open air (aft. 52 h.). [*Lr.*]

240. Tearing and partly sharp cutting pains in the limbs, the head, and the jaws, often only momentary. [*L. Rkt.*]

After a meal—where during the first days the symptoms are always most severe—stretching tearing pain in the scapulæ, upper arms, head and nape, increased by touching. [*L. Rkt.*]

Twitchings and distortions of the limbs. [PELARGUS, l. c., t. i.]

Paralytic twitching on various parts of the body, especially in the limbs. [*Gss.*]

Epileptic convulsions with consciousness (eclampsia).

245. In the afternoon (4 p.m.) an attack of spasmodic extension of the body, then trembling in the whole body, with blue lips and lachrymose complaints of pain in the chest, neck, and all the limbs.

Paralytic pain in the arms and legs (for several days). [*L. Rkt.*]

The child is very weak and ill.[1] [PELARGUS, l. c., t. ii.]

Grunting, groaning, and croaking (in the afternoon).

Painful sensitiveness of all the joints of the body when moved or laid hold of. [*Gss.*]

250. The attacks are worst in the morning and evening. [*L. Rkt.*]

Frequent yawning as though he had not slept enough (aft. 5 h.). [*Lr.*]

While sitting, great drowsiness ; he must lie down (aft. 6½ h.). [*Lr.*]

In the afternoon he is overtaken by unusual drowsiness. [*Gss.*]

Drowsiness all day. [*Ar.*]

255. Irresistible drowsiness, in the evening (for several days). [*L. Rkt.*]

---

1 The next morning after S. 285.

Nocturnal restlessness, frequent turning from one posture to another, on account of discomfort. [*Gss.*]

The child tosses about uneasily even when awake. [*Stf.*]

Sleeplessness.

Tossing about in sleep and piteous howling and crying owing to belly-ache (aft. 8—12 h.).

260. Awakes with piteous weeping, groaning and hiccup, with restless movements (aft. 2 h.).

Many, absurd dreams.

Sleep in an upright position, with the head leant backwards or to the right side (aft. 2 h.).

Frequent waking out of disagreeable or busy dreams. [*Gss.*]

Anxious dreams. [*Gss.*—*Lr.*]

265. Sleep full of tiresome dreams. [*Gss.*]

After sleep, flushes of heat and glowing redness of the cheeks, without thirst. [*Lr.*]

When yawning, trembling of the body with shuddering feeling. [*Gss.*]

Shudder over the upper part of the body up to the head, as if the hair would stand on end, even when near the warm stove (immediately. [*Gss.*]

Febrile rigor all over (aft. ½ h.). [*Lr.*]

270. Shudder moving over the trunk so that he trembles (even beside the warm stove). [*Gss.*]

Coldness of the face with warm hands. [*Stf.*]

Pale, cold face.

Cold cheeks.

Cold frontal sweat.

275. Cold sweat on the forehead and hands.

Cold sweat on the forehead, nose, and hands (aft. 12, 20 h.),

Fever : vomiting of the ingesta, then chill all over, and then heat with great thirst (aft. a few h.).

Quotidian fever at the same hour : chill, then heat without thirst (aft. 24 h.).

Quotidian fever at the same hour, with very short breath (aft. 48 h.).

280. Fever : every day in the afternoon (from 1 p. m. onwards) several attacks of chill with thirst, with cold hands and feet : afterwards heat of the pale face, but especially heat of hands and feet, with cutting pain in the abdomen.

In the morning, even beside the warm stove, cold hands, and rigor running over him without thirst. [*Gss.*]

Strong fever and heat.[1] [ANDRY, *De Generatione Vermium*, p. 182.]

Febrile rigor all over the body, with hot cheeks, without thirst. (aft. 25 h.). [*Lr.*]

Strong fever with vomiting and diarrhœa.[2] [PELARGUS, l. c., t. i.]

---

1 Observations.

2 In several children.

285. Heat in the evening and throughout the night. [PELARGUS, l. c., t. ii.]
Heat in the fever, chiefly in the head, with yellow colour of the face, and blue rings round the eyes

(Heat with redness of face, immediately accompanied by perspiration, without thirst (aft. 8 h.).

Hot feeling and heat and redness in the face (aft. 2 h.). [*L. Rkt.*]

Burning heat over all the face with redness of the cheeks and thirst for cold drink (aft. 35 h.). [*Lr.*]

290. Trembling of the heart. [*Gss.*]

Talking nonsense. [PELARGUS, l. c., t. i.]

When walking in the open air great anxiety and anguish about the heart, as if he had done something bad (aft. 37 h.). [*Lr.*]

The child is very lachrymose and complaining. [*Stf.*]

Weeps piteously when one attempts to touch or lead him (aft. 3 h.).

295. Great seriousness and sensitiveness ; he takes the slightest joke in bad part. [*Lr.*]

Indifference ; nothing either agreeable or disagreeable could make the slightest impression on him. [*Lr.*]

Restlessness.

Incessant restlessness.

Longs for many different things.

300. Refuses everything offered to him, even what he used to like best.

Cannot be quieted by any persuasion ; insensible to caresses.

COCCULUS.[1]

(Menispermum cocculus.)

(The tincture prepared by macerating the powdered seeds at a moderate temperature in twenty parts of spirits of wine.)

This vegetable substance, hitherto only used for the purpose of destroying some noxious vermin and for stupefying fish so that they may be taken by the hand, was (like staphisagria) first employed by myself as a medicine after I had ascertained its dynamic effects on the healthy human body. It possesses many curative virtues, as the following symptoms produced by it show, and the tincture prescribed according to the similarity of effect in high attenuation and potency is indispensable for the cure in many cases of common human diseases, more especially in some kinds of lingering nervous fevers, in several so-called spasms in the abdomen, and so-called spasmodic pains of other parts, where the mental state is one of extreme sadness, particularly in the female sex, in not a few attacks of paralysis of the limbs, and in the emotional derangements resembling those that cocculus can itself produce.

Camphor is its principal antidote.

The duration of its action depends on the nature of the disease in which it is used ; it quickly passes in acute, but lasts many days in chronic diseases.

[HAHNEMANN was helped in this proving by BAEHR, FLAMING, GROSS, HAYNEL, HORNBURG, LANGHAMMER, TRINKS and HARTLAUB (from their 'R.A.M.L.'), WAHLE.

The old-school authorities quoted are :

AMATUS LUSITANUS, Cent. iv.

JOHN HILL, *Hist. of the Mat. Med.*

RUMPF, *Ambcin.*, v.

In the *Fragmenta* there are 162 symptoms of cocculus, in the 1st edit. of the R.A.M.L. 230, in the 2nd edit. 554, and in this last edition 557.]

COCCULUS.

Vertigo as of intoxication and stupid feeling in the forehead, as if he had a board before the head. [*Gss.*]

Attack of vertigo as from intoxication (when sitting) (aft. 1¾ h.). [*Lr.*]

Tendency to vertigo (the 8th d.). [*Hnl.*]

Vertigo for six hours.

5. When he rises up in bed, there occur whirling vertigo and sickness, which compel him to lie down again.

A sick headache, just as if he had taken an emetic, with nausea.

---

1 From vol. i, 3rd edit., 1830.

Stupid in the head.

Stupidity in the head with cold sweat on the forehead and hands and aversion from food and drink.

Distraction (want of memory) ; he easily forgets something he had just thought of.[1] [*Gss.*]

10. Stupidity and confusion of the head, increased by reading, so that he must read a passage several times over in order to understand it. [*Hnl.*]

Heaviness in the head. [*Hnl.*]

Feeling as if something heavy lay on the head, but without pain. [*We.*]

Thinking tries his head much. [*Hnl.*]

In the morning confusion of the head ; there is a humming in it, as after a debauch the previous night.

15. Heaviness and confusion of the head, as after a debauch the day before.

Cloudiness of the head, chiefly aggravated by eating and drinking.

Pain in the head as if it were bound up.

Headache as if the brain were constricted.

Headache in the temples, as if the head were screwed in.

20. (Painful shock in the brain when walking, moving the head and speaking.)

A headache compounded of constriction, burning, tearing, digging and boring.

A violent aching through the whole head, chiefly in the forehead (in the forenoon), which increases to unconsciousness by reading and thinking (aft. 60 h.).

Aching headache in the sinciput. [*We.*]

Aching headache in the vertex (aft. 10 h.). [*Hbg.*]

25. Dull compression in the right half of the forehead. [*Gss.*]

Pressive pain in the head, as if the brain were compressed (aft. 5 h.). [*Lr.*]

In the right temple a pressing inwards as from a blunt body slowly pressed deep into the brain. [*Gss.*]

In the left temple, a pressing inwards. [*Gss.*]

Violent pressing downwards in the whole head, especially in the forehead, increased by walking (aft. 6½ h.). [*Lr.*]

30. In the left half of the forehead, a dull undulating compression. [*Gss.*]

Tearing throbbing headache in the forehead in the evening (from 7 to 9 o'clock) (aft. 38 h.).

Frequent attacks of headache lasting some minutes on a small spot in the left frontal protuberance, at first of raging, throbbing shooting pain, which then spreads to the right frontal protuberance as a formication and there goes off.

A fine shooting in the temples.

A severe stitch in the head above the right eye (aft. 12 h.).

1 This S. occurs almost identically in *Hb.* and *Ts.* 'R.A.M.L.'

35. Several stitches in the right side of the brain (aft. 24 h.) [*Hnl.*]

Intermitting boring needle-pricks in the right frontal region. [*Lr.*]

Fine needle-pricks in the left temple (aft. 6 h.). [*Lr.*]

Headache as if the eyes would be torn out.

Cramp-like pain in the left temporal muscle (aft. 1½ h.). [*Lr.*]

40. Headache as if something closed the eyes forcibly.

Convulsive trembling of the head.

Shuddering on the left side of the occiput as if the hair would stand on end.[1] [*Gss.*]

On the outer border of the orbit obtuse pressure (immediately). [*Gss.*]

Aching in both eyes, as if dust had got into them (aft. 7 h.). [*Lr.*]

45. Aching pain in the eyes with inability to open the eyelids, at night.

Bruised pain in the eyes with inability to open the eyelids, at night (aft. 5 h.).

Stitches in the eyes from within outwards (aft. 24 h.).

(After severe nocturnal headache, in the morning swelling of one eye and of half of the nose.)

Dryness of the eyelids.

50. **Dimness of sight.**

Flies and dark spots float before the eyes, as if amaurosis were coming on.

She sees a black figure before the eyes that receded from her; when she turns it turns along with her, and yet she saw everything clearly.

Contracted pupils (aft. 5 h.). [*Lr.*]

Blue rings round the eyes. [*Bhr.*]

55. A kind of pressive sensation, more stupefying than painful, in the left zygomatic process. [*Gss.*]

Cramp in the zygomatic process, in the masseter muscles (aft. 2 h.).

Cramp-like pain in the masseter muscles *per se*, but increased by opening the jaws (aft. 3 h.).

(Heat in the right ear externally and internally, in the morning in bed).

A sensation alternately in either ear, as if they were stopped up and deaf.

60. Rushing sound in the ear, as when hearing through a tube. [*Hbg.*]

Noise in the ears like the rushing of water, with hardness of hearing (aft. 1 h.).

It seems to him as if he were hard of hearing in the right ear.

Swelling of the right half of the nose.

Stitches externally in the skin and muscles of the cheek.

65. Flying heat of the cheeks, without thirst (aft. 27 h.). [*Lr.*]

Redness of the cheeks and heat in the face, without thirst, in a cold room. [*Hbg.*]

1. This S. is also in *Hb.* and *Ts.* 'R.A.M.L.'

A pustule under the right outer angle of the mouth, with a red areola, with tensive pain on touching it (aft. 24 h.). [*Lr.*]

Swelling of the parotid gland.

Fine stitches in the external parts of the throat (aft. 1 h.).

70. Swollen hard glands under the lower jaw and lumps on the fore-arm, which are painful when stroked.

Painless glandular swellings under the chin (aft. 8 h.). [*Lr.*]

Paralytic drawing on the side of the neck and other parts, sometimes almost like intermittent paralytic pressure. [*Gss.*]

When moving the neck and yawning stiff pain in the cervical muscles. [*Gss.*]

Fine stitch externally on the right side of the neck. [*Hnl.*]

75. Pulsating stitches externally on the left side of the neck. [*Hnl.*]

Weakness of the cervical muscles with heaviness of the head for several days; the cervical muscles seemed unable to support the head; he must lean his head in one direction or another, otherwise the cervical muscles were painful; what gave him most ease was leaning backwards. [*Hnl*]

Tearing digging pain in the lower jaw.

Smarting sensation in the upper and lower molars, as after taking a quantity of sea-salt; biting the teeth together causes an aggreeable sensation.. [*We.*]

The incisors are as if lifted out and seem to her to be so heavy they must fall out. [*Bhr.*]

80. The decayed tooth seems to have become longer; it is loose; the gum around it is swollen (aft. 12 h.).

The hollow tooth is painful only when eating even soft food, as if it were quite loose, and yet not on merely closing the teeth when not eating.

(The gums are sensitive and as if sore.)

(When speaking she has a sort of contraction in the mouth and must speak more slowly.)

In the morning, rough tongue.

85. Dryness in the mouth, at night, without thirst.[1]

Dryness of the tongue, with whitish-yellow fur, without thirst (aft. $\frac{1}{4}$ h.). [*We.*]

Dry feeling in the mouth with frothy saliva and violent thirst. [*Bhr.*]

Water runs into his mouth without sickness (aft. $1\frac{1}{2}$ h.). [*Hnl.*]

Sensation as if water collected in the mouth for a long time, without sickness. [*Hnl.*]

90. If he puts out his tongue far, he feels pain at the back of it as if bruised. [*Gss.*]

Dryness and roughness in the fauces and œsophagus, especially observed when swallowing, without thirst (aft. 2 h.). [*Lr.*]

In the throat scraping, scratching, which goes off on swallowing. [*Ts. Hb.*]

Great sensitiveness n the interior of the throat; all the food

1 This S., without "at night," is also in *Hb.* and *Ts.* 'R.A.M.L.'

seems sharp and stinging, as if it contained too much salt and pepper, [*Bhr.*]

Dryness at the back and upper part of the throat, as if it and the tongue were rough.

95. **Dryness in the œsophagus.**

Dryness in the throat, with hot sensation in the œsophagus and stomach (aft. 2 h.).

Burning in the palate.

Burning like fire in the œsophagus up to the palate, in the evening, and at the same time shuddering round about the head.

Pain at the top of the œsophagus with sensation of swelling at the root of the tongue, which is painful on swallowing.

100. Aching pain in the tonsils, much worse on swallowing the saliva than on swallowing food.

A kind of choking constriction in the top of the œsophagus, which impedes respiration and at the same time excites coughing (aft. 1 h.).

A kind of paralysis of the gullet; the œsophagus is unable to swallow.

Taste in the mouth as if he had fasted a long time.

Metallic taste posteriorly on the root of the tongue.

105. Coppery taste in the mouth.

Metallic taste in the mouth, with loss of appetite. [*Gss.*]

After eating sourish taste in the mouth. [*Gss.*]

When coughing he has a sour taste in the mouth. [*Bhr.*]

Tobacco tastes bitter when smoking. [*Hbg.*]

110. Slimy tastes in the mouth ; the food however has the right taste. [*We.*]

The food has not its right taste, as if tasteless and unsalted. [*Bhr.*]

Sensation in the mouth as if he smelt badly from his mouth (aft. 6 h.).

A bitter taste comes on the root of the tongue.

Frequent empty eructation (aft. $3\frac{1}{2}$ h.). [*Lr.*]

115. Bitter eructation (aft. $\frac{1}{4}$ h.). [*Hnl.*]

Very bitter eructation (immediately). [*Hnl.*]

Acrid, scraping eructation, especially in the evening. [*Ts. Hb.*]

Empty eructation, which leaves a bitter taste in the mouth and throat (aft. 24 h.).

Eructation with taste of food (aft. 18 h.).

120. In the forenoon he has putrid eructation.

Eructation of musty, foul air (aft. 8 h.).

Attempts to eructate, which cause pain in the stomach (aft. $\frac{1}{2}$ h.).

At every eructation, a pain in the scrobiculus cordis, as if he had got a blow or knock there.

When eructating a pain in the scrobiculus cordis, almost like a stitch. [*Fz.*]

125. When she eructates, she has a pressure on the chest.

First attempts to eructate, and imperfect, baulked eructation, causing hiccup, that lasts for an hour (aft. 3 h.).

Hiccup (aft. 10 m.). [*Hbg.*]

Hiccup (immediately). [AMATUS LUSITANUS,[1] Cent. iv, Curat. 79.]

Inclination to hiccup.

130. Hiccup (aft. $\frac{1}{8}$ h.).

No appetite for breakfast ; he feels quite full.

Extreme loathing at food, the very smell of food irritates him, and yet he is hungry. [*Bhr.*]

Feeling of hunger in the scrobiculus cordis, little relieved by eating, almost all day. [*Hnl.*]

Great thirst at all times of the day, but especially when eating. [*Bhr.*]

135. Aversion from food and drink.

Want of appetite, and what he eats has no taste.

When smoking the tobacco tastes bitter (aft. 2 h.).

He is very sensitive to sour things ; he has an aversion for sour things ; bread tastes sour (aft. 3 h.).

In the stomach a feeling as if a worm moved therein. [*Bhr.*]

140. Nausea as from over-eating. [*Hbg.*]

Nausea while smoking tobacco (to which he is accustomed), going the length of vomiting (aft. 4 h.). [*Lr.*]

Nausea (immediately). [AMATUS LUSITANUS, l. c.—JOHN HILL,[2] *Hist. of the Mat. Med.*, p. 504.]

Excitation to vomit. [*Hbg.*]

When she eats, she becomes sick and inclined to vomit.

145. After each time she drinks, in the afternoon, nausea, that seems to be chiefly in the mouth.

Frequent inclination to vomit (aft. several h.).

When driving in a carriage unusual nausea and inclination to vomit (aft. 48 h.).

In the morning she cannot raise herself up in bed on account of feeling poorly and inclined to vomit (aft. 48 h.).

When he becomes cold, or catches cold, there occurs an inclination to vomit, causing a copious flow of saliva.

150. **Inclination to vomit in connexion with headache, and a pain as if bruised in the bowels** (aft. $\frac{1}{2}$ h.).

(Vomiting about midnight with attacks of suffocation, he vomits food and mucus, during which he has a bitter and sour taste in the throat.)

Sensation in the stomach as if he had eaten nothing for a long time and his hunger had gone off.

Immediately after eating pain under the stomach.

Gurgling under (in) the scrobiculus cordis. [*Gss.*]

155. Pecking and gnawing under the scrobiculus cordis. [*Gss.*]

After eating, aching in the stomach. [*Hbg.*]

Aching in the scrobiculus cordis. [*Hbg.*]

Aching pain in the stomach, scrobiculus cordis, and hypochondria some hours after a meal or at night in bed.

---

1 Poisoning of a man by four grains.

2 General account of effects of C.

A pressure in the scrobiculus cordis, that takes away the breath (aft. 1 h.).

160. Squeezing and tension in the scrobiculus cordis when walking.
Violent spasm in the stomach, clutching in the stomach.
Spasm in the stomach, squeezing in the stomach.
Constrictive pain in the stomach, that prevents him sleeping.
A pinching together in the epigastrium, that takes away the breath.

165. Squeezing, constrictive pain in the epigastrium after a meal, which extends to the left side of the abdomen and the chest (aft. 100 h.).

Aching in the epigastrium.

Under the last true rib of the right side an extremely violent aching pain, increased by bending the body forwards, by coughing and on inspiration, but not by external touch.

(Pain in the hypochondria as if bruised (aft. 12 h.).

Continued fine stitch in the skin of the left gastric region, that went off on rubbing. [*Hnl.*]

170. On the left, near the navel, intermittent obtuse stitches. [*Gss.*]
On the right, above the navel, fine nipping. [*Gss.*]
Pinching pain in the abdominal muscles of the left side. [*We.*]
She feels empty and hollow in the abdomen, as if she had no intestines. [*Bhr.*]
Squeezing in the abdomen (aft. $\frac{3}{4}$ h.). [*Hbg.*]

175. Audible rumbling in the abdomen. [*Hnl.*]
Drawing pain in the bowels.
Drawing pain in the abdomen from the right to the left side (aft. 4 d.). [*Hnl.*]
Violent cutting in the abdomen after dinner while walking, with feeling of cold and vertigo (8th d.). [*Hnl.*]
Cutting in the hypogastrium up to the epigastrium, alleviated by standing.[1] [*Hnl.*]

180. Continued stitch in the right side of the abdomen. [*Hnl.*]
In the left side of the abdomen, several needle-pricks. [*We.*]
Stitches in several parts of the abdomen, only when stooping (aft. 15 h.). [*Hnl.*]
Tearing in the bowels.
Burning in the abdomen.

185. Great distension of the abdomen.
Soon after supper, flatulent sufferings; the flatus distends sometimes one, sometimes another part of the bowels, and is expelled with difficulty (aft. 5 h.).
Flatulent colic about midnight; he awakes and flatus is incessantly generated, which distends the abdomen, causing aching pain here and there and passing off singly without much relief, whilst new flatus continues to form again for several hours; he must turn in bed from side to side in order to obtain ease (aft. 20 h.).

---

1 In the original "stechen," evidently a misprint of "stehen."

In the lumbar and renal regions, in the morning in bed, whilst lying, a sharp hard pressure, that goes off after getting up.

The flatulence presses upwards.

190. A constrictive pain in the abdomen with pressing towards the genital organs (female), and at the same time a qualmishness in the scrobiculus cordis with tendency to water-brash.

Nausea (without inclination to vomit) spreading up from the right side of the abdomen towards the navel (immediately). [*Gss.*]

Constipation for several days.

A hard stool only every other day, that comes away with great effort.

After the passage of a motion violent tenesmus in the rectum causing faintness.

195. There occur tendency to and premonitory signs of inguinal hernia (aft. 8 h.).

Dilatation of the left inguinal ring and tendency to the protrusion of inguinal hernia, with sore-pain (aft. 14 h.).

Continued stitch in the right inguinal region. [*Hnl.*]

Painful tendency to inguinal hernia, especially on rising up from a seat. [*Gss.*]

In the right inguinal ring paralytic pain, as if something would be forced out there; a rupture-pain only whilst sitting, going off by rising up. [*Gss.*]

200. Forcing pain in the flanks, as if the catamenia were coming on. [*Ts. Hb.*]

In the flanks internally all is full and swollen as if stuffed full; only in both sides, not in front; especially when stepping forwards, when it feels as if the swelling was pushed along and as if everything came asunder (aft. some h.). [*Ts. Hb.*]

Soft stool, diarrhœa (aft. ½ h.).

Frequent small evacuations by stool (aft. several h.).

(Every day several bright coloured, pale motions.)

205. (Slimy stools.)

Discharge of hot flatus before the fæculent diarrhœa. [*Gss.*]

Urging to stool, thin fæculent diarrhœa of a fœtid odour. [*Gss.*]

Soft, thin motion (aft. 1 h.). [*Hbg.*]

Urging to pass a motion and break wind at the same time, and with the latter there rapidly occurs in short fits diarrhœic fæcal evacuations in small quantities. [*Gss.*]

210. Ineffectual urging to stool with constipation for three days; the fourth day hard stool passed with effort. [*Hnl.*]

Excitation to stool in the rectum; but the peristaltic movement is deficient in the upper intestines; hence the stool is delayed for 36 hours (aft. ½ h.). [*We.*]

Creeping and itching in the rectum, as from ascarides.

Contractive pain in the anus, that prevents him sitting, in the afternoon (aft. 20 h.).

Burning itching in the anus.

215. (Retention of the urine for 10 minutes.)

Watery urine (aft. 2½ h.).

(He passes at very short intervals a great quantity of watery urine and the urging is constantly renewed, on account of fulness of the bladder.) [*Gss.*]

Frequent urging to urinate, every quarter of an hour, with discharge of very little urine, for 30 hours (aft. 4 h.). [*Lr.*]

During the urging to pass water, pain in the urethra. [*Hbg.*]

220. Pricking itching in the fore part of the urethra (aft. 13 h.). [*We.*]

Tensive aching pain in the urethral orifice when not urinating (aft. 1 h.).

Shooting pain in the urethra (aft. 12 h.).

Shooting pain at the end of the prepuce.

Itching on the scrotum.

225. **Itching in the scrotum.**

Itching burning in the scrotum. [*Hnl.*]

Violent pains in both testicles as if bruised, especially when touched (8th d.). [*Hnl.*]

Shooting pain in one of the testicles.

Drawing pains in the testicles.

230. Catamenia seven days too soon, with distension of the abdomen, and cutting contractive pain in the abdomen at every movement and every breath ; at the same time a contraction in the rectum (aft. 48 h.).

Catamenia eight days too soon with distension of the abdomen and a pain in the epigastrium, not only at every movement—every step gives pain—but also while sitting, as if the internal parts suffered a sharp pressure from a stone ; the parts are painful on external pressure as if there was an ulcer internally.

(Metrorrhagia.)

Leucorrhœa.

The catamenia, which had ceased for a year, come on immediately in 2 cases. [*Ts. Hb.*]

235. Excitation of the genitals and inclination for coitus.

Increased sensitiveness of the genital organs. [*Hnl.*]

Nocturnal emission of semen (aft. 6 h.).

In the night relaxed genital organs and prepuce retracted behind the glans (aft. 12 h.).

* * *

Sneezing. [*Gss.—We.*]

240. Sneezing.

When walking in the open air, he cannot sneeze.

(She blows bloody mucus from the nose.)

Pain in the anterior angle of the nostril at the point of the nose, especially on touching it.

Severe coryza all day. [*Lr.*]

245. In the left nostril pain as from an ulcer, when not touched.

Violent coryza for four days.

Viscid mucus adheres to the larynx and compels him to cough and hawk.

Irritation to cough in the upper part of the larynx.

Cough that strains him much on account of an oppression of the chest, that comes on every time when he begins to cough (in 48 h.). [*Fg.*]

250. In the evening in bed irritation to cough in the back of the larynx; the cough always consists of two impulses.

In a quartan type, every fourth night, about 12 o'clock, also at 2 o'clock, a cough wakes him up, with dryness of the mouth; on coughing it feels as if the glottis were not wide enough.

A suffocating sensation, taking away the breath and contracting the wind-pipe, which almost always excites coughing.

In the pit of the throat a sensation, as if something were there that takes away the breath; the glottis is constricted. [*Ts. Hb.*]

Audible rattling as if in the left side of the chest, as from an emptiness there, especially perceptible on walking (aft. 3 h.). [*Lr.*]

255. She has no breath, must always breathe short, gasp. [*Ts. Hb.*]

Tightness of the chest and difficult respiration. [*Hbg.*]

Tensive constriction of the right side of the chest, which oppresses the breathing (aft. ½ h.).

Oppression of the chest especially in the upper part of the sternum, which impedes respiration (aft. 4 h.).

A whistling, snoring breathing, oppressed almost to suffocation, especially the inspiration; very slow breathing alternates with complete cessation of respiration, and the face is swollen as in apoplexy.

260. (Rawness and sore feeling in the chest.)

Aching pain in the middle of the sternum with anxiety, afterwards shooting pain in the sternum (aft. 3 h.).

In the middle of the sternum a pain as if a blunt instrument were pressed on it. [*Gss.*]

In the sternum a sudden pressure, as if from a push with the fist. [*Hbg.*]

On bending the body towards the right side, when sitting and standing, a dull drawing pain in the right side of the chest as long as the bending is continued. [*Hnl.*]

265. Reading aloud fatigues his chest to such a degree that he cannot continue reading without great effort. [*Hnl.*]

Stitches in the interior of the chest synchronous with the pulse, when sitting, lasting continuously for a quarter of an hour. [*Bhr.*]

When walking, an extraordinarily violent stitch through the left side of the chest as far as the back. [*Hnl.*]

Anteriorly on the right false ribs intermittent blunt stitches. [*Gss.*]

Fine shooting pains in the left side of the chest during inspiration. by paroxysms. [*Fg.*]

270. Some stitches in the right side of the chest (aft. 2 h.). [*Hbg.*]

Fine shooting pain in the sternum when walking (aft. 48 h.).

Stitches in the right side (aft. 1 h.).

Stitches in the left side (aft. 3 h.).

Fine stitches in both nipples (aft. ½ h.).

275. Shudder over the breasts (aft. ⅛ h.).

Some stitches in the left side of the chest, near the scrobiculus cordis, in the evening (aft. 24 h.).

In the articulations of the thorax, and in all the vertebræ, a penetrating pain, as if they were dislocated or spasmodically contracted, particularly when moving (aft. 20 h.).

A paralytic pain in the sacrum like weak back.

A paralytic pain in the sacrum with spasmodic drawing over the hips, which hindered him greatly when walking, with anxious timid disposition.

280. In the lumbar region, paralytic aching pain. [*Gss.*]

Bruised pain in the bones of the sacrum, not increased by touching.

Through the abdomen out to the lower part of the back, several stitches in the morning in bed.

Trembling in the back.

An itching in the back, in the evening after undressing, with an eruption of red pimples.

285. In the side through to the back a drawing pain when talking, walking, and stooping ; when lying the drawing becomes worse for a few minutes, then goes off completely.

Aching pains in the back, especially on his left side (when sitting) (aft. 5 h.). [*Lr.*]

Drawing pains in the back.

Tearing pains in the back.

Boring pains in the back.

290. Pain in the back when standing, as if over-tired or sprained (aft. 12 h.).

Pain in the spine as if it were broken.

Tearing pain betwixt the shoulders and spine, in the evening before going to bed. (aft. 36 h.).

Immediately beneath the left scapula, drawing pains when standing and lying, worst in the morning (aft. 6 h.). [*Fg.*]

Under the left scapula intermittent aching paralytic pain, when at rest. [*Gss.*]

295. When he moves the shoulders, his back feels stiff and painful. [*Gss.*]

Shooting pain in the nape on moving the head backwards and forwards. [*Hnl.*]

Stitches in the scapulæ from right to left.

Pressure in the scapulæ and nape.

Painful cracking of the cervical vertebræ when moving the head.

300. After a meal, on raising the arm, a very severe drawing pain in the shoulder-joint and the shafts of the bones of the arm ; on touching the parts they pain as if bruised and crushed.

In the shoulder-joint and in the muscles of the upper arm single stitches when at rest (aft. 1 h.).

Itching pricking in the left axilla, as from a flea. [*Hnl.*]

Under the shoulder a pimple which itches under the bed-clothes [*Hbg.*]

Under the right shoulder, a sort of living crawling and throbbing, and a burning which extends to the fingers (aft 1 h.).

305. In the shoulder and elbow-joints, as also in the shaft of the humerus between them, a pain compounded of crushing, tearing, and shooting, which is intolerable when at rest, with a sensation of heaviness ; he dreads moving the arm and yet the pain is alleviated by moving (aft. 5 h.).

Paroxysms of burning pain in the left arm.

Convulsions of the arms with the thumb turned into the fist.

During and after a meal, sufferings in the arms as if asleep and paralysed (aft. 3 h.).

The arm as if asleep with formicating sensation. [*Hbg.*]

310. Whilst writing, a kind of paralysis of the arm ; he could scarcely hold the pen (aft. 4 h.). [*Hbg.*]

During violent movement of the arms an acute paralytic pain, as if its bones were broken in two. [*Gss.*]

When he raises the upper arm it pains as if it was broken. [*Gss.*]

The shafts of the humeri, just above the elbows, are as if bruised and have paralytic pains when moved. [*Gss.*]

The arm on which he lies in bed pains as if bruised. [*Gss.*]

315. In the shaft of the left humerus, a digging (undulatory drawing) bruised pain. [*Gss.*]

Drawing in the humerus with bruised pain. [*Gss.*]

Twitching in the muscles of the left upper arm. [*Hnl.*]

Pulse-like visible twitchings in the muscles of the left upper arm, and immediately afterwards above the elbow of the right arm. [*Hnl.*]

Stitches in the right upper arm. [*Hbg.*]

320. On the outer side of the left upper arm below the head of the humerus, intermitting, obtuse stitches (like blows). [*Gss.*]

While eating the right arm gives him great pain, it is very heavy and tired, when he tries to raise it up high.

Sudden ; paralytic pain in the bend of the right elbow. [*Gss.*]

Continued shooting in the left elbow (4th d.) [*Hnl.*]

Shooting pain in the outer side of the left forearm down to the little finger. [*We.*]

325. Pressive pain on the right forearm. [*We.*]

In the anterior muscles of the forearm, intermitting, very acute, almost tearing, paralytic aching, especially when at rest.

In the radius of the forearm, a pain as from dislocation, when moved or touched.

The forearm gone asleep, with a sensation in the hand, as if it were swollen, and a constrictive pain in the muscles ; the fingers are cold, with an internal sensation of icy coldness (aft. 3 h.).

Cold sweat now on one, now on the other hand.

330. Sweaty hands (immediately).

Sometimes one hand, sometimes the other, is as if insensible and asleep.

Sometimes one hand, sometimes the other, is alternately hot and cold (aft. $\frac{1}{4}$ h.).

On the border of the hand where the little finger ends, a blister, which comes on in the night, and the following day bursts (aft. 5 d.).

Her hand trembles while eating, and all the more the higher she raises it. [*Bhr.*]

335. Spasmodic pain on the outer side of the right hand and of the four fingers, with some heat of the hand. [*We.*]

Cramp-like contraction of the finger. [*Gss.*]

Cramp-like pain in the right little finger when writing. [*Lr.*]

Cramp-like shooting pain from behind forwards in the right index. [*We.*]

Painful paralytic twitching through the fingers (6th. d.). [*Gss.*]

340. Tearing, boring, drawing pain in the fingers.

A deep, penetrating, tickling itching on the ball of the thumb, not alleviated by scratching and rubbing (aft. 16 h.).

In the right nates a nipping when sitting ; it afterwards changes into obtuse blows. [*Gss.*]

Shooting pain in the left hip-joint, when walking (5th d.). [*Hnl.*]

On turning the thigh, a cracking and painful sensation in the left hip-joint, especially observed when walking (aft. 24 h.). [*Hnl.*]

345. Repeated stitches on the outside of the left hip-joint. [*Hnl.*]

Twitching in the muscles around the right hip-joint. [*Hnl.*]

In the left hip-bone, intermitting aching, paralytic pain. [*Gss.*]

In the middle of the left thigh, intermitting aching bruised pain. [*Gss.*]

Shooting pain in the bone of the whole right thigh, only when walking. [*Hnl.*]

350. When sitting violent pulsating stitches on the outer side of the left thigh, that caused involuntary movements. [*Hnl.*]

Paralytic numb feeling traverses in paroxysms the left leg from the middle of the thigh downwards.

Numb feeling from the thigh over the knee downwards. [*Gss.*]

Paralytic drawing in the thighs with weakness in the knees, as if they would bend under him. [*Gss.*]

Paralytic feeling in the left thigh, worst when at rest. [*We.*]

355. The thighs feel paralysed and bruised. [*Gss.*]

When he walks round in a circle towards the left, the inner side of the left thigh pains as if bruised. [*Gss.*]

When he lifts up the thighs they pain as if broken. [*Gss.*]

On commencing to walk after sitting, the thighs pain as if bruised. [*Gss.*]

When he raises the legs while sitting, the thighs are very acutely painful as if bruised. [*Gss.*]

360. Constrictive not painful sensation down the thigh, sometimes attended by a sensation as if it would become rigid ; the constriction then extends downwards in the muscles of the leg below the hough. [*Gss.*]

Drawing pains in the feet.

Tearing pains in the feet.

Boring pains in the feet.

Paralytic insensibility of the lower extremities (aft. 24 h.).

365. A boil on the inner side of the thigh (aft. 12 h.).

(On kneeling down, a trembling in the thighs.)

Cracking of the knee when moving (immediately).

On rising up after sitting, an intolerable drawing pain in the knee.

Stitches in the knee.

370. In the patella, a drawing, tearing pain.

Violent stitch in the left knee-joint (aft. 27 h.). [*Hnl.*]

In the outer side of the left knee-joint, a continued stitch, while walking (6th d.). [*Hnl.*]

At night when bending the knees, cramp in the calves.

Tensive pain in the calves while moving.

375. While sitting, violent stitches in the skin of the left knee, so that at every stitch he must move the leg involuntarily. [*Hnl.*]

Itching in the bend of the left knee, the calf and the ankle-joint, when walking; it went off when standing, but returned when walking. [*Hnl.*]

Great lassitude in the knees, as if after a long walk, frequently recurring (immediately). [*We.*]

Under the left knee, feeling as if he had tied his garter too tightly on the leg. [*Gss.*]

Constrictive sensation on the outer side of the left leg, more numb than painful. [*Gss.*]

380. On the outer side of the left leg downwards, a dull, undulating paralytic pain. [*Gss.*]

While walking after sitting, the left foot falls asleep, and he has pricks in it as with many pins. [*Gss.*]

While sitting both feet fall asleep. [*Gss.*]

Swelling of the feet in the evening.

Cold sweat on the feet.

385. Heat and swelling of the feet, with incessant eroding itching.

Itching in the ankle-joint.

Violent pain as if dislocated, in the ankle-joint, when moving.

Bruised pain on the dorsum of the foot, when bending the foot upwards, and when touching it (aft. 3 h.).

Tearing jerks and tearings in the hitherto painless corn, when at rest in the evening.

390. Pain in the proximal joint of the big toe, as if a chilblain were about to come there, and like a boil; painful also when touched.

Tearing pain in the big toe, even when at rest.

Drawing pain in the right toes (aft. 4 h.). [*Hbg.*]

Eroding pain in the toes (aft. 3 h.).

Pain on the inner part of the heel, as if in the heel-bone, just as though it was bruised (aft. ½ h.).

395. The muscles of the limbs are painful when touched (aft. 24 h.).

Here and there burning obtuse stitches. [*Gss.*]

Here and there in the skin, burning itching pricks as if from fleas. [*Hnl.*]

When he touches with the fingers the affected part (that was previously swollen and inflamed) he has fine pricks in it, as if he pressed upon it with a pin's point.

Itching on the skin of the body, especially in the evening, when undressing.

400. When undressing, violent smarting itching, as after profuse sweat, in the skin of the whole body, compelling him to scratch (aft. 16 h.). [*Lr.*]

Itching in the skin under the bed-clothes ; after scratching it becomes more tickling. [*Hbg.*]

Itching and burning here and there in the skin, especially on the inner side of the thighs, as if from nettles ; also eruption of pimples there, which have shooting pain when touched.

At night itching on various parts ; after scratching these parts are painful.

At night an itching sometimes on the chest, from the scrobiculus cordis to the neck, sometimes on the tibia and under the shoulders ; after scratching serum exudes from the parts (aft. 4 h.).

405. Single pimples which fill with pus and afterwards dry up and disappear, above the nose, on the temples, on the chest and between the scapulæ.

Eruption of red miliary papules on the face, on the back and on the chest, which itch in the warmth (not when taking off the clothes).

Pimple-like, hard pustules, which contain no fluid, have a red areola, and all day itch with burning pain, on the limbs, wrist, and back of the fingers.

Eruption of red, shapeless spots on the skin, as if coloured with red wine, over the whole of the chest, and on the sides of the neck behind the ears, without heat or other sensation.

Excites tearing pain in indurated glandular swellings.

410. **Excites shooting pains and heat, in cold glandular swellings, at least when they are touched.**

All the symptoms and sufferings, especially in the head, are aggravated by drinking, eating, sleeping, and speaking.

The symptoms are exceptionally aggravated by smoking tobacco.

The symptoms are increased by coffee.

After drinking, flying heat in the face.

415. The symptoms, especially the headache, are much aggravated by cold air.

Hæmorrhages. [RUMPF, *Amboin.*,[1] v, p. 35.]

He shuns the open air.

The open air feels too cold to him.

Intolerance of cold and warm air.

420. Intolerance of the open air, with heat and redness of the cheeks (aft. 4 h.).

Pain of the limbs when moving, as if they were crushed or broken.

Subsultus (palpitation) of single muscular parts, especially on the lower extremities, as after a long journey on foot. [*Gss.*]

---

1 General statement of effects of C. This symptom not found.

Here and there in the limbs an acute paralytic drawing, continuous and in jerks, as if in the bone. [*Gss.*]

Internal digging pain in the bones of the limbs. [*Gss.*]

425. Internal pain of the limbs, increased by touching and external presture (aft. 24 h.).

Drawing pain in the limbs of the left side.

Drawing pain in the limbs and abdominal muscles, as after taking cold.

Cracking and creaking in the joints.

The joints crack when walking. [*Hbg.*]

430. Painful stiffness of all the joints, at one time in the hands and fingers, at another in the knees and ankle-joints, for two days (aft. 24 h.). [*Fg.*]

Painful stiffness of the joints (aft. 1 and 8 h.).

Falling asleep of the feet and hands alternately, in short paroxysms.

Tendency to tremble (aft. 1 and 6 h.).

Trembling in all the limbs.

435. Want of vital spirits.

The limbs are as if paralysed.

Paralytic immobility of the limbs with drawing pains, apparently in the bones.

Attacks of paralytic weakness with backache.

Hemiplegia of the left side.

440. A kind of epilepsy: he comes into the room with a cheerful countenance and sits down, when he feels as if intoxicated; thereupon he becomes quiet and stares long at one point, not replying to questions; he then falls unconscious to the ground and curls himself up with unintelligible whinings: "Ah! au! au! ah! brr," &c. The urine comes away involuntarily; the limbs and all the body are shaken by spasmodic starts, and the outstretched hands are bent convulsively inwards; at the same time he has choking of a jerking and spasmodic character in the throat, with mouth half open, as if he were about to vomit, with frothy foam at the mouth; the hands are cold, the face covered with cold sweat and spasmodically contorted, the eyes glassy and protruded. He then stands up, but does not answer questions, but shows his teeth and bellows at those questioning him; will not allow himself to be touched, but endeavours to strike those about him and to wrestle with them; the expression of the countenance is that of furious rage; at last he grunts and groans, until after a quarter of an hour he gradually recovers and regains consciousness. This is followed by disinclination for all food, even such as he formerly liked best (aft. $\frac{1}{4}$ h.). [*Gss.*]

The slightest movement causes loss of strength; the least thing fatigues him.

Very exhausted by a short walk.

She is so weak that she must sit down to an easy work she used to do standing. [*Bhr.*]

The knees are like to give under him from weariness; when walking he staggers and would fall to one side. [*We.*]

445. Painful paralytic feeling in the arms and legs; she can hardly rise from the seat; at the same time loss of appetite. [*Gss.*]

Exhaustion of the body, especially when sitting. [*Hnl.*]

Extraordinary weakness of the body when walking. [*Hnl.*]

Great exhaustion of the body, so that it was an exertion to him to stand steady. [*Hnl.*]

In the morning, about 9 o'clock, such heaviness in the limbs, and such great fatigue in the whole body, that she cannot ward off sleep—for several days at the same time. [*Bhr.*]

450. Syncope.[1] [JOHN HILL, l. c.]

On moving the body, syncope, with spasmodic distortion of the facial muscles.

Extreme weakness.

Laziness with silence.

The slightest interruption to sleep causes loss of strength; he misses every hour of sleep.

455. Desire to lie down.

After lying down in bed, constant yawning and stretching of the limbs. [*Hbg.*]

Interrupted, short yawning, for which he cannot draw sufficient breath.

Much yawning towards evening.

Violent yawning.

460. Forcible yawning with a cracking in the internal ear.

Somnolence (sopor).

Unconquerable, waking sleepy stupefaction (coma vigil).

(Whilst sleeping he lies prone on the abdomen.)

When asleep he lays one arm under the head (aft. 4 h.).

465. Frequent waking out of sleep.

Frequent waking out of sleep, as from fright. [*Lr.*]

He frequently wakes up at night with a sensation of being too warm.

At night sleepless, restlessness in the whole body; pricking and stinging here and there.

Many ideas about his daily business prevented him sleeping for an hour; he woke about 1 o'clock and could not go to sleep again. [*Hnl.*]

470. He wakes up at night with fear, as if he were afraid of ghosts.

Very vivid, fear-exciting dreams (aft. 2 h.).

Dreams of dying and of death.

Dream of having done something bad.

Vivid, unremembered dreams. [*Lr.*]

475. He dreams that his knees are swollen and painful. [*We.*]

She cries out anxiously in her sleep, calls her mother and sisters, with rapid, anxious respiration; she clutches with her hands about the bed, and strikes out with her hands; at the same time she opens her

---

1 Not found.

eyes and distorts them, without waking up, and moves her head about constantly, especially towards the left side. [*We.*]

The sleep is interrupted by frequent starting up and waking.

Frightful anxiety like a dream, which frustrates every attempt to fall sleep.

He would like to sleep until the day is advanced, and is also very sleepy by day.

480. He sleeps in the morning until late in the day; the eyes will not open in the morning; he is awake but cannot get up nor open the eyes.

In the morning after waking laziness and disinclination to speak. [*Hbg.*]

In the morning he has not slept enough and yawns incessantly. [*Hbg.*]

Shivering in the evening in the back.

Chill in the back, as if it was touched here and there with ice, which is not removed by the warmth of the stove.

485. Shivering on the lower part of the body (very soon).

In the afternoon rigor over the whole body.

In the morning (about 8 a. m.) rigor for half an hour, without thirst and not followed by heat.

General coldness, without rigor, with bluish hands (the first h.).

Repeated though short shiverings, especially through the lower extremities (immediately). [*Gss.*]

490. Shiver running through the whole body. [*Gss.*]

In the evening, along with longing for stimulating strengthening food, he is suddenly affected with internal chilliness, so that he trembles, and yet he is not externally cold to the touch. [*Gss.*]

The hands feel cold when held to the face, but warm to one another. [*Gss.*]

Trembling in all the limbs, always with chilliness, which does not go off in the warm room, especially in the evening. [*Fg.*]

He has a cold shiver over the back, although sitting near the warm stove (8th d.). [*Hnl.*]

495. Chilliness and cold feeling on the back. [*Hnl.*]

Chilliness which does not go off with the heat of the stove, with violent cutting in the abdomen (8th d.). [*Hnl.*]

Severe chilliness over the whole body, in the evening (7th d.). [*Hnl.*]

Cold feeling without perceptible external coldness, on the shoulder (aft. 4 h.).

Fever: frequent rigor, followed by flying heat on the head.

500. Fever: alternate heat and chill of the body (aft. some h.).

(Fever: gradually increasing chilliness, with little or no thirst, warm forehead, cold cheek bones, cold nose, and icy-cold hands; then heat with great anxiety, as if he could not get breath enough, with nausea and great thirst, until perspiration came on; the perspiration was slight, quite cool, almost confined to the head and hands, the anxiety continuing all the time.)

Fever: frequently during the day he begins shuddering, as when one warms oneself at the fire in the cold ; he then again becomes hot, exhausted, must lie down, but all without thirst and without perspiration.

Fever : in the afternoon (6 p.m.) hot hands, with sensation of dry heat all over the body ; sleeplessness until 4 a.m., then shivering and cold hands all day.

(External heat of the body, without feeling hot and without thirst) (aft. 5 h.).

505. Burning heat in the cheeks with quite cold feet.

The pulse is not quicker, but very small and hard.

Heat in the forehead.

Increased feeling of heat, quick pulse (aft. 24 h.). [*Hnl.*]

Redness of the left hand with drawing in the middle finger (4th d.). [*Hnl.*]

510. Glowing heat of the cheeks, at the same time chilliness of the whole body. [*Hnl.*]

Rapid alternation of heat and chill ; she is suddenly attacked by great heat rising up from the feet and spreading all over the body ; at the same time a sensation as if the blood rushed into the face ; but withal she is more pale than red ; after a few minutes she is overrun by icy coldness from the head down to the feet, and the heat is momentarily suppressed—attacks which come on several times during the day. [*Br.*]

Quick and severe flushes of heat.

Frequent transient attacks of a disagreable burning heat and redness of the cheeks, such as are wont to occur when one gets angry or receives disagreeable news.

Heat and redness in the face with thirst.

515. Thisrt for cold drinks, **especially beer.**

Perspiration on the body (immediately) from evening till morning, with cold sweat on the face.

General perspiration in the morning, chiefly on the chest and the part affected.

Transpiration and slight perspiration over the whole body on the slightest exertion (aft. 1 h.).

Dejection,

520. **The thoughts are fixed on a single disagreeable subject ; she is absorbed in thought and notices nothing about her.**

He is sunk in the saddest thoughts, and insults he has received he takes deeply to heart.

She sits in deep reverie.

Time passes too rapidly with him, several hours appear to him as short as one hour.[1] [*Gss.*]

Continual sad thoughts, just as if he had received insults. [*Fg.*]

525. He has no inclination to do anything, and finds no pleasure in anything.

Weeping.

1, This S. also appears in *Hb.* and *Ts.* 'R.A.M.L.'

He has no desire for any work.

He has no pleasure in anything, and no inclination to do anything.

Great discontent with himself. [*Hbg.*]

530. He is extremely serious, afterwards he breaks out in complaints.

Serious, and though caring little about his own health, he is very anxious about the illness of others.

She dawdles ; in business she cannot accomplish anything nor finish anything, with contracted pupils (aft. 12 h.).

Busy restlessness.

Anxiety.

535. In the morning, anxiety respecting the incurability of a trifling malady.

Anxiety as if she had conmmitted a great crime.

Great anxiety as if he had done something bad (aft. 29 h.). [*Lr.*]

Cardiac anxiety, mortal anguish[1] (immediately). [AMATUS LUSITANUS., l. c.]

Palpitation of the heart.

540. **Sudden, extreme anxiety.**

Despairing disposition.

Hypochondriacal, especially in the afternoon.

Over sensitiveness (aft. 24 h.).

A slight noise goes through all his limbs.

545. He dreads any sudden surprise.

He is easily startled.

Great sensitiveness of disposition ; everything offends him.

He cannot bear any interruption in coversation, nor any noise.

Too great irritability of disposition ; every trifle makes him angry. [*Hnl.*]

550. Everything angers and vexes him ; after a few hours he becomes lively and disposed to make jokes. [*Hbg.*]

Easily annoyed ; he takes everything in bad part (aft. 24 h.).

Extreme inclination to be annoyed and to take every trifle in bad part (aft. 1 h.).

She is annoyed at the merest trifle even to weeping, when the pupils are contracted ; after the weeping want of appetite.

He is very indignant and annoyed at slight faults and fibs of others.

555. Joyous, contented, merry ; he becomes witty and makes jokes* (aft. 3 h.).

Happy humour, and contended with himself.† [*Lr.*]

Irresistible inclination to trill and sing ; like a kind of madness.

* Partly curative action.
† Curative action.

---

1 The original is simply "anxietas."

COLOCYNTHIS.[1]

(Cucumis Colocynthis, Colocynth.)

(The dry fruit reduced to powder and digested with alcohol, in the proportion of 20 grains of the powder to 400 drops of alcohol, without heat, for a week, two succussions being given every day so as to form a tincture, twenty drops of which contain one grain of colocynth-powder.)

The older physicians brought colocynth into disrepute by giving it in large dangerous doses as a purgative. Their successors, terrified by this dreadful example, either rejected it entirely, whereby the curative power it possessed was lost to mankind, or they only ventured to employ it on rare occasions, and then never without previous alteration and weakening of its properties by silly procedures, which they called ***correction***, whereby its pretended poisonous character was said to be tamed and restrained. With the aid of mucilage they mixed up with it other purgative drugs, or they partially destroyed its power by fermentation or by prolonged boiling with water, wine, or even urine, as had already been stupidly done by the ancients. But even after all this mutilation (their so-called *correction*) colocynth always continued to be a dangerous remedy in the large doses in which physicians prescribed it.

It is really wonderful that in the medical school there has always been such an absence of reflection, and that in regard to matters like this the obvious simple thought never occured to any one that, if the heroic medicines acted too violently in a certain dose, this was owing less to the drug itself than to the excessive magnitude of the dose, which yet may be diminished to any extent required ; and that such a diminution of the dose, whilst leaving the drug unaltered in its properties, only reduces its strength so as to make it innocuous and capable of being employed with advantage, and hence must be the most natural and appropriate *corrigens* of all heroic medicines. It is obvious that if a pint of alcohol drunk all at once can kill a man, this is owing not to the absolute poisonousness of the alcohol but to the excessive quantity, and that a couple of drops of alcohol would have been harmless to him. It is obvious that whilst a drop of strong sulphuric acid immediately produces a blister and erosion on the part of the tongue to which it is applied, on the other hand, when diluted with 20 or 100,000 drops of water it becomes a mild, merely sourish fluid, and that hence the most natural, the simplest, *corrigens* of all heroic substances is to be found only in the dilution and the diminution of the dose until it becomes only useful and quite innocuous.

---

1 From vol. vi, 2nd edit., 1827.

In this way, and in this way only, can the inestimable curative powers for the most incurable diseases that have hitherto lain concealed in the heroic—much less in the weaker—medicines (called *poisons* by those afflicted with intellectual poverty) be elicited in a perfectly sure and mild manner to the advantage of suffering humanity. By means of the knowledge so obtained we may effect results in the treatment of acute and chronic diseases such as the whole medical school has hitherto failed to effect. This method, so childishly simple, of rendering the strongest medical substances mild and useful never occurred to the minds of physicians, and they were consequently forced to dispense with the aid of the grandest and most useful remedies.

Guided by the following peculiar pathogenetic effects produced in the healthy by colocynth, I have been enabled by means of it to perform extraordinary cures on the homœopathic principle by the administration of a small portion of a drop of the octillion- or decillion-fold dilution of the above tincture as a dose.

Thus, to mention only a single example, many of the most violent colics may, under the guidance of symptoms 69 to 109, be often very rapidly cured, when at the same time the other characteristic symptoms of the disease, or a portion of them, are to be found in similarity among the symptoms of colocynth.

The action of colocynth is of long duration.

[HAHNEMANN was assisted in this proving by GUTMANN, FR. HAHNEMANN, HORNBURG, LANGHAMMER, L. RUCKERT, STAPF.

The following old-school authorities furnished some of the symptoms:

ALIBERT, in *Med. Nat. Zeit.*, 1799.
Breslauer Sammlungen, 1727.
HOFFMANN, J. M., in *Ephem. Nat. Curios.*, Cent. x.
HOYER, in *Misc. Nat. Cur.*, Dec. iii, Ann. 7, 8.
KOLPIN, in *Hufel. Journ.*, iii.
PLATER, *Obs.*, Lib. iii.
SALMUTH, *Obs.*, Cent. iii.
SCHENCK, *Obs.*, Lib. vii.
SCHNEIDER, in *Annal. d. Heilk.*, 1811, April.
STALPAART VAN BER WIEL, Cent. i.
TULPIUS, *Obs.*, Lib. iv.
VALENTINI, in *Eph. Nat. Cur.*, Ann. 3.
ZACUTUS LUSITANUS, in *Pharmac.*

In the 1st edit. Colocynth has 227 symptoms, in this 2nd edit. 250; 33 additional symptoms appear in the *Chr. Kr.*]

COLOCYNTHIS.

On turning the head quickly, vertigo apparently arising in the left temple, as if he would fall, with a giving way in the knees. [*Stf.*]

Dazedness and confusion of the head. [ALIBERT, in *Med. Nat. Zeit.*, 1799.[1]]

Confusion of the head, especially in the sinciput. [*Gn.*]

---

1 Not accessible.

Head dazed and empty, as after a noisy nocturnal debauch. [*Hbg.*]

5. Vertigo and stupid feeling in head, at the commencement of the bellyache. [*Fr. H—n.*]

Violent pains in the head, as from a draught of air, which go off when walking in the open air (aft. 3 h.). [*Lr.*]

Single, slight pressure here and there in the interior of the head.* [*L. Rkt.*]

Pressing, aching pain in the sinciput, most violent on stooping and when lying on the back, for six hours. [*Gn*]

Aching pain along the sagittal suture, worse on moving and shaking the head and on stooping forwards. [*Stf.*]

10. Pressing squeezing pain in the upper part of the brain. [*Gn.*]

Digging pressive pain in the left temple. [*Gn.*]

Pressing drawing headache on the left side of the forehead. [*Gn.*]

Drawing, semilateral headache (aft. $1\frac{1}{2}$ h.). [*Hbg.*]

Tearing pain in the whole brain, which became a pressure in the forehead, as if it pressed out the forehead—more violent on moving the eyelids. [*Gn.*]

15. In the morning after rising, a dull pricking pain on the forehead, as if externally (aft. $\frac{1}{4}$ h.). [*Lr.*]

Burning pain in the skin of the forehead, above the eye brows. [*Gn.*]

Boring stitches in the right temple, which went off on touching (aft. $8\frac{1}{2}$ h.). [*Lr.*]

Smarting burning pain on the hairy scalp, left side. [*Gn.*]

Burning sensation in the right upper eyelid (aft. 34 h.). [*Gn.*]

20. Burning pain in the whole of the right eye-ball. [*Gn.*]

Sharp cutting pain in the right eye-ball (aft. 7 h.). [*Gn.*]

Sparks before the eyes. [SCHNEIDER, in *Annal. d. Heilk.*, 1811, April.[1]]

Prickling burning pain in the right inner canthus. [*Gn.*]

Burning cutting pain in the right lower eyelid, when at rest. [*Gn.*]

25. Severe itching in the right eyeball, rendering rubbing necessary. [*Gn.*]

Paleness and relaxation of the facial muscles; the eyes looked sunk in. [*Gn.*]

Eruption of a pimple on the left cheek, which smarts when touched, and after scratching discharges a watery fluid (aft. $4\frac{1}{2}$ h.). [*Lr.*]

* The following peculiar varieties of headache, which colocynth causes explain the homœopathic cures effected by the Swede DALBERG (*Vetensk. Acad. Handl.*, 1785, p. 146) from the administration of tincture of colocynth in some chronic headaches, especially in those called gout in the head.

1 From colocynth given in apoplexy.

Digging burning pain in the cheek worse when at rest than when moving. [*Gn.*]

Eruption of white pimples on the face, especially betwixt eye and ear, on the forehead and chin, which itched a little, but smarted when touched (aft. 4 h.). [*Lr.*]

30. Tearing and tension on the left side of the face to the ear and into the head.

Earache in the right ear, not going off by introducing the finger. [*Gn.*]

Cutting shooting pain in the lower cavity of the right auricle that goes off on introducing the finger. [*Gn.*]

Deep in the ear an itching shooting pain which extends from the Eustachian tube to the membrana tympani, and is momentarily removed by boring in the finger (aft. 1½ h.). [*Stf.*]

Formicating sensation in the inner ear which goes off on introducing the finger. [*Gn.*]

35. Painful long-continued drawing behind the left ear. [*Hbg.*]

Aching behind the left ear. [*Hbg.*]

Throbbing and digging pain from the middle of the left side of the nose to the root of the nose. [*Gn.*]

In the evening, a violent itching in the left nostril, compelling him to scratch, as irritating as if coryza were coming on (aft. 15 h.). [*Lr.*]

Burning pain in front of the right commissure of the mouth (aft. 12 h.). [*Gn.*]

40. A suppurating pimple on the left commissure of the mouth (aft. 2 h.). [*Lr.*]

Quivering in the muscles of the chin, only when the parts are at rest. [*Gn.*]

Pain in the lower row of teeth, as if the nerve were tugged and stretched. [*Hbg.*]

(A shooting throbbing pain in the right lower molars, as if struck with a metal wire.) [*Stf.*]

In the morning, white tongue with rough sensation upon it as from too much tobacco-smoking (aft. 1¼ h.). [*Lr.*]

45. Rough tongue as if sand were strewed upon it (aft. 36 h.). [*Fr. H—n.*]

On the upper surface of the tip of the tongue, a metallic astringent taste. [*Stf.*]

Smarting pain on the inside of the right cheek and side of the tongue. [*Gn.*]

A scraping feeling on the palate, also when not coughing. [*Stf.*]

In the throat, a fine pricking as with needles, or as if an awn of an ear of corn were sticking there, on the upper part of the velum pendulum palati. [*Stf.*]

50. Fine smarting stitches in the fauces, not observed when swallowing. [*Gn.*]

Frequent hiccup (aft. 1¼ h.). [*Lr.*]

A disgusting putrid taste, stronger in the fauces than in the mouth. [*Gn.*]

Bitterness in the mouth, for four hours (immediately). [*Fr. H—n*]

After drinking beer, bitter taste in the mouth, which increases for several minutes (aft. 27 h.). [*Gn.*]

55. Anorexia. [ALIBERT, l. c.]

Diminished appetite, though the food tastes all right. [*Fr. H—n.*]

Much desire to drink. without thirst ; the mouth is always watery, the liquid drunk tastes very good, but immediately after every draught a flat taste comes into the mouth.

Feeling of thirst in the gullet. [*L. Rkt.*]

Eructation of a bilious fluid.

60. **Empty eructation.** [*Hbg.*]

Nausea. [SCHNEIDER, l. c.]

Nausea for two hours (immediately). [*Fr. H—n.*]

Nausea for six hours, until he falls asleep at night ; in the morning after waking the nausea returns. [*Fr. H—n.*]

Nausea for eight hours. [*Fr. H—n.*]

65. Vomiting twice of food only, without nausea and without bad taste (aft. 10 m.). [*Fr. H—n.*]

Very frequent vomiting. [J. M. HOFFMANN, in *Ephem. Nat. Curios.*, Cent. x, Obs. 30.[1]]

A pressure in the stomach, as from a stone. [*Hbg.*]

Violent stomach-ache, precordial pressure (immediately). [HOFFMANN, l. c.]

After eating particularly, an aching sensation in the gastric region, with sensation as of hunger, not relieved by eating more—every day. [*L. Rkt.*]

70. Cutting pressure in the epigastrium, as from flatulence, on inspiring. [*L. Rkt.*]

Transient cutting in the epigastrium. [*L. Rkt.*]

Single stitches under the last ribs. [*L. Rkt.*]

Pressure in the bowels, which seems to come sometimes from emptiness, but is rather increased than diminished by eating, especially by bending forwards when sitting, for about six successive days, particularly in the evening. [*L. Rkt.*]

Great distension of the abdomen occasionally.

75. Pressure as from fulness in the abdomen. [*Hbg.*]

Along with some distension colic-like pain in the abdomen and discharge of flatus. [*Stf.*]

Colic. [TULPIUS, *Obs.*. Lib. iv, Cap. 25.[2]—ALIBERT, l. c.]

Continued pain in the abdomen through all the bowels, compounded of bruised pain and aching.

In the hypogastrium, a sore cutting pain, which commenced when walking and increased in violence at every step (aft. 5 d.). [*L. Rkt.*]

---

1 Poisoning by a whole apple. 2 Poisoning.

80. Cutting pains in the abdomen. [*Breslauer Sammlungen*, 1727, p. 148.[1]]

Continued cutting in the hypogastrium, at last so violent that he must walk in a bent-forward attitude; at the same time weakness in the whole body, so that walking was a trouble to him, with dread of the work he had to do. [*Gn.*]

The most violent pains in the abdomen. [HOFFMANN, l. c.]

Indescribable belly-ache. [STALPAART VAN DER WIEL, *Cent.* i, Obs. 41.[2]]

Excessive pain in the abdomen, on a small spot below the navel, which, after the night-sweat, spread through the whole abdomen. [*Fr. H—n.*]

85. At each attack of pain in the abdomen, restlessness in the whole body, whereby a kind of shudder rushes through both cheeks, which gradually rises up from the abdomen, and after a more severe pain immediately goes off. [*Hbg.*]

Movement in the abdomen, as if he were still fasting, in the afternoon (aft. 8 h.). [*Lr.*]

Emptiness in the abdomen, as if there were nothing in it (aft. 10 h.). [*Hbg.*]

An emptiness in the abdomen, as though he had had a severe diarrhœa. [*Stf.*]

pains in the abdomen, as if from catching cold, or from having eaten a variety of incongruous articles of food. [*Hbg.*]

90. Alleviation of the violent belly-ache by smoking tobacco, but a sensation long remains in the abdomen as if he had taken cold. [*Fr. H—n.*]

Pinching sensations in the abdomen, which terminate above the pubes. [*Hbg.*]

Pinching in the abdomen, without evacuation of the bowels (aft. 34 h.). [*Gn.*]

Pinching and grasping pains in the abdomen (aft. 21 h.). [*Hbg.*]

Acute pains, as if severely clawed in the abdomen—a grasping in the bowels; on account of these pains he can neither lie quiet nor sit, and can only walk bent double; by lying still these pains were not allayed, but they were when he had moved quickly or tossed about (aft. 6 h.). [*Hbg.*]

95. Shooting pain in a small spot in the umbilical region, which compels him to bend and stoop forwards, and is increased to the severest degree by lifting anything, for eighteen hours (aft. $\frac{3}{4}$ h.). [*Fr. H—n.*]

Belly-ache, which compels him to crouch and bend together. [*Fr. H—n.*]

Dull tensive pain in the abdomen, which went off by pressure. [*Gn.*]

Pains as if the bowels were squeezed in and pressed; at the same time cutting pain towards the pudendum; below the navel the

1 Nothing about colocynth can be found here.

2 Poisoning.

pains were so violent that the facial muscles were much distorted and the eyes closed ; this pain was only allayed by pressing with the hand on the abdomen and bending in the abdomen (aft. 8 h.). [*Hbg.*]

Constriction of the bowels in the hypogastrium always gradually increasing every ten to twenty minutes, which goes off by strong pressure with the hand (aft. 24 h.). [*Hbg.*]

100. Forcing together of the abdominal intestines, especially round about the pudendum. [*Hbg.*]

Sensation in the whole abdomen as if the bowels were squeezed between stones and threatened to burst out, sometimes so severe that the blood mounted to the upper parts, the face and head, with outbreaks of perspiration on these parts ; the face and head felt as if a cool air blew on them when the cramp-like pains declined (aft. 7 h.). [*Hbg.*]

Cramp-like belly-ache, so that he can neither sit still, nor lie, nor walk ; after a meal there ensued immediately an almost resultless urging to stool, tenesmus (aft. 10 h.). [*Hbg.*]

A forcing from both sides of the hypogastrium towards the middle of the pelvic cavity, like flatulence which will not come away (compelling emission of semen).

Boring pain in the left illiac region, close to the bones of the pelvis (aft. 12 h.). [*Gn.*]

105. Digging, tearing pain in the umbilical region, more violent when expiring and laughing loud. [*Gn.*]

All the abdominal pains from colocynth went off on drinking a cup of coffee ; but he must then go immediately to stool. [*Hbg.*]

After eating a single potato, violent pain in the abdomen and hurried evacuation of the bowels. [*Fr. H—n.*]

Violent urging to stool, which consisted of copious yellowish-brown, semi-fluid fæces, as from a purgative, of sourish-putrid smell : after this evacuation the belly-ache seemed to disappear, but soon returned (aft. 9 h.). [*Hbg.*]

Greenish-yellow diarrhœic stools, with sensation as if he had taken cold. [*Fr. H—n.*]

110. Quite thin, frothy stool of saffron-yellow colour and mouldy smell, almost like burnt grey blotting-paper (aft. 12 h.). [*Hbg.*]

Diarrhœa ; fifteen motions in eighteen hours, by which the bellyache was gradually allayed (aft. 1 h.). [*Fr. H—n.*]

Day and night, diarrhœa with nausea, without being able to vomit. [*Fr. H—n.*]

Frequent urgent call to stool ; at the same time sensation at the anus and in the lower part of the rectum, as if these parts were weakened by long-continued diarrhœa and had lost their tone. [*Hbg.*]

He must keep back the evacuation by a great effort, in order that it should not come away involuntarily before reaching the night-chair (aft 10 h.). [*Hbg.*]

115. Small fæcal evacuation which was viscid and slimy. [*Hbg.*]

Hard stool with little pressing (aft. 48 h.). [*Gn.*]

Very hard stool, which comes away in pieces* (aft. 5, 6 d.). [*L. Rkt.*]

First watery and slimy, then bilious, at last bloody stools. [HOFFMANN, l. c.]

Bloody stools. [HOYER, in *Misc. Nat. Cur.*, Dec. iii, Ann. 7, 8. Obs. 178;[1] and *Bresl. Samml.*, l. c.]

120. Hæmorrhage from the anus. [TULPIUS, l. c.]

Excites dysentery. [ZACUTUS LUSITANUS, in *Pharmac.*, p. 208.[2]]

Fatal dysentery.† [PLATER, *Obs*, Lib. iii, p. 858.]

Hæmorrhage from the anus, some hours after death.‡ [SCHENCK, *Obs.*, Lib. vii.]

Pain in the lower part of the rectum from swollen hæmorrhoidal venous lumps, when sitting, walking, and during stool.

125. Blind hæmorrhoids.

A constant grumbling and croaking in the abdomen, as if frogs were in the bowels.

Grumbling and creaking in the abdomen, with cutting pains. [*Hbg.*]

Frequent noisy discharge of flatus (aft. ½ h.). [*Lr.*]

Illusory desire to discharge flatus for some minutes; after that some came away with great violence. [*Hbg.*]

130. In the whole abdomen, flatulence, which is not discharged.§ [*Hbg.*]

Retained flatus.‖ [*Hbg.*]

Pain above the hips with nausea and chilliness (aft. 3 h.). [*Fr. H—n.*]

Tensive shooting pain in the right loin only felt on inspiration, and most violent when lying on the back.¶ (aft. 54 h.). [*Gn.*]

Constant pressure in the pubic region (aft. 8, 10 h.). [*Hbg.*]

135. Tensive pain in the right iliac region worse when pressed on. [*Gn.*]

A violent itching stitch in the anus, not connected with the evacuation of the bowels. [*Gn.*]

Pressure on the pubic[4] region, with call to urinate (aft. 8 h.). [*Hbg.*]

* Secondary effect.

† From a whole gourd macerated in wine.

‡ From a drachm in a clyster.[3]

§ Apparently secondary action.

‖ Apparently secondary action.

¶ Note to 132 and 133. This lumbago, which colocynth is apt to produce in the healthy, explains how DALBERG (*Konigl. Vetensk. Handl.*, 1785, p. 146) was able to effect such happy homœopathic cures with this plant in some kinds of lumbago. The symptoms 184, 185, point to the curative power of colocynth in affections of some parts near the hip.

---

1 From the decoction.

2 From an enema containing colocynth.

3 Administered for apoplexy.

4 In the original "Schienbein-Gegend" (region of the tibia), evidently a misprint for "Schambein-Gegend" (region of the os pubis). (Corrected thus in *Chr. Kr.*, S. 160.)

Some minutes after passing urine, an aching pain at the end of the urethra, as if it were bruised (aft. 14½ h.). [*Lr.*]

Urine seems to be secreted sparingly. [*Hbg.*]

140. Frequent strangury, with scanty discharge of urine (aft. 1 h.). [*Lr.*]

Strangury, with inability to pass urine, which as a rule was passed very sparingly. [*Hbg.*]

Urine, immediately, of intolerable odour; in the utensil it became at once thick, gelatinous, viscid, like coagulating albumen. [SCHNEIDER, l. c.] [1]

Complete impotence; the prepuce, that at other times always covered the glans, remained retracted behind the glans, though he was not deficient in sexual desire.

* * *

In the morning, fluent coryza, without sneezing (aft. 1½ h.). [*Lr.*]

145. In the morning, when inspiring, a whistling in the chest (aft. 1¾ h.). [*Lr.*]

In the evening **short cough when smoking tobacco** (aft. 15 h.). [*Lr.*]

Frequent irritation to dry cough in the larynx, like a tickling (aft. 1 h.). [*Stf.*]

The place in the larynx where it scrapes and tickles so as to cause cough, becomes more scrapy during inspiration. [*Stf.*]

Pressure in the middle of the sternum, as if something lay on the lung. [*L. Rkt.*]

150. For several days, breathing twice as short as normal, without tightness of chest or heat.

In the night, an attack of tightness of chest with slow difficult breathing, which forces him to cough.

Oppressive pressure anteriorly on the chest; it seems to be much too narrow—also compression on the sides, especially when sitting bent forwards, and in the evening, for six days (aft. 2¼ h.). [*L. Rkt.*]

Increased oppression of the chest: on inspiring the lung feels as if squeezed by a pressure from without, but on inspiring there are stitches in it (aft. 6 d.). [*L. Rkt.*]

A running and creeping in the skin of the left side of the chest and abdomen, as if insects were running about in it (aft. 6 d.). [*Gn.*]

155. Pressure with obtuse stitches in the scrobiculus cordis, which compels rapid breathing; the lung appears to be unable to expand itself sufficiently. [*L. Rkt.*]

Obtuse stitches in the right side of the chest, on inspiring, but on expiring a slight pressure, for six days (aft. 1 h.). [*L. Rkt.*]

Muscular twitching in the right intercostal muscles, which went off on raising himself up (aft. 5 h.). [*Gn.*]

---

1 Not found.

Single stitches in the chest and under the ribs, here and there every day. [*L. Rkt.*]

A grasping pain in the right intercostal muscles (aft. 2 h.). [*Gn.*]

160. Betwixt the scapulæ a shooting tensive pain, chiefly when walking, so that he must walk for some time crooked.

An aching bruised pain in the lower part of the back, with, at the same time, hard pressure in the scrobiculus cordis, equally felt when at rest and when moving.

Obtuse stitch under the right scapula, during inspiration. [*L. Rkt.*]

Sore pain in the left scapula, when at rest. [*Gn.*]

In the region of the right scapula, an internal drawing sensation, as if the nerves and vessels were stretched. [*Hbg.*]

165. From the right side of the neck to down over the scapula, severe pain, as if the nerves were forcibly opened out and tugged, or as if bruised. [*Hbg.*]

A drawing pain, like a violent concraction in the left sternocleido-mastoideus muscles, when at rest ; on moving and walking it extends towards the back part and goes off entirely (aft. ½ h.). [*Stf.*]

Stiffness of the left side of the neck, painful on moving. [*Hbg.*]

Severe drawing, sharp pain in the left cervical muscles, still more severe on movement (aft. 1 h.). [*Hbg.*]

Painful drawing in the nape, even when at rest ; soon afterwards stiffness of the nape, which is painful even without movement, but most so on turning the head. [*Hbg.*]

170. In the nape, towards the protuberance of the occipital bone, a feeling as if a heavy pressing weight lay across it, as acute when turning the head as when at rest. [*Hbg.*]

Sensation behind the right scapula, as if the arms were sprained when at rest and when moving. [*Hbg.*]

A suppurating boil in the glands of the axilla. [KOLPIN, in *Hufel. Journ.*, iii, p. 575.[1]]

Prickling burning pain in the right upper arm, when moving. [*Gn.*]

Occasional stitches in the arms, here and there (aft. 4 h.). [*L. Rkt.*]

175. Fine, itching stitch in the bend of the right elbow, when at rest. [*Gn.*]

Paralytic pain, as if bruised, in the arms, occasionally (aft. 5 d.). [*L. Rkt.*]

Aching, drawing pain in the shafts of the arm-bones, when at rest, especially under the head of the humerus and above the wrist-joint, where it pains as if in the periosteum on raising the arm.

Tensive pain in the right forearm (aft. 27 h.). [*Gn.*]

Violent drawing pains in the thumb of the right hand, feeling as if in the tendons, which commenced in the ball and terminated in the tip of the thumb (aft. 5 h.). [*Lr.*]

---

1 Critical phenomena in a rheumatic paralysis getting well under colocynth.

180. Spasmodic pain in the right palm, so that he could only open the fingers with difficulty; the pain was more severe when at rest than when moving. [*Gn.*]

A burning painful point in the right middle finger. [*Hbg.*]

In the gluteal[1] muscles of the left side, a tickling itching when sitting. [*Hbg.*]

On the right thigh a drawing tension.

Only when walking, pain in the right thigh, as if the psoas muscle that raises it were too short; on standing it ceased, but on walking it returned (aft. 32 h.). [*Gn.*]

185. Shooting tearing pain in the right thigh, when standing and sitting (aft. 2 d.). [*L. Rkt.*]

In the muscles of the thigh tearing stitches, when sitting. [*L. Rkt.*]

Trembling of the feet, as after a severe fright, with rigor for a quarter of an hour (aft. 1 h.). [*Fr. H—n.*]

(Cold sensation on the knees, which, however, are warm.)

Paralytic pain in the knee when walking, as if the joint were tightly bound.

190. Only when moving, pains like needle-pricks in the left hough, which at length changed into itching pricking. [*Gn.*]

In the evening a violent itching in the left hough, which compelled him to scratch; after scratching there ensued a smarting sensation (aft. 14 h.). [*Lr.*]

Tensive pressure on the tibiæ, even when sitting. [*L. Rkt.*]

Itching prick in the right tibia, most severe when at rest (aft 2½ h.). [*Gn.*]

Itching prick in the right leg, continuing also when moving. [*Gn.*]

195. Weakness, chiefly of the legs, as from fatigue.

Pain in the hitherto painless varicose knots of the right leg. [*Gn.*]

Quivering in the right calf, when at rest, which went off on movement. [*Gn.*]

Sharp cutting pain in the inner side of the left calf, when at rest. [*Gn.*]

In the calves sometimes a tearing pain, when sitting and standing. [*L. Rkt.*]

200. Itching prick in the right calf, which was not removed by rubbing. [*Gn.*]

Aching tearing pain in the ankle-joint, when sitting. [*L. Rkt.*]

Going to sleep of the left foot [*Hbg.*]—when at rest. [*Gn.*]

Aching boring prick on the dorsum of the right foot, most severe when at rest (aft. 25 h.). [*Gn.*]

Severe tearing on the dorsum of the left foot upwards (aft. 4 h.). [*Lr.*]

205. **Tearing pain in the sole of the right foot, most violent when at rest** (aft. 35 h.). [*Gn.*]

Twitching of some muscular parts of the limbs. [J. M. Hoffmann, l. c.]

---

1 "Gesichtsmuskeln," in place of "Gesassmuskeln" in original. This mistake is corrected in *Chr. Kr.*

All the limbs are drawn together, so that he resembles a hedgehog. [STALPAART, l. c.]

Tearing stitches lengthways on the whole body, on the forehead, temples, back, upper and lower extremities, side of the abdomen, and chest (aft. 6 h.). [*Lr.*]

An itch-like eruption. [KOLPIN, l. c.]

210. In the evening in bed a smarting itching here and there on the body, which is removed only momentarily by scratching, and at last develops into a restlessness, during which he must constantly move the limbs, and is unable to get to sleep (aft. 32 h.).

Troublesome itching, in the afternoon and evening, followed by perspiration. [KOLPIN, l. c.]

In the morning, on waking and after rising, a violent itching, as after profuse perspiration all over the body, but especially on the chest and abdomen (aft. 26 h.). [*Lr.*]

The skin of the whole body desquamates. [SALMUTH, *Obs.*, Cent. iii, Obs. 2.[1]]

Forces completely sunk. [HOYER, l. c.]

215. Syncope. [VALENTINI, in *Eph. Nat. Cur.*, Ann. 3, Obs. 78.[2]]

Syncopes, with coldness of the external parts. [HOFFMANN, l. c.]

Fatal syncope. [HOYER, l. c.]

When walking in the open air weariness of all the limbs, as after a long journey on foot; in the lower extremities he felt as if he had to drag a great weight along with them, and, especially in the right leg, a trembling, so that the perspiration broke out all over his body (aft. 11 h.). [*Lr.*]

Drowsiness and disinclination for intellectual work. [*Gn.*]

220. Restless sleep, he tosses from one side to the other (aft. 30 h.). [*Hbg.*]

Very vivid, anxious dreams.

Extremely vivid, but not anxious, dreams, which gradually become so excessively vivid that he wakes up with them.

At night sleep disturbed by many dreams (aft. 29 h.). [*Lr.*]

He dreams much, and of many different things. [*Hbg.*]

225. When lying on the back lascivious dreams and emission of semen, without erection of the penis. [*Gn.*]

At night sleep interrupted by voluptuous dreams, without pollution (aft. 20 h.). [*Lr.*]

Lascivious dreams, with uncontrollable erection of penis, without seminal emission. [*Gn.*]

Voluptuous dreams and seminal emission (aft. 8 h.). [*Hbg.*]

In his sleep he lies almost always on his back, with one hand under the occiput, and the other arm laid above the head.

230. When he lies still he feels the beating of his heart and arteries through the whole body. [*L. Rkt.*]

Slow, but full pulse, from the commencement until the tenth hour. [*Hbg.*]

---

1 Poisoning. This desquamation occurred during convalescence.

2 Not found.

Quick, full pulse. [SCHNEIDER, l. c.]

Violent thirst. [HOFFMANN, l. c.—*Bresl. Samml.*, l. c.]

Violent chill (aft. 5 h.). [*Fr. H—n.*]

235. In the morning, after rising, shivering through the whole body, with cold hands, whilst the face and the rest of the body were hot, without thirst (aft. ½ h.). [*Lr.*]

(Feeling of icy coldness in the soles of the feet, though they are not cold.)

Coldness of the whole body.

Feeling of warmth rapidly rushing over the whole body, but soon passing off, without thirst (aft. 2 h.). [*L. Rkt.*]

At night profuse sweat on the head, hands, legs, and feet, of a urinous smell.

240. In the morning, on waking, he found himself perspiring on the legs (aft. 24 h.). [*Lr.*]

Night-sweat. [*Fr. H—n.*]

Sensation of heat in the interior of the whole body, and also externally warm to the touch (aft. 10 h.). [*Hbg.*]

In the morning after rising, warmth of the face, whilst the hands and especially the tips of the fingers were cold (aft ¾ h.). [*Lr.*]

Febrile heat. [HOFFMANN, l. c.]

245. Palpitation of the heart. [SCHNEIDER, l. c.]

Great anxiety. [HOYER,—and *Bresl. Samml.*, l. c.]

All day long, disinclination to speak. [*Lr.*]

Dejected, joyless, not inclined to speak. [*Gn.*]

Discomfort ; he wishes and asks for many things. [*L. Rkt.*]

250. Morose disposition ; he takes everything in bad part and does not answer willingly. [*L. Rkt.*]

CONIUM.[1]

(Hemlock.)

(The freshly expressed juice of the Conium maculatum obtained from the whole plant at the commencement of flowering, mixed with equal parts of alcohol.)

Hemlock is one of those medicines whose primary and secondary actions are most difficult to be ascertained, and respecting which it is most difficult to form a judgement. Among its symptoms we find several of a somewhat opposite character which should only be regarded as alternating actions (perhaps as a transient secondary action suppressed for some time by the repeated attack of the medicine). On the other hand the sad effects resulting from the long-continued employment of hemlock in increasing doses, as we observe in the results of STOERCK's, LANGE's, EHRHARDT's, GREDING's, BAYLIES', REISMANN's, COLLIN's, and TARTREUX's disastrous treatments, are true secondary actions of the depressed vitality overpowered by the repeated attacks of such large doses of hemlock: a dissolution of all the connexions of the fibres combined with asthenic inflammation and the most painful sensitiveness—see 264 to 273, 276, 342 to 345, 349, 350, 205, 207, 209. The opposite of this seems to lie in the primary action of hemlock, which appears to indicate a tension, condensation, contraction of the fibres (and glandular swellings), with suppression of the sensibility—compare 28, 60, 127, 147, 148, 178, 179, 212, 215 216, 225, 238, 249, 253, 254, 286. These are primary actions which seem to be corroborated by some of my own homœopathic cures (glandular indurations on the lip, the breasts, &c., arising *from a bruise*, and two cases of cataract produced *by an external blow*). These recorded primary actions of hemlock (especially 127, 286), together with the symptoms 10, 11, 115, 117, 293, 333, 359 to 367, point to it as an excellent remedy for that bad kind of hypochondriasis which is sometimes observed in unmarried males who are strictly chaste, where it does not depend on a miasmatic cachexia.

Experience must decide as to the value of hemlock in the morbid long-sightedness (presbyopia) of elderly persons, as indicated in 38, and perhaps it will confirm the curative power here hinted at.

The homœopathic practitioner will know how to make use of the curative indications given in the other symptoms of the primary action of hemlock.

Coffee has been found to be the antidote of hemlock.

---

1 From vol. iv, 2nd edit., 1825.

[HAHNEMANN was assisted in this proving by FRANZ, LANGHAMMER, WISLICENUS.

The following old-school authorities furnished symptoms :

AMATUS LUSITANUS, *Cent.* v. ANDREE, *Obs. upon a Treatment by Stoerck*, London, 1761. ANDRY, *Quæst. med. an cancer ulceratus cicutam eludat*, Paris, 1763.

BAYLIES, *Essays on Med. Subjects*, London, 1773. BIERCHEN, *Tal om Kraftskador*. BŒRHAVE, *Præl. ad Instit.*, vi.

CLARK, *Essays and Obs Phys. and Liter.*, iii, Edinb., 1771 COLLIN, *Annus med.*, iii, Vindob., 1764. CULLEN, *Materia Medica*, ii

EHRHARDT, *Diss. de Cicuta*, Argent., 1763.

FOTHERGILL, *Med. Obs. and Enq.*, iii.—*Works*.

GATAKER, *Essays on Med. Subj.* GREDING, *Vermischte Schriften*.

HALLE, in *Samml. f. pr. Aerzte*, xv, iii. HALLER, in *Gotting. Anzeigen*, 1775.

KALTSCHMIDT, *Progr. de Cicuta.*, Jen., 1768.

LANDEUTTE, *Journal de Medecine*, xv. LANGE, *Dubia cicutæ vexata*, Helmst., 1764. LIMPRECHT, *Acta Nat. Cur.*, i.

Med. Obs. and Enq., ii, Lond., 1771.

OBERTEUFFER, in *Hufel. Journal*, ix.

PAULLI, SIM., *Quadrip. Botan. Pharm. Helv.*

REISMANN (reference not given). ROWLEY, W., *Seventy-four cases*, London, 1779.

SCHMUCKER, *Chir. Wahrnehm.*, ii. STOERCK, *Lib. de Cicuta.—Lib. de Colchico.—Lib. de Stram. Hyos. et Acon.*

VALENTINI, in *Hufel. Journ.*, xxix.

TARTREUX, *Epist. apol.*

VAN EEMS, in *Bœrhave Prælect. de m. n.*, *i.*

WATSON, *Philos. Transact.*, No. 473, 1744. WHYTT, *on Nervous Disorders*.

Zurcher Abhandlungen, tom. ii.

The 1st edit. gives 373 symptoms ; only two more are added in this 2nd edit. ; the *Chr. Kr.* gives 912 symptoms.]

CONIUM.

Vertigo. [BAYLIES, *Essays on Med. Subjects*, London, 1773.[1]—ANDRY, *Quæst. med. an Cancer ulceratus cicutam eludat*, Paris, 1763.[1]—ANDREE, *Obs. upon a Treatment by Stoerck*, Lond., 1761.[2]—WATSON, *Philos. Transact.*, No. 473, 1744.[3]—LANGE, *Dubia cicutæ vexata*, Helmst.; 1764, pp. 12, 20.[4]—*Pharm. Helv.*, p. 50.[5]—SCHMUCKER, *Chir. Wahrnehm.*, ii, pp. 82,84.[6]—WHYTT, *on Nervous Disorders*, p. 22.[7]—GATAKER, *Essays on Med. Subjects*, Introd., p. 8.[8]—FOTHERGILL, *Med. Obs. and Inqu.*, iii, p. 400, and *Works*, ii, p. 58.[8]

1 Not accessible.
2 Symptoms observed in patients taking conium.
3 Case of poisoning.
4 Not accessible ; probably as in note[2].
5 General statement from experience.
6 As in note[2].
7 Observed in self.
8 General statement from observation.

—OBERTEUFFER, in *Hufel. Journal*, ix, iii, p. 77.[1]—CULLEN, *Materia Medica*, ii, p. 300.[2]]

Vertigo that affects the head. [FOTHERGILL, l. c.]

Vertigo round in a circle, when he rises from a seat.

Vertigo, so that all seemed to go round in a ring with him. [BOERHAVE, *Præl. ad Instit.*, vi, p. 255.[3]]

5. Staggering. [VAN EEMS, in *Bœrhave Prælect. de m. n.*, i, p. 236.[4]].

Intoxication. [BIERCHEN, *Tal om Kraftskador.*[5]]

Heaviness of the head.[6] [WATSON, l. c.]

Want of memory.

Loss of memory. [W. ROWLEY, *Seventy-four cases*, London, 1779.[7]]

10. Stupidity, the head is confused; difficulty of comprehending what he reads.

Stupefaction; he understands with difficulty what he reads.

After drinking he becomes stupid in the head.

Apoplexy. [LANGE, l. c., p. 20.]

Serous apoplexy. [COLLIN, *Annus Med.*, iii, Vindob., 1764, p. 104.[8]]

15. When walking in the open air, simple headache; he feels stupid; also in the morning till break-fast.

Violent headache, with vertigo, owing to which she remains seated in one spot, sad and speechless, for three or four days. [LANGE, l. c., p. 12.]

Sensation in the right half of the brain, as if a large foreign body were therein.

Gradually increasing, semilateral headache, like a pressing downwards, as from something heavy therein, and as if bruised, aggravated by moving the eyes towards the affected side of the head (aft. 2, 3. h.).

On the left side of the occiput (when walking) slow tearing (aft. $\frac{1}{4}$ h.). [*Fz.*]

20. In the morning, tearing pain through the temple (4th d.). [*Fz.*]

Tearing pain in the temporal region and aching in the forehead, after a meal (3rd d.). [*Fz.*]

Tearing pain in the temples when eating. [*Fz.*]

Drawing pain in the temples on touching them. [*Fz.*]

When sitting bent forward, there occurs from time to time a sensation of weight in the occiput, that often goes off and recurs; it went off every time he raised himself up (aft. $2\frac{1}{2}$ h.). [*Ws.*]

25. Stitches in the forehead.

---

1 Observation.
2 From thirty grains of the powder in an adult.
3 Observed on self.
4 Effects of Cicuta aquatica.
5 Observation.
6 During convalescence.
7 Not accessible.
8 Symptoms observed in patients taking conium. This occurred in an old woman of 80, ten days after leaving off the medicine.

(At noon) shooting pain out at the forehead.

Pressive headache above the eyes from within outwards (aft. 4 h.). [*Ws.*]

Headache (externally), as if contracted, on the upper part of the frontal bone, which goes off by stooping and applying his own hand to the part, with chilliness, vertigo, and peevish want of recollection (aft. $1\frac{1}{2}$ h.). [*Fz.*]

Aching pain externally on the forehead (aft. 3 h.), [*Lr.*]

30. Aching stupefying pain externally on the forehead (aft. 11, 54 h.). [*Lr.*]

On the frontal bone superiorly, pressive pain as from a stone [*Fz.*]

Sharp pressure on a small spot of the integuments of the head.

A pimple on the forehead with tensive pain *per se*, touching it causes tearing pain round about it (2nd and 3rd d.). [*Fz.*]

Pimple on the forehead with tensive drawing pain *per se* (4th d). [*Fz.*]

35. Itching erosion on the forehead, that goes off, but only for a short time, by rubbing (aft. $\frac{1}{2}$ h.). [*Ws.*]

Dilated pupils (aft. 1 h.). [*Fz.*]

Contracted pupils (curative action) (aft. $3\frac{1}{4}$ h.). [*Lr.*]

Longsightedness (in a shortsighted person) : he could see distinctly objects at a considerable distance (aft. $3\frac{1}{2}$ h.). [*Lr.*]

Greater shortsightedness than usual : he could only see distinctly very near objects (secondary action) (aft. 29 h.). [*Lr.*]

40. (Illusion of vision : objects appear red.) [GREDING, *Vermischte Schriften*, p. 118.[1]]

Weak sight. [GATAKER, l. c.]

Dimness of vision.[2] [BAYLIES,—ANDREE, l. c.]

Blindness, immediately after sleeping, exposed to the sun's heat. [AMATUS LUSITANUS, *Cent.* v, Cur. 93.[3]]

Red eyes. [BAYLIES, l. c.]

45. (Drawing pain in the eyes, with redness of the eyes.)

Trembling of the eyes. [WHYTT,—OBERTEUFFER, l. c.]

Projecting eyes.

Movement of the eyes, as if they were pressed out. [FOTHERGILI, l. c.]

(In the morning) shooting in the inner canthus of the eyes, the lids of which are stuck together.

50. **Itching pricking in the inner canthus, not removed by rubbing** (aft. $1\frac{1}{2}$ h.). [*Ws.*]

Smarting pain in the inner canthus, as if something corrosive had got in : the eye waters (aft. $4\frac{1}{2}$ h.). [*Ws.*]

Aching in the eyes as from a grain of sand, especially in the forenoon ; the white of the eye is red and inflamed ; the tears forced out make the eyelids smart.

---

1 Symptoms observed in patients taking conium. This symptom occurred in a case of cataract, while the sight was improving under the drug.

2 In Andree's case, with giddiness.

3 Not found.

Burning on the inner surface of the eyelids.

Long continued, pricking itching in the right cheek and down the left side of the face, which only goes off by repeated scratching (aft. 2½ h.). [*Fz.*]

55. A fine stitch darts through the right side of the face, near the zygoma (aft. 2½ h.). [*Ws.*]

Fine stitches dart through the right cheek, towards the commissure of the mouth (aft. 56 h.). [*Ws.*]

Swelling of the face. [LANDEUTTE, *Journal de Medecine*, xv.[1]]

Bluish, swollen face. [STOERCK, *Lib. de Cicuta*, Cap. 6.[2]]

Blue colour of the face. [SIM. PAULLI, *Quadrip. Botan., Cicuta major.*[3]]

60. Behind the ears and on the mastoid process, painful tension of the skin, even when not moved (aft. ½ h.). [*Ws.*]

Stitches behind both ears, especially in the mastoid process, followed by obtuse pains in that part (aft. 5 h.).

Sharp blows outwards in the inner ear, especially and more severe when swallowing (aft. ¾ h.). [*Ws.*]

Violent itching in the external ear (aft. 1 h.). [*Ws.*]

In the external ear, pain partly drawing, partly tearing.

65. Noise in the ear, as if the blood rushed through the brain.

When she blows her nose, she feels a dart in the ears, and then they seem to be stopped up.

Sensation as if the inner ear were forced asunder.

Twitching in the nose.

Formication on the dorsum of the nose (aft. 1½ h.). [*Ws.*]

70. Itching formication on the point of the nose and in the nostrils (aft. 3½ h.). [*Ws.*]

Itching formication in the nose (aft. 1½ h.). [*Ws.*]

Frequent bleeding of the nose.

Hæmorrhage from the nose. [EHRHARDT, *Diss. de Cicuta*, Argent., 1763[4]—LANGE, l. c., p. 15.]

Trembling of the under lip.[5] [STOERCK, l. c.]

75. Itching on the upper lip (aft. ½ h.).

Ulceration of the lips after fever.[6] [GREDING, l. c.]

On the chin, fine stitches up through the jaw (aft. ½ h.). [*Ws.*]

Soon after drinking a drawing from the jaws towards the ears and head, not exactly painful.

Lock-jaw (trismus). [EHRHARDT, l. c.]

---

1 Symptoms observed in patients taking conium. This, with S. 146, 172, 200, 234, 336, occurred shortly before death in a man convalescing from suppurative pneumonia, and treated by conium for splenic cancer.

2 Symptoms observed in patients taking conium. This, with S. 74, 103, 174, 328, 339, 362, arose from overloading the stomach. All disappeared after an emetic.

3 Not found.

4 A list of symptoms from authors.

5 See note to S. 58.

6 Should be, "breaking out on the lips, following slight fever."

80. Grinding of the teeth. [*Medic. Obs. and Inq.*, iv, Lond., 1771, p. 44.[1]]

On moving the lower jaw, boring needle-pricks between the left teeth-rows (aft. 42 h.). [*Lr.*]

When eating cold food (not when drinking cold fluids) drawing in the hollow tooth and through the temple (aft. 3 h.). [*Fz.*]

Impeded swallowing. [EHRHARDT, l. c.]

Spasms in the œsophagus. [EHRHARDT, l. c.]

85. Pain in the tongue. [SIM. PAULLI, l. c.]

Stiff, swollen, painful tongue.[2] [STOERCK, l. c., cap. i.]

Difficult speech. [ANDREE, l. c.]

Speechlessness.[3] [STOERCK.—EHRHARDT, l. c.]

Dry tongue. [BAYLIES, l. c.]

90. Dryness of the mouth. [STOERCK, l. c., cap. ii.]

Thirst.[4] [BAYLIES—FOTHERGILL, l. c.]

Excessive thirst, without heat, all day (aft. 74 h.). [*Lr.*]

Ptyalism.[5] [BIERCHEN, l. c.]

Great flow of saliva. [VALENTINI, in *Hufel Journal*, xxix, iii.[6]]

95. Immediately diminished appetite for food and tobacco-smoking.

Loss of appetite. [ANDRY,—*Pharm. Helv.*—LANGE, l. c., p. 25.—LANDEUTTE, l. c.]

Complete loss of appetite and great weakness of stomach. [LANGE, l. c., p. 9.]

Frequent eructation.

Incomplete eructation, which causes pain in the stomach.

100. Putrid eructation.[7] [SCHMUCKER, l. c.]

Eructation and inclination to vomit. [GREDING, l. c.]

Inclination to vomit and eructation, with exhaustion [GREDING, l. c.]

Nausea, inclination to vomit. [STOERCK.[8]—FOTHERGILL,—SCHMUCKER, l. c.]

Frequent nausea and total loss of appetite. [LANGE, l. c., pp. 14, 37.]

105. Inclination to vomit. [CULLEN, l. c.]

Violent vomiting. [EHRHARDT, l. c.]

Frequent vomiting, with total loss of appetite. [LANGE, l. c., p. 33.]

Sometimes there occurs spontaneously a bitter taste in the throat (aft. 11 h.). [*Fz.*]

---

1 Symptoms occurring after the application of conium to a cancerous breast. The patient had attacks of this, with S. 175 and 360, till she died. The reporter has no thought of ascribing them to the conium.

2 From touching the tongue with the juice of the root.

3 In Stoerck's case, as with S. 86.

4 According to Fothergill, with S. 121 and 346.

5 In cases of cancrum oris

6 Symptoms observed in patients taking conium.

7 Not found.

8 See note to S. 58.

After eating, inclination to vomit and hiccup thereafter, yet he has a proper taste and good appetite.

110. After eating, the drawing in the head and the numbness of the brain diminishes (aft. $4\frac{1}{2}$ h.). [*Fz.*]

After eating, oppression and hard pressure externally on the sternum (aft. $4\frac{1}{2}$ h.). [*Fz.*]

After eating (in the evening), pain in the umbilical region, as if the bowels were bruised (aft. 12 h.). [*Fz.*]

Half an hour after eating, drawing pain in the abdomen, in the umbilical region. [*Fz.*]

Every time after eating, pinching deep in the hypogastrium, with good appetite.

115. After dinner drawing pain in the hypogastrium when sitting (3rd d.). [*Fz.*]

After drinking, a drawing sensation in the abdomen.

In the morning, after eating, belly-ache, and all day a great fullness in the stomach and on the chest (4th d.). [*Fz.*]

Cardialgia. [*Pharm. Helv.*, l. c.]

A pressure in the scrobiculus cordis, like a drawing about in it, and then in the side of the chest some stitches, also in the morning.

120. Fine stitches in the scrobiculus cordis (aft. $\frac{1}{2}$ h.). [*Ws.*]

Spasmodic pinching in the stomach. [FOTHERGILL, l. c.]

Shooting in the epigastrium, in the morning on awaking, aggravated by movement.

Pinching pain in the abdomen, but not immediately before, and not immediately after, the stool.

Cutting pain deep in the hypogastrium, with appetite and sleep at night.

125. Belly-ache. [*Zurcher Abhandlungen*, tom. ii.[1]]

In the morning, after rising, drawing pain in the umbilical region (3rd d.). [*Fz.*]

Oppression in the abdomen.

Pressure and clawing in the abdomen.

When walking he has pains above the hips.

130. When laughing he has pain in the abdomen.

When walking drawing pain in the abdomen (aft. 3 h.). [*Fz.*]

Pain in the abdomen : drawing bruised pain in the bowels when sitting (aft. $9\frac{1}{2}$ h.). [*Fz.*]

Violent pains in the abdomen with chilliness.[2] [STOERCK, l. c.]

The most violent colic pains. [STOERCK, *Lib. de Colchico*, p, 89.[3]]

135. Extremely violent pains in the abdomen. [KALTSCHMIDT, *Progr. de Cicuta.*, Jan., 1768, p. 5.[4]]

---

1 Not accessible.

2 A patient under treatment by conium for a mammary scirrhus had a chill in the streets ; got this and S. 144 ; and died with dysentery.

3 A woman could not take more than four grains a day (of the extract) without having this.

4 Not accessible.

When not eating, constant pressure deep in the hypogastrium as from something heavy.

In the morning when sitting, drawing in the hypogastrium and pressure up to the epigastrium.

In the abdominal muscles, on the left of and below the navel, sharp stitches dart upwards in short fits (aft. 3 h.). [*Ws.*]

Fine pinching in the abdominal muscles above the navel on bending the body forwards (aft. 3 h.). [*Ws.*]

140. Tearing in the pubes, when sitting. [*Fz.*]

Immediately slight discharge of flatus.

Constant call to stool; but he can only evacuate twice daily, and the motion is thin.

Diarrhœa. [LANDEUTTE—EHRHARDT, l. c.]

Weakening diarrhœa.[1] [STOERCK, *de Cicuta*, cap. ii.]

145. Constipation.[2] [ANDREE, l. c.]

Swelling of the abdomen. [LANDEUTTE,[3]—EHRHARDT, l. c.]

Swollen mesenteric glands.* [KALTSCHMIDT, l. c.]

An extremely contracted place in the colon.* [KALTSCHMIDT, l.c.]

(Burning in the rectum during stool.)

150. Red urine. [BAYLIES, l. c.]

(Burning in the urethra, in the morning, immediately after urinating; for half an hour.)

(Violent stitch in the urethra, extending forwards to its orifice.)

Burning in the urethra. [STOERCK, l. c.]

Suppression of urine, ischuria. [BAYLIES, l. c.]

155. Strangury. [LANGE, l. c., p. 16.—EHRHARDT, l. c.]

Diuresis. [BIERCHEN,—GATAKER, l. c.]

Cramp-like pressure in the region of the neck of the bladder, from without inwards, with sharp stitches, soon after urinating, which lasts many hours, worse when walking than when sitting (aft. 48 h.). [*Ws.*]

Great pains in the urethra when urinating, which always brings along with it turbid, viscid mucus. [LANGE, l. c., pp. 28, 30.]

(A sharp pressure on the bladder.)

160. Diuresis with great pains. [LANGE, l. c.]

After urinating, a smarting urging to urinate (aft. ½ h.). [*Fz.*]

Hæmaturia.[4] [HALLER, in *Gotting. Anzeigen*, 1775, p. 62.]

Frequent hæmaturia with tightness of chest. [LANGE, l. c., p. 15.]

When not urinating, tearing through the penis (4th d.). [*Fz.*]

165. Itching on the penis, mostly on the glans.

Pain as if a knife were cutting through the middle of the

* Observed after death from a short employment of hemlock in large doses.

1 See note to S. 133.
2 In the original, "irregular stools, attended with griping."
3 See note to S. 57.
4 In a gouty subject.

scrotum, between the testicles up to above the root of the penis, often returning for a short time (aft. 50 h.). [*Ws.*]

Uncontrollable sexual desire. [LIMPRECHT,[1] *Acta Nat Cur.* i, Obs. 52.]

Leucorrhœa of white acrid mucus, which causes burning.* [BAYLIES, l. c.]

Suppression of the menses.[2] [ANDRY,—ANDREE,—GREDING, l. c.]

* * *

170. Frequent sneezing, without coryza (aft. 57 h.). [*Lr.*]

Frequent discharge of nasal mucus, for several days, as in coryza.

Difficult respiration.[3] [LANDEUTTE, l. c.]

Slow respiration.

Short, panting respiration.[4] [STOERCK, l. c.]

175. Tightness of chest. [*Medic. Obs. and Inquir.*[5]—LANGE, l. c., p. 21.]

Frequent tightness of chest. [LANGE, l. c., p. 21.]

Difficult respiration and violent pains in the chest (after taking it for three or four weeks). [LANGE, l. c., p. 11.]

His breathing, especially inspiration, is very difficult; it feels as if the chest did not expand sufficiently (aft. 4 h.). [*Fz.*]

In the evening in bed, extremely difficult respiration, slow, difficult inspiration (aft. 17 h.). [*Fz.*]

180. In the evening, when lying on the side in bed, oppression of the breathing, with much pain in the chest, a drawing and tearing through the whole chest, and hard pressure on the upper part of the sternum, which takes away the breath during inspiration (3rd d.). [*Fz.*]

Severe stitches in the chest, like knife thrusts, with loud lamentations over it.

All day, pain in the chest, pressure on the sternum, and a pain, at one time tearing, at another shooting, round the nipple and the mammæ, with frequent oppression and shortness of breath (4th d.). [*Fz.*]

Agreeable but violent itching on both nipples (aft. 4 h.).

In the region of the heart, occasional pressure as if the heart would be pressed down, with oppression of the breathing (3rd d.). [*Fz.*]

185. Pressive cutting on both sides of the chest, aggravated by inspiration (aft. 14 h.). [*Ws.*]

In the morning, pressive pain on the sternum, with dyspnœa, when standing (3rd d.). [*Fz.*]

* Is a very good remedy for the same symptoms.

---

1 Poisoning by "cicuta" root, but of what species is doubtful.—Inordinate excitement was present, but nothing is said as to its being sexual.

2 Checked while on her in Andree's case; in Greding's delayed.

3 See note to S. 57.

4 See note to S. 58.

5 See note to S. 80.

Cramp-like tearing on the right side of the chest (aft. 3 h.). [*Lr.*]

Burning in the sternal region.[1] [STOERCK, l. c.]

On walking in the open air, needle-pricks in the right side of the chest (aft. 12 h.). [*Lr.*]

190. Shooting itching all over the chest, which was always removed for a short time only by scratching (aft 1 h.). [*Ws.*]

On both sides of the chest, fine shooting pressure, worst when he lies in the prone position (aft. 9 h.). [*Ws.*]

Stitch in the side.[2] [STOERCK, l. c.]

Violent pains in the chest. [LANGE, l. c., p. 34.]

Violent pain in the chest, with very severe cough.* [LANGE, l. c., p. 16.]

195. (There is a scraping and crawling in the chest, that causes a dry almost continual cough.)

Dry short cough.[3] [STOERCK, l. c.]

Nocturnal cough.[4] [STOERCK, l. c.]

Violent cough. [LANGE, l. c.]

Whooping cough, with tightness of chest. [LANGE, l. c., p. 22.]

200. Nocturnal whooping cough.[5] [LANDEUTTE, l. c.]

Whooping cough, with bloody mucous expectoration.† [LANGE, l. c., p. 11.]

The most violent cough, that made him keep his bed.[6] [STOERCK, *Lib. de Stram., Hyos. et Acon.*, p. 93.]

Cough as from a tickle behind the middle of the sternum, without expectoration (aft. 24 h.). [*Lr.*]

More severe cough, as from a tickle in the middle of the sternum, with expectoration (aft. 24 h.). [*Lr.*]

205. Purulent expectoration from the chest.[7] [STOERCK, *Lib. de Cicuta*, cap. ii.]

Dryness of the chest.[8] [STOERCK, l. c.]

(Inflammation of the scirrhous mamma.) [LANGE, l. c., p. 33.]

Fine stitches in the chest under the left axilla (aft. $\frac{1}{4}$ h.). [*Ws.*]

Caries of the sternum. [KALTSCHMIDT, l. c.]

210. Drawing on the right side of the neck down to the shoulder-joint, when at rest (3rd d.). [*Fz.*]

When walking in the open air, drawing in the nape (aft. 1 h.). [*Fr.*]

(Increased swelling of the goitre.)

* Relieved by opium.

† After taking it for several weeks.

---

1 From injecting a solution of conium into a penetrating fistula in the neck.

2 In a case of caries of the ribs.

3 In a case of suppurating mammary scirrhus, this and S. 206 coincided with the expectoration becoming thin.

4 Not found.

5 In the original, simply "urgent cough". See note to S. 57.

6 This supervened in a case of tubercle of the breast while taking conium.

7 In a case of mammary scirrhus, when the lungs were found cancerous after death.

8 See note to S. 196.

Stitches in the sacrum and drawing through the lumbar vertebræ when standing (aft. 3½ h.). [*Fz.*]

Drawing through the lumbar vertebræ, when standing (aft. ½ h.). [*Fz.*]

215. Tensive pain in the back.[1] [STOERCK, l. c.]

Under both scapulæ, painful tension in the muscles, when at rest that is very much increased by raising up the arms (aft. 24 h.). [*Ws.*]

In the nape where it passes into the right shoulder, throbbing drawing (aft. 8 h.). [*Fz.*]

In the upper arm, paralytic drawing pain, when at rest (aft. 1½ h.). [*Fz.*]

Tearing through the upper arm, in the evening in bed (the first evening). [*Fz.*]

220. Alternate tearing and shooting in the upper arm, when at rest which goes off by movement, but comes back again (aft. 3 d.). [*Fz.*]

Heaviness in the elbow-joints, with fine stitches.

Cutting pain in the bend of the left elbow, from within outwards, when at rest (aft. 50 h.). [*Ws.*]

Dull drawing in the forearms, more severe when at rest than when moving (aft. 72 h.). [*Ws.*]

On the outside of the left forearm, bruised pain, most severe when touched (aft. 62 h.). [*Ws.*]

225. In the muscles of the forearm, cramp-like pain, especially when leaning on the arms (aft. ½ h.). [*Ws.*]

Itching formication on the foreasm, that goes off only for a short time by rubbing (aft. 1 h.). [*Ws.*]

In the wrist-joint, paralytic drawing pain, when at rest (aft. 1½ h.). [*Fz.*]

Fine stitches in the wrist-joints (aft. 10 m.). [*Ws.*]

(Shooting dislocation-pain in the articulation of the metacarpal bone of the left thumb with the wrist, especially on bending it inwards.)

230. Sharp stitches in the middle joints of the fingers (when at rest). (aft. 8 h.). [*Ws.*]

Cutting blows in the proximal joint of the thumb (aft. 48 h.). [*Ws.*]

Long-continued, deep stitch superiorly at the insertion of the right gluteus maximus (aft. 3½ h.). [*Fz.*]

While sitting, some obtuse stitches on the upper end of the left thigh, near the trochanter, that do not interfere with walking (aft. ¼ h.). [*Ws.*]

Swollen thighs.[2] [LANDEUTTE, l. c.]

235. When sitting, needle-pricks in the muscles of the left thigh (aft. 26 h.). [*Lr.*]

Itching needle-pricks on the posterior aspect of the thigh, most severe when sitting (aft. 8 h.). [*Ws.*]

---

1 See note to S. 188.
2 See note to S. 57.

Dull drawing in the right thigh, when at rest, which was alleviated by movement (aft. $1\frac{1}{4}$ h.). [*Ws.*]

When walking in the open air, cramp-like pain in the anterior muscles of the right thigh (aft. 13 h.). [*Lr.*]

Fine clawing-in on the posterior aspect of the thigh (aft. 12 h.). [*Ws.*]

240. Tearing around the patella, when sitting (aft. $2\frac{1}{2}$ h.). [*Fz.*]

When walking, and even when standing in the open air, extreme pain, causing him to cry out, round the whole left knee, as if the patella were bruised and smashed, from which when he makes an effort to walk he became hot all over, like the heat of anguish (aft. 10 h.). [*Lr.*]

Tearing pain around the knee-joint.

When walking in the open air, stitches on the outer tendon of the flexor muscle in the right hough (aft. 1 h.). [*Fz.*]

Tearing on the tibia, in the evening in bed (the first evening). [*Fz.*]

245. Cramp like tearing now on the right, now on the left tibia, when walking in the open air (aft. 37 h.). [*Lr.*]

The tibia pains as if bruised (4th d.). [*Fz.*]

On stretching out the leg, when sitting, a throbbing pressure on the tibia (aft. $3\frac{1}{2}$ h.). [*Fz.*]

A spot on the leg that had been injured (twelve days before by a blow), and was hitherto painless, becomes blue and spotted, and on the slightest movement gets pain like knife thrusts, but when walking and when touched it pains as if bruised.

Tensive stiff pain in the calves.

250. Drawing on the inner side of the left calf, and on the dorsum of the right foot (aft. 8 h.). [*Fz.*]

At first a fine, then a severe, shooting on both ankles of the right foot, which lasted two days, and woke him up at night ; it went at last to the calf also ; when sitting they were slower, when walking more frequent and severer stitches.

At night a twitching and uneasiness in the feet, and, after every twitch in them, shivering.

Numbness and insensibility of the feet.

Numbness and insensibility of the feet. [HALLE, in *Samml. f. pr. Aerzte*, xv, iii.]

255. Brings on podagra. [CLARK, in *Essays and Obs. Phys. and Liter.*, iii, Edin., 1771[1]]

Tearing on the dorsum of the foot, in the evening in bed (the first evening). [*Fz.*]

In the morning tearing in the ball of the big toe, when standing and sitting (third day). [*Fz.*]

On treading the sole of the foot is painful like formication ; on walking the pain is more shooting.

Tearing in the soles when walking.

260. Itching on the limbs. [STOERCK, l. c.]

---

1 Observation.—In gouty subjects, the author says.

Bruised sensation in all the joints, when at rest, but little or not at all when moving.

Formication and disagreeable itching in the glands.[1] [STOERCK, l. c.]

Formication in the affected part. [COLLIN, l. c.]

In the evening the glands are painful.[2] [STOERCK, l. c.]

265. Increased intolerable pains in the affected part. [LANGE, l. c., pp. 9, 25, 33.]

Fœtid ichor from the ulcer.[3] [STOERCK, l. c.]

The borders of the ulcer become blackish and discharge a fœtid ichor.[3] [STOERCK, l. c.]

Bleeding of the ulcer.[4] [GREDING, l. c.]

Increased pain in the ulcer.[3] [STOERCK, l. c.]

270. Tensive pain in the ulcer.[3] [STOERCK, l. c.]

Coughing causes pain in the ulcer.[5] [STOERCK, l. c.]

Sphacelus of a part of the ulcer.[6] [GREDING, l. c.]

In the bones, especially in the middle of the bone-shafts, concealed caries, with burning, gnawing pain.[7] [STOERCK, l. c.]

Here and there on the body, slow, itching, smarting (burning) stitches.

275. In the evening in bed, an eroding itching, always commencing with a prick, only on the right half of the body, especially when he lies on it, which causes a restlessness in all the limbs, is readily allayed by scratching, but soon reappears on another spot.

Inflammation of the skin of the whole body, with burning pain. [BAYLIES, l, c.]

Tearing through various parts of the body (4th d.). [*Fz.*]

Blue colour of the whole body. [EHRHARDT, l. c.]

Dropsy. [TARTREUX, *Epis. Apol.*, p. 51.[8]]

280. Petechiæ. [SIM. PAULLI, l. c.]

Putrid dissolution of the juices. [REISMANN, l. c.[9]]

Consumption. [REISMANN,—COLLIN, l. c.[10]]

The pains from hemlock mostly occur when at rest and, only as a rare alternating action, during movement. [*Fz.*]

Nervous weakness.[11] [SCHMUCKER, l. c.]

285. Illusion of sensation : when walking he feels as if something opposed his steps, and yet he walked very quickly (aft. 8 h.). [*Fz.*]

A kind of stiffness of the body ; moving the joints of the nape, &c., causes a disagreeable sensation.

Great exhaustion.

---

1 Not found.
2 In a case of scirrhous mamma.
3 Variations of an open cancer of the face while the patient took conium.
4 In mammary cancer.
5 See note to S. 205.
6 Not found ; but if there, probably as in note[4].
7 Not found.
8 Observations on patients.—This was the end of a case of mammary cancer.
9 Not traceable for want of reference.
10 In Collin's case the end of mesenteric disease.
11 After taking conium for seven months.

In the evening and morning, a remarkable exhaustion in the whole body.

In the morning on waking, exhaustion, that goes off after getting up.

290. Weakness of the whole body. [WHYTT, l. c.]

Sinking of all the forces.*[1] [STOERCK, l. c.]

Paralysis. [ANDRY,—ANDREE, l. c.]

After a short walk he feels very exhausted and fatigued, and is as if paralysed, whereupon the peevish, hypochondriacal humour comes on again (aft. 10 h.). [*Fz.*]

Syncopes. [LANGE, l. c., p. 9.—*Pharm. Helv.*, l. c.]

295. Pulselessness. [SIM. PAULLI, l. c.]

The strongest and most active persons, when taking hemlock for a length of time, lost all strength and had to keep their bed. [LANGE, l. c., p. 9.]

Loss of all strength (even to death). [LANGE, l. c.]

Laziness combined with insensibility (torpor). [SIM. PAULLI, l. c.]

Obtuseness of all the senses. [SIM. PAULLI, l. c.]

300. Frequent yawning, as if he had not slept enough (aft. 72 h.). [*Lr.*]

When he gets up in the morning, he is sleepy.

Sleepiness by day : he cannot keep awake while reading (aft. 3, 8 h.). [*Ws.*]

Somnolence.[2] [WATSON,—SIM. PAULLI, l. c.]

Drowsiness (in the afternoon) : **with all his efforts he could not keep off sleep, he must lie down and sleep** (aft. 54 h.). [*Lr.*]

305. In the evening great drowsiness and disinclination for everything (the 3rd evening). [*Fz.*]

In the evening in bed, tearing now in one now in another limb (the first evening). [*Fz.*]

Dreams of serious diseases.

Dream full of being made ashamed.

In sleep, vivid, voluptuous dream-pictures (the first night). [*Lr.*]

310. Vivid anxious dreams (the second night). [*Lr.*]

Sleep at night full of frightful dreams (the third night). [*Fz.*]

Sleep towards morning full of frightful dreams (the first night). [*Fz.*]

Sleep. [CULLEN, l. c.—(immediately) AMATUS LUSITANUS, l. c.]

Stupefied, too deep sleep, after which the headache, which previously was scarcely noticed, becomes always increased (aft. 2 h.)

315. Sleep quiet, especially in the morning very profound and longer than usual† (the second night). [*Fz.*]

* For which STOERCK found cinchona-bark useful,

† Curative reaction ?

---

1 In case described in note to S. 196. This and S. 334 supervened on free purulent discharge setting in.

2 In Watson's case this represents "coma" in the original.

Interrupted sleep.

He only gets to sleep after midnight.

He wakes up earlier in the morning.

She becomes peevish and falls asleep (aft. ½ h.). ; during sleep twitchings in the arms and hands, the eyes are staring open and roll about.

320. Sleeplessness. [REISMANN,—LANGE, l. c., p. 9.]

Trembling. [BAYLIES,—CULLEN,—EHRHARDT, l. c.]

Trembling of all the limbs[1] [FOTHERGILL.—SCHMUCKER,* l. c.]

Constant trembling. [ANDRY, l. c.]

Subsultus tendinum. [EHRHARDT, l. c.]

325. Convulsions. [ANDRY,—WATSON,—CULLEN, l. c.]

Convulsions of the affected part and of all the body, with danger of suffocation. [LANGE, l. c., p. 14.]

Shivering (immediately).

Shivering.[2] [STOERCK, l. c.]

Chilliness, with trembling in all the limbs, so that she must always remain in the sun.

330. On several successive days, in the morning (about 8 o'clock), shivering for half an hour.

Rigor all over the body, without either accompanying or subsequent heat (aft. 15 h.). [*Lr.*]

Rigor all over the body, without heat or thirst (aft. 50 h.). [*Lr.*]

In the morning, coldness and chilliness of the body, with giddy constriction of the brain, and indifferent, dejected humour (aft. 2, 3 h.). [*Fz.*]

From time to time shivering all over the body, followed by quick pulse with heat and thirst.[3] [STOERCK, l. c.]

335. Fever. ANDREE,—COLLIN, l. c.]

Fever for one day. [LANDEUTTE, l. c.]

Large, slow pulse, betwixt which several small quick beats follow without regularity.

Slow, weak pulse. [SIM. PAULLI, l. c.]

Pulse irregular as to strength and rapidity.[4] [STOERCK, l. c.]

340. Quick pulse. [EHRHARDT, l. c.]

Several fits of fever.[5] [TARTREUX, l. c.]

Lingering fever with complete anorexia. [LANGE, l. c., p. 25.]

Acute (fatal) fever. [LANGE, l. c., p. 32.]

Fever: great heat, with profuse sweat and thirst, with loss of appetite, diarrhœa, and vomiting. [GREDING, l. c.]

345. In the afternoon flush of warmth all over the body, without thirst. [*Fz.*]

* Sometimes life-long.

1 Not found in Schmucker.

2 See note to S. 58.

3 See note to S. 291.

4 See note to S. 58.

5 See note to S. 279. The words of the original are, "after various fevers the woman died dropsical.

Heat. [BAYLIES,—FOTHERGILL, l. c.]

Sensation of internal and external heat (after sleep.)

Continual heat.

Great heat. [STOERCK, l. c.]

350. Internal heat, especially in the face, and redness of it, without thirst (aft. ¼ h.). [*Ws.*]

He became red in the face and all over the body, without particular heat, but perspired all over, especially on the forehead.

Excessive heat. [BAYLIES, l. c.]

In the afternoon (5 to 6 hours after rigor and coldness) a feeling comes over him of growing heat in all the limbs, whereupon the numbness of the head and the different sad humour goes off, and in place thereof he takes the liveliest interest in all around him (aft. 7, 8 h.). [*Fz.*]

Transpiration.[1] [GATAKER, l. c.]

355. Night sweat.

On awaking from sleep he finds himself in a gentle perspiration all over the body (the third night). [*Lr.*]

Profuse sweat after midnight.

Local, fœtid, pungent perspiration, with eruption of white, transparent papules, which, filled with an acrid fluid, change into a scab, like scabies.[2] [STOERCK, l. c.]

Anxiety.[3] [SCHMUCKER, l. c.]

360. Hysterical anxiety.[4] [*Medic. Obs. and Inquir.*, l. c.]

Attack of hysteria, with chilliness and a kind of spasmodic movements.[5] [GREDING, l. c.]

Anxiety in the region of the scrobiculus cordis.[6] [STOERCK, l. c.]

Extremely peevish and anxious thoughts after a meal, in the morning, with confusion of the head in the forehead (aft. 29 h.). [*Fz.*]

When walking in the open air, hypochondriacal indifference and dejection (aft. 1 h.). [*Fz.*]

365. Sunk in deep thought, he cogitated timorously about the present and the future and sought solitude. [*Lr.*]

Cross temper : everything about him made a disagreeable impression on him. [*Lr.*]

Peevish disposition ; he knows not what to occupy himself with, the time appears to pass too slowly (aft. 8 h.). [*Ws.*]

Constant ill-humour and crossness.

Disposition devoid of all agreeable feelings.

370. Cheerful disposition ; he was inclined to speak* (aft. 10 h.). [*Lr.*]

* The previous opposite state of the disposition went off by the curative reaction of the organism.

---

1 *i.e.* Slight perspiration.
2 Critical, in a gouty patient.
3 Not found.
4 See note to S. 80.
5 Not found.
6 See note to S. 58.

In the morning, well, cheerful and strong* (aft. 24 h.). [*Fz.*]
Disposition cheerful and free† (3rd, 4th d.). [*Fz.*]
Confused thoughts. [VAN EEMS, l. c.]
Delirium. [ANDRY, l. c.]
375. Mania, delirium. [CULLEN, l. c.].

* Alternating curative reaction of the organism.
† Curative reaction of the vitality.

CYCLAMEN EUROPÆUM.[1]

(Sowbread.)

(The expressed juice of the fresh root, obtained in autumn, mixed with equal parts of alcohol.)

From the earliest times this valuable plant has lain under the unfounded suspicion of acting violently and uncertainly. Even should we grant that Discorides really referred to this plant, still all he says about it was only from hearsay. The Arabians employed this root under the name of *Arthanita* as one of the ingredients of a purgative ointment for rubbing in (*unguentum de Arthanita*), which contains a number of the most powerful purgative remedies, and in this dangerous combination they brought it into the unmerited reputation of a drastic purgative medicine, which it is far from being.

Modern physicians know nothing more respecting it, scarcely as much as the ancients romanced about it.

But as our new (homœopathic) medical art takes nothing on the authority of unintelligent tradition, and neither accepts anything because it has been praised, nor rejects it because it has been condemned, without having first subjected it to impartial trial, I undertook the investigation of this much decried root.

Just as the virtue of a man cannot be determined by the deceptive appearance of his outward form, nor by the colour of his coat, nor by the shallow gossip of the multitude, but as it assuredly displays itself in no doubtful manner to the honest observer in the goodness of his conduct, so, truly, the real value of a medicine can be determined neither by its outward appearance, nor by any unfounded reputation it may have obtained. It is only by our own careful proving of medicines on healthy persons that we can truly learn what are the peculiar qualities of a medicine, what changes it can produce in the health, and thence the similar changes in the sick it can cure.

And so from the following few pure symptoms we may learn that cyclamen is one of the most excellent remedies in the most desperate morbid states.

Hitherto I have given it in a very small portion of a drop of the million-fold dilution of the juice, but even this I have found to be a too strong homœopathic dose for many cases.

[HAHNEMANN (who only contributed five symptoms) was aided in this proving by FRANZ, HARTUNG, HERRMANN, LANGHAMMER.

He only cites one old-school authority for one symptom.

ABANO, PETRUS DE, *De Venenis*.

The 1st edition has 200 symptoms, only two more appear in this 2nd edition.]

1 From vol. v, 2nd edit., 1826.

CYCLAMEN.

The memory is sometimes very obtuse, and he can hardly recollect what has occurred quite recently; but sometimes it is very active—in quick alternation. [*Fz.*]

His mind is in a constant state of stupefaction, all its powers are in abeyance; he can neither rejoice nor be sad, although he is always as if after some great (though passed) sorrow; only when he is excited his head becomes somewhat clearer, and he behaves like a person wakened up from sleep, having only half understood what has happened about him (2nd d.). [*Fz.*]

Obtuseness of the mind; he is neither inclined for, nor capable of any work (3rd d.). [*Fz.*]

Vertigo: on standing still when he leans against something, he feels as if the brain moved in the head, or as if he was riding in a carriage with his eyes shut. [*Fz.*]

5. Dizziness in the head. [*Hrr.*]

Continual stitches in the fore part of his brain, on stooping.

When lying in bed in the evening, perceptible pulsation in the brain and delay in falling asleep.

Dull pain in the occiput. [*Htg.*]

Painful drawing in the brain from the left side of the occiput forwards, through the left temple to the forehead, in a line (aft. 1 h.). [*Hrr.*]

10. Slight pressure in the vertex, as if the brain were enveloped in a cloth, and he were thereby deprived of consciousness (2nd d.). [*Fz.*]

Aching pain in the middle of the vertex, that sometimes causes dizziness. [*Fz.*]

Aching drawing pain from the right side of the forehead to the left, and then back again to the right side; then in the left temple; the pain went off on touching (aft. 9 h.). [*Lr.*]

Dull stitches in the right temporal region in all position (aft. 3 h.). [*Lr.*]

Some drawing stitches in the left temporal region, that went off on touching (aft. 16 h.). [*Lr.*]

15. Twitching stitches, first in the left, then in the right temporal region. [*Htg.*]

Pains in the head with yawning, without drowsiness (aft. 5 h.). [*Lr.*]

Tearing pressive pain, externally on the head. [*Fz.*]

Fine, sharp, itching pricking on the hairy scalp, which, when he scratches, always recommences on another spot. [*Fz.*]

Breaking out of an eruption of pimples on the hairy scalp of the occiput, without sensation, and painless even when touched (aft. 1½ h.). [*Lr.*]

20. **Dilatation of the pupils** (aft. 1½ h.). [*Lr.*]

Extreme dilatation of the pupils, especially of the right eye (aft. 15½ h.). [*Lr.*]

Aching stupefaction of the whole head with dimness of vision; there seemed to be a mist before the eyes and the eyes were as if forcibly closed (aft. 1 h.). [*Lr.*]

Dimness of vision* (aft. 1½ h.). [*Lr.*]

Swelling of the upper eyelids (without dilatation of the pupils) (aft. 1 h.). [*Lr.*]

25. The eyes lie deep in the orbits and have a dull appearance (aft. 1½ h.). [*Hrn.*]

Dryness and aching in the eyelids, as if they were swollen, with violent itching pricking in them and in the eye-balls (aft. 7 h.). [*Fz.*]

Obtuse stitches on the right eye-ball and the upper eyelid (aft. 4 h.). [*Hrn.*]

In the eyes and lids a fine pricking, penetrating itching. [*Fz.*]

Fine tearing in the interior of the left meatus auditorius. [*Hrn.*]

30. **Drawing pain in the interior of the right meatus auditorius**; he then hears less distinctly with this ear (aft. ½ h.). [*Hrn.*]

The right ear feels as if stopped up with cotton wool, or as if something were held before the ear, so that the sound cannot properly penetrate into it (aft. 36 h.). [*Hrn.*]

Itching pricking in the right cheek, that becomes always stronger, then goes off of itself and leaves behind it a burning on the spot. [*Fz.*]

Diminished power of smelling. [*Fz.*]

Dry lips, without thirst. [*Htg.*]

35. In the upper lip, numb sensation, or as if there were an induration in it. [*Fz.*]

Violent stitches in the farthest back hollow molar of the upper jaw (aft. 15½ h.). [*Lr.*]

Tearing pain in the three left molars, as if the teeth were being drawn out. [*Htg.*]

(An existing, dull drawing toothache, that had lasted all night, went off in a minute.†) [*Fz.*]

Very white furred tongue, for three days (aft. 8 h.). [*Lr.*]

40. Fine stitches on the tongue (aft. 2 h.). [*Fz.*]

Drawing bruised pain deep in the muscles of the throat, which spreads internally down to the œsophagus and there causes a feeling of tension (aft. 10 h.). [*Fz.*]

Aching drawing pain in the submaxillary gland, when he bends his neck forwards. [*Fz.*]

Nausea, with flow of water into the mouth, like water-brash (aft. 1 h.). [*Lr.*]

In the evening and all day, very frequently accumulation of water in the mouth and imperfect eructation with the taste of food. [*Fz.*]

* Hence this root has proved serviceable in dimness of vision from cold, SIMON PAULLI, JOS, LANZONI, in *Misc. Nat. Cur.*, Dec. ii. An. 10, Obs. 133.

† Reaction of the organism, secondary action.

45. Nausea and running of water out of the mouth, like water-brash (aft. 5 h.). [*Lr.*]

In the evening great dryness in the palate, with thirst and hunger. [*Fz.*]

In the mouth a continual rough, slimy feeling, as if he had not rinsed his mouth out in the morning. [*Fz.*]

Empty eructation, soon after a meal (aft. 7¾ h.). [*Lr.*]

Frequent, sometimes acid, eructation. [*Hrn.*]

50. Eructation, in the morning after a meal, that always ended with a hiccup, and during which a fluid with burnt taste rises up into the fauces. [*Fz.*]

In the morning after the (accustomed) tobacco-smoking, nausea and fulness in the chest, attended by unusual hunger (aft. 3 h.). [*Fz.*]

Little hunger and little appetite. [*Hrn.*]

No appetite for breakfast. [*Hrn.*]

If he takes but a small quantity of food, the remainder is repugnant to him and excites loathing, and he feels nausea in the palate and throat (aft. 27 h.). [*Hrn.*]

55. **Complete anorexia ; he has no relish especially for breakfast and supper ; as soon as he commences to eat at these times he is immediately satiated** [*Hrn.*]

Fulness in the stomach, as if it were overloaded, and six hours after a meal, incomplete eructation with the taste of the food. [*Fz.*]

For eight days he could eat but little and felt always satiated. [*Hrn..*]

Sudden bad, putrid taste in the mouth. [*Fz.*]

He has dislike to bread and butter ; warm food goes down better. [*Hrn.*]

60. His food has a good taste, but whilst eating and some time thereafter he gets hiccup—a hiccupping eructation. [*Fz.*]

Food has for him a flat, almost no, taste. [*Hrn.*]

Adipsia, for four days. [*Hrn.*]

After four days the thirst returned and was sometimes more intense than in his normal condition. [*Hrn.*]

After dinner and supper nausea with inclination to vomit, squeamishness and qualmishness in the gastric region, as from eating too much fat.

65. Drowsiness after a meal (aft. 6½ h). [*Lr.*]

After dinner great drowsiness and weariness. [*Fz.*]

Hiccup after a meal (aft. 14½ h.). [*Lr.*]

All day long, pressure and fulness in the scrobiculus cordis, as from overloaded stomach. [*Fz.*]

Tearing stitches penetrating through and through in the epigastrium below the stomach, on moving. [*Fz.*]

70. **Immediately after a meal rumbling in the hypogastrium, and this recurred every day** (aft. 24 h.). [*Hrn.*]

Discomfort in the hypogastrium with some nausea therein. [*Hrn.*]

Bellyache (aft. 14 h.). [*Lr.*]

Pinching pain in the hypogastrium (aft. ½ h.). [*Hrn.*]

Pinching, cutting pain in the hypogastrium ; it comes on suddenly at various periods and goes off quickly (aft. 2 h.). [*Hrn.*]

75. Obtuse shooting pains in the bowels under the hepatic region. [*Htg.*]

In the epigastrium a paralytic, aching sensation, as if one portion of the bowels were loose and a tension occurred in the neighbouring parts. [*Fz.*]

Squeezing and pressive pain from without inwards in the hypogastrium. [*Htn.*[1]]

Single stitches dart through the abdomen, when he moves (4th d.). [*Fz.*]

Pinching in the epigastrium, as if diarrhœa would ensue, and shortly afterwards a yellow, soft stool, with recurring persistent pinching in the abdomen (aft. ¼ h.), whereupon constipation lasting three days ensued. [*Fz.*]

80. The right side of the abdomen beneath the navel seems to him swollen and distended in the morning ; an illusory sensation. [*Fz.*]

The hypogastrium is painful on the slightest touch, sometimes with an aching, sometimes a pinching pain, sometimes with a mixture of the two. [*Hrn.*]

After discharge of flatus, rumbling in the hypogastrium (aft. 1 h.). [*Lr.*]

Pappy stool (aft. 15 h.). [*Lr.*]

Frequent evacuation of hard stool (aft 10 h.). [*Lr.*]

85. No stool the second day. [*Fz.*]

Inside and outside the anus and in the perinæum drawing aching pain, as if a part there were gathering, when walking and sitting. [*Fz.*]

Frequent call to urinate, without pains (aft. 1 h.). [*Lr.*]

Frequent copious discharge of a whitish urine (aft. 4 h.). [*Fz.*]

The second day he only urinated twice. [*Fz.*]

90. Frequent urging to urinate with scanty flow of urine (aft. 15 h.). [*Lr.*]

Shooting pain in the front of the urethra when urinating (aft. 7½ h.). [*Lr.*]

* * *

Sneezing from the smell of the juice (aft. ½ h.). [*Lr.*]

Sudden violent fluent coryza (aft. 1½ h.). [*Lr.*]

Fluent coryza and several times sneezing therewith (aft. 7 h.). [*Lr.*]

95. Short cough (aft. ½ h.). [*Lr.*]

Oppression of chest with difficult respiration. [*Htg.*]

Suffocation, strangulation. [Petrus de Abano, *de Venenis*, cap. 22.[2]]

---

1 In original "*Hartmann,*" but this is apparently a misprint for *Hartung* or *Herrmann*, as Hartmann is not credited with any other symptom.

2 Statement from observation.

In the evening great exhaustion and shortness of breath ; he feels as if he had not strength enough to draw a full breath (aft. 8½ h.). [*Fz.*]

Pressive pain in the left side of the chest, especially about the precordial region, as if too much blood had accumulated there, with perceptible palpitation of the heart. [*Htg.*]

100. When sitting still, paralytic pressure on the chest, upper arm and tibia (aft. 8 h.). [*Fz.*]

On the upper part of the sternum sharp, broad stitches, recurring at irregular intervals (aft. 32 h.). [*Hrn.*]

On the chest, while moving and when at rest, tearing stitches, with tightness of the chest and dyspnœa, the second day. [*Fz.*]

Tearing stitches on the last true rib on bending the body forwards. [*Fz.*]

Rheumatic drawing in the left side of the nape, only whenever he bends back his head (aft. ½ h.). [*Fz.*]

105. Externally and internally on the nape, sore excoriated sensation. [*Fz.*]

Aching paralytic pain in the nape, which goes off on bending back the head. [*Fz.*]

In the evening, drawing (rheumatic) pain on the left side of the neck, on moving the head, whilst there was a sensation of heat in the cervical muscles and on the left ear. [*Fz.*]

Some deep penetrating, pinching, obtuse stitches which recur in equal periods of a few seconds (on the right side near the spine, betwixt the os innominatum and the last false rib), in the renal region, more severe on inspiration, which is impeded by the excessive pain (aft. 28 h.). [*Hrn.*]

When sitting stitch-like pains in the back on the left side in the region of the false ribs, which go off on touching (aft. 15 h.). [*Lr.*]

110. Drawing down the back, which is alleviated by drawing back the scapulæ, but increased by drawing the shoulders forwards (aft. 7 h.). [*Fz.*]

Rheumatic drawing in the left gluteus maximus, at its superior insertion in the os ilii towards the sacrum, when sitting, which goes off on standing up (aft. 7 h.). [*Fz.*]

Tearing ending in a stitch over the scapulæ with paralytic pain in the arm. [*Fz.*]

A kind of paralytic, hard pressure on the right upper and fore-arm, feeling as if in the periosteum and quite in the interior of the muscles ; it extends thence into the fingers and hinders him in writing (aft. 37 h.). [*Hrn.*]

Drawing pain on the left arm extending into the fingers.

115. Pain over the outer aspect of the elbow-joint, as from a blow, or contusion, or as if bruised, still more painful when moving the arm and when touching the part, for three days (aft. 25 h.). [*Lr.*]

Painful drawing in the inner aspect of the shaft of the ulna and in the wrist-joint (aft. 38 h.). [*Hrn.*]

A kind of paralytic, hard pressure, which commences only feebly in the forearm, but thence extends into the fingers, where

it becomes so violent that it is only with the greatest effort he can write. [*Hrn.*]

Stitch-like pain in the muscles of the right forearm, during rest and motion (aft. 2 h.). [*Lr.*]

Fine tearing on the left radius near and in the wrist-joint, feeling as if in the periosteum (aft. ¾ h.). [*Hrn.*]

120. Aching on the back of the left hand. [*Fz.*]

Tearing in the little, middle and ring fingers of the left hand, feeling as if in their periosteum (aft. ¾ h.). [*Hrn.*]

Spasmodic slow bending of the right thumb and index, the points of which approach one another, and which must be extended by force (aft. 5½ h.). [*Lr.*]

Between the fingers a quick and fine pricking itching as with needles, which goes off immediately by scratching entirely and without any after-sensation (aft. 6 h.). [*Fz.*]

After severe itching a red vesicle appears on the middle joint of the little finger of the left hand (aft. 15½ h.). [*Lr.*]

125. After violent itching that compelled him to scratch, there appeared a red pimple on the proximal joint of the ring-finger, which soon became white like a blister, surrounded by a red areola (aft. 1½ h.). [*Lr.*]

Weakness in the thighs and legs; on standing a long time they totter hither and thither (aft. ½ h.). [*Hrn.*]

Cramp-like pain in the thigh posteriorly above the right hough (aft. 8 h.). [*Hrn.*]

Spots half an inch in diameter of deep red colour, like burns, on both thighs (aft. 10½ h.). [*Lr.*]

Internal twitching under the left knee. [*Fz.*]

130. Sometimes on one knee, sometimes on the other, a pressive bruised pain, which goes off on moving the knee (aft. 11 h.). [*Fz.*]

In the ligaments of the knee-joint a stretching, aching drawing, when sitting and standing. [*Fz.*]

In the evening, heat in the whole of the left leg and drawing pain in it when sitting. [*Fz.*]

Stitch-like pain in the muscles of the right calf, when at rest and when moving (aft. 2 h.). [*Lr.*]

Itching in the skin of the calf (aft. 6 h.). [*Lr.*]

135. Severe itching in the skin of the right calf, so that he must scratch till the blood came, whereupon the part had hot burning pains, in the evening (aft. 6½ h.). [*Lr.*]

In the morning, great itching of the right calf, with swelling of its blood-vessels down to the foot; he must scratch till the blood came, whereupon the part remained red and bloody (aft. 23 h.). [*Lr.*]

When moving, tearing, aching, paralytic pain on the tibiæ, with powerlessness and unsteadiness in the knees (2nd d.). [*Fz.*]

Drawing pressure in the tibiæ, sometimes when sitting, sometimes when walking; it goes off by walking if it came on when sitting, and goes off by sitting if it came on when walking; but the pain is more frequently felt when sitting (aft. 9 h.). [*Fz.*]

Drawing pressure on the dorsum of the feet when sitting, which goes off on rising up. [*Fz.*]

140. **A pain, like dislocation, in the foot**, especially beside the heel and in the ankles, when sitting and standing, but increased when walking (aft. 3 h.). [*Lr.*]

In the ankle-joint, aching, dislocation pain, when walking and standing, which goes off on sitting down (aft. 4½ h.). [*Fz.*]

Dislocation pain in the right foot, which, however, goes off when touched and when walking (aft. 4½ h.). [*Lr.*]

A dislocation pain in the foot only when walking (aft. 6 h.). [*Lr.*]

Itching above the ankles and on the toes, which recommences suddenly with a fine prick, is sometimes stronger, sometimes weaker, and when it has ceased leaves behind it a sensation sometimes of warmth, sometimes of numbness of the skin on the part (aft. 3 h.). [*Fz.*]

145. Violent itching on the dorsum of the right big toe, which compels him to scratch, after which white pustules break out that itch still more violently; the itching only declines when he has rubbed the toe raw (aft. 5 h.). [*Hrn.*]

When walking in the open air, a burning sore pain on the heels, which was also still perceptible when standing and when sitting (aft. 24 h.). [*Lr.*]

Violent itching, not only on the skin, but also as it were on the bones of the toes of the left foot, in the evening (aft. 16½ h.). [*Lr.*]

After walking the toes are as if dead, and yet when walking, and still more when leaping, he feels a sore pain on them. [*Fz.*]

Ill-smelling perspiration between the toes of the left foot, for several successive days (aft. 16 h.). [*Lr.*]

150. Hard pressure on the left big toe. [*Hrn.*]

Drawing pain on the big toe. [*Fz.*]

Hard, drawing pressure on the left little toe, towards the outside —feeling as if in the periosteum. [*Hrn.*]

A drawing from without inwards where the left big toe is connected to the metatarsal bone (aft. 30 h.). [*Hrn.*]

Itching on various parts of the body, consisting of a rapidly occurring, sharp, throbbing continued prick, and when it went off a numb sensation remained for some time. [*Fz.*]

155. Itching erosion on many parts of the body; it excites scratching, whereby it is removed for some time, but then recurs. [*Hrn.*]

On various parts of the body, where the bones are immediately covered by the skin, *e g.* on the tibiæ and clavicles, pressive, drawing or tearing pains, more when moving than when at rest. [*Fz.*]

In the evening, in bed, he can scarcely bear the pricking itching on all parts of the body. [*Fz.*]

Itching (sometimes in the forenoon) on various parts of the body, consisting of coarse pricks, which then changes into drawing and tearing pain there (2nd d.). [*Fz.*]

The child always wants to go to bed and lie down.

160. As long as he is moving he feels nothing but exhaustion; but on

sitting down there occurs an itching and many other sufferings (towards evening). [*Fz.*]

Sometimes great peevishness and lethargy of the mind, with bodily exhaustion, which latter only goes off as soon as he moves about. [*Fz.*]

Great weakness of the body, especially in the knees, though he feels strong in his mind and is lively (aft. 1½ h.). [*Fz.*]

He is fatigued in all his limbs, as if their mobility were hindered. [*Fz.*]

Relaxed feeling of the whole body ; it was a trouble to him to move even one limb. [*Htg.*]

165. In the evening extraordinary fatigue ; he must lie down and slumber ; on rising up again the lower extremities are as if bruised and stiff, with drawing aching pains in the thighs and knees. [*Fz.*]

Drowsiness when sitting (aft. 3½ h.). [*Lr.*]

Great inclination to slumber all the forenoon. [*Fz.*]

In the evening great inclinatlon to sleep ; he cannot resist it. [*Fz.*]

In the evening, he had scarcely fallen asleep when he had nightmare ; he could not cry out even when he was awake. [*Fz.*]

170. Restless sleep, dreams about money (aft. 22 h.). [*Lr.*]

Frequent waking at night, as from sleeplessness. [*Lr.*]

Sleep towards morning, with slight dreams. [*Fz.*]

The sleep at night is broken, only towards morning many dreams and a seminal emission (3rd night). [*Fz.*]

In the morning he awakes very early ; he cannot get to sleep again, and when he wishes to get up he cannot do so on account of weariness and sleepiness. [*Fz.*]

175. In the evening he cannot refrain from sleep, with constant chilly feeling. [*Fz.*]

All the forenoon continued chilliness and coldness of the whole body, renewed by every dose ; after the chill had passed off and the normal warmth had ensued, at first only the nose still remained cold, but when it again got warm the hands, which had previously got warm, became again cold (aft. ½ h.). [*Hrn.*]

In the evening sometimes, along with chilly feeling, sudden shuddering. [*Fz.*]

Shivering all through the body, with yawning, without coldness or goose-skin, in the morning (aft. 24 h.). [*Lr.*]

Towards evening, great chill, without thirst ; at the same time great sensitiveness to cold, during which he often shakes and shivers, then heat on various parts, with anxiety, as if some misfortune threatened him. [*Fz.*]

180. Coldness of the hands, whilst the face and hands were warm, without thirst, in the morning (aft. ¾ h.) [*Lr.*]

Towards evening, first for some minutes chilliness and great sensitiveness to cold, then heat in some parts of the body, the backs of the hands and the nape, but not in the face. [*Fz.*]

In the morning hot feeling on the hands, face and whole body without particular elevation of temperature, and without thirst (aft. ¾ h.). [*Lr.*]

Heat of single parts of the hands, nape, and neck under the jaw, and an hour afterwards dryness of the palate and thirst. [*Fz.*]

Feeling of heat, and externally perceptible heat of the hands, with swelling of the veins; whilst the rest of the body and the forehead are only warm, the cheeks are cold. (aft. 15½ h.). [*Lr.*]

185. Each time he wakes from sleep at night, slight sweat all over the body (aft. 10 h.). [*Lr.*]

Out of the febrile chill and coldness, gradually occurring thirstless heat all over the body, especially in the face, with redness, that was increased after a meal. (aft. 2 h.). [*Hrn.*]

All day long he had no thirst, but in the evening, when the face and hands became warm, thirst came on. [*Fz.*]

He is always in a reverie, and not inclined to speak. [*Hrn.*]

In fits of two hours and longer, disinclination to speak; talking is a trouble to him. [*Hrn.*]

190. Disinclination for all work, until towards evening; he cannot make up his mind to do the least thing. [*Fz.*]

In fits of two hours and longer, disinclination to work, and then, again, inclination for it. [*Hrn.*]

Previously cheerful, he suddenly became very grave, and to a certain degree peevish (aft. 2 h.); after some time he again became cheerful, and then again peevish. [*Hrn.*]

Peevish, morose disposition; he easily takes every trifle in bad part, and gets angry over it. [*Lr.*]

Sunk in deep thought, he sought solitude and thought about his future fate (aft. 1 h.). [*Lr.*]

195. Deep thought about the present and future, so that he almost wept (aft. 12 h.). [*Lr.*]

Inward grief and anxiety of conscience, as if he had not done his duty or had committed a crime (aft. 1 h.). [*Lr.*]

Excessive sadness, as if he had done something bad and had neglected his duty (aft. 10 h.). [*Lr.*]

Calm, contented with himself* (aft. 3 h.). [*Lr.*]

Tranquillity of mind.* [*Htg.*]

200. Sometimes he is quite peevish and ill-humoured; but soon there occurs again a strange happy feeling, which shows itself by a slight trembling in the joints. [*Fz.*]

All day long he is peevish, not disposed to talk, and insensible, so that he feels little in his body. [*Fz.*]

Towards evening there suddenly occurs a strange happy feeling and lively fancy, which conjures up agreeable picture. [*Fz.*]

* Secondary and curative action.

DIGITALIS.[1]

(Foxglove.)

(The fresh expressed juice of the leaves of *Digitalis purpurea* mixed with equal parts of alcohol.)

From the following symptoms, which are by no means complete as to their number, it is undeniably evident that the morbid conditions of a chronic character, physicians have sometimes hitherto cured with foxglove, were all, without exception, cured homœopathically, although they were unaware of the fact. But the much more numerous instances of unsuccessful treatment with this extremely powerful plant, belong to those employments of foxglove which were, as is usually the case, directed against mere pathological names (not the totality of the symptoms), and were effected with a medicine (foxglove), which was estimated, in hap-hazard fashion, only in accordance with conjectures respecting its general mode of action deduced from hypothesis (not known from its pure effects, *i.e.* from the morbid states it developed in the healthy body). As long as this theoretical blindness is persisted in, much more harm than good will be done with this great gift of God. The true physician, who selects his remedy homœopathically in accordance with its pure pathogenetic effects for very similar cases of disease, will never give foxglove except where it can, will, and *must* do good, and will never fail to prescribe it in such suitable cases. Such treatment is immensely superior to the deplorable treatment of the ordinary practitioner. The homœopathic practitioner, besides, will find in the following few symptoms the means of affording homœopathic relief for many more morbid states than have hitherto been cured by it.

A very small portion of a drop of the quintillion-fold or, still better, the decillion-fold dilution of the juice, will often be found to be a too powerful dose for homœopathic treatment.

The action of such a small dose lasts several days, that of an excessively large dose several weeks.

[HAHNEMANN was assisted in this proving by BECHER, FRANZ, GROSS, HORNBURG, LANGHAMMER, J. G. LEHMANN, MEYER, E. F. RUCKERT, STAPF, TEUTHORN.

Symptoms are borrowed from the following old-school authorities :

BAIDON, in *Edinb. Med. and Surg. Journal*, vol. iii, pt. 11, No 4.

BAKER, in *Med. Essays of the London Coll. of Phys.*, pt. iii.

BAYLIES, *Practical Essays on Medical Subjects*. London, 1773.

BEDDOES. in *Med. Facts and Obs.*, v. London, 1794.

BOERHAVE, *Hortus Lugd. Batav.—Rar. Morb. Historiæ.*. Jenæ, 1771.

BRANDIS, in *Schiemann, Diss. de Digit. purp.* Gott., 1786.

---

1 From vol. iv, 2nd edit., 1825.

DRAKE, in *Phys. Med. Journ.*. 1802, Feb.
Edinburgh Med. Comment., vol. x.
HALLER, VON, in *Vicat's Mat. Med.*, i.
HENRY, W., in *Med. and Chir. Journ.* Edinb., 1811.
HORN, *Neues Archiv*, v.
KINGLAKE, ROB., in *Beddoes' Med. Facts and Obs.*, vol. v. London, 1794.
LENTIN, *Beobachtungen einiger Krankheiten*, 1774.
LETTSOM, *Mem. of the Med. Soc. of London*, vol. ii.
MACLEAN, in *Phys. Med. Journ.*, 1800, Aug., 1802, Feb.
MANGOLD, in *Horn's Archiv f. pr. Med.*, iii.
MEYER, in *Richter's Chir. Bibl.*, v.
MONRO, DON, in *Samml. f. pr. Aerzte*, xiii.
MOSSMANN, G., in *Phys. Med. Journ.*, 1801, July.—*Essay to Elucidate the Scrophula.* London, 1800.
PENKIVIL, J., in *Phys. Med. Journal*, 1801.
QUARIN, *Animadvers. pract.*
REMER, *Annalen der Klin. Anstalt*, i.
SACKREUTER, in *Annalen der Heilkunde*, 1811, March.
SCHIEMANN, in *Diss. de Digit. purp.* Gott., 1786.
WARREN, in *Samml. br. Abh. f. pr. Aerzte*, vol. xi.
WITHERING, *Abhan. uber den Fingerhut.* Lpz., 1786.

The 1st edit. gives 418 ; 10 additional symptoms appear in the 2nd edit. ; in the *Chr. Kr.* the symptoms are increased to 702.]

DIGITALIS.

Vertigo. [QUARIN, *Animadvers. pract.*, pp. 118—120[1]—MACLEAN, in the *Phys. and Med. Journ.*, Lpz., 1800, Aug., p. 585.[2]—WITHERING, *Abh. ub. den Fingerhut*, Lpz., 1786.[2]—J. PENKIVIL, in *Phys. and Med. Journ.*, 1801, Aug.[3]—LETTSOM, *Mem. of the Med. Soc. of London*, vol. ii.[4]]

Vertigo so that she fell when going upstairs. [PENKIVIL, l. c.]

Vertigo and trembling. [DRAKE, in *Phys. and Med. Journ.*, 1802, Febr.[5]]

Confusion of the whole head and sensation as if the brain beat like water on both sides of the skull and would burst it, in a pulsating manner. [*Trn.*]

5. Undulating headache, like the beating of waves, from within towards both sides, that is relieved by lying and stooping forwards, but increased when standing and bending back (aft. 2 h.). [*Trn.*]

Painful confusion of the head. [*Stf.*]

Gloomy in the head, as if hypochondriacal.

He is at first quite unable to collect his thoughts and giddy in the head. [*Fz.*]

Weakness of memory. [LETTSOM, l. c.]

10. The head is affected. [WITHERING, l. c.]

---

1 Effects of digitalis when given for scrofula.
2 Effects on patients.
3 Effects of digitalis when given for phthisis.
4 Effects of digitalis when given to dropsical patients.
5 Effects of digitalis when given for phthisis. This symptom occurred after each dose.

Headache. [QUARIN,—LETTSOM, l. c.]

Headache for several days.* [SCHIEMANN, *Diss. de Digit. purp.*, Gott., 1786, pp. 34, 41.[1]]

Headache, pressure and heaviness, as from rush of blood to the head.

Giddy drawing in the sides of the head. [*Gss.*]

15. Tearing in the left side of the head. [*Gss.*]

Tearing in the right temporal region, close to the ear. [*Gss.*]

Pressure and stretching in the sides of the head (aft. 10 m.). [*Gss.*]

Contractive and pressive pain in the forehead and temples which is increased by thinking. [*Fz.*]

Anteriorly in the forehead, pressive tensive pain. [*Hbg.*]

20. In the middle of the forehead, superiorly, pressure as from a hard weight on exerting the thoughts. [*Fz.*]

Sharp pressive pain in the forehead, on a small spot above the eye (aft. $\frac{1}{2}$ h.). [*Stf.*]

In the evening and at night in sleep, single obtuse stitches in the left temple, which darted through the whole brain.

Shooting now in the right, now in the left temporal region, but transient. [*Myr.*]

Aching headache in jerks, now in the temples, now in the whole head. [*Rkt.*]

25. Throbbing pain in the forehead or in the fundus of the orbits. [MACLEAN, l. c.]

When he turned the eyes to the right or left side, in order to look to right or left, without moving the head, there occurred an uncomfortable tensive sensation in the sinciput (aft. 30 h.). [*Bch.*]

For several hours, every time he stooped forward, in the side of the brain, on a small spot, a stitch-like tension, which extended to a left upper tooth, but which went off every time he raised himself up. [*Stf.*]

On bending the head forward, sensation as if something fell forwards in it, frequently recurring. [*Rkt.*]

Headache on one side, like an internal itching. [*Ln.*]

30. At the occipital protuberance an aching pain as from a blow or fall (aft. $1\frac{1}{2}$ h.). [*Hbg.*]

Aching stitches externally on the left side of the forehead (aft. 4 h.). [*Lr.*]

Tearing stitches externally on the left temple (aft. 34 h.). [*Lr.*]

On the middle of the forehead, a red pimple with burning smarting pain, increased by touch. [*Hbg.*]

Single stitches in the left frontal region (aft. 84 h.). [*Lr.*]

35. Swollen head.[2] [QUARIN, l. c.]

Heat in the whole head, externally and internally ; thinking was

* From the emanations from the juice.

---

1 Not accessible.

2 This was only a sensation as of being swollen.

difficult for him, and he forgot everything immediately (aft. 1 h.). [*Myr.*]

The head always falls backwards, when sitting and walking, as if the anterior cervical muscles had no power (as if paralysed). [*Trn.*]

Paleness of face.[1] [WITHERING, l. c.]

Convulsions on the left side of the face. [G. MOSSMANN, in *Phys. and Med. Journ.*, 1801, Jul.[2]]

40. **Burning pain in the right eye-brow, with dimness of vision, as if a veil were before the eyes** (aft. 5 and more h.). [*Myr.*]

Pressive pain on the right eye-brow, towards the external canthus of the eye (aft. 52 h.). [*Lr.*]

Tendency of both eyes to turn towards the left side; when he forced them to turn to the right they were painful, and he then saw all near objects double or threefold; at the same time the face was puffed (aft. 29 h.). [*Bch.*]

Pain of the eyes, excessive pain in the eye-balls on touching them.

Aching pain in the eye-balls.

45. An aching in the right eye-ball, rapidly coming and going off (aft. 2 h.). [*Stf.*]

Violent inflammation of the eyes.

(Very contracted pupils) (aft. ½ h.). [*Stf.*]

Great dilatation of the pupils (aft. 1 h.). [*Trn.*]

Dimness of vision. [QUARIN, l. c.]

50. Weak sight, imperfect vision. [PENKIVIL, l. c.]

Slight dimness of vision. [MOSSMANN, *Essay to elucidate the Scrophula*, London, 1800.[3]]

He sees objects only darkly.[4] [WITHERING, l. c.]

Dimness of vision. [WITHERING, l. c.]

Blindness.[5] [LETTSOM, l. c.]

55. Blindness, amaurosis, for three days. [REMER, *Annalen d. Klin. Anstalt*, B. i.[6]]

Imperfect vision, as if a cloud or a mist hung before the eyes. [MACLEAN, l. c.]

When he wishes to look at distant objects, dark bodies hover before his eyes, like flies. [BAKER, in *Medical Essays of the London College of Physicians*, iii.[7]]

All sorts of figures hover before the eyes. [PENKIVIL, l. c.]

Appearances before the eyes.[8] [LETTSOM, l. c.]

---

1 Not found.
2 Effects of digitalis given in pneumonia.
3 Not accessible.
4 Not found.
5 Lasting for a month after omitting the medicine, with throbbing pain and sense of fulness in the eye-balls.
6 Not accessible.
7 Effects of digitalis in a case of anasarca. The "dark bodies like flies" represent "muscæ volitantes" in the original.
8 "Fiery appearances" in the original.

60. When he covers up the eyes, bright bodies seem to dance before his eyes.[1] [BAKER, l. c.]

In the morning, on awaking, all objects seem as if covered with snow. [MOSSMANN, in *Phys. Med. Journ.*, l. c.]

The flame of the candle appears to him larger and brighter[2] than natural. [BAKER, l. c.]

In the dusk he saw glittering colours, red, green and yellow, before his eyes, like flickering light (aft. 8 h.). [*Ln.*]

The faces of persons coming into the room appeared to him deadly pale. [BAKER, l. c.]

65. Illusion of vision: **objects appear of a green or yellow colour.** [WITHERING, l. c.]

Objects appear yellow to him, even silver. [PENKIVIL, l. c.]

The eyes water. [WITHERING, l. c.]

The tears running from his eyes smart.

In a moderately warm room, less in the open air, the eyes become full of water; they are dim, hot, full of red blood-vessels, with aching pain, and the canthi are full of mucus (as in severe coryza). [*Stf.*]

70. In the inner canthus a painful scraping sensation, as if coarse dust had got into it. [*Hbg.*]

(Swelling of the lower eyelid, which interferes with his looking down.)

The edges of the eyelids are painful, as if excoriated, when they are shut (in the evening in bed). [*Rkt.*]

Inflammation of the Meibomian glands on the borders of the eyelids.

Paralytic drawing beneath the left zygomatic process in front of the ear. [*Gss.*]

75. Cramp-like drawing pain on the zygoma, which goes off by strong pressure. [*Fz.*]

Cramp under the right zygomatic arch on moving the lower jaw, which, when he bites, is closed spasmodically, and more strongly than he wished. [*Fz.*]

An erosion and itching on the cheek and chin, worst at night.

In the ears a sensation as if they were contracted internally; he hears the pulse in them (the hearing remained good). [*Fz.*]

A tensive pressure in the left ear. [*Stf.*]

80. Hissing before both ears, like water boiling. [*Trn.*]

Single stitches behind the ear, externally. [*Trn.*]

A large pimple with smarting pain under the left nostril.

Epistaxis; bright blood from both nostrils (aft. 1 h.). [*Trn.*]

Drawing pain in the muscles under the mastoid process. [*Fz.*]

85. Under the right mastoid process, a drawing, which goes off by strong pressure. [*Fz.*]

Aching drawing on the occiput at the seat of the insertion of the cervical muscles, on bending back the head. [*Fz.*]

---

1 The muscæ of S. 57 become these when the eyes are covered and pressed upon.

2 In the original "whiter."

Stiffness of the posterior and lateral cervical muscles, with pressive pain like blows (aft. 10 h.). [*Hbg.*]

Shooting pains externally in the cervical muscles on moving the neck. [*Bch.*]

A painful stiffness and tension in the cervical muscles and nape, especially on moving. [*Stf.*]

90. Eruption on the neck.

Swelling of the lips and tongue.* [W. HENRY, in *Med. and Chir. Journal*, Edinb., 1811.]

In the morning, white coated tongue (aft. 48 h.). [*Lr.*]

Excoriation internally in the mouth, on the tongue and gums, with flow of saliva, for three days. [BAYLIES, *Practical Essays on Med. Subjects*, London, 1773, pp. 39, 41.[1]]

Excoriation of the inside of the mouth, fauces, œsophagus, stomach. [BOERHAVE, *Hortus Lugd. Batav.*, p. 308.[2]]

95. Collection of saliva in the mouth (aft. ¼ h.). [*Bch.*]

Flow of saliva.

Flow of saliva. [WITHERING, l. c.—LENTIN, *Beobachtungen einiger Krankheiten*, 1774, p. 167.[3]]

Accumulation of saliva, as after vinegar. [*Hbg.*]

Collection of watery saliva in the mouth, which at first tastes sweet, but afterwards very salty, in frequent fits (aft. ½ h.). [*Stf.*]

100. Collection of very sweet saliva. [SCHIEMANN, l. c.]

Collection of saliva in the mouth, with spitting of it out, and great nausea on swallowing the saliva (aft. ¼ h.). [*Bch.*]

Profuse flow of saliva of a fœtid smell.[4] [HENRY, l. c.]

Bad smell from the mouth (aft. 4 h.).

Flat, slimy taste, and a soft flossy feeling in the mouth, as if it were lined inside with velvet. [*Trn.*]

105. Rough palate, as if he had smoked too much tobacco, without thirst. [*Fz.*]

A scrapy, rough feeling in the palate. [*Stf.*]

(Painfulness of the front teeth.) [*Stf.*]

After smoking tobacco, taste in the mouth as from sweet almonds. [*Fz.*]

Spasmodic constriction of the throat. [LENTIN, l. c.]

110. Sore throat ; shooting (also) when not swallowing.

Stitches in the back part of the palate and in the commencement of the gullet, not observable when swallowing. [*Rkt.*]

Little appetite, he is immediately satiated. [*Stf.*]

* In a woman from an ounce of the decoction, in whom the swelling of the lips and tongue was accompanied by fœtid salivation and suppression of urine.[5]

---

1 Not accessible.

2 Observed effects. This ascribed by the owner to the acrimony of the plant.

3 From an overdose.

4 For "fœtid smell" read "viscid consistence."

5 The patient was ascitic. There is no mention in the original of fœtor about th salivation. (See S. 102.)

Very little appetite on account of nausea. [*Bch.*]

Anorexia, with indescribable emptiness in the stomach. [ROB. KINGLAKE, in *Beddoes' Med. Facts and Obs.*, vol. v, Lond., 1794.[1]]

115. **Anorexia, with clean tongue.** [PENKIVIL, l. c.]

With good appetite bread tastes bitter. [*Trn.*]

Appetite for bitter food. [*Bch.*]

Thirst for sour drinks. [*Trn.*]

Sour eructation after eating. [*Trn.*]

120. Nausea.

Nausea. [BAYLIES, l. c.]

Nausea in the gastric region, without retching and vomiting (aft. 11 h.). [*Bch.*]

Nausea after a meal. [*Ln.*]

Nausea for three days without cessation. [MACLEAN, l. c., 1802, Febr.]

125. Deadly nausea. [WARREN, in *Samml. br. Abh. p. fr. Aerzte*, vol. xi. p. I.]

In recurring fits, deadly sickness, with extreme depression of the mind and anguish.* [WITHERING, l. c.]

Vomiting.

Nausea of the worst kind and vomiting. [MACLEAN, l. c., 1800, Aug., p. 585.]

Excessive nausea, with inordinate vomiting, coldness of the limbs, and cold sweats, for two days. [BAKER, l. c.]

130. With excessive nausea, vomiting of green bile. [BAKER, l. c.]

Increased nausea, with vomiting of the food he had eaten, which was enveloped in white tasteless mucus, whereupon the bellyache that was present went off (aft. 8½ h.). [*Bch.*]

Violent vomiting, for four hours. [BAYLIES, l. c.]

Nocturnal vomiting.[2] [PENKIVIL, l. c.]

Morning vomiting. [MOSSMANN, l. c., 1801, Jul.—PENKIVIL, l. c.]

135. Excessive vomiting. [LENTIN, l. c]

Long-continued vomiting. [WITHERING, l. c]

Uncontrollable vomiting, for six days, until death ensued.† [*Edinburgh Med. Comment.*, vol. x.]

Bilious vomiting for several days. [BEDDOES, in *Med. Facts and Obs.*, v, London, 1794.[3]]

Hiccup, that did not rise quite up into the throat, six or seven times (aft. 21 h.). [*Bch.*]

* This lasted every time several, often four, hours, and came on sometimes before, sometimes after the diuresis.

† In a woman who in two days had taken twelve leaves in six doses; she died the seventh day. In the ileum was found inflammation, and an almost complete adhesion and union of the walls of some parts of this intestine.

---

1 Not found.

2 This and the following symptom do not mean vomiting recurring each night or morning, but simply that the vomiting caused by the drug came on on the following night or morning.

3 From overdosing.

140. Hiccup. [LENTIN, l. c.]

Disagreeable sensation in the gastric region. [MOSSMANN, *Essay*, l. c.]

A weakness of the stomach, like a sinking of the stomach, as if life would be extinguished.*[1] [MACLEAN, l. c., 1800, Aug.]

Cardialgia.[2] [WITHERING, l. c.]

Weight in the stomach. [PENKIVIL, l. c.]

145. A feeling of constriction over the gastric region, towards the liver. [*Hbg.*]

(Anxious tension and constriction under the short ribs.)

After a meal the food presses in the scrobiculus cordis, when he is seated, but not when he is standing. [*Fz.*]

Weight in the stomach, alternating with exhaustion. [MOSSMANN, in *Phys. and Med. Journ.*, l. c.]

Pressure, as from a hard weight, in the scrobiculus cordis, on raising up the body. [*Fz.*]

150. Cutting aching in the scrobiculus cordis, with feeling of nausea there. [*Gss.*]

In the scrobiculus cordis squeezing stitches, unaffected by breathing, increased by touching, only when standing not when sitting (aft. 24 h.). [*Gss.*]

Aching and burning in the gastric region. [HORN, *Neues Archiv*, v. i, p. 104.[2]]

Stomachache, and at the same time sensation of great heat in the stomach and bowels. [WITHERING, l. c.]

Sensation in the bowels as if they were twisted together and the gastric region were retracted.[3] [DRAKE, l. c.]

155. Pinching contraction in the abdomen, as from a severe chill, when sitting, but of which he feels nothing when walking (aft. 3, 4 d). [*Fz.*]

Sharp stitches in the navel. [*Gss.*]

A persistent stitch in the left infracostal region, with sensation, especially during expiration, as if the surrounding parts were gone asleep. [*Fz.*]

(While eating) above and to the right of the navel obtuse, as it were, squeezing stitches. [*Gss.*]

Single stitches and pinching in the abdomen, sometimes with paroxysms of sick feeling (aft. 24 h.). [*Rkt.*]

160. Pinching in the hypogastrium, as from a purgative (aft. ½ h.) [*Myr.*]

Flying needle-pricks in the whole abdomen. [*Gss.*]

Fine stitches in the right side of the abdomen on expiration, when standing and walking (aft. 58 h.). [*Lr.*]

Stitches in the right side of the abdomen, during expiration, while sitting, in the morning (aft. 75 h.). [*Lr.*]

* All the patients complained of this in the same terms.

1 Literally, "a faintness or sinking at the stomach, as if life were going from them."

2 Not found.

3 Literally, "sensation of twisting in the bowels after each dose, and of much sinking at the pit of the stomach."

Single fine shooting in the left side of the abdomen, when at rest and during movement, which was increased on expiration (aft. 88 h.). [*Lr.*]

165. Just above the umbilical region digging, aching, shooting internally (aft. 10 m.). [*Gss.*]

Shooting in the bend of the groin when walking. [*Fz.*]

Tearing pains about the navel, in the morning (aft. 8 h.).

When walking shooting tearing in the umbilical region. [*Fz.*]

In the evening cutting tearing in the abdomen, as from a chill, especially when rising up from a seat, with aching pain in the vertex. [*Fz.*]

170. Cutting in the whole of the epigastrium and hypogastrium. [*Gss.*]

Under the third left false rib a part that is painful, as if all inside were lacerated. [*Fz.*]

Twitching tearing from the pubes to the left groin, on leaning the body backwards. [*Fz.*]

Simple pain, as from excoriation, in the left inguinal ring, as if a hernia would come out (aft. 6 h.).

In the bend of the groin (in the tendon of the psoas muscle that becomes prominent on moving), almost only when walking, pressive tension ; when pressed on it is painful, as if a hard body lay under the skin, which increased the pressure. [*Fz.*]

175. Drawing cramp anteriorly in the bend of the right groin, which after moving the tendon of the psoas muscle is increased, and becomes, as it were, throbbing, and then continues even when sitting. [*Fz.*]

Aching, rumbling, gurgling in the abdomen. [*Gss.*]

Colic-like rumbling and rolling in the abdomen, for half an hour.

Flatulence and discharge of flatus. [*Rkt.*]

Noises in the abdomen, without sensation of flatulence therein, and without discharge of flatus. [*Bch.*]

180. Tension of the skin on the abdomen when he raises himself up. [*Fz.*]

The abdomen is painful, as if ulcerated, when moving, but not when touched. [*Fz.*]

Forcing downwards and boring anteriorly in the left side of the abdomen. [*Fz.*]

In the left side of the abdomen sensation as if something were forcing itself through. [*Fz.*]

Urging to stool. [*Hbg.*]

185. Before stool, chilliness.

After constipation for forty-eight hours there occurred a quite soft, yellow stool, without suffering. [*Fz.*]

Ash-coloured diarrhœa, as in jaundice. [SCHIEMANN, l. c.]

After vomiting four times, faintness, followed by violent diarrhœa of an ash-coloured, pappy matter, as in jaundice. [MEYER, in *Richter's Chir. Bibl.*, v, p. 532.[1]]

---

1 Effect of digitalis given for mammary scirrhus.

Jaundice.[1] [WITHERING, l. c.]

190. Diarrhœa.

Purging. [WITHERING, l. c.]

Thin stool. [*Hbg.*]

First two or three thin stools (aft. 24 h.), then constipation in the morning; and only in the evening evacuation with many thread-worms (aft. 55 h.). [*Stf.*]

After seventy-two hours the stool became quite soft and liquid and also much more frequent. [*Fz.*]

195. For several days two or three stools. [*Lr.*]

Violent diarrhœa. [LENTIN,—BAYLIES, l. c.]

Painful purging for three or four days. [WITHERING, l. c.]

Bellyache, more tearing than shooting, in the morning in bed, followed by two attacks of diarrhœa and thereafter urging to stool in the rectum.

Diarrhœa with cutting in the abdomen. [*Bch.*]

200. Several diarrhœic stools, preceded by cutting in the abdomen (aft. 8 h. and longer). [*Bch.*]

Diarrhœa of fæces mixed with mucus, preceded by bellyache, sometimes pressive, sometimes cutting (aft. 6—8 h.), which went off each time he went to stool. [*Bch.*]

Almost incurable dysenteries.[2] [BOERHAVE, *Rar. Morb. Historiæ*, Jenæ, 1771, hist. 308.]

He passes stool and urine involuntarily.

In the left renal region a fine shooting, when sitting. [*Hbg.*]

205. Urging to urinate (aft. ½ h.). [*Hbg.*]

Retention of urine.[3] [HENRY, l. c.]

Straining, ineffectual urging to pass urine. [MANGOLD, in *Horn's Archiv f. pr. Med.*, iii, 1, p. 141.[4]]

A contractive pain in the urinary bladder, whilst urinating; the urine was evacuated with difficulty owing to this pain. [*Ln.*]

The first day he only passes urine twice and but little, but without suffering; after forty-eight hours the urine becomes much more copious and accompanied by cutting drawing in the bladder. [*Fz.*]

210. Diuresis.

She must get up every night to pass urine.

Frequent urging to urinate; the urine only comes away by drops, with burning sensation in the urethra and the region of the glans; the urine had a reddish appearance (aft. 3 h.). [*Myr.*]

The urine commences to be passed less frequently, but in greater quantity and with less burning (aft. 20 h.). [*Myr.*]

At night constant urging to urinate, and when he got up to make water, he had dizziness and vertigo (aft. 12 h. and beyond till morning). [*Myr.*]

---

1 This indeed occurred in several of Withering's patients, but always in the natural sequence of their maladies, and never traceable to digitalis.

2 As in note to S. 94.

3 Rather, "suppression." It lasted nearly three days.

4 Not accessible.

215. Without urging to urinate, dark urine, which on standing grew redder and cloudy (aft. 14 h). [*Bch.*]

After the diuresis, retention of urine, then nausea, vomiting and diarrhœa.* [WITHERING, l. c.]

Frequent passing of a watery urine. [*Stf.*]

Frequent urging to urinate, and he passed much water of a healthy colour (aft. 8, 9, 10 h.). [*Bch.*]

Increased discharge of urine, with increased urging thereto, and inability to retain it. [WITHERING, l. c.]

220. Inability to retain the urine. [WITHERING, l. c.]

After the diuresis, nausea. [WITHERING, l. c.]

While urinating, in the middle of the urethra, a pressing (burning) sensation, as if the urethra were too narrow, which, however, goes off on continuing to urinate.

During the diuresis and diarrhœa small quick pulse, whilst the hands and feet are icy cold. [WITHERING, l. c.]

The urine is acrid.[1] [WITHERING, l. c.]

225. Inflammation of the neck of the bladder. [DON. MONRO, in *Samml. f. pr. Aerzte*, xiii, p. 2.[2]]

Several times in the night sensation as if pollutions would occur, but none came ; in the morning a sticky moisture at the mouth of the urethra.

In the right testicle a pain as if contused.

* * *

In the morning, with some coryza, stoppage of the nose (aft. 73 h.). [*Lr.*]

Coryza and cough to a great degree ; he could scarcely speak for coryza.

230. In the morning he is hoarse.

After a night-sweat, in the morning such great hoarseness, that he could not speak.

In the morning mucus adheres in the larynx, which is easily detached, but when he wishes to cough it up it generally gets into the fauces, so that he must swallow it. [*Gss.*]

In the morning expectoration of mucus by voluntary hacking cough, (aft. 73 h.). [*Lr.*]

The irritation to cough extends to the palate.

235. A dry dull cough, as from tickling in the trachea. [*Stf.*]

* This is a very rare alternating action of foxglove, and only happens from excessive doses. Much more frequent and usual is the difficulty of urinating in the primary action of this medicine, see—205—209, 212, and 222, owing to which it can be not unfrequently of great use homoeopathically in dropsical diseases, which are accompanied by similar difficulty with regard to the urinary secretion and other symptoms of a similar character only observed in the primary action of foxglove, The copious, often involuntary, passing urine occurring during the use of foxglove, see 213, 214, 217 to 220, and diuresis 210, are only secondary action and reaction of the organism after the above-mentioned primary action.

1 Not found.

2 Effect of digitalis given for dropsy.—Literally, "urging to urinate even to inflammation of the bladder."

(After a meal the cough is so severe that he vomits his food.)

(About 12 p.m. cough and sweat.)

Dry cough which excites tensive aching pains in the arm and shoulder (aft. 36 h.). [*Stf.*]

Pain in the chest, which makes the cough difficult. [BRANDIS, in *Schiemann*, l. c., p. 6[1].]

240. In the morning, after rising, tightness of the chest, with dry cough.

Hæmoptysis.

Expectoration from the lungs coloured with blood.[1] [PENKIVIL, l. c.]

At every breath sensation as if he were electrified. [SACKENREUTER, in *Annalen der Heilkunde*, 1811, March.[2]]

Palpitation of the heart.

245. Almost audible, strong heart's beats, with anxiety and contractive pains under the sternum. [*Bch.*]

Aching (pressing contractive) heart's beats, with anxiety and spasmodic pains in the sternum and under the ribs, which are increased by bending forward the head and upper part of the body (aft. ½ h.). [*Bch.*]

In the right side of the chest a strong perceptible beating as from an artery synchronous with the pulse (aft. ½ h.). [*Hbg.*]

Painful suffocating constriction of the chest, as if its internal parts were all grown together, especially in the morning on awaking, owing to which he must quickly sit upright.

Contractive pains in the sternum itself; they are increased by bending forward the head and upper part of the body (aft. 2½ h.). [*Bch.*]

250. Sensation as if raw in the chest and stitches in it.

When raising up the body tension on the left side of the chest, as if that part were contracted. [*Fz.*]

When sitting in a bent position pressure on the lower part of the chest; the breathing is shorter and not enough; he cannot hold his breath long but must quickly breathe again. [*Fz.*]

Breath drawn with difficulty, slowly and deeply. [*Rkt.*]

Tension on the chest and pressure in the scrobiculus cordis, which often forces him to take a deep inspiration. [*Rkt.*]

255. For many days a painful tightness of chest; he must often draw a deep breath, and yet he felt as if he had not breathed in sufficient air, especially when sitting. [*Stf.*]

Drawing pain in the middle of the sternum when walking. [*Fz.*]

Pressive drawing on the chest when coughing. [*Fz.*]

From violent exertion of the arm he gets immediately cutting pressure on the opposite side of the chest, anteriorly in the region of the third rib, externally. [*Fz.*]

Great heat on the chest, as if he stood undressed in front of the warm stove, soon followed by coldness about the chest. [*Hbg.*]

---

1 A standing symptom with the patient.

2 Not accessible.

260. On the right, above the scrobiculus cordis, sharp stitches. [*Gss.*]

Eroding, itching pricking synchronous with the pulse in the left side, close above the scrobiculus cordis. [*Gss.*]

Below the right axilla, under the ribs, obtuse (squeezing) stitches. [*Gss.*]

On blowing the nose, pain in the sacrum as if bruised.

In the left side of the loins eroding itching, compelling him to scratch. [*Gss.*]

265. In the left side, in the region of the lumbar vertebræ, drawing cutting pain, which is relieved by pressing on it with the hand. [*Fz.*]

Drawing in the spine, the limbs, and fingers as sometimes after a chill. [*Rkt.*]

In the first dorsal vertebræ a sensation like a blow (aft. 2 h.). [*Hbg.*]

In the junction of the first dorsal and last cervical vertebræ, the joint pains as if excoriated on bending forward the neck, but not on touching.

(Eruption of pimples on the back.)

270. Cutting pain, with numbness of the skin, in the upper part of the nape, which compels the head to be drawn backwards, whereby it appears to him as if a soft dead part were jammed in between the joint, that did not allow the head to be bent backwards. [*Fz.*]

Tearing under the right scapula. [*Gss.*]

Obtuse stitches betwixt the scapulæ.

Voluptuous itching in the axilla. [*Fz.*]

On moving the arms tensive aching pain of the muscles of the arm and shoulder. [*Stf.*]

275. Paralytic weakness in the left arm ; he could scarcely raise it up or close the fingers to make a fist without pain. [*Hbg.*]

On the right arm a sore burning.

Heaviness in the left arm, also felt when at rest.

In the left upper arm a burning shooting sensation. [*Hbg.*]

A painful twitching beating in the flesh of the upper arm and thigh.

280. Tearing stitches on the right upper arm when walking (aft. 74 h.). [*Lr.*]

Needle-pricks on the lower part of the left upper arm, continuing on moving it. [*Rkt.*]

Tingling sensation on the inner side of the right elbow-joint, as if the arm would go to sleep, and as if the nerve were somewhat pressed (aft. ½ h.), and the same sensation there on touching this part (aft. 18 h.). [*Rkt.*]

In the middle of the shaft of the ulna paralytic pain, on extending the arm and when it lies outstretched. [*Fz.*]

The right hand, together with the fingers, greatly swollen at night ; the swelling lasted three hours (aft. 22 h.). [*Myr.*]

285. Above the right wrist-joint on the back of the ulna, a pinching and squeezing sharp shooting. [*Gss.*]

Severe stitches in the muscles of the right forearm (aft. ½ h.). [*Lr.*]

Paralytic tearing in the bones of the right wrist. [*Gss.*]

Severe tearing on the right forearm, more externally, when at rest and when moving (aft. 32 h.). [*Lr.*]

On the back of the hand a kind of miliary eruption without sensation.

290. An itching on the back of the hand, mostly at night.

Paralytic tearing in the right metacarpal bones (aft. 8 h.). [*Gss.*]

Spasmodic stitches in the ball of the left thumb, when at rest and when moving (aft. 6 h.). [*Lr.*]

Twitching paralytic tearing in the right index, front and back. [*Gss.*]

Paralytic tearing in the finger-joints, when at rest and when moving. [*Gss.*]

295. Involuntary twitching of the left index, which is drawn outwards by it. [*Fz.*]

Burning shooting on the left thumb just above the nail, which is much aggravated by pressing on it. [*Fz.*]

The nates go to sleep in the evening when sitting, and become as if quite dead. [*Fz.*]

Slow drawing above the nates. [*Fz.*]

After sitting (in a carriage) great stiffness in the joints of the lower extremities, which went off by walking.

300. On the upper anterior part of the thigh an eroding itching. [*Gss.*]

On the thigh, somewhat above the left knee towards the outside, sharp stitches (aft. ½ h.). [*Gss.*]

Aching drawing in the anterior muscles of the thigh. [*Fz.*]

Drawing on the inside of the thigh, when sitting, and on the inner side of the left foot, when it hangs free and is not supported. [*Fz.*]

Pressure in the right thigh on its anterior aspect of a pressive drawing character, that gradually increased and then diminished. [*Hbg.*]

305. On crossing the lower extremities one over the other, cutting sensation in the thigh, which goes off on uncrossing them. [*Fz.*]

Cramp-like drawing in the muscles above the hough when sitting, which goes off after walking a little. [*Fz.*]

When he moves the knees after lying, on commencing to move, the thighs and legs and sacrum are painful, as if bruised.

Painless stiffness on the outer condyle of the knee-joint, as from internal swelling, with sensation of coldness. [*Fz.*]

On going upstairs a sensation in the knees as from great fatigue. [*Bch.*]

310. Under the left knee, on the outer side of the tibia, sharp stitches, during movement and when at rest (aft. 1 h.). [*Gss.*]

When walking tired pain in the knees and tibiæ, as after a long walk. [*Bch.*]

Prostration in all the limbs, especially the feet, in the joints, as after a long journey.

Twitching of the muscles under the left hough synchronous with the pulse, which goes off on touching. [*Fz.*]

Tension in the houghs, which does not permit them to be straightened. [*Fz.*]

315. In the left leg a heaviness, just as if it were in the shaft of the tibia, that hinders him in walking.

Drawing on the shaft of the left tibia, as if a part were torn out there. [*Fz.*]

Constant stretching of the legs, compelled by the weariness. [*Hbg.*]

When standing the left leg has sore pain, and as if shattered. [*Fz.*]

Burning in the right calf as soon as he lays it over the other leg. [*Fz.*]

320. The ankle-joint pains on extending it, as if over-stretched. [*Fz.*]

Eroding itching above the outer ankle of the foot. [*Gss.*]

An itching on the dorsum of the right foot, chiefly at night.

In the evening painful sharp stitches in the right sole, so that the whole lower extremity twitches. [*Fz.*]

Penetrating pain in the joints.

325. After the midday sleep all the joints are painful, as if broken on the wheel.

General soreness of the whole body. [PENKIVIL, l. c.]

(In the warm room the sufferings seem to be increased.) [*Stf.*]

The epidermis of the body scales off. [VON HALLER, in *Vicat's Mat. Med.*, i, p. 112.[1]]

Tearing, burning (and slightly itching), slow stitches on various parts of the body.

330. Eroding itching on various parts of the body, which compelled him to scratch, whereby it remits somewhat, but soon recurs. [*Gss.*]

When, during the eroding itching on almost all parts of the body he does not scratch, it usually becomes ever more severe, and at last develops to intolerable burning needle-pricking, that at one time declines, at another returns in greater intensity. [*Gss.*]

Pain on the affected part. [QUARIN, l. c.]

Tickling on the affected part. [QUARIN, l. c.]

Weakness and weariness of the lower extremities, with a trembling sensation. [*Rkt.*]

335. Exhaustion, powerlessness, and paralytic weakness of the lower extremities, without pain. [*Hbg.*]

Laziness and heaviness of the limbs. [MOSSMANN, *Essay*, l. c.]

On rising from bed in the morning, lazy and tired. [*Ln.*]

Sinking of the vital powers.

Weakness, sinking of the strength. [WITHERING, l. c.]

---

1 Statement from authors.

340. Sudden sinking of the strength, with general sweat, and, some hours afterwards, cough.

Sudden extreme exhaustion, as if he should lose consciousness (after the midday meal) with general heat and perspiration, without thirst.

All his muscles are relaxed ; he feels as if he had not slept enough. [*Fz.*]

Frequent exhaustion ; she must go to bed because sitting up fatigues her. [PENKIVIL, l. c.]

Extreme languor. [MACLEAN, l. c.]

345. Considerable degree of languor and vertigo, with intermitting pulse. [DRAKE, l. c., p. 132.]

General loss of power. [LETTSOM, l. c.]

General weakness, as if all parts of the body were exhausted (aft. 2 h.). [*Hbg.*]

(Fatal) apoplexy. [SHERWIN,[2] in *Phys. Med. Journ.*, 1801, Jul.]

350. Weakness almost to death*[3] [MACLEAN, l. c., 1802, Febr.]

Constant inclination to syncopes. [MACLEAN, l. c., 1800, Aug.]

Great inclination to syncopes. [DRAKE, l. c., p. 126.]

Tendency to faint, and relaxation of the vital power. [DRAKE, l. c., p. 124.]

Syncopes. [WITHERING, l. c.]

355. Syncope during the sickness.[4] [WITHERING, l. c.]

He feels as if the body were very light (aft. 4 h.). [*Fz.*]

Frequent yawning and stretching. [*Stf.*]

Frequent drowsiness to a considerable degree. [MACLEAN, l. c.]

Drowsy fatigue, slumber (aft. 8 h.).

360. Frequent drowsiness. [DRAKE, l. c., p. 128.]

A deep sleep.[5] [MACLEAN, l. c.]

Sleep with many not disagreeable dreams. [*Hbg.*]

At night sleep disturbed by disagreeable dreams of miscarriage of his projects (aft. 23 h.). [*Lr.*]

At night merely slumber in place of sleep, half consciousness, without being able to get to sleep.

365. Restless sleep with tossing about in bed at night, and comical dreams. [*Frn.*]

At night restless sleep on account of constant urging to urinate. [*Myr.*]

* Opium proved to be the antidote.

---

1 Literally, "much languor and sense of faintness ; the patient says he would rather die than endure it."

2 From an overdose. The reporter writes : "he was suddenly and unexpectedly carried off with all the dreadful distress and jactitation which an overdose of digitalis sometimes produces. His death was pretty generally ascribed to apoplexy, and was indeed truly apoplectic."

3 Rather, "as if to death."

4 Rather, between the attacks of sickness.

5 Curative effect.

Nocturnal restlessness and tossing about, half awake and not fully conscious. [*Rkt.*]

He woke up frequently at night as from anxiety, and with the impression that it was time to get up.

At night frequent waking, as from fright (aft. 47 h.). [*Lr.*]

370. **At night frequent waking in a fright, as from a dream, as if he fell from a height or into the water** (aft. 24, 72 h.). [*Lr.*]

Restless sleep ; he could not lie on one spot, and could only lie on his back. [*Ln.*]

At night violent pain in the left shoulder and elbow-joints, in half sleep, in which the consciousness was not quite clear, whilst he lay on his back with the left arm above the head. [*Rkt.*]

Convulsions. [WITHERING, l. c.]

Epileptic convulsions, then blindness and amaurosis, for three days. [REMER, l. c.]

375. Febrile state.[1] [QUARIN, l. c.]

Slow pulse.[1] [LENTIN, l. c.]

The pulse for twenty-four and even forty-eight hours was much slower, but thereafter all the quicker and suppressed.[2]* [LETTSOM, l. c., p. 172.]

Pulse 40 beats per minute. [WITHERING, l. c.]

Pulse slower, but stronger. [*Hbg.*]

380. Along with weakness and laziness of the whole body, diminution of the pulse-beats from 82 to [illegible] beats ; in longer or shorter intervals it made short pauses ; the beats were feeble. [*Bch.*]

The pulse at first slow, then suddenly commences to make a couple of beats, or the finger placed on it now and then loses a whole beat.[3] [MACLEAN, l. c.]

The pulse sank from 65 to 50 beats, which were quite irregular, always between three or four soft beats a fuller and harder one, on the first day ; on the third day it was 75. [*Fz.*]

Diminution of the pulse from 100 beats down to 40. [MOSSMANN, *Essay*, l. c.]

The pulse sinks to 50 and finally to 35 beats. [WITHERING, l. c.]

385. Pulse slower by one half, for several days.

Pulse beats diminished to almost half their number. [BAKER, l. c.]

When the pulse has become slow, it is increased in quickness by the slightest corporeal exertion. [MACLEAN, l. c., 1800, Aug.]

* This is the most usual phenomenon from foxglove, that after the preliminary slowness of the pulse (primary action), after some days it is the reverse (reaction or secondary action), a much quicker and smaller pulse is permanently induced ; see also 383. From this we see how wrong the ordinary physicians are who endeavour to produce a permanently slower pulse by means of foxglove.

---

1 Not found.

2 Rather, "but thereafter quicker and proportionately weaker."

3 Literally, "pulse suddenly quickened for a few beats, then slow again ; or it loses a whole beat."

Irregular pulse, from 40 to 58 beats.[1] [BAKER, l. c.]

The number of the pulse beats diminishes scarcely at all when standing, little when sitting, most when lying, when the number sinks to 60,[2] whereas it is 100 when he stands. [BAIDON, in *Edinb. Med. and Surg. Journal*, vol. iii, pt. 11th, No. iv.]

390. Hard, small, quick pulse.

Before death, 100 pulse beats in a minute.[3] [WITHERING, l. c.]

Frequent yawning and stretching with chilliness. [*Stf.*]

Internal coldness in the whole body (aft. 5 m.). [*Gss.*]

Shivering all over the back (aft. 1 h.). [*Myr.*]

395. In the afternoon, three or four times shivering, and in the night, profuse sweat, even on the hair.

Slight rigor in the back (aft. 30½ h.). [*Bch.*]

By day, internal chilliness without shivering; when walking in the open air he was chilly so that he could not get warm.

Constant chilliness, chiefly in the back. [*Stf.*]

Coldness first of the fingers, hands and feet, then of the palms and soles, then of the whole body, especially the limbs.

400. Feeling of coldness and actual coldness, first in the hands and arms, then through the whole of the rest of the body down into the feet (aft. ½ h.). [*Bch.*]

Coldness of the body with sticky sweat. [MACLEAN, l. c.]

Cold sweats. [WITHERING, l. c.]

Coldness and chill internally and externally in the whole body (aft. 36 h.). [*Gss.*]

Internal chill in the whole body with unusual warmth perceptible externally (aft. 14 h.). [*Gss.*]

405. Cold feeling through the whole body at once; the body felt cooler, the face excepted, which had no sensation of coldness and remained warm (aft. ½ h.). [*Bch.*]

One hand was cold, the other warm. [*Ln.*]

A suddenly arising warmth through the whole body, which just as suddenly went off again, and left behind a weakness of all the parts (aft. 25 h.). [*Bch.*]

Fever: succession of shivering, heat and strong transpiration. [MOSSMANN, in *Phys. Med. Journ.*, l. c.]

Frequent warmth all over the body, but in the forehead cold sweat—thirteen or fourteen hours after the coldness. [*Bch.*]

410. Along with slight chilliness in the back, burning of the head, face and ears, with red cheeks; at the same time the left eye seems much smaller (after a meal in a moderately warm room). [*Stf.*]

Redness and heat of the whole face, with chilliness over the rest of the body (aft. 3 h.). [*Trn.*]

The inner surface of the hands is warm and perspiring. [*Hbg.*]

In the morning on waking he found himself in slight perspiration (aft. 24 h.). [*Lr.*]

---

1 Rather, "from 48 to 56."
2 Should be "40." This is a statement from observation.
3 Subsequent to S. 384.
4 Accompanying purulent expectoration.

Perspiration in sleep at night.

415. Great desire for work (aft. 1½ h.).

Disposed for mental work and for all kinds of business.* [*Hbg.*]

Indisposed to speak. [*Hbg.*]

Gloominess and peevishness. [*Hbg.*]

Gloomy, morose humour ; he scolds about everything. [*Rkt.*]

420. Lachrymose sadness about many things in which he has been unsuccessful (aft. ½ h.).

He is sad and has a feeling of being very ill ; all objects appear to him as in fever, just as if he had a perversion of the visual faculty as in fever.

Dejection of the mind and apprehensiveness.[1] [WITHERING, l. c.]

Dispirited.[2] [PENKIVIL, l. c.]

Fear of death.

425. An anxious feeling as if he had done something bad. [*Ln.*]

(Secret mania with disobedience and obstinacy ; he tries to run away).

Mind indifferent, as insensible to surroundings, as if he had not slept enough, but without sleepiness. [*Trn.*]

The disposition is sociable and in other respects tranquil, except that he has very lively fancies.† [*Fz*]

* Curative action.

† Mostly secondary and curative action.

1 Not found.

2 On account of the apparent inefficiency of the medicine.

DROSERA ROTUNDIFOLIA.[1]

(Sundew.)

(The freshly expressed juice of this lowly plant, which grows on peaty soil [Hb. Rorellæ, Roris solis], mixed with equal parts of alcohol.)

This plant, one of the most powerful medicinal herbs in our zone, was used by the older physicians mostly as an external remedy—in cutaneous eruptions—but not with the best effects. They also gave it internally, and sometimes, as it would seem, with advantage. The moderns who, guided by tradition, had no knowledge of any other than large doses, knew not how to employ this uncommonly heroic plant without endangering the life of their patients, hence they rejected it altogether.

I first employed it in the trillion-fold dilution of the juice, but laterly in still higher potency, and at last in the 30th (decillion-fold) dilution (each diluting phial getting only two succussion), and of this I gave as a dose only the smallest portion of a drop, to wit, one, or at most two, globules the size of a poppy-seed (of which from 200 to 300 can be completely moistened with a drop of the dilution) in morbid conditions similar to the characteristic effects produced by the plant on healthy persons.

Thus, for example, a single such dose is quite sufficient for the homœopathic cure of epidemic whooping-cough,* according to the indications given by symptoms 135, 137, 144, 149, but especially 145 and the second part of symptom 143.

Allopathy, as may easily be understood, could hitherto do nothing for this formidable disease, which does not pass off by itself like other acute diseases, without terminating fatally or tormenting its victim for twenty or twenty-two weeks. In consequence it allowed many children to die of the disease where it did not hasten death by large doses of unsuitable drugs.

He who fails to perceive that in this as in other similar cases homœopathy is the only perfect, true medical art, let him continue blindly to employ unknown drugs to the injury of sick mankind!

Drosera requires further provings of its pure effects on the healthy human subject.

Camphor alleviates and antidotes its effects.

* The cure takes place with certainty in from seven to nine days, under a non-medicinal diet. Care should be taken not to give a second dose (or any other medicine) immediately after the first dose, for that would inevitably not only prevent the good result, but do serious injury, as I know from experience.

---

1 From vol. vi, 2nd edit., 1827.

[HAHNEMANN was aided in this proving by GUTMANN, FRIEDRICH HAHNEMANN, LANGHAMMER, WISLICENUS.
A few symptoms are derived from :
BONFIGLI, in *Vicat's Matiere Medicale*, i.
HALLER, *Ibid.*
NICOLAUS, *Ibid.*
In the *Fragmenta*, Drosera has 40 symptoms, in the 1st edit. of the 'R. A. M. L.' 279, and in this 2nd edit., 287.]

DROSERA.

When walking in the open air, vertigo (aft. 4 d.).

When walking in the open air, attack of vertigo ; he felt always as if he would fall to the left side (aft. 9 h.). [*Lr.*]

Whirling and giddy, with disinclination for work (aft. 33 h.). [*Gn.*]

The head is confused and heavy.

5. **Aching pain in the head.**

Out-pressing pain in the right temple. [*Gn.*]

On stooping, headache above the orbits, which goes off on walking.

After strong exercise and when walking, a headache in the forehead, like the confusion of the head that comes from much speaking.

Out-pressing pain in the forehead and zygomatic processes (aft. 7½ h.). [*Gn.*]

10. Aching pain above the right temple (aft. 3½ h.). [*Gn.*]

Pain boring out at the forehead, only on stooping while writing (aft. 7 h.). [*Gn.*]

A dull drawing pain in the left side of the brain towards the temple (aft. 28 h.). [*Gn.*]

In the right half of the brain, drawing pain towards the occiput (aft. 9 h.) [*Gn.*]

Tearing tensive pain in the forehead, more violent on stooping (aft. 11 h.). [*Gn.*]

15. Sharp cutting needle-pricks in the right side of the forehead (aft. 33 h.). [*Lr.*]

Tearing pain in the brain, more towards the forehead, worse on moving the eyes, but relieved by supporting the head on the hand (aft. 10 h.). [*Gn.*]

Heaviness of the head when held upright, but not when stooping (aft. 37 h). [*Gn.*]

Painfulness of the whole brain ; he feels every step in it (aft. 8 h.). [*Gn.*]

Burning sore pain on the right side of the hairy scalp ; it went off each time it was touched (aft. 6½ h.). [*Gn.*]

20. Smarting burning pain in the hairy scalp at the crown (aft. 10 h.). [*Gn.*]

Sore pain on the hairy scalp, above the right side of the forehead (aft. 32 h.). [*Gn.*]

Sore pain on the left frontal protuberance. [*Gn.*]

Sore sensation in the skin of the right temple. [*Gn.*]

Itching gnawing on the hairy scalp anteriorly, which went off on rubbing. [*Ws.*]

25. Eroding itching on the whole hairy scalp, but especially on the sides, which compelled scratching (aft. 12 h.). [*Lr.*]

Aching, sometimes combined with gnawing, externally on the top of the head (aft. 2 h.). [*Ws.*]

Obtuse boring pain externally on the crown (aft. 10 h.). [*Ws.*]

Aching gnawing pain externally over the eyebrows, with drawing thence into the cerebellum, in the morning (aft. 28 h.). [*Ws.*]

On pressing on the left eyebrow and eyelid, they pain as if festering (aft. 3 d.). [*Gn.*]

30. Drawing burning pain on the superciliary arch, more towards the temple (aft. 25 h.). [*Gn.*]

Contracted pupils.

Contracted pupils (aft. 1, 2 h.). [*Lr.*]

Dilated pupils (aft. 25 h.). [*Lr.*]

Long sight (presbyopia) and weakness of the eyes ; when he tries to see small objects, he has flickering before the eyes.

35. Like a veil before the eyes ; on reading the letters run together.

In the evening (7 o'clock), when he comes from a walk in the open air in the room, he is affected with dimness of vision, without vertigo, and there is flickering before the eyes.

Bright glittering playing before the right eye, rather above and to the side ; if he directs his sight towards the glittering, it recedes always more out of the line of sight ; it hinders him in reading (aft. 48 h.). [*Ws.*]

Tensive burning transversely across in the left eye and eyelids (aft. 13 h.). [*Gn.*]

The eyelids stick together as if with matter.

40. His eyelids itch (aft. 24 h.).

Sore pain in the right lower lid, worse when touched (aft. 11 h.). [*Gn.*]

A cutting pain transversely across the whole of the left eye. [*Gn.*]

Obtuse tearing transversely across the left eyeball (aft. 32 h.). [*Gn.*]

Severe stitches out at the eyes, especially when stooping.

45. A sharp stitch in the left eyeball, when at rest. [*Gn.*]

When he strains the eyes to look, he gets a pain in them, which is more smarting than aching.

Burning pain in the right eyeball, and fine stitches in the left internal ear (aft. 9 h.). [*Gn.*]

Broad, slow stitches through the left ear inwards (aft. 2 h.). [*Ws.*]

Squeezing and shooting in the left middle ear (aft. 30 h.). [*Gn.*]

50. Obtuse stitch in the right ear, not quite externally (aft. 3 h.). [*Gn.*]

A tickling prick in the innermost part of the right ear. [*Gn.*]

A pain in the right inner ear, as if all were compressed, almost cramp-like (aft. 7½ h.). [*Gn.*]

Drawing pain in the right ear-lobe and in a portion of the cartilage (aft. 31 h.). [*Gn.*]

Sharp gnawing beneath both aural cartilages (aft. ½ h.) [*Ws.*]

55. Tearing and twitching pain anteriorly in the orifice of the left ear (aft. 35 h.). [*Gn.*]

Tensive shooting in the left ear, more externally than internally (aft. 12 h.). [*Gn.*]

Pecking and burning pain externally in the whole right ear; soon followed by a dull drawing from without inwards (aft. 57 h.). [*Gn.*]

(Behind and beneath the left ear, a pimple painful when touched.)

Roaring and buzzing before the ears, or like a distant drum, which continues when moving and when at rest.

60. Hardness of hearing with increased buzzing before the ears.

Prickling burning pain in the skin of the cheek, below the left eyelid (aft. ¾ h.). [*Gn.*]

Drawing pressure on the upper jaws (aft. 2 h.). [*Ws.*]

Sudden, fine twitching in the left cheek, which makes him start (aft. 8 h.). [*Ws.*]

Digging aching in the right maxillary joint, and in the neighbouring bones, persisting when at rest and when moving—aggravated every time the mouth is opened (aft. 52 h.). [*Gn.*]

65. Severe aching pain in the right maxillary joint, when at rest and when moving (aft. 26 h.). [*Gn.*]

Prickling on the left side of the nose and formication in the left ear. [*Gn*]

Bleeding from the nose when stooping.

Bleeding from the nose in the morning and evening.

When washing his face in the morning he blows blood from his nose (aft. 4 d.). [*Gn.*]

70. Great sensitiveness to sour smells (aft. 3 d.). [*Gn.*]

The lower lip chapped in the centre.

Red pimple in the middle of the chin, close below the lower lip, its apex covered with a white scaly skin, without sensation even when touched (aft. 27 h.). [*Lr.*]

Here and there in the face small pimples with fine shooting pain only when touched, in the centre of which a pustule is formed, which dries up after some days. [*Ws.*]

Shooting tearing on the left lower jaw as if in the periosteum (aft. 8 h.). [*Ws.*]

75. Burning pain in the skin before the right oral commissure. [*Gn.*]

Causes pain in the teeth. [HALLER, in *Vicat's Matiere. Med.*, i, pp. 313, 314.[1]]

Shooting pain in the teeth, in the morning, after warm drinks.

(Looseness of the teeth.)

---

1 From its acridity.

Sensation of coldness in the crown of an incisor (aft. 56 h.). [*Gn.*]

80. Fine pecking pricks on the dorsum of the tongue (aft. 25 h.). [*Gn.*]

On the tip of the tongue there appears a whitish ulcer.

Shooting smarting pain in right side and tip of the tongue. [*Gn.*]

A small, round, painless swelling in the middle of the tongue (aft. 48 h.).

Smarting pain on the inside of the left cheek (as from pepper) (aft. 2 h.). [*Gn.*]

85. **Copious discharge of watery saliva—water-brash.**

Lips always dry and little taste.

Thirst.

Food is quite without any taste for him.

Bread tastes bitter.

90. In the morning, bitter taste in the mouth until he dines.

On the soft palate and deep down in the fauces, a rough, scraping dry sensation, which causes short cough. [*Ws.*]

Creeping, smarting sensation in the fauces, on the right side, when not swallowing (aft. 35 h.). [*Gn.*]

(Frequently during the day ravenous hunger, without appetite; when he thought he had appeased it, it returned after one and a half or two hours.)

Frequent hiccup (aft. 28 h.). [*Lr.*]

95. Something bitter rises from the stomach and comes into his mouth.

Something bitter and sour rises from the stomach and comes into his mouth.

(Nausea comes on by mere imagination.)

After a meal nausea with inclination to vomit.

Nausea with aching stupefying pain in the head, especially in the forehead (aft. 4 h.). [*Lr.*]

100. Nocturnal vomiting.

Vomiting before dinner.

In the morning, vomiting, mostly bile.

Vomiting of blood.

Shooting and throbbing in the scrobiculus cordis.

105. Squeezing tension in the scrobiculus cordis, as if all were drawn inwards there, especially on inspiring deeply (aft. 10 h.). [*Ws.*]

Fine, transient clutching together in the scrobiculus cordis (aft. 4 h.). [*Ws.*]

The region below the ribs (hypochondria) is painful on being touched and when coughing, and when he coughs he must press on the spot with his hand, in order to mitigate the pain.

Tensive pain in the epigastrium before and after stool, when he kept in his breath; he felt nothing when inspiring and expiring; when sitting and stooping the pain in the epigastrium becomes very violent; the stool is softer than usual (aft. 50 h.). [*Gn.*]

From the right side of the abdomen an obtuse drawing stitch darted across to the left side, which almost took away his breath, when walking (aft. 5 d.). [*Gn.*]

110. Pinching and clawing in the abdomen, with diarrhœa.

A twisting pain in the abdomen.

A shooting in the right side of the abdomen, when sitting.

Cutting in the abdomen (aft. 3 h.).

Nipping, cutting pinching in the abdomen, as if caused by displaced flatulence (aft. 13 h.). [*Lr.*]

115. Cutting blows in the abdominal and pectoral muscles, more severe when sitting than when moving (aft. 8 h.). [*Ws.*]

Boring stitches in the right side of the abdominal integuments (aft. 13 h.). [*Gn.*]

Obtuse stitch in the right iliac fossa (aft. 51 h.). [*Gn.*]

Out-pressing pain in the rectum, independent of stool (aft. 6 h.). [*Gn.*]

Cutting in the abdomen, not followed by stool (aft. 5 h.). [*Gn.*]

120. Frequent stools, with cutting in the abdomen.

Bloody mucus comes away with the stool, followed by pains in the abdomen and pain in the sacrum.

The first days thin stool, then somewhat harder, but after the evacuation there remained still fruitless call to stool.

A stool always becoming softer as it passes (aft. 1 h.). [*Gn.*]

Stool consisting of much pappy fæces (aft. 14 h.). [*Lr.*]

125. Scanty stool of hard fæces, with pressing (aft. 38 h.). [*Lr.*]

Watery, inodorous urine, with white, slimy fœtid stools (aft. 24 h.).

Frequent urging to urinate, with very scanty urine, often only passed by drops (aft. 2 h.). [*Lr.*]

Diuresis. [NICOLAUS,[1] in *Vicat*, l. c.]

Frequent copious flow of urine, all day (aft. 48 h.). [*Lr.*]

130. Itching obtuse prick in the glans penis, lasting some minutes (aft. 33 h.). [*Gn.*]

* * *

Crawling sensation in the right nostril, provoking sneezing (aft. 26 h.). [*Gn.*]

Frequent sneezing, with or without fluent coryza (aft. 13, 24 h.).

Painful sneezing and a cough, during which he must support the chest with his hand laid on it.

Severe fluent coryza, especially in the morning. [*Lr.*]

135. When coughing, pain in the hypochondria, as if that region were forcibly constricted.

Pain across the lower part of the chest and hypochondria.

Across the chest a violent pain when sitting, also independently of the cough, which is composed more of pressure than shooting, and goes off on moving ; the part also aches when touched.

The region beneath the short ribs (hypochondria) suffers from a contractive pain, which hinders the cough ; he cannot cough on account of pain unless he presses his hand on the scrobiculus cordis.

Deep breathing.

1 Observation.

140. Dyspnœa.

Tightness of chest, especially whenever he speaks, even at every word—the throat was contracted ; he felt no tightness of chest when walking.

Crawling in the larynx, which provokes coughing, with sensation as if a soft body was located there, with fine shooting therein to the right side of the gullet (aft. 4 d.). [*Gn.*]

Deep down in the fauces (and on the soft palate) a rough, scraping sensation of dryness exciting short cough, with yellow slimy expectoration and hoarseness of the voice*, so that it is only with an effort that he can speak in a deep bass tone ; at the same time he feels an oppression of the chest, as if something there kept back the air when he coughed and spoke, so that the breath could not be expelled (lasting several days). [*Ws.*]

Cough coming from quite deep down in the chest.

145. Cough, the impulses of which follow one another so violently, that he can hardly get his breath

Cough in the evening, immediately after lying down.

Nocturnal cough.

He wakes up at night (about 2 a.m.) for a short time to cough and then falls asleep again.

In the evening, while lying in bed, when he breathes out, a sudden contraction of the hypogastrium, which makes him heave as though he would vomit, and excites coughing.

150. The cough, when expectoration did not properly occur, affected the abdomen, like a clawing together and retching.

The cough makes him like to vomit.

On coughing, he vomits water, mucus and food.

On coughing, the breath he brings up from his lungs has a smell of burning.

Cough in the morning with expectoration.

155. (The taste of what he coughs and hawks up is salt.)

What is coughed up in the morning tastes bitter.

What is coughed up has a disgusting taste in the morning—not during the day.

Shooting in the chest when coughing.

From the morning onwards, intolerable stitches when coughing and breathing deeply in the upper part of the side of the chest, near the axilla, which is somewhat alleviated only by pressing the hand on the painful part—with expectoration intimately mixed with

* Very similar to this must be the state, where, in some kinds of so-called laryngeal phthisis (provided that no specific cachexy of a syphilitic, psoric, &c. kind is at the bottom of it), sundew is so peculiarly useful. This plant also excites a very violent cough in sheep (see BORRICHIUS, in *Act. Hafne.*, vol. iv, p. 162). Several of the older physicians found this plant useful in some kinds of malignant cough, and in phthisical persons, thus confirming its (homoeopathic) medicinal power ; but the moderns (vide MURRAY, *Apparat. Med.*, vol. iii, p. 501), in conformity with their antipathic theories, warned against its use on account of its supposed acridity.

blood, and coloured red ; but the part is not painful to external touch (aft. 24 h.).

160. Hæmoptysis.

When coughing and breathing, stitches in the pectoral muscles.

A burning rough sensation deep down in the throat, immediately after dinner (aft. 29 h.). [*Gn.*]

Tensive pain in the pectoral muscles, lasting several hours, when inspiring and expiring (aft. 8 h.). [*Gn.*]

Burning sensation in the middle of the chest, without thirst. (aft. 4 h.). [*Gn.*]

165. Creeping sensation in the left costal muscles, with a pressing headache in both temples, especially the right (aft. 8½ h.). [*Gn.*]

A hot, obtuse stitch in the muscles of the right true ribs, continuing on inspiration and expiration. [*Gn.*]

Obtuse stitches in the left costal muscles, so violent that they almost take away his breath, continuing on inspiration and expiration (aft. 3 d.). [*Gn.*]

Itching stitch in the coccyx, when sitting (aft. 29 h.). [*Gn.*]

On walking quickly, a clawing-together pinching in the left lumbar region, which tightens the breath, relieved by pressing with the hand (aft. 1 h.), [*Ws.*]

170. Drawing stitch in the left loin down into the penis (aft. 6 h.). [*Gn.*]

Shooting tearing from the spine to the anterior process of the left os ilii, when sitting (aft. 8 h.). [*Ws.*]

An obtuse stitch in the left dorsal muscles (aft. 12 h.). [*Gn.*]

Here and there pain in the back as if bruised.

The back is painful as if it were beaten (broken on the wheel), in the morning (aft. 12 h.).

175. Drawing pain in the back and shoulders, when at rest and when moving (aft. 6 h.). [*Fr. H—n.*]

During movement, rheumatism felt between the scapulæ, which extends to the sacrum.

The nape is stiff, and painful on movement.

Quivering on the right shoulder, only when at rest (aft. 52 h.). [*Gn.*]

In the shoulder-joint pain as if bruised, when he bends the arm backwards, or raises it, or lies on it, or only touches the joint.

180. Pain in the shoulder-joint, as if the arm would go to sleep, and were tired and weak—it goes off on continuing to move.

When walking or standing dislocation pain in the left axilla, which however, is alleviated by touching (aft. 11 h.) [*Lr.*]

Sharp pressure from within outwards in the axilla, when at rest (aft. 7 h.). [*Ws.*]

The arm is painful on movement, as if the flesh of the muscles were detached from the bones.

Shooting in the right arm, and there occurs a pain from the shoulder to the elbow, even when at rest ; the elbow-joint is painful when touched, as if gathering.

185. Pain as if contused, first in the bend of the elbow-joint, then in that of the shoulder-joint.

Squeezing tension in the bend of the elbow on flexing the arm, felt but little on extending it (aft. 24 h.). [*Ws.*]

Severe, very acutely painful stitches through the middle of the left forearm (aft. 12 h.). [*Ws.*]

On the wrist-joint, where the heads of the ulna and radius touch one another, pain on bending and turning the hand, and on touching.

Pain as if beaten and contused in the hands, up to the elbow-joints.

190. Sudden cutting behind the wrist-joint, between the shafts of both bones, at the same time with paralytic weakness of the arm (aft. 48 h.). [*Ws.*]

On the back of the hand and behind the wrist-joint, two red, raised spots the size of lentils, at first painful, afterwards, in one of them, itching pricks, which are more violent on being rubbed. [*Ws.*]

Stitches into the fingers and out at their tips, also when at rest.

Inclination of the fingers to draw themselves spasmodically together, and when grasping anything a stiffness in the middle finger-joints, as if the tendons would not yield, sometimes in the right, sometimes in the left hand.

Spasmodic contraction of the flexor tendons of the fingers, so that he could only extend them with difficulty, when he held something in the hand (aft 8 h.). [*Ws.*]

195. A deeply eroded little ulcer on the back of the right hand, with an itching sensation, which on rubbing changes into burning, whereupon a bloody watery discharge comes out (aft. 24 h.). [*Lr.*]

He feels pulsation in a blood-vessel of the back of the left hand, together with an out-pressing pain in the forehead (aft. 7 h.). [G*n.*]

In the ball of the left thumb a tearing pain, lasting some minutes, when at rest and when moving (aft. 28 h.). [*Gn.*]

A violent, sharp stitch in the tuberosity of the ischium, on rising from a seat (aft. 55 h.). [*Gn.*]

Paralytic pain in the right hip-joint and thigh, and in the ankle-joint, but in the latter rather as if dislocated, when walking, when he must limp on account of the pain (aft. 11 h.). [*Gn.*]

200. (After a meal tearing pain in the thigh, with heaviness of the legs.)

At night aching pain in the posterior muscles of the left thigh, increased by pressing on it and stooping; he could not lie on it at night; it went off after getting up.

Acute pain in the bones of the right thigh and leg, coming on at night during sleep, so that on waking she must stretch out the limb immediately in order to allay the pain, for 18 hours. [*Fr. H—n.*[

A single cutting stitch in the middle of the anterior aspect of the left thigh, recurring from time to time (aft. 24 h.). [*Ws.*]

Cutting pinching on the posterior aspect of the left thigh (aft. 2 h.). [*Ws.*]

205. Pain in the left thigh and in the knee-joint, as if both were broken, only when walking (aft. 1½ h.). [*Gn.*]

Painful stiffness of the houghs ; he could scarcely bend the knees.

Trembling of the knees when walking, even in the room, chiefly when going up stairs.

Stitches in the shaft of the fibula upwards towards the calf, when at rest ; the pain woke her up at night from sleep.

A fine cutting stitch in the right calf, which comes on when sitting, and goes off on walking. [*Gn.*]

210. He cannot extend the leg without great pain, and must limp.

Paralytic tearing in both ankle-joints, worst when keeping the feet at rest (aft. 8 h.). [*Ws.*]

Tearing pain in the right ankle-joint, as if it were dislocated, only when walking (aft. 34 h.). [*Gn.*]

Tearing pain in the ball of the right big toe on one point, when at rest (aft. 26 h.). [*Gn.*]

Fine stitch-like pains in the three middle toes, so violent that he must limp, only observable when walking (aft. 4½ d.). [*Gn.*]

215. Staggering unsteady gait from weakness of the feet, on commencing to walk, which goes off on continuing to walk.

Inflexibility of the ankle-joints—they are very stiff.

(Shooting and throbbing about the right ankle-joint, worst when lying, at night.)

Drawing pain up and down in the feet to the calves.

Tearing pain in the heel during movement (when walking).

220. An itching prick in the left sole, in the balls of the toes, when sitting (aft. 1½ h.). [*Gn.*]

A pain compounded of gnawing and shooting in the shafts of the bones of the arms, thighs and legs, particularly severe in the joints, with severe stitches in the joints, less felt when moving than when at rest. [*Ws.*]

Cramp-like pressure now in the upper, and now in the lower extremities, when at rest and when moving (aft. 18 h.). [*Lr.*]

Painful shooting pressure in the muscles of the upper and lower extremities at the same time, in every position (aft. 4½, 30 h.). [*Lr.*]

On turning the head and trunk, in order to look about him, painful cramp in the dorsal and abdominal muscles, which lasted a long time.

225. (A twitching or twitching sensation in the limbs.)

All the limbs are as if bruised and are also painful externally.

All his limbs feel paralyzed.

Pain in all the limbs—he feels as if all were paralyzed.

Soreness of all the limbs on which he lies, as if the bed were too hard, and he had not enough mattresses under him.

230. When applied externally the plant erodes the skin. [HALLER, in *Vicat.*, l. c.]

He is weak in the whole body, with sunken eyes and cheeks (aft. 8 h.). [*Gn.*]

Frequent stretching, and yawning, as if he had not slept enough (aft. 30 h.). [*Lr.*]

At night she often starts up in sleep, as from fright or fear, but when awake she is not anxious.

Frequent waking from sleep, as if he had already slept enough and it were time to get up. [*Lr.*]

235. Frequent violent starting up in affright, in the evening, in sleep.

At night anxious dreams.

Sleeplessness.

In the morning, extreme weariness, he is unwilling to get out of bed.

So exhausted, in the morning on waking, that he can scarcely open his eyes.

240. He snores in his sleep when lying on his back. [*Lr.*]

Vivid dreams, sometimes pleasant, sometimes anxious. [*Lr.*]

Vivid vexatious dream about the ill-treatment of others, [*Lr.*]

Frequent nocturnal waking, each time on the commencement of a breaking out of perspiration (the first night). [*Lr.*]

He dreamt of thirst and drinking and awoke thirsty and must drink (the second night). [*Gn.*]

245. Fever: confused heavy head, constant chilliness, he cannot get warm, food has no taste—then comes on thirst and heat of head, with flow of watery saliva.

Quotidian intermittent fever: in the forenoon before 9 o'clock, chilliness with icy cold hands and blue nails (he must lie down) until noon, after the chill, thirst—thereafter heaviness in the head, throbbing pain in the occiput and heat in the face, with normal temperature of the rest of the body, until 3 p.m.—in the evening well; at night profuse sweat, especially on the abdomen; after the heat, inclination to vomit.

Fever, qualmish nausea, which seemed to arise out of the stomach. with feeling of heat in the face and rigor all over the body, with icy cold hands (aft. 27½ h.). [*Lr.*]

When at rest, shivering; when moving, no shivering.

While at rest and though the body is normally warm to the touch, still he shivers, and even in bed he cannot keep off of the shivering and feeling of coldness.

250. He always feels too cold; he cannot get warm.

He has a feeling of coldness at night in bed, but without shivering.

Febrile rigor all over the body, without heat or thirst (aft. 12½ h.). [*Lr.*]

Face, nose and hands are cold.

Febrile rigor all over the body, with heat in the face, but icy cold hands, without thirst. (aft. 3, 27 h.). [*Lr.*]

255. (Coldness of the left half of the face, with shooting pains in it, whilst the right side of the face is hot and dry, after midnight.)

(In the evening, cold cheeks and hot hands.)

In the afternoon, frequent attacks now of chilliness, now of heat, accompanied by inclination to vomit.

Rigor all over the body, with warm forehead, hot cheeks, but cold hands, without thirst (repeated the following day) (aft. 34 h.). [*Lr.*]

During the febrile chill vomiting, when at last bile is thrown up.

260. All day, chilliness; all night, heat (aft. 36 h.).

Warmth of the upper part of the body, towards evening.

Heat in the head.

Heat and redness in the face (aft. 5 h.).

For three successive nights, sweat only on the face.

265. (Heat and sweat on the chest, thighs and houghs, with thirst, all day and night.)

Night-sweat.

Sweat, immediately after midnight.

Sweats.[1] [Bonfigli, in *Vicat*, l. c.]

Anxiety with feeling of heat quickly running all over the body, but especially all over the face, as though he were about to receive bad news (aft. 3½ h.), and again (aft. 27 h.) rigor all over the body, without heat and without thirst. [*Lr.*]

270. **Restlessness; when reading he could not stick long to one subject—he must always go to something else** (aft. 36 h.). [*Gn.*]

All day long, uneasiness of disposition and anxiety, full of mistrust, as if he had to do with none but false people (aft. 38 h.). [*Lr.*]

Extremely uneasy, sad disposition, all day—he imagined he was being deceived by spiteful, envious people. [*Lr.*]

Silent and reserved, with anxiety—he always feared he was about to learn something disagreeable. [*Lr.*]

Anxiety, as if his enemies would not leave him quiet, envied and persecuted him. [*Lr.*]

275. He is sad and dejected about the ills of life, which people cause one another and himself, respecting which he is anxious and concerned; at the same time want of appetite (aft. 5 h.). [*Gn.*]

He is dejected about the malice of others on all hands, and at the same time disheartened and concerned about the future (aft. 4 d.). [*Gn.*]

Anxiety, especially in the evening (about 7 or 8 o'clock), as if he were impelled to jump into the water in order to take his own life by drowning—he was not impelled to any other mode of death. [*Lr.*]

Anxiety in solitude—he wished to have someone always near him, could not bear to be without companions, and was quieter when he had someone to speak to; but when they again left him in

1 Observation.

solitude, he was all the more anxious, until he fell asleep ; on awaking the anxiety returned (for six successive evenings). [*Lr.*]

The anxiety appeared to rise up from the subcostal region. [*Lr.*]

280. Very peevish ; a trifle puts him out of humour.

He takes insults very resentfully, not without vexation.

Unhappy, obtuse of sense and disinclined for manual and intellectual work (aft. 33 h.). [*Gn.*]

An unimportant circumstance excited him so much, that he was beside himself with rage (aft. 4½ h.). [*Gn.*]

Obstinate prosecution of resolutions he had formed.

285. He feels an inner tranquillity and cheerfulness* (aft. 12 h.). [*Gn.*]

Tranquillity of disposition.* [*Lr.*]

Happy, steadfast disposition ; he dreaded no evil, because he was conscious of having acted honourably.* [*Lr.*]

* Reaction of the vital power, secondary action, curative action.

DULCAMARA.[1]

(Solanum dulcamara, Woody Night-shade.)

(The juice freshly expressed from the young stalks and leaves of this shrub-like plant before its flowering time, mixed with equal parts of spirits of wine. Two drops of the clear fluid lying over the sediment are added to 98 drops of spirits of wine, the phial shaken with two strokes of the arm, and in this way diluted through 29 phials (filled two thirds full with 100 drops of spirits of wine), and each potentized with two succussions up to the decillion-fold development of power ; one or two smallest globules moistened with this serve for a dose.)

It is very probable, as experiments have indeed partly proved. that this very powerful plant belongs to the *antipsorics*, as the following pure effects of it seem also to show ; still, I shall try to obtain more accurate corroboration of this.

It will moreover be found specific for some epidemic fevers, as also for various acute diseases the result of a chill.

Its long duration of action is shown in its trials on healthy persons.

[AHNER, CUBITZ, GROSS, MULLER, of Treuen, NENNING (in HARTLAUB and TRINKS' *Mat. Med.*), E. F. RUCKERT, STAPF, TRINKS and HARTLAUB (in their *Mat. Med.*), GUST, WAGNER, WAHLE, aided HAHNEMANN in this proving.

Symptoms quoted from the following old-school authorities :

ALTHOF, in *Murray*, *Appar. Med.*

CARRERE, *Ueber das Bittersuss*, 1789.

FRITZE, *Annal d. Klin. Ins. in Berlin*, iii.

GOUAN, *Memoires de la Soc. de Montpellier.*

HAEN, DE, *Ratio Medendi.*

LINNÆUS, *Diss. de Dulcamara.* Upsal., 1753.

PIQUOT, *Samml. br. Abh. f. pr. A.*, ii.

STARCKE, in *Carrere*, l. c.

TODE (reference not given).

In the 1st edit. of the 'R.A.M.L.' dulcamara had 123 symptoms, in the 2nd edit. 349, and in this last edit. 401 ; the *Chr. Kr.* gives 409.]

DULCAMARA.

A transient slight vertigo. [*Ng.*]

At noon before eating, whilst walking, giddy, as if all objects remained standing before him, and as if it became black before his eyes.

Momentary vertigo. [PIQUOT,[1] in *Samml. br. Abh. f. pr. A.*, ii, 4.]

Vertigo [ALTHOF,[2] in *Murray, Appar. Med.*, i, p. 621.]

5. When he wanted to get up out of bed in the morning, he almost

[1] From vol. i, 3rd edit., 1830.
[2] Statement from observation

fell from vertigo, general weakness and trembling of all the body (aft. 24 h.). [*Mr.*]

Stupefaction. [CARRERE,[1] *Ueber das Bittersuss, v. Starcke*, Jen., 1786.]

Great stupefaction of the head. [STARCKE,[2] in *Carrere*, l. c.]

Dull stupefying headache.

Headache in the morning in bed, aggravated by rising. [*Mr.*]

10. Headache, lassitude, icy coldness of all the body, and inclination to vomit. [*Mr.*]

Heaviness of the head. [CARRERE, l. c.]

Heaviness in the forehead (aft. 12 h.). [*We.*]

Heaviness in the forehead for several days, at the same time frequent darts from within outwards in the temporal region. [*We.*]

Heaviness in the occiput, for three days. [*We.*]

15. Heaviness of the whole head all day, as if the integuments of the head were stretched, especially in the nape, where the sensation becomes a kind of formication. [*We.*]

Heaviness of the head, with out-boring pain in the temple and forehead, as after a debauch overnight. [*Wr.*]

Stupid feeling in the head, as after intoxication, which went off in the open air. [*Wr.*]

Stupid and empty in the head, in the afternoon about 6 o'clock. [*Ng.*]

Stupid feeling in the head and slight drawing in the left frontal protuberance. [*Ng.*]

20. The stupid headache lasted for 10 days. [*Ng.*]

Giddiness in the head with warmth rising up into the whole face. [*Ng.*]

Heat in the head. [CARRERE, l. c.]

Digging aching in the whole of the forehead. [*Gss.*]

Violent headache like a digging in the middle of the brain in the sinciput, like dulness, and a sensation as if the brain were swollen, a pain that came on early in bed, and was not diminished or increased either by rest or movement; but it was worse on getting up. [*Mr.*]

25. Out-boring headache at one time in the forehead, at another in the temples (aft. 15 h.). [*Wr.*]

Before midnight boring headache from within. [*We.*]

Boring headache in the right temple (aft. 23 h.). [*We.*]

The headache never involves the whole head, but only quite a small spot, where it shows itself as pressure as with a blunt instrument. [*Gss.*]

1 Carrere's original work is "Traite des proprietes, usages, et effets de la Douceamere," Paris, 1789. The citations have been corrected from this treatise. They consist of effects of dulcamara when given for chronic rheumatism, suppressed secretions, and cutaneous diseases. The author says that he has, after seventeen years' experience with the drug, seen no inconvenience result from full doses save those described in S. 88 and 278; 199; 395, 358 (sometimes the precursors of a new eruption, and then associated with 341 and 342); 11 and 65; and 94.

2 Carrere's German translator. Additional observations (of the same kind) by him.

All the afternoon a dull headache, especially in the left frontal protuberance. [*Ng.*]

30. In the evening the dull pressive headache became more severe, with increasing coryza. [*Ng.*]

Painful stupefying aching in the left side of the vertex (aft. 3 h.). [*Ng.*]

Aching stupefying pain in the occiput, from the nape upwards. [*Rkt.*]

In the temples a pressure, as with a blunt instrument, at one time on the right, at another on the left side. [*Gss.*]

Dull feeling in the forehead and root of the nose, as if he had a board in front of the head. [*Gss.*]

35. Towards evening, when walking in the open air, headache like a pressing outwards. [*We.*]

Quite late in the evening out-pressing pain in the left frontal protuberance. [*Ng.*]

Out-pressing pain in jerks in the sinciput, worse when moving. [*Ng.*]

Drawing pressure in the left frontal protuberance (6th d.) [*Ng.*]

Aching drawing in the left temporal region, in the afternoon. [*Ng.*]

40. Headache, drawing from both temples inwards. [*We.*]

Aching tearing in the temples in fits. [*Gss.*]

Aching beating pain in the left side of the forehead with whirling feeling. [*Ng.*]

Tearing compression in the top of the head. [*Gss.*]

Intermitting tearing in the left temple. [*Gss.*]

45. Stitches in the head, so that she got angry over it, mostly in the evening ; relieved when lying.

A very slow pricking in the occiput, as with a needle, that was always drawn back again. [*We.*]

Deep in the brain violent shooting in the sinciput, with nausea. [*Mr.*]

Intermitting pressure on the left of the crown, as if a blunt instrument were preseed into the head. [*Gss.*]

Sensation as if the occiput were enlarged. [*We.*]

50. Pressing pain in the left occipital bone. [*We.*]

Headache in the occiput, in the evening in bed. [*We.*]

Slow drawing pain through the whole brain, especially in the evening (aft. $\frac{1}{4}$ h.).

In the evening when eating a drawing pain on the skull to the nasal bones, where it became contractive. [*We.*]

From the frontal protuberance there is a drawing down to the tip of the nose in rapid jerks. [*Gss.*]

55. A slight drawing in the left frontal protuberance, especially on stooping forwards. [*Ng.*]

On the head, just over the left ear, a stupefying pain, as if some one pressed with a blunt instrument into the head. [*Gss.*]

On the forehead lumps, touching which causes shooting pain.

Aching tensive pain over the right eye (aft. 3 h.). [*Wr.*]

Boring pain over the right palpebral arch from within outwards.

60. Contractive pain at the supra-orbital border. [*Gss.*]

Aching in the eyes when reading and at other times, but aggravated by reading. [*Rkt.*]

When she walks in the sun it is as if fire flew out of the eyes, as also in the room.

Sparks before the eyes. [PIQUOT, l. c.]

Commencement of amaurosis and such weakness of the eyes that he saw all objects, both near and distant, as if through a veil; the upper lid was as if half paralysed, as if it would fall down. [*Mr.*]

65. Dim vision.[1] [CARRERE, l. c.]

Inflammation of the eyes (chemosis). [TODE,[2]—STARCKE, l. c.]

Painless pressure on the left zygoma (immediately). [*Gss.*]

Ringing in the ears. [*Rkt.*]

Ringing in the ears.

70. Clear ringing in the ears (aft. 4 to 8 d.). [*Stf.*]

A kind of prickling in the left ear and then in the right, as if very cold air had penetrated into the ear. [*We.*]

Tearing in the left ear intermingled with shootings from within outwards; a drumming and bubbling before the ear, he does not hear well afterwards; on opening the mouth a crackling in the ear as if something broken were in it. [*Ts. Hb.*]

Squeezing pain in the left ear, at the same time great nausea. [*Ts. Hb.*]

Frightful earache all night, he cannot sleep on account of it. In the morning the pain ceased all at once, but there remained a roaring before the ear for some time. [*Ts. Hb.*]

75. In the left ear, a pinching stitch towards the membrana tympani. [*We.*]

Fine pricks in the meatus auditorious and parotid gland. [*Rt.*, senr.]

Squeezing, accompanied by small pricks, in the right ear. [*We.*]

Transient drawing in the external meatus. [*Gss.*]

Below the left ear, towards the ramus of the lower jaw, a cramp-like contraction. [*Gss.*]

80. There occurred such a violent bleeding of the nose that the blood lost amounted to four ounces; it was bright red, flowed very warm out of the left nostril, with a pressure in the region of the longitudinal sinus, which pressure continued after the profuse hæmorrhage. [*Ng.*]

Epistaxis. [STARCKE, l. c.]

In the inside of the left ala nasi, a pimple with ulcerative pain. [*We.*]

Eruption in both angles of the nose, a pimple.

Drawing and tearing in the whole cheek.

---

1 With S. 11.

2 Cannot be traced for want of reference.

85. Itching on the cheeks, close to the alæ nasi (aft. ½ h.).

A humid eruption on the cheek.[1] [CARRERE, l. c.]

On the inside of the upper lip, on the anterior part of the palate, also externally round the mouth, pimples and small ulcers, which on moving give rise to tearing pain.

Twitching movements of the lips and eyelids (in cold air). [CARRERE, l. c.]

Under the chin, a pinching on a small spot. [*Gss.*]

90. Itching pimples on the chin.

A drawing pain in the right cervical muscles. [*Mr.*]

Obtuseness of the teeth, as if they were insensible. [*Mr.*]

Pressure in the throat, as if the uvula were too long.

Pains in the throat. [CARRERE, l. c.]

95. Flow of saliva.[1] [CARRERE, l. c.]

Flow of saliva with loose, spongy gums. [STARCKE, l. c.]

Flow of saliva, what is called waterbrash.

Flow of much viscid, soapy saliva. [STARCKE, l. c.]

Itching crawling on the tip of the tongue. [*We.*]

100. Dry tongue. [CARRERE, l. c.]

Dry rough tongue.[5] [CARRERE, l. c.]

Paralysis of the tongue, which hindered her in speaking (when using dulcamara in cold wet weather). [CARRERE, l. c.]

Paralysis of the tongue after taking it for a long time. [LINNÆUS,[3] *Dis de Dulcamara*, Upsal., 1753.]

Paralysis of the tongue. [GOUAN,[4] *Memoires de la Soc. de Montpellier.*]

105. Much eructation. [*Mr.*]

Very scrapy fauces, with constant hawking up of very viscid mucus. [*Ng.*]

Four times eructation, with scratching in the œsophagus and heartburn. (aft. 9 h.). [*Ng.*]

Empty eructation, with shuddering as from disgust. [*Ng.*]

Frequent empty eructation. [*Gss.*]

110. Eructation combined with hiccup. [*Gss.*]

Flat, soapy taste in the mouth, and hence want of appetite. [STARCKE, l. c.]

While eating repeated eructation, so that the soup comes up again into the throat immediately after it is swallowed. [*Gss.*]

Hunger, with repugnance to all kinds of food.

He has a good appetite and eats with relish, yet he soon becomes satiated and full, with much rolling and rumbling in the bowels. [*Gss.*]

115. While eating repeated pinching in, and distension of, the abdomen. [*Gss.*]

---

1 Not found.

2 See note to S. 343.

3 Not accessible. According to Murray, Linnæus is only citing Gouan (see next symptom).

4 Not accessible.

Nausea. [ALTHOF, in *Murray*, *Appar. Med.*, i, p. 621.—LINNÆUS. l.c.]
Nausea and disgust. [CARRERE, l. c.]
Nausea, vomiting, heat, and anxiety. [STARCKE, l. c.]
Disgust with shuddering, as though about to vomit [*Ng.*]

120. Great nausea, as if he would vomit, with rigor. [*Ts. Hb.*]

Actual vomiting of nothing but viscid mucus, but not of the medicine (aft. ½ h.). [*Ng.*]

Warmth rises up and there then occurs vomiting of mucus, in the morning.

Retching. [ALTHOF, l. c.]

Feeling of increased warmth in the fauces. [*Rkt.*]

125. Vomiting. [LINNÆUS, l. c.]

After a moderate meal, distension of the abdomen as if it would burst. [*Gss.*]

Feeling of distension in the pit of the stomach, with a disagreeable feeling of emptiness in the abdomen. [*Ng.*]

In the left side, below the short ribs, sudden contraction, almost like cutting. [*Gss.*]

On going to sleep continual pinching in the region of the stomach, until he fell asleep (2nd d.). [*Ng.*]

130. Uneasiness in the abdomen, like flatulent distension, with frequent eructation only of air (3rd d.). [*Ng.*]

Tensive pain on the right near the scrobiculus cordis, as if he had strained and injured himself. [*We.*]

An acute aching pain in the scrobiculus cordis, as if he had received there a blow with a blunt instrument, which becomes more painful by pressing on it (aft. 35 h.). [*Ar.*]

To the left of the scrobiculus cordis an obtuse stitch, that rapidly went off, returned again soon, and then went off gradually (aft. ¼ h.). [*Ar.*]

A shooting pain in the scrobiculus cordis (aft. 9½ h.). [*Ar.*]

135. In the umbilical region a shooting pain, that did not go off by pressure (aft. 1 h.). [*Ar.*]

Under the ribs on the right side, obtuse stitches that take away the breath. [*Gss.*]

In the left side of the abdomen, intermittent obtuse stitches ; pressing with the finger just upon the painful spot causes pain, and the shooting becomes worse. [*Gss.*]

Short obtuse stitches to the left of the navel, in the evening. [*Ng.*]

Obtuse stitches outwards in rapid succession on a small spot on the left of the abdomen, which take away his breath ; when he presses on it with the finger, the place is painful ; he feels as if something would force itself through from within. [*Gss.*]

140. Single pulsating stitches under the left short ribs, when sitting, which went off on rising up (aft. 6 d.). [*Ar.*]

Pinching shooting pain to the right of the navel, which did not go off by pressure (aft. 4¼ h.). [*Ar.*]

On the left above the navel a fine pinching in a small spot of the abdomen. [*Gss.*]

Violent pinching in abdomen, as if a long worm crept about and gnawed and pinched in the bowels (aft. 31 h.). [*Ar.*]

Obtuse pinching in the abdomen, as if diarrhœa were about to come on (aft. 2 h.). [*Ng.*]

145. Just under the navel, a pinching pain on sitting in a bent-forward attitude, but on stretching himself out it dimished, and soon afterwards ceased (aft. 4½ d.). [*Ar.*]

Quite early, a pinching pain around about the umibilical region, as if he must go to stool, but without urging. [*Ar.*]

Transient pinching and cutting in the abdomen and chest, as from incarcerated flatulence. [*Gss.*]

Bellyache (immediately).

Bellyache as from a chill.

150. Rumbling in the abdomen (immediately).

Each time he leans forward a gushing round about in the bowels as if he had taken a purgative. [*Ng*]

Rumbling in the bowels, as if a stool would ensue, with some sacral pain. [*Ng.*]

Bellyache as though he had caught cold (aft. 23 h.). [*We.*]

Bellyache such as usually occurs during cold wet weather. [*We.*]

155. He has pinching and cutting and digging round about in the abdomen, as if diarrhœa were coming on. [*Gss.*]

In the morning, without having eaten anything, flying pinching and cutting in the bowels, with distension of the abdomen. [*Gss.*]

Twitching cutting and pinching here and there in the abdomen, that soon goes off. [*Gss.*]

A twisting, digging pinching pain round about the umbilical region (aft. 10 h.). [*Ar.*]

A forcing out pain on the left above the navel, as if a rupture would occur there. [*Mr.*]

160. A gnawing beating pain just above the navel. [*Gss.*]

Aching pain now in the left, now in the right inguinal gland.

Swelling of the left inguinal gland as large as a walnut.

(In the inguinal swelling, severe burning (mingled with shooting) on the slightest movement; also on touching it burning mingled with shooting.)

Swelling of the glands of the groin.[1] [CARRERE, l. c.]

165. Swollen hard inguinal glands of the size of a haricot-bean, but without pains. [*We.*]

Pinching pain in the umbilical region and above the left hip, that compels him to go to stool; after the passage of some flatus, in spite of strong straining, there only passes a little hard fæces, but the pain after this was somewhat lessened (aft. 2½ d.). [*Ar.*]

Pain in the abdomen, as if diarrhœa were about to ensue; after the passage of some flatus the bellyache ceased. [*We*]

---

1 During treatment of scrofula by D., there supervened S. 378 going on to 376, and followed by this swelling of the inguinal glands, and also of those of the neck and axillæ. The continued use of the medicine removed all.

In the evening, in the whole abdomen, pinching with call to stool; after having previously had in the afternoon his usual stool, though it was very hard and difficult, he had a large moister stool, and at last a copious, quite thin, sour smelling motion, whereupon he felt relieved but exhausted. [*Gss.*]

Very slight sensation of cold on the back, with rumbling in the bowels and pain in the left groin, not increased by touch (aft. 12 h.). [*Ng.*]

170. Tension in the region of the os pubis on rising up from the seat.

Soft stool in small pieces. [*We.*]

Mucous diarrhœa, alternately yellow and greenish.[1] [CARRERE, l. c.]

White mucous diarrhœa.[1] [CARRERE, l. c.]

Mucous diarrhœa with prostration.[1] [CARRERE, l. c.]

175. Soft stool (immediately).

Several successive afternoons thin evacuations with flatus (aft. 3 d.).

Normal stool, but with some straining (aft. $\frac{1}{4}$ h.). [*Ng.*]

He had a rapid call to stool which he could scarcely retain, although only little and hard fæces came away (aft. $\frac{1}{2}$ h.). [*Ar.*]

Along with nausea he had frequent call to stool, and yet all day long he could pass nothing (aft. 2 h.). [*Mr.*]

180. He has pinching in the bowels and must go to stool, but he is costive and but little passes with much straining (aft. 8 h.). [*Ar.*]

Pressure in the abdomen and colic before the stool, not during the evacuation, afterwards recurring with rumbling in the bowels. [*Rkt.*]

Difficult, dry, rare stools. [CARRERE, l. c.]

Suddenly a dreadful pressing on the rectum, so that he can scarcely keep back the motion, and when he gets to the night-stool, there comes away slowly, after a while, with some straining, very hard fæces, along with transient pinching and cutting here and there in the abdomen. [*Gss.*]

Rare, slow and hard stool; even when he wants to go there is no urging in the rectum, and it is only by a great effort that a very large hard motion comes slowly away. [*Gss.*]

185. Great discharge of flatus. [*We.*]

Flatus smelling of asafœtida. [*Mr.*]

Turbid whitish urine.[1] [CARRERE, l. c.]

Copious discharge at first of clear and viscid, then of thick and milk-white urine.[1] [2] [CARRERE, l. c.]

Urine at first clear and viscid, then white, then turbid, then clear, with white sticky sediment.[1] [CARRERE, l. c.]

190. Turbid, ill-smelling urine and ill-smelling perspiration.[1] [CARRERE, l. c.]

Urine reddish and scalding.[3] [CARRERE, l. c.]

---

1 All these symptoms are critical discharges, coinciding with improvement in the patient's malady.

2 For "viscid", read "limpid."

3 See note to S. 343.

Urine with mucous sediment, at one time red at another white.[1] [CARRERE, l. c.]

Turbid urine.[2] [CARRERE, l. c.]

Turbid whitish urine.[3] [CARRERE, l. c.]

195. Pulsating[4] outwards in the bladder. [*We.*]

Strangury, painful micturition. [STARCKE, l. c.]

Burning in the orifice of the urethra while urinating.

Tetter-like rash on the labia majora.[5] [CARRERE, l. c.]

Heat and itching on the genitals, and inclination for coitus. [CARRERE, l. c.]

200. Increase and anticipation of the menses.[6] [CARRERE, l. c.]

Increased menstrual flux.[6] [CARRERE, l. c.]

Diminished menstruation.[6] [CARRERE, l. c.]

Menstruation delayed several, even as many as 25, days.[7] [CARRERE, l. c.]

* * *

Stuffed coryza, with confusion of head and a single sneeze. [*Ng.*]

205. Very dry nose, in the evening. [*Ng.*]

Sneezing. [*We.*]

Short hacking cough, that seems to be produced by deep inspiration. [*Gss.*]

Hæmoptysis.[8] [CARRERE, l. c.]

A very acute undulatory pain, almost like tearing pressure, darts through the left side of the chest in fits. [*Gss.*]

210. Numbing, obtuse stitch under the right clavicle into the chest. [*Gss.*]

To the left above the xiphoid cartilage (when sitting bent forward) a painful pressure, as with a blunt instrument, afterwards it comes even in an erect posture of the body in long fits, and develops into blows penetrating deep into the chest. [*Gss.*]

External tension and drawing on the front of the chest. [*Ng.*]

Intermittent pain in both sides below the shoulders, as though the fists were knocked violently in there from both sides. [*Gss.*]

A twitching pain in the right axilla (aft. 3 d.). [*Ar.*]

215. A pulsating pain in the left axilla, going off by movement (aft. 9 h.). [*Ar.*]

Twitching and drawing under the sternum. [*Gss.*]

Intermitting aching under the whole extent of the sternum. [*Gss.*]

On breathing deeply tension on the chest. [*We.*]

---

1 This symptom is a critical discharge, coinciding with improvement in the patient's malady.

2 Critical phenomenon.

3 Repetition of S. 187.

4 The corresponding symptom in the *Chr. Kr.* stands thus : "Pulsating (stitches ?) in the urethra."

5 During treatment of "dartrous" vagina and uterus by D.

6 Curative effect.

7 Ascribed to abundant evacuations.

8 Not found.

Under the sternum superiorly, on a small spot, intermitting squeezing [*Gss.*]

220. Oppression of the chest. [*We.*]

Painful shooting on the sternum (aft. ½ h.). [*Ar.*]

On the sternum a thrust-like, rather obtuse stitch (aft. 8 h.). [*Ar.*]

Obtuse shooting pain in the right side in the region of the third rib, especially when pressing on it;, then the pain spread to the sacrum, and then mounted upwards to between the shoulders: a shooting on the inner border of the left scapula on inspiring. [*Ts. Hb.*]

In the left side of the ribs slow, intermitting, obtuse stitches. [*Gss.*]

225. On the middle of the sternum a shooting tearing pain that went through the whole chest to the spine, when sitting, and went off on rising up (aft. 7 d.). [*Ar.*]

A digging pain in the right side of the chest, going off when pressed upon (aft. 8½ h.) [*Ar.*]

Pain in the chest, like digging or as if he had hurt (sprained) himself. [*Gss.*]

In the right side, between the fourth and sixth ribs, a suddenly coming, and rapidly departing, painful shoot (aft. 8½ h.). [*Ar.*]

In the left side of the chest, in the region of the fifth and sixth ribs, a painful stab as from a rather blunt knife (aft. 4½ h.). [*Ar.*]

230. Shooting pain in the left side of the chest in the region of the sixth rib. [*Ar.*]

Violent shooting in the chest, now on the right, now on the left side; he must cough much, and expectorate a viscid mucus (aft. 4 d.). [*Ar.*]

A deep cutting pain in the left side of the chest, close under the clavicle, that went off on pressure (aft. 30 h.). [*Ar.*]

Pinching pain in the whole chest, increased by inspiration (aft. 14 h.). [*Ar.*]

Oppression of the chest, as after sitting bent forwards. [*We.*]

235. **Great oppressive pain in the whole chest, especially on inspiration and expiration.** [*Ar.*]

He feels as something were forced out on the left side of the chest. [*Gss.*]

Palpitation of the heart; strong beating of the heart, felt externally, especially at night.

Strong palpitation of the heart; it seemed as though he felt the heart beating outside the thoracic cavity. [*Stf.*]

A digging shooting pain on the left side near the sacrum (aft. 10 h.). [*Ar.*]

240. Sacral pains, as after stooping long. [*We.*]

Under the left crista ilii a digging pain, that went off by pressing on it (aft. 6 h.). [*Ar.*]

On sitting in a bent position (after a short walk) every time he inspires, an obtuse stitch outwards—a kind of forcing out—in both lumbar regions. [*Gss.*]

Above the left hip, quite close to the lumbar vertebræ, pain as if he had previously received a blow there (aft. ½ h.). [*Ar.*]

In the loin, over the right hip, a deep cutting pain, that went off by pressure, but soon afterwards returned, and then went off gradually of its own accord (aft. 4 d.). [*Ar.*]

245. Pain as if the body were cut off in the lumbar region above the hips ; owing to the pain he moved to and fro, unable to sit still, but this gave him no relief. [*Gss.*]

In the loin, above the left hip, a digging shooting pain, that went off on walking, but came again when sitting (aft. 4½ d.). [*Ar.*]

Close to the lumbar vertebræ, above the right hip, severe single stabs in jerks, as with a fork (aft. 6 d.). [*Ar.*]

Posteriorly on the left side on the loin, just above the hip, an obtuse stitch outwards at every breath. [*Gss.*]

Single painful stitches on inspiring in the middle of the spine (aft. 29 h.). [*Ar.*]

250. Intermittent, obtuse stitches, like a painful beating, in the left side of the back near the spine. [*Gss.*]

Intermittent pressure on the left side close to the spinal column, at the commencement of the back up near the nape, in the morning in bed when lying on the back. [*Gss.*]

An agreeable tickling sensation on the outer border of the right scapulæ. [*Ar.*]

In the middle of the right scapula a tickling prick. [*Ar.*]

Drawing tearing pain on the outer border of the right scapula (aft. 6 d.). [*Ar.*]

255. Drawing tearing in the right shoulder, above the right hip-joint, and above and below the right knee-joint. [*Ts. Hb.*]

Intermitting tearing blows on the outer side of the left scapula. [*Gss.*]

Stiff pain in the nape-muscles on turning the head to one or both sides. [*Gss.*]

Stiffness in the nape-muscles. [*Rkt.*]

Pain in the nape, as if the head had been in a wrong position. [*We.*]

260. In the nape-muscles contractive pain as if the neck were twisted round. [*Gss.*]

In the whole of the right arm a dull violent pain, as from an apoplectic attack, combined with heaviness like lead, immobility, and cold feeling ; the arm was icy cold to the touch, the muscles felt as if stretched, even when at rest : the arm was almost completely paralysed, he could not bend it voluntarily, nor lift it up, nor hold a pen ; on trying to do so he felt a sharp pain as if bruised in the elbow-joint. which is also painful to the touch as if bruised (aft. ½ h.). the same icy coldness of the right arm came again next morning (aft. 24 h.). [*Mr.*]

When she wishes to bring the arms forward or backwards she cannot do it, as that brings on jerks in the arms.

When she bent the arm and moved it backwards she had twitchings in the flesh of the upper arm ; when she extended it it did not twitch, but the fingers then became stiff so that she could not close them.

In the evening in bed and in the morning after rising, pain in the upper arm.

265. Burning itching externally on the right upper arm, that compelled him to scratch ; the part was red and had a vesicle on it, with burning sensation. [*Wr.*]

The left arm pains as if paralysed, as from a bruise, almost only when at rest, little when moving, it is not painful to the touch ; but the arm had its proper strength.

A paralytic sensation in the right upper arm, which went off on moving it strongly (aft. 4½ d.). [*Ar.*]

On the outside of the right elbow an eroding gnawing pain in short fits. [*Gss.*]

A drawing pain in the right forearm (aft. 3¼ d.). [*Ar.*.]

270. Dull drawing from the left elbow to the wrist, especially noticed on pronation, in the evening (aft. 9 d.). [*Ng.*]

In the shaft of the left ulna a repeated acute drawing. [*Gss.*]

A sudden, jerking, pinching tearing in the middle of the left forearm (aft. 12 h.). [*Ar.*]

In the right forearm, from the elbow-joint to the wrist, a slow, down-drawing, twisting, boring pain, which went off by moving the arm, but immediately returned when at rest (aft. 4 h.). [*Ar.*]

The left forearm powerless, as if paralysed, with a paralytic feeling in the elbow-joint (aft. 36 h.). [*We.*]

275. Disagreeable itching on the middle of the right forearm that compelled scratching, whereby it was removed, but it soon returned (aft. 36 h.). [*Ar.*]

In the bend of the elbow eruption of red pimples, visible morning and evening in the warm room, that caused a fine pricking itching, and burning after scratching, for twelve days.

On the right wrist a prick, as with a blunt point, which went off by movement (aft. 1 h.). [*Ar.*]

Trembling of the hands (in cold wet weather when taking dulcamara). [CARRERE, l. c.]

Tetter-like eruption, especially on the hands.[1] [CARRERE, l. c.]

280. Much perspiration of the palms. [*We.*]

The hands are covered with a kind of warts, such as he had never had before (aft. 21 d.). [*Stf.*]

On the back of the hand a redness, which causes burning pain, when he becomes warm by walking in the open air.

In the ball of the left thumb cramp-like drawing, so that he scarcely dares to move the thumb. [*Gss.*]

Cramp-like twitching pain in the first joint of the right middle finger. [*Gss.*]

285. Single small stitches on the right buttock (aft. 8½ d.). [*Ar.*]

Drawing tearing pain in the left hip (aft. 14 h.). [*Ar.*]

Drawing pinching pain in the right hip (aft. 26 h.). [*Ar.*]

---

1 Critical eruption.

Drawing shooting pain in the left hip-joint extending to the groin, only when walking, at every step, with the sensation as if the head of the hip-bone would be dislocated ; stretching it out forcibly diminished the pain, and caused the feeling as if the femur were thereby put into place ; but a bruised pain remained for some time in the parts, which made him limp (for 14 d.). [*Ctz.*]

Pain in the thigh.

290. Shooting tearing pain in the whole right thigh, that did not go off by pressure. [*Ar.*]

Fine pricking pain as with needles in the back of the left thigh close to the knee (aft. 81 h.). [*Ar.*]

Continued sometimes shooting, sometimes beating, sometimes pinching pain in both thighs, which went off on walking, but then developed into weariness ; when sitting it immediately returned (aft. 3½ d.). [*Ar.*]

Drawing tearing pain in both thighs, which went off on walking, but changed into weariness and returned immediately when sitting (aft. 12, 14 h.). [*Ar.*]

Here and there drawing in the flesh of the thighs. The parts were painful to the touch. [*Ng.*]

295. A drawing sensation on the front of the right thigh (aft. 36 h.). [*Ar.*]

A drawing tearing pain on the back of the right thigh, extending from its middle into the knee-joint (aft. ¼ h.). [*Ar.*]

A drawing paralytic sensation on the front of the right thigh (aft. 8⅓ d.). [*Ar.*]

Shooting tearing pain from the knee-joint up into the thigh, when walking in the open air. [*Rkt.*]

Burning itching sensation externally on the thighs, that compels scratching (aft. 7 h.). [*Wr.*]

300. Falling asleep and weakness of the lower limbs. [CARRERE, l. c.]

Great weakness of the knees, as after a long walk (3rd day.). [*Ng.*]

Twitching of the inferior extremities.[1] [CARRERE, l. c.]

Tearing in the knee-joint, when sitting. [*Rkt.*]

On the inside of the knee regularly recurring undulatory aching pain. [*Gss.*]

305. On the outside of the right leg, itching, ending in an itching prick (aft. ¼ h.). [*We.*]

On the outside of the left leg, itching, going off on scratching, but soon recurring (aft. ¼ h.). [*We.*]

Cramp-like drawing (almost cutting) pain down through the left leg. [*Gss.*]

Puffiness and swelling of the leg and calf (but not of the foot) with tensive pain and feeling of extreme weariness towards evening.

Slight tearing upwards in the right tibia (2nd d.). [*Ng.*]

---

1 Not found.

310. Pain in the tibia, as from being tired by a long walk (aft. 36 h.). [*We.*]

A pain draws downwards from the back of the left calf, as if some one slit him inwardly (aft. ½ h.). [*Ar.*]

Tearing pain in the back of the left calf, that went off on moving the foot (aft. ⅓ h.). [*Ar.*]

A sudden prick as from a needle in the left calf followed by the sensation as if warm blood or water flowed down out of the part. [*Ar.*]

Numb sensation in the calf, in the afternoon and evening.

315. Painful cramp in the left calf when walking (aft. 9 h.). [*Wr.*]

Burning in the feet.

He woke up at night from severe cramp on the inner right ankle, he must get up out of bed and walk about, whereupon it went off.

Drawing tearing near the inner ankle of the right foot (aft. 12 h.). [*Ng.*]

Tearing in the left leg from the outer ankle to the front of the foot. [*Ng.*]

320. A cutting pain in the middle of the right sole, that did not go off by treading (aft. 27 h.). [*Ar.*]

Pulsating tearing pain in the big and second toes of the left foot. [*We.*]

On the toes, intermitting, shooting burning. [*Gss.*]

Slight twitchings on the hands and feet. [CARRERE, l. c.]

Convulsions first in the facial muscles, then in the whole body. [FRITZE,[1] *Annal. d. Klin. Inst. in Berlin*, iii, p. 45.]

325. Cramp-pain here and there in the limbs, especially in the fingers. [*Gss.*]

The symptoms appear to occur by preference chiefly towards evening. [*Ng.*]

Violent trembling of the limbs.[2] [CARRERE, l. c.]

Obtuse stitches here and there in the limbs and on the rest of the body, generally outwards. [*Gss.*]

Pain in the limbs.

330. On various parts of the body pains as if these parts had caught cold. [*We.*]

Burning itching here and there, running quickly to and fro, like vermin ; he must scratch violently, after which it at first increased, and then declined ; by day the itching is but slightly felt ; only at night and then worst from 12 till 3 o'clock ; after a short sleep he is wakened by this sensation (aft. 14 d.). [*Stf.*]

Itching pinching pricks on various parts of the body. [*We.*]

Violent itching all over the body.[3] [CARRERE, l. c.]

Pricking itching on various parts of the body. [CARRERE, l. c.]

335. A violently itching eruption of red spots with vesicles.[4] [CARRERE, l. c.]

---

1 Statement from observation.
2 Not found.
3 See note to S. 343.
4 On parts affected by "dartres,"

Eruption on the arms and thighs, like white lumps (wheals) surrounded by a red areola; there was itching pricking only in the wheals and, after rubbing, burning in them.

Eruption of small papules on the chest and abdomen, with moderate itching. [*Stf.*]

Eruption of a tetter-like scab all over the body.[1] [CARRERE, l. c.]

Bright red pointed elevations on the skin which filled with pus after five or six days. [STARCKE, l. c.]

340. Red elevated spots as from nettles.[2] [CARRERE, l. c.]

Red places on the body. [CARRERE, l. c.]

Red, flea-bite-like spots. [CARRERE, l. c.]

Dryness, heat and burning in the skin.[3] [CARRERE, l. c.]

Dryness and heat of the skin, constipation and painful retention of urine, with soft, full, slow pulse with jerking beats. [CARRERE, l. c.]

345. Sudden swelling of the body and puffiness of the limbs, sometimes painful or accompanied by a feeling of being asleep. [STARCKE, l. c.]

Emaciation.

Lassitude; he shuns movement.

Weariness.

Lassitude, heaviness and weariness in all the limbs which compels him to sit or lie down (aft. 12 h.). [*Wr.*]

350. In all the limbs a feeling of great bruisedness, lasting almost all day. [*Ar.*]

Heaviness in the thighs and arms. [*Rkt.*]

Great, persistent weakness.[4] [CARRERE, l. c.]

Attack of sudden weakness, like faintness.

He must lie down.

355. All day long he is very drowsy and must yawn much. [*Ar.*]

Great sleepiness, laziness, yawning. [*Mr.*]

Frequent great yawning. [*Gss.*]

Restlessness, twitching, sleeplessness. [CARRERE, l. c.]

Sleeplessness, [CARRERE, l. c.]

360. Restless sleep, disturbed by confused dreams, with profuse perspiration during sleep. [*Wr.*]

Restless, disturbed, anxious sleep, full of heavy dreams. [STARCKE, l. c.]

In the evening, just when going to sleep, he leapt up high as if from fright. [*Gss.*]

Sleep with loud snoring with open mouth (immediately).

After midnight, anxiety and fear of the future.

365. Frightful dreams that compelled him to jump out of bed (the first night). [*Wr.*]

---

1 Critical. See note to S. 343.

2 On seat of vanished "dartres."

3 A youth, hereditarily "dartrous," and in bad health, after taking D., had S. 395, 333, 191, 101, with hard and tense pulse. Then came S. 338, with relief to all symptoms. The medicine was continued, and he got well.

4 After much sweating.

After 4 a. m. the sleep becomes very restless, whatever way he lies. [*Ar.*]

Tossing about in bed all night, with stupid feeling in the head. [*We.*]

Unquiet sleep ; he tossed about uncomfortably in bed. [*Stf.*]

He woke very early and could not go to sleep again ; he stretched himself with great weariness, and lay first on one side and then on the other, because the muscles at the back of the head were as if paralysed and he could not lie on it. [*We.*]

370. She wakes early as if she had been called, sees a ghostly figure that always grows bigger and seems to vanish upwards.

Towards morning a kind of wakefulness with closed eyes. [*We.*]

Towards morning no sleep, and yet in all the limbs tired as if paralysed, as after exposure to great heat. [*We.*]

Sleeplessness, ebullition of blood, shooting and itching in the skin. [CARRERE, l. c.]

(At night, no sleep, on account of itching in the front of the body, from the chest over the abdomen and thighs, like flea-bites ; at the same time he was hot and transpired, without being wet ; the transpiration had a disagreeable smell.)

375. Shivering as from nausea and chilliness combined with cold feeling and coldness all over the body ; he could not get warm at the hottest stove ; at the same time occasional shuddering and shaking (immediately). [*Mr.*]

Double tertian fever.[1] [CARRERE, l. c.]

He is chilly and uncomfortable in all his limbs. [*We.*]

Frequent rigor, heaviness of head, general prostration[1] (after a chill when taking dulcamara). [CARRERE, l. c.]

In the open air, especially when exposed to a draught, chilliness on the back without thirst. [*Ng.*]

380. Towards evening chilliness over the back, the nape, and the occiput, with a feeling as if the hair of the head stood on end (3rd d.) [*Ng.*]

For several evenings slight but disagreeable chilliness from the back over the occiput. [*Ng.*]

The chilliness on the back towards evening lasted for more than ten days, recurring daily. [*Ng.*]

Dry heat at night.

Hot, dry skin, ebullition of blood. [CARRERE, l. c.]

385. Burning in the skin all over the back, as if he were sitting near a hot stove, with perspiration on the face and moderate heat. [*We.*]

Heat, restlessness. [CARRERE, l. c.]

Violent fever, with great heat, dryness of skin and delirium daily ; recurring every 15, 16 hours.[2] [CARRERE, l. c.]

Heat and feeling of heat all over the body, especially in the hands, the pulse equable, slow, but full ; at the same time thirst, afterwards rigor. [*Rkt.*]

---

1 See note to S. 164.

2 Critical. S. 384 and 386 probably belong to this observation.

Heat of the body, burning in the face, constipation. [CARRERE, l. c.]

390. General perspiration, especially in the back.

Perspiration for five days and more.[1] [CARRERE, l. c.]

Perspiration all over at night, by day under the shoulders and in the palms. [CARRERE, l. c.]

In the morning profuse perspiration all over, but chiefly over the whole head (aft. 20 h.).

Ill-smelling perspiration, and at the same time copious discharge of clear urine. [CARRERE, l. c.]

395. Restlessness. [CARRERE, l. c.]

Talking nonsense. [DE HAEN,[2] *Ratio Medendi*, iv, p. 228.]

Increased pain at night with delirium.[3] [CARRERE, l. c.]

Wandering, delirium, a kind of insanity. [STARCKE, l. c.]

In the morning, very impatient; he stamped his feet, wished to throw away everything, commenced to wander in his mind; followed by weeping. [STARCKE, l. c.]

400. Very much out of humour, inclined for nothing, for several days. [*Ng.*]

In the afternoon a peculiar humour, he must quarrel with every one, but he is not angry. [*Ng.*]

---

1 Critical, in rheumatism. S. 392 and 394 cannot be found, but they are probably of the same nature.

2 Observation in disease.

3 Not found.

EUPHRASIA OFFICINALIS.[1]

(*Eye-bright.*)

(The freshly expressed juice of the whole plant mixed with equal parts of alcohol. The juice in the latter part of summer is often so viscid, that after pounding the plant to a fine pap of uniform consistence, it must generally be mixed up and diluted with some of this alcohol, in order to allow of the juice being expressed.)

From the following few observations, it may be seen that the ancients did not give it either its German[2] or its Latin name without reason, and that this plant does not merit the neglect with which modern physicians treat it.

The homœopathic physician, who for the cure of a case of disease only selects a medicine proved to cause similar symptoms in the healthy, will find the smallest portion of a drop of this juice generally too strong a dose.

[HAHNEMANN was assisted in this proving by FR. HAHNEMANN, LANGHAMMER, WISLICENUS.

Symptoms were obtained from the following old-school authorities :

BONNET, *Merc. Compil.*, 13.

LOBELIUS, *Advers.*, 210.

PAULLI, SIM , *Quadripart. Bot.*, class. 3.

In the 1st edit. of the 'R.A.M.L.' euphrasia had 115 symptoms, in this 2nd edit. 127.]

EUPHRASIA.

(Confusion and pressure externally on the top of the head.)

Much heat in the head, with aching.

Heat in the forehead with headache in the temple.

In the evening such violent dazed and bruised headache (with fluent coryza) that he was compelled to go to bed earlier than usual, and yet the headache was increased by lying (aft. 14 h.). [*Lr.*]

5. A long-continued, penetrating needle-prick in the right temple (aft. 7 h.). [*Lr.*]

Fine needle-pricks externally on the left temple (aft. ½ h.). [*Lr.*]

Some sharp stitches on the right side of the forehead (aft. ½ h.). [*Lr.*]

Sharp tearing stitches on the left side of the occiput, when at rest and when moving, in the afternoon (aft. 6½ h.). [*Lr.*]

A pressive pain externally on the head, but especially on the forehead (aft. 2 h.). [*Lr.*]

---

1 From vol. v, 2nd edit., 1826.

2 Augentrost, *angl.*, eye-comfort.

10. On blowing the nose a sensation of painful dazedness in the head and painfulness of the interior of the nose, so that he can only blow his nose gently (aft. 15 h.). [*Lr.*]

The candle appeared to him dimmer.

The candle seemed to be unsteady, and to burn at one time more brightly, at another more dimly.

The eyes are painful from the glare of light, as though he had not slept enough.

Dimness of vision on looking at distant objects (short sight) all day. [*Lr.*]

15. On walking in the open air dimness of vision for distant objects (short sight), for three days (aft. 1½ h.). [*Lr.*]

Vessels in the sclerotic run close up to the cornea.* [*Lr.*]

Painful aching in the left inner canthus; the eye waters (aft. 24 h.). [*Ws.*]

Aching in both eyes, as if he would go to sleep. [*Fr. H—n.*]

Aching sensation in both eyes, as if he were trying to keep awake (aft. 2 h.). [*Fr. H—n.*]

20. Sleepy dry aching in both eyes, not aggravated by the brightest daylight nor by looking at the fire. [*Fr. H—n.*]

Tiresome dryness in the eyes, just as if he had had no sleep. [*Fr. H—n.*]

In the evening a sensation of contraction from both sides in the eyes, especially in the upper eye-lids, which compelled him to wink frequently (aft. 10 h.). [*Lr.*]

Contractive aching in the eye, when walking in the open air.

Sometimes a smarting in the eyes; scalding water runs from them.

25. Very fine pricks in the eye-ball (aft. 11 h.). [*Fr. H—n.*]

In the inner canthi eye-gum, even during the day.

Eye-gum in the canthi (aft. 13 h.). [*Lr.*]

Twitching together of the upper and lower lids.

Flux of the eyes, so that he almost became blind.† [LOBELIUS, *Advers.*,[1] 210.]

30. Sore eyes; he almost became blind. [BONNET,[2] *Merc. Compil.*, 13—SIM. PAULLI,[3] *Quadripart. Bot.* class. 3.]

Very violent boring pain in the interior of the right ear, in the region of the membrana tympani, as from within outwards (aft. 7 h.). [*Ws.*]

Painful tension in the interior of the left ear (aft. 6 h.). [*Ws.*]

Stiffness of the left cheek when speaking and chewing, with sensation of heat and single flying stitches in it (aft. 6 h.). [*Ws.*]

Eruption of pimples, containing pus, in the alæ nasi (aft. 1½ h.). [*Lr.*]

* At the same time an aching he had long felt in the eyes and dark spots on the cornea disappeared in two days. [*Lr.*]

† After using the plant for a quarter of a year.

---

1 From three months' internal use of euphrasia for an ophthalmia with lachrymation.

2 Not accessible.

3 Only a citation of Lobelius (S. 29.)

35. A drawing pain transversely across in the upper jaw (aft. 2½ h.). [*Lr.*]

At noon, when eating, needle-pricks penetrating forwards in the left lower jaw, which even prevented chewing (aft. 7 h.). [*Lr.*]

Violent stitches from behind forwards, under the right lower jaw near the neck, which quickly went off on touching (aft. 8½ h.). [*Lr.*]

Fine stitches on the chin, with sensation of internal heat on that part (aft. ½ h.) [*Ws.*]

Shooting in the lower teeth.

40. (A throbbing in two teeth, after eating and at other times)

Great bleeding of the gums (aft. 1 h.). [*Fr. H—n.*]

He repeats frequently when speaking, both at the first word (a kind of stuttering), and also often repeating sentences frequently in order to express himself differently—whereas he formerly spoke correctly. [*Fr. H—n.*]

Insipid taste in the mouth.

In the morning bitter taste from tobacco-smoking (aft. 52 h.). [*Lr.*]

45. He became qualmish and sick from (accustomed) tobacco-smoking, which tastes to him bitter pungent (aft. 14 h.). [*Lr.*]

At noon hunger without appetite (aft. 54 h.). [*Lr.*]

Hiccup (aft. 5 m.). [*Lr.*]

Eructation with the taste of food.

During inspiration and expiration some fine pricks beneath the scrobiculus cordis, in the evening, when sitting (aft. 15 h.). [*Lr.*]

50. Distension of the abdomen, as if without flatulence, before dinner.

Painless rumbling in the abdomen, as when hungry and empty (aft. 1½ h.). [*Lr.*]

A kind of oppression in the abdomen, a burning pressing pain going across when at rest and when moving (aft. 5½ h.). [*Lr.*]

Pinching in the abdomen in short fits (aft. 3, 4 h.). [*Fr. H—n.*]

Bellyache for seven hours (aft. 2 h.). [*Fr. H—n.*]

55. Stool every day, but only hard and scanty.

A pressure on the anus, when sitting.

Frequent micturition (aft. ¾ h.). [*Lr.*]

Frequent discharge of clear urine (aft. 2 h.). [*Ws.*]

A voluptuous itching on the seam of the prepuce compelling scratching, after the scratching and on pressing on it the part is painful (aft. 2 h.). [*Lr.*]

60. Several needle-pricks on the point of the glans penis (aft. 1½ h.). [*Lr.*]

When sitting voluptuous itching needle-pricks on the glans penis, which is painful after scratching (aft. 10 h.). [*Lr.*]

(In the condylomata a shooting, even when sitting, still more severe when walking; on touching them they pain as if sore and burning.)

(In the condylomata an itching sensation.)

The testicles are drawn up, and there is formication in them (aft. 12 h.). [*Ws.*]

65. Spasmodic retraction of the genitals, with aching above the os pubis, in the evening in bed. [*Ws.*]

* * *

Sneezing with severe fluent coryza, during which much mucus passes through the nostrils anteriorly and also through the posterior nares (aft. 9 h.). [*Lr.*]

In the morning copious fluent coryza, and severe cough with expectoration (aft. 46 h.). [*Lr.*]

For several days, copious mucous expectoration by voluntary hacking cough. [*Lr.*]

Cough most severe by day, with phlegm on the chest, which can not be detached.

70. Cough only during the day ; at night he has no cough.

During the cough he loses his breath, almost as in whooping-cough.

Laboured breathing, even in the room.

He has difficulty in drawing a deep breath, even when sitting.

Single fine stitches under the sternum, especially during inspiration (aft. 10 h.). [*Ws.*]

75. Cramp-like backache (aft. 1 h.). [*Fr. H—n.*]

Continued aching pains in the back when sitting and walking (aft. 54 h.). [*Lr.*]

Intermittent cramp-like backache, for half an hour (aft. 1 h.). [*Fr. H—n.*]

Sensation in the arms as if they had gone asleep.

A numbing stitch in the left upper arm (aft. ½ h.). [*Lr.*]

80. Single obtuse stitches anteriorly on the left forearm, close to the wrist (aft. 13 h.). [*Lr.*]

In the right forearm and in the hand, pain as if gone asleep (aft. 1½ h.). [*Fr. H—n.*]

Dull tearing in the elbow and wrist-joints (aft. 2 h.). [*Ws.*]

Pain like cramp in the wrists for half an hour (aft. 24 h.). [*Fr. H—n.*]

Cramp-pain in the metacarpus. [*Fr. H—n.*]

85. In the metacarpus, pain like cramp, alternately stronger and weaker for half an hour (aft. 1 h.). [*Fr. H—n.*]

Cramp-like aching pain in the left hand, after which the squeezing aching pain went into the fingers. [*Fr. H—n.*]

Very penetrating pinching pain on the back of the hand (aft. 3 h.). [*Fr. H—n*]

Pinching pain in the proximal phalanx of the index (aft. 3 h.). [*Fr. H—n.*]

In the knuckles of the fingers and finger-joints, more towards their outer side, pain as if gone asleep (aft. 1½ h.). [*Fr. H—n.*]

90. Cramp-pain in the fingers, especially the finger-joints of the left hand (aft. 1½ h.). [*Fr. H—n.*]

Shooting in the left hip-joint, when walking.

A violent needle-prick in the posterior muscles of the right thigh, only when standing (aft. ½ h.). [*Lr.*]

Violent needle-pricks in the anterior muscles of the right thigh, when standing (aft. ½ h.). [*Lr.*]

Shooting drawing from the upper part of the thigh to the groin, most severe when sitting (aft. 48 h.). [*Ws.*]

95. Only when walking in the open air a voluptuous itching on the front of the thigh, that compels scratching, whereupon the part is painful (aft. 9½ h.). [*Lr.*]

Twitching shooting in the left knee, when walking.

Weariness in the knees, as from a long walk (aft. 4 h.). [*Ws.*]

Whilst walking, painful tension in the tendons of the hough, as if they were too short, whereby walking is difficult (aft. 3 h.), [*Lr.*]

Continued boring stitches upwards in the shaft of the tibia, (aft. 1½ h.). [*Lr.*]

100. When sitting, an up-and-down drawing pain anteriorly in the periosteum of the shaft of the left tibia (aft. 2½ h.). [*Lr.*]

On standing long, a cramp-like pain in the calves, with sensation of heaviness (aft. 2½ h.). [*Ws.*]

In the evening when walking, a voluptuous itching in the right, calf, that compels scratching (aft. 12 h.). [*Lr.*]

When walking and sitting, a tension from the outer ankle near the tendo Achillis towards the calf.

On the left outer ankle a cracking when treading. [*Lr.*]

105. A tickling formication on the left toes ; the part is painful after rubbing (aft. 2 h.). [*Lr.*]

All through the night, flying, itching pricks here and there ; he tosses about uneasily in bed and cannot get warm enough. [*Ws.*]

Such great exhaustion in the whole body, especially the lower extremities, that he must make a great effort to walk—all the third day. [*Lr.*]

By day very tired, and yet the ensuing night when he lay in bed he could not fall asleep till about 2 a.m.—for three successive nights.

Uncommon yawning, on walking in the open air.

110. Very sleepy by day, and yet he had slept all through the previous night.

Drowsiness, which begins as it were in the eyes, for ten hours (aft. ½ h.). [*Fr. H—n.*]

Drowsy yet busy. [*Fr. H—n.*]

Drowsiness without being able to sleep, with much yawning. [*Fr. H—n.*]

At night frequent waking as if from fright.

115. At night horrible dreams of fire and burning by lightning (the 2nd night). [*Lr.*]

Attack for three successive mornings : he wakes up at night after 3 a.m. every instant, then about 6 a.m. falls into a stupefied sleep, without dreams, and on awaking from this, he has pressure on the upper part of the chest, the head is giddy and heavy ; at the same time he feels sick and perspiration breaks out all over him ; at every, even the slightest movement, the vertigo increases, inclining him to fall sideways ; all the limbs are at the same time weak and trembling ; the upper part of his body seems heavy on rising, as if his legs could not support him ; the attack gradually declines till noon, with loss of cheerfulness.

Paleness of face—for an hour (immediately). [*Fr. H—n.*]

Always chilly.

All the forenoon, internal chilliness, but in the afternoon (after 2 o'clock), great chilliness in both arms, which were quite cold.

120. Febrile rigor all over (aft. ½ h). [*Lr.*]

Redness and heat of the cheeks—for an hour (aft. ¼, ½ h.). [*Fr. H—n.*]

Red, hot face—for an hour and a half (aft. ¼ h.). [*Fr. H—n.*]

Sudden flush of heat and redness of face, with coldness of hands (without thirst) (aft. ¼ h.). [*Lr.*]

Sweat at night in sleep, which went off on awaking—for two successive nights.

125. For three successive nights, sweat all over, in sleep, of a strong smell, chiefly on the chest (on rising from bed, chilliness).

Silent, wrapped up in himself and disinclined to speak, all day. [*Lr.*]

Lazy, hypochondriacal ; external objects had no charm, no life for him.

FERRUM.[1]

(Iron.)

(Filings of soft iron are powdered by sufficient trituration in a cast iron mortar, then sifted through linen, and of this dust-like iron powder (in the pharmacopœias called *errum pulveratum*) one grain is triturated for three hours with milk-sugar (in the manner taught for arsenic) up to the million-fold or third attenuation, and then brought to the thirtieth potency (x̄) through 27 dilution phials.)

Although most of the following medicinal symptoms were observed from the employment of a solution of acetate of iron, it is beyond doubt that they correspond essentially with those of metallic iron as exactly as do the symptoms obtained from dry calcareous earth with those of acetate of lime.

This metal is said by ordinary physicians to be a strengthening medicine *per se*, and not only innocuous, but entirely and absolutely wholesome.

How far from being true is this dictum pronounced without consideration and testing, and handed down by teachers to their disciples equally without consideration and testing, we are taught by the reflection that, if iron possess medicinal power it must also for that very reason alter the health of human beings, and make the healthy ill, and the more ill the more powerfully curative it is found to be in disease.

Nil prodest, quod non lædere possit idem.

The actual sanitary condition of persons residing near waters impregnated with iron might have taught them that this metal possesses strong pathogenetic properties. The inhabitants of chalybeate* watering places, where all the springs and wells in the neighbourhood usually contain some of this metal, show marked signs of its morbific influence.

In such localities there are few persons who can resist the noxious influence of the continued use of such waters and remain quite well, each being affected according to his peculiar nature. There we find, more than anywhere else, chronic affections of great gravity and peculiar character, even when the regimen is otherwise faultless. Weak-

* It is mere charlatanry to call solutions of iron *steel-drops*, and chalybeate mineral waters *steel-waters*, *steel-baths*. By these expressions it is intended to convey the notion that they indubitably possess an absolute strengthening power in a high degree; for *to steel* is a metaphorical expression for *to strengthen*. But iron only becomes steel when its peculiar elasticity and hardness are developed. In its solution by acids the steel disappears; the solution then only contains a substratum of iron, and the oxyde (iron ochre) collected from chalybeate waters, when smelted, produces nothing but ordinary *iron*.

1 From vol, ii, 3rd edit., 1833.

ness, almost amounting to paralysis of the whole body and of single parts, some kinds of violent limb pains, abdominal affections of various sorts, vomiting of food by day or by night, phthisical pulmonary ailments, often with blood-spitting, deficient vital warmth, suppressions of the menses, miscarriages, impotence in both sexes, sterility, jaundice, and many other rare cachexies are common occurrences.

What becomes of the alleged complete innocuousness, let alone the absolute wholesomeness of this metal? Those who are constantly drinking chalybeate waters, called *health-springs*, and the other iron-impregnated waters of the neighbourhood, are mostly in a sickly state!

What prejudice, what carelessness has hitherto prevented physicians from observing these striking facts, and referring them to their cause, the pathogenetic property of iron?

How can they, ignorant as they are of the action of iron and its salts, determine in what cases chalybeate waters are of use? Which of their patients will they send thither for a course of treatment? Which will they keep away? What, in short, seeing that they know nothing accurately concerning the peculiar effects of this metal on the human body, leads them to determine the cases suitable for chalybeate waters? Is it blind fancy? Hap-hazard conjecture and guess work? Fashion? Do not, indeed, many of their patients come back from the chalybeate springs in a more miserable* and diseased condition, showing that iron was an unsuitable remedy for them? God preserve patients from a doctor who does not know, and can give no satisfactory reasons, why he prescribes this or the other drug, who cannot tell *beforehand* what medicine would be beneficial, what injurious to the patient!

Only a thorough knowledge of the characteristic primary effects of medicines, and whether they present a great similarity to the symptoms of the disease to be cured (as homœopathy teaches), could protect patients from such fatal mistakes.

The following list of morbid symptoms which iron causes is far from being as complete as it might be, and yet it will contribute not a little to prevent such mistakes being made by those who will refrain from prescribing medicines in a hap-hazard manner, and from feeling no scruples of conscience whether they draw death or life for their patients in the lottery.

Large and oft-repeated doses of iron, as also frequent baths in chalybeate waters, have a very long duration of action, extending to months even. Doses of even the thirtieth potency ($\bar{X}$), such as the homœopathic physician now gives in ordinary cases, act for a good many days.

* The attempt of the common run of practitioners to produce a purely *strengthening* effect is a capital mistake. For why is the patient so weak? Obviously because he is ill! Weakness is a mere consequence and a single symptom of his disease. What rational man could think of strengthening his patient without first removing his disease? But if his disease be removed, then he *always*, even during the process of the removal of his disease, regains his strength by the energy of his organism freed from its malady. There is no such thing as a strengthening remedy as long as the disease continues; there can be none such. The homœopathic physician alone knows how to cure, and in the act of being cured the convalescent regains his strength.

Chronic ailments caused by iron are mostly ameliorated by (calcareous) hepar sulphuris (($\frac{1}{100}$th or $\frac{1}{1000}$th of a grain in one or several doses), and most of the remaining sufferings by pulsatilla, when the symptoms are not (as sometimes happens) of such a kind and complexity as to require some other medicine according to the rule of similarity of action.

[HAHNEMANN was aided in this proving by GROSS, FRIEDRICH HAHNEMANN, ROSAZEWSKY.

Symptoms are derived from the following old-school sources :

HARCKE, in *Hufel. Journ.*, xxv.

LENTIN, *Beitr.*

NEBEL and WEPFER, *Diss, de Medicamentis Chalybeatis*. Heidelb., 1711.

RITTER, in *Hufel Journ.*, xxvi, 1.

SCHERER, in *Hufel. Journ.*, iii.

SCHMIDTMULLER, in *Horn's Archiv*, ix, 2.

ZACCHIROLI, in *Kuhn's Magazin fur Arzneimittellehre*, i, St. Chemnitz, 1794.

In the 1st edition ferrum has 264 symptoms, in the 2nd edit. 290, and in this 3rd edit. 295.]

FERRUM.

Confusion and stupefaction of the head. [RITTER,* in *Hufel. Journ.*, xxvi, 1.]

On lying down a vertigo as if he were knocked forwards, or driving in a carriage (especially when the eyes are shut).

Vertigo on going down hill, as if she would fall forwards.

When walking staggering and as if intoxicated, as if she would fall down.

5. When walking, very whirling and sick : he feels as if the head inclined always to hang to the right side.

On looking at running water she becomes reeling and giddy in the head, as if all went round with her.

Great rushing up to the head.

Intoxication.[1] [RITTER, l. c.]

Undulating headache, like waves, for an hour (aft. ½ h.). [*Rz.*]

10. Drawing headache. [*Rz.*]

A rush of blood to the head ; the blood-vessels of the head were swollen for two hours, with severe flushes of heat in the face.

A momentary, giddy blow in the brain (immediately).

The cool open air gives her a peculiar pressure on the top of the head, which gradually went off in the room.

Disinclination to think and confusion of the head.

15. Headache every evening ; dulness about the root of the nose.

In the morning very dull in the head.

Headache, as if the brain were lacerated (also in the morning during slumber before awaking).

Empty feeling in the head.

* Observations referring to the employment of the waters of Pyrmont and Schwalbach, in which the carbonic acid is to be taken into account.

1 Not found.

The head is dull and stupid.

20. The head is dazed and stupid.

Heaviness of the head.

(Pressive headache in the forehead, as if it would burst.)

A cutting shooting in the forehead.

Violent shooting pain in the left side of the head, in the afternoon, for five hours.

25. (Every two or three weeks, for two, three, or four days, headache, hammering and beating, so that she must sometimes lie down in bed : then loathing of food and drink.)

Falling out of the hair, whereby the scalp is painful, with formication.

A drawing from the nape up into the head, in which there is then shooting, roaring, and rushing.

In the evening darkness before the eyes ; he got an aching pain over the orbits, and some blood dropped out of the nose.

Pain externally on the head, as if blood were extravasated ;the hairs are painful to the touch.

30. Earthy complexion, with blue spots on the face.

Earthy jaundiced complexion.

Paleness of the face and lips.[1] [RITTER, l. c.]

In the evening itching in the eyes and aching as from a grain of sand in them.

For five days, red eyes with burning pains (aft. 3 d.).

35. Burning in the eyes.

The eyes are painful, as when one is very sleepy, and they tend to close ; also burning in them.

An aching in the right eye ; the eyelids stick together at night.

When he writes for only a couple of hours, he is unable to open the eyes wide ; they become watery, as if he had not slept enough.

Redness and swelling of the upper and lower eyelids ; on the upper a kind of stye filled with pus ; the lower eyelids are full of eye-gum (purulent mucus).

40. (Shooting in the left eye.)

The pupils are only capable of slight dilatation.

In the evening on stooping some bleeding from the nose.

Bleeding from the left nostril (four times in ten hours.)

Painfulness of the left auricle, as if there were an ulcer on it. (aft. 12 h.).

45. Stitches in the right ear, in the morning (aft. 12 h.).

Rushing in the ears, which, as well as the disagreeable feeling in the brain, is relieved by laying the head down on the table.

Singing before the ears, as from crickets.

Pale lips.

At the back and on the middle of the tongue a continued painfulness, like fine uninterrupted pricks, which is aggravated by the contact of the food and drink ; when not eating and drinking

1 Effects of uterine hæmorrhage induced by iron, not of the metal itself.

the part has the feeling as if it had been burnt, and is numb and stiff.

50. (Swelling of the gums and cheeks.)

(Rough and sore throat, with hoarseness.)

(On swallowing, an aching with sore sensation in the gullet, as if blisters had been crushed there and so the part had become sore.)

(Sometimes a sensation as from a plug in the throat, when not swallowing, not whilst swallowing.)

On swallowing, aching pain in the throat, with heat in the fauces; the cervical muscles feel stiff, and are painful when moved.

55. Sensation as of constriction in the throat.

Chronic glandular swelling in the neck.

Very great nausea in the throat, as if vomiting would ensue; it ended with eructation. [*Gss.*]

As soon as she eats something it is ejected by vomiting.

Vomiting only of food, immediately after eating, for eight days.

60. When she eats something she heaves, like nausea from loathing.

The vomiting is before midnight, worst when she is lying, and especially when she lies on the side.

Vomiting of food, immediately after midnight, whereupon there follow dislike to food and repugnance to the open air (aft. 6 h.).

She vomits every morning and after eating, only mucus and water (not food); a kind of water-brash; the water runs from the mouth and the throat feels as if drawn together.

She has always loathing and nausea.

65. Inclination to vomit for three hours.

Everything she vomits is sour and acrid.

She vomits much after taking acids and beer.

After sourish beer (in the evening) heart-burn.

Beer gets into her head.

70. From beer-soup, heat and anxiety.

Anorexia without bad taste and without thirst.

(She became pale, had rumbling in the abdomen; the chest was squeezed together, a rushing up to the head; she got spasmodic violent eructation, then heat in the face, especially in the right cheek, and pain in the crown of the head like shooting.)

Constant eructation, as soon as she has eaten anything.

Little appetite, least of all for meat; he felt full.

75. He eats with normal appetite and taste at noon; but after eating there comes eructation in jerks and the food is belched up, without nausea or inclination to vomit.

After a walk such a feeling of fulness, as though he would eructate; this went off after eating.

As soon as she eats anything it oppresses her.

Aching, very acute pain in the stomach. [SCHMIDTMULLER,* in *Horn's Archiv*, ix, 2.]

Violent stomachache and extraordinary tension. [ZACCHIROLI,† in *Kuhn's Magazin fur Arzneimitellehre*, i, St., Chemnitz, 1794.]

* From very fine iron powder. † From some grains of iron filings.

80. Distension of the gastric region. [SCHMIDTMULLER, l. c.]

Spasms in the stomach. [NEBEL and WEPFER, *Diss. de Medicamentis Chalybeatis*, Heidelb, 1711.[1]]

An aching in the abdomen, immediately below the stomach, as soon as she has eaten or drunk anything.

After drinking and eating violent stomachache.

Cramp-like pain in the stomach.

85. Stomachache from eating butcher's meat.

He can only eat bread and butter ; butcher's meat does not agree with him.

Solid foods taste too dry, as if they had neither juice nor strength in them ; they have, certainly, the natural taste, but it is not pleasant ; he prefers thin warm articles of food.

He has no appetite, because he always feels satiated ; but drinks taste well, and are taken with relish.

Even when she has appetite, she can eat but little ; she is immediately full, and food oppresses her.

90. After dinner he is thirsty ; but he does not know for what.

Complete adipsia.

He feels very full.

(In the morning, sourish taste in the mouth.)

Everything she eats tastes bitter.

95. Sweetish taste in the mouth, as of blood.[2] [RITTER, l. c.]

Sometimes an earthy taste in the mouth.

In the afternoon, a putrid taste rises up into the mouth, which destroys all his appetite.

When he has slept an hour before midnight, a heat rises as from his abdomen ; the mouth becomes dry, and a nauseous vapour and putrid taste rise up into his mouth.

(Burning in the stomach.)

100. The scrobiculus cordis is painful when touched.

Some stitches in the abdomen.

Fine shooting pain in the abdomen.

A severe stitch in the side, beneath the ribs (aft. 24 h.).

Quiet swelling of the abdomen, without flatulent sufferings.

105. Great rumbling in the abdomen by day and night.

Hard distension of the abdomen.

Distension of the abdomen. [SCHMIDTMULLER l. c.]

A quantity of flatus passes away. [LENTIN, *Beitr.*, p. 75.[3]]

Violent contractive pains in the abdomen and back. [RITTER, l. c.]

110. Colicky pains (immediately). [RITTER, l. c.]

(On touching the abdomen, and on coughing, the bowels are painful as if bruised, or as if they were irritated by purgatives.) (aft. 36 h.).

Especially when walking, painful heaviness of the hypogastric intestines, as if they would fall down.

Contractive spasm in the rectum, for some minutes.

---

1 Not accessible. 2 With SS. 157 and 181. 3 Symptoms not found.

Itching and erosion in the rectum, and thread-worms pass away in the slimy stool.

115. **The thread-worms seem to be increased by it**; he cannot sleep at night on account of itching in the rectum; the worms crept out at the anus at night.*

Obstinate constipation. [RITTER, l. c]

Constipation and piles, which cause painful pressure during stool.

Tearing in the rectum.

With every stool mucus, and also some discharge of blood.

120. Protrusion of large piles at the anus.

Violent discharge of blood from piles. [RITTER, l. c.]

Frequent urging to stool with burning at the anus and backache during movement.

Frequent diarrhœa.

Diarrhœic stool. [*Fr. H—n.*]

125. Diarrhœa with nervous spasmodic pains in the abdomen, back and anus. [RITTER, l. c.]

Severe diarrhœa. [LENTIN, l. c.]

Frequent, diarrhœic stools. [RITTER, l. c.]

Violent purging. [RITTER, l. c.]

Involuntary emission of urine, especially by day.

130. Erections of the penis.

Erections of the penis by day, almost without cause.

Nocturnal seminal emission.

(When urinating, burning pain in the urethra, as if the urine ran out hot.)

(Clap) discharge of mucus from the urethra after a chill.

135. Leucorrhœa, like milky water, which (at first) scalded and excoriated.

A previously painless leucorrhœa became painful, as if the parts were excoriated.

Before the occurrence of the menses, discharge of long strings of mucus from the womb, during which she had pain going about in the abdomen, such as usually occurred during the menses.

Painfulness of the vagina during coitus.

Before the appearance of the menses, shooting headache and singing in the ears.

140. In the morning bearing-down pains in the abdomen, as if the menses were coming on (aft. 12 h.).

The menses, which were due, came on immediately after the chalybeate bath, and twice as profusely as usual.†

The menses cease for two or three days and then reappear.

Metrorrhagia. [RITTER, l. c.]

The menses come on one day later, little and watery blood comes away with severe cutting in the abdomen (aft. 6 d.).

145. Menses delayed some days beyond the proper time.

* From drinking Pyrmont waters,

† This is the primary action of iron; the following symptoms are secondary actions, hence it is only in those cases of suppressed menstruation, in which the other symptoms are in homœopathic accordance with iron, that this metal can be curative.

The menses are delayed for eight weeks.

The menses are absent for three years.*

Prolapsus of the vagina, only during pregnancy, not otherwise.

Abortion.

150. Sterility without abortion.

* * *

A hot vapour rises up from his wind-pipe.[1] [RITTER, l. c.]

Sensation of dryness and phlegm on the chest; the dryness is diminished for a short time only by drinking.

On the chest fulness and tightness.

Oppression on the chest, as if it were constricted. [RITTER, l. c.]

155. Tightness of the chest. [RITTER, l. c.]

Tightness of the chest; difficult slow respiration, diminished by walking or speaking, or by being continually engaged in reading or writing; it is worst when sitting quitely doing nothing, and still worse when lying, especially in the evening; he must take several breaths before he can fill the lungs with air. [*Rz.*]

Rush of blood to the chest. [RITTER, l. c.]

Tightness of chest and weariness of the limbs, generally worst in the forenoon; often better when he has walked a little; only sometimes it becomes intolerably bad when walking in the open air.

He cannot get his breath; even when sitting he has dyspnœa.

160. (The child's chest is oppressed; it wheezes.)

In the evening in bed her larynx is closed, the blood rushes to the head, she feels a burning externally on the neck and between the scapulæ, and generally on the upper part of the body, whilst the feet are cold; in the morning, sweat.

In the morning in bed (about 6 o'clock) all is drawn painfully together in the scrobiculus cordis, then there occurs a kind of spasmodic cough with mucous expectoration.

Tightening of the chest as if it were constricted; severe anxious asthma, which is aggravated by walking.

Contractive spasm on the chest.

165. Difficult respiration and oppression of the chest, as if it were pressed on by the hand.

A pressure superiorly, beneath the sternum, with catarrh and cough.

Sometimes he must sit up in bed after midnight, owing to tightness of the chest.

A kind of asthma; an anxiety in the scrobiculus cordis, that impedes inspiration.

During corporeal exertion heat from the scrobiculus cordis upwards, like an anxiety; she must lie down.

170. At night in bed shooting in the sternum.

During bodily exercise stitches in the side.

Pain in the chest and shooting and tension between the scapulæ; he could not stir.

* During continued use of chalybeate water.

1 With SS. 157 and 181

Pain on the chest as if it were beaten.

Contractive spasm on the chest and **cough, only when moving and walking.**

175. (Increased dry cough.) [RITTER, l. c.]

Dull cough without expectoration, and when coughing she feels as if she could get no air.

In the evening after lying down the cough is dry, but on walking it is attended with expectoration.

Cough more when moving than when at rest.

A burning in the upper part of the sternum after the cough.

180. Nocturnal coughing up of blood followed by increased tightness of chest.

Hæmoptysis.[1] [RITTER, l. c.]

Scanty, thin, frothy expectoration with streaks of blood. [RITTER, l. c.]

Coughing up of blood on rising from bed in the morning.

By hacking cough he expectorates bloody mucus (aft. 5 d.).

185. Whilst suckling, cough with expectoration of blood.

Copious white purulent expectoration after slight coughing, which is increased by smoking tobacco and drinking brandy.

In the morning he expectorates a great deal of pus (of a putrid taste).

In the morning on waking much greenish purulent expectoration of a sickly taste.

Cough all day long, and some cough also in the evening after lying down.

190. A kind of tearing in the back, even when sitting and lying.

When she works a little with her arms she has a shooting in the scapulæ.

Betwixt the scapulæ a kind of tearing, even when sitting, which becomes worse on walking.

Whilst walking stitch-like jerks in the sacrum, which extend more towards the hips than upwards, more painful after sitting or standing, almost as if he had strained himself.

Pains in the sacrum on rising from a seat.

195. Bruised pain in the sacrum.

Pain in her left clavicle as if it had gone to sleep.

Creaking in the shoulder-joint, which pains as if bruised on touching it.

Pain, shooting and tearing from the shoulder-joint into the upper arm and farther down, which made it impossible for him to lift up the arm.

Shooting and tearing in the upper arm proceeding from the shoulder-joint, so that he could not raise the arm.

200. A kind of paralysis; inability to raise the arms on account of painful tension between the scapulæ and on the sternum.

Drawing in the arm, from which it becomes heavy and as if paralysed.

---

1 With SS. 151, 154, and 157.

He had no rest in his arms, and must flex and extend them by turns.

He cannot raise the right arm up ; there is shooting and tearing in the shoulder-joint—which pains as if bruised when touched—down through the upper arm, with creaking in the shoulder-joint.

Swelling of the hands ; afterwards the epidermis desquamates.

205. Hands and legs up to the knees swollen.

Coldness of the hands and feet. [RITTER, l. c.]

Cramp in the fingers, and numbness and insensibility of them.

In the morning, when she attempts to work a little, she feels trembling in the hands.[1]

A kind of paralysis ; a tearing with severe stitches from the hip-joint downwards to the tibia and foot (the ball of the foot is always very painful to the touch, as if bruised) ; by day he cannot tread for pains, which, however, are ameliorated by walking ; in the evening after lying down it is worst, he must get up and walk about in order to allay the pain, until midnight.

210. Shooting and tearing in the hip-joint—which pains as if bruised on touching—down over the tibia ; in the evening in bed it is worst, compelling him to get up and walk about.

Paralytic pain in the thigh, also when sitting ; when she has sat for some time doubled up, she must extend the limb in order to relieve herself ; when she gets up from her seat the paralytic pain is worst, but it is relieved by walking.

Numbness on the thigh.

After rising from a seat, relaxation and weariness in the houghs, especially when walking* after standing still.

Weakness of the knees so as to sink down (immediately).

215. Swelling of the knees and ankle-joints, and pain in them, especially on straightening the knee in bed.

A contractive pain in the knee and ankle-joint.

On account of pains as if they were over-tired, he must alternately flex and extend the knees ; he had no rest in them.

In the morning on rising from bed, painful cramp in the calf (aft. 16 h.).

Tonic spasm† of the thigh and leg. [SCHERER, in *Hufel. Journ.*, iii.]

220. In the evening when walking‡ contractive pain like cramp in the tibia and calves.

When standing, cramp in the calves, that goes off when walking (aft. 28 h.).

A painful drawing in the legs.

Bruised pain of the legs, in the morning in bed, which is allayed soon after rising.

* On commencing to walk.
† From iron applied to the soles.[1]
‡ On commencing to walk.

1 In a case of chorea.

The legs are disposed to tremble, and on walking they are painful as if bruised.

225. The thighs feel as if gone to sleep.

After resting from a walk, stiffness in the feet, when she wishes to move again.

Varicose veins on the feet.

Swelling of the foot up to the ankles.

Painful cramp in the soles of the foot.

230. Frequent cramp in the toes and sole of the foot.

The cramp draws the fingers and toes crooked with great pain.

Very cold feet, which he could hardly drag along for weariness.

After a meal, weariness in the feet.

Her feet cannot bear her.

235. Parts of the skin (*e.g.* on the back of the thumb, the toes, &c.) have burning pain when not touched, but intolerable sore pain when touched ever so slightly.

Dark liver-spots (*e.g.* on the back of the hand) inflame and suppurate.

Easily tired by walking.

He is very exhausted and emaciated.

Very exhausted and drowsy. (aft. 2 h.)

240. Very great weakness, like fatigue (immediately).

Heaviness of the limbs, for forty-eight hours.

Heaviness, exhaustion and relaxation of the limbs.

A general weakness caused even by speaking.

Great weakness. [HARCKE, in *Hufel. Journ.*, XXV.[1]]

245. Great trembling on the whole body, which lasts several weeks. [HARCKE, l. c.]

Fainting fits. [RITTER, l. c.]

Fainting fits, which leave weakness all the rest of the day. [RITTER, l. c.]

Weakness of fatigue, alternating with an anxious trembling.

Frequent attacks of trembling all over body.

250. The symptoms are aggravated by sitting, and ameliorated by gentle movement.

Walking in the open air fatigues her.

When walking feeling of faintness; it became black before her eyes; she felt as if she were going to have a fit of apoplexy; at every step roaring in the ears and head.

Inclination to lie down.

Irresistible inclination to lie down (aft. 1 h.).

255. Constant weariness and day-drowsiness (for which sleep procures only transient relief).

After dinner, drowsiness and dulness, also some headache above the root of the nose; he could not engage in any mental work.

---

1 Not found.

When sitting, she could immediately go to sleep, at any time of the day.

Light, not sound, slumber-like sleep.

She lies long before going to sleep.

260. He lies for half and a whole hour before he falls asleep.

She must lie two or three hours before she falls asleep.

He wakes up at night every hour, and then goes off only into a slumber.

She falls asleep tired, and **sleeps** though uneasily, and **is long awake before she falls asleep again**, and yet on rising in the morning she is not tired.

At night she must lie only on the back, she cannot sleep on either side.

265. Nocturnal flatulent colic ; much flatulence is formed in the abdomen, which causes pain, although much flatus escapes.

At night unquiet sleep.

At night very vivid dreams.

At night disturbed by many dreams ; in the morning on rising great weariness.

Restless, dreamful sleep, accompanied by emissions of semen.

270. Dreams that he is in battle, that he has fallen into the water, &c.

Anxious tossing about in bed, after midnight.

Anxiety at night, as if she had done something bad ; she could not sleep, tossed about in bed.

Heavy sleep in the morning until 9 o'clock, from which he can with difficulty rouse himself.

He sleeps with half-open eyes.

275. In the evening in bed he became cold all over, in place of becoming warmer.

After the midday sleep, heat.

Much perspiration when walking and sitting, by day.

Perspiration by day, when walking.

About midnight, frequently perspiration during slumber.

280. Morning perspiration, for a long period.

In the evening before going to sleep, rigor, without external coldness ; in bed he felt chilly all night.

Nocturnal perspiration with exhaustion.

In the morning at break of day, perspiration until about noon, on alternate mornings, immediately preceded every time by headache.

In the morning, attack of stretching and yawning, during which the eyes fill with water (aft. 8 h.).

285. (In the morning heat in the face.)

(Chilliness, and during the chill his face became glowing hot.)

During the day ebullition in the blood, and heat in the evening, especially in the hands.

Heat on the body with redness of cheeks, during which the head is free (aft. 24 h.).

Scarcely perceptible pulse.[1] [RITTER, l. c.]

---

1 As S. 32.

290. (Low spirits as if from the bowels being too relaxed.)
Violence, quarrelsomeness, positiveness (aft. 4 h.).
Alternately one evening excessively merry, the next sad and melancholy.
Anxiety. [NEBEL and WEPFER, l. c.—RITTER, l. c.]
From slight cause, anxiety, with throbbing in the scrobiculus cordis.
295. Anxiety, as if she had done something bad.

GUAIACUM.[1]

(The alcoholic solution of the inspissated juice of the West Indian tree *Guaiacum officinale*, which consists chiefly of resin.)

The homœopathic physician will find even in these few symptoms a sufficient guide to enable him to make a sure curative employment of this vegetable substance in morbid states for which it is suitable by similarity, and to prevent him from being misguided by the vague and misleading recommendations of it in gout and rheumatism by the ordinary works on materia medica, into prescribing it for some imaginary name of a disease, instead of attending only to the similarity of the symptoms of the disease to be cured on the one hand, with those of the remedy on the other.

One drop of the alcoholic tincture stirred up in one ounce of water, in which the small quantity of resin it contains is completely dissolved by shaking, is quite sufficient for a dose ; in some cases, indeed, it will be found rather too strong.

[HAHNEMANN'S fellow-provers were HARTMANN, LANGHAMMER, TEUTHORN.

He obtained a few symptoms from the following old-school authorities :

BANG, *Tagebucher des frid. Krankenhauses in Copenhagen*, 1784, Sept. 13.

MATTHIOLI, *de Morbo Gallico*, 1537.

WHITE, WILL., in *Edinb. Med. Comment.*, iv.

In the 1st edit. guaiac has 142 symptoms, in this 2nd edit. 3 additional symptoms ; the *Chr. Kr.* gives 160.]

GUAIACUM.

Weakness of memory ; what he has just read he knew nothing about ; old names he completely forgot. [*Trn.*]

In the morning when standing (during breakfast) absence of thought ; he remains standing at one spot, and stares right in front of him without thinking. [*Trn.*]

Violent coarse stitches outwards in the brain (aft. 2 h.).

Nocturnal headache, like a pressure from below upwards in the brain.

5. In the morning headache, as if the brain were loose, and moved at every step.

Painless pressure in the left temple. [*Htn.*]

Painful pressure, as with something broad, in the right temple. [*Htn.*]

---

1 From vol. iv, 2nd edit., 1825.

Aching and pressing in the anterior part of the forehead. [*Htn.*]

From the left side of the nape to over the vertex an obtuse aching pain going up obliquely and terminating superiorly in a stitch (aft. 1 h.). [*Htn.*]

10. A dull aching pain in the head, that ends with a sharp stitch in the right frontal eminence. [*Htn.*]

Aching headache across the forehead (aft. 10 h.). [*Lr.*]

Aching, drawing, tearing stitch in the right side of the head going towards the frontal bone. [*Htn.*]

Dull, stitch-like pressure in the right frontal eminence. [*Htn.*]

Dull drawing stitches from the left parietal bone to the left frontal eminence, which at last terminate together in a single stitch, after having taken in a greater extent. [*Htn.*]

15. Drawing pain from the middle of the frontal bone down into the nasal bones. (aft. 2½ h.). [*Htn.*]

Drawing pain in the anterior part of the forehead. [*Htn.*]

Drawing tearing in the occiput and forehead. [*Htn.*]

Tearing in the whole of the left side of the head. [*Htn.*]

Tearing in the right side of the occiput. [*Htn.*]

20. An external headache, as if there were too much blood in the external blood-vessels of the head, and the head were swollen (when sitting). [*Trn.*]

External pulse-like throbbing headache, with shooting on the temples, which goes off by external pressure, but returns afterwards, is relieved by walking, but aggravated by sitting and standing (aft. 3 h.). [*Trn.*]

A tearing externally on the left temple (aft. ¾ h.). [*Htn.*]

Tearing ftom the left side of the frontal bone downwards into the cheek muscles. [*Htn.*]

Acute sharp stitches in the left side of the head at the junction of the parietal and frontal bones. [*Htn.*]

25. Obtuse painful stitches on the left side of the occiput. [*Htn.*]

In the right eye-brow a hard pimple with a white apex, which is very painful when touched as if sore, and as when a wound is touched.

Eye-gum in both canthi of the right eye (aft. 1 h.). [*Lr.*]

Dilatation of the pupils (aft. 3 h.). [*Trn.*]

Amaurosis for some days. [WILL. WHITE,[1] in *Edinb. Med. Comment.*, iv, p. 327.]

30, **All day long he felt as if he had not slept enough, combined with yawning and stretching, and with sensation of swelling of the eyes, and as if the eyes would be driven out of the head ; the eyelids seemed as if they were not able to cover the eyes.** [*Trn.*]

---

1 Observation.—The writer is speaking of a hysterical patient. He states that any sudden surprise will make her speechless for an hour or so, and that guaiacum always causes loss of her sight for some hours (not "days").

Single, painful stitches in the right zygomatic process. [*Htn.*]

Painful, red swelling of the face, for some days.[1] [BANG, *Tagebucher des frid. Krankenhauses*, 1784, Sept. 13.]

Dull, almost spasmodic drawing in the right cheek muscles (in the morning on rising). [*Htn.*]

Knife thrusts in the right cheek muscles (aft. 1 h.). [*Lr.*]

35. Tearing in the outer border of the left ear cartilage. [*Htn.*]

Tearing in the left ear. [*Htn.*]

Earache in the left ear. [*Htn.*]

In the nose a pimple with sore pain.

(Dull, aching pain in the left lower jaw.) [*Htn.*]

40. On the left side of the lower jaw, a drawing pain that ended in a stitch. [*Htn.*]

Tearing in the upper molar teeth of the left side. [*Htn.*]

On biting an aching pain in the left upper molars. [*Htn.*]

Great hunger, in the afternoon and evening (aft. 7½, 9 h.). [*Lr.*]

Anorexia from disgust at everything, eructation of wind, and flat taste in the mouth, together with a mucous expectoration by hawking and hacking cough. [*Trn.*]

45. Eructation (immediately). [*Htn.*]

Eructation of wind, empty eructation. [*Htn.*]

Constrictive sensation in the region of the stomach, which impedes the breathing and causes anxiety (aft. 19 h.). [*Htn.*]

In the scrobiculus cordis, a feeling of frequently recurring pressure, which impedes breathing and causes oppression and anxiety (aft. 1 h.). [*Htn.*]

Stitches in the left subcostal region. [*Htn.*]

50. Single dull stitches in the left epigastrium. [*Htn.*]

Rumbling with dull pinching pain in the abdomen, which always extends more backwards, whereupon flatus is discharged (aft. 1 h.). [*Htn.*]

Grumbling in the abdomen, as from emptiness, in the afternoon (aft. 5 h.). [*Lr.*]

Rumbling in the abdomen (aft. 10 h.). [*Lr.*]

Dull, pinching pain in the hypogastrium, that always sinks deeper backwards ((aft. ¼ h.). [*Htn.*]

55. **Pinching in the abdomen, as from displaced flatulence, which extended backwards, whereupon flatus was discharged.** [*Htn.*]

Pinching in the abdomen on the left side of the navel, on a single point (aft. 3½ h.). [*Htn.*]

Pinching in the abdomen followed by thin, slimy stool (immediately). [*Htn.*]

During inspiration, pinching cutting bellyache transversely through the abdomen. [*Htn.*]

---

1 In a woman aged 48, affected with arthritis of hands and feet, from a tablespoonful of the aqueous solution every 3 hours for a month ; as the arthritis improved this symptom appeared, followed by S. 70.

A constant quivering in the inner abdominal muscles of the right side, close to the os ilii. [*Htn.*]

60. Pain in the groin as from an inguinal hernia.

The first day, constipation; the second and third days, costiveness. [*Trn.*]

Rather soft, broken up stool [*Htn.*]

Frequent urging to urinate with scanty discharge of urine at a time (aft. 5½ h.). [*Lr.*]

Constant urging to urinate, and every time he passes much urine. [*Htn.*]

65. He had frequent calls to pass water, and immediately after doing so he had again urging to urinate, and after the urine was passed stitches in the neck of the bladder followed. [*Trn.*.]

He must urinate every half hour, and he passes much urine, and when he has passed it he has again urging to urinate for fully a minute, whereby only a few drops come away. [*Trn.*]

Cutting during micturition, as if something acrid came away.

At night, emission of semen without voluptuous dreams (aft. 20 h.). [*Lr.*]

Increased flow of mucus from the vagina.

* * *

70. Profuse discharge of a watery fluid from the nose, for a month. [BANG, l. c.]

A crawling in the chest.

Stitches in the left side of the chest, more towards the back, under the true ribs. [*Htn.*]

Shudder in the breasts.

On the chest, in the region of the scrobiculus cordis, a sort of stoppage or stagnation seizes her suddenly, even in the night during sleep, as if she could not get her breath well; this brings on an almost dry cough, which recurs until some expectoration is brought up.

75. A constant shooting, which seemed at last to change into a single continuous stitch, close under the right scapula, which seemed to arise from the middle of the right thoracic cavity, considerably aggravated during inspiration (aft. 36 h.). [*Htn.*]

Drawing and tearing posteriorly under the axilla down the right side of the spine to the last true rib. [*Htn.*]

Tearing stitches on the posterior border of the right scapula (aft. 10 h.). [*Htn.*]

Tearing stitches on the posterior border of both scapulæ, followed by a constrictive sensation in the dorsal muscles (aft. 3 h.). [*Htn.*]

Eroding itching on the back by day.

80. In the left side of the nape and the left side of the back down into the sacrum, a rheumatic stiffness; when not moving at all there was no pain, nor yet when touched, but on the slightest movement and on turning the parts the pain was intolerable.

Betwixt the scapulæ, contractive pain. [*Htn.*]

Violent long-continued stitches in the left clavicle, which commenced from the larynx (aft. 9½ h.). [*Htn.*]

When moving, as also when holding the head stiffly, frequent, continued stitches on the left side of the neck, from the scapula to close to the occiput (aft. 1½ h.). [*Htn.*]

Painful aching in the cervical vertebræ on the right and left sides (aft. 4 h.). [*Htn.*]

85. **Frequently recurring, sharp stitches on the top of the right shoulder.** [*Htn.*]

Severe painful stitches in the right upper arm, chiefly in its middle (aft. 2 h.). [*Htn.*]

Painful drawing tearing in the left upper and forearm into all the fingers, but particularly continued and permanent in the left wrist-joint (aft. 2 h.). [*Htn.*]

Frequent drawing tearing stitches from the left elbow into the wrist-joint. [*Htn.*]

Tearing in the right forearm extending into the wrist-joint. [*Htn.*]

90. Pressive-like tearing in the left wrist-joint. [*Htn.*]

Single violent stitches in the thumb-muscles of the right hand (aft. ½ h.). [*Htn.*]

In the nates, needle-pricks when sitting down (she feels as if she sat on needles), sometimes when walking.

When walking in the open air, bruised pain in the left thigh (aft. 8 h.). [*Lr.*]

An aching drawing pain from the middle of the femur to the knee, when extending the right leg; on drawing up and flexing it the pain goes off again (aft. 2 h.). [*Htn.*]

95. Formication throughout the thighs and legs to the toes, as if the limbs would go to sleep, when sitting.

In the right thigh from its middle to the knee a formicating aching pain in the bone, when sitting still (aft. ¼ h.). [*Htn.*]

Weakness of the thighs, especially the right thigh, when walking, as if the muscles were too short and stretched; on touching the pain was increased, but when sitting it was allayed. [*Trn.*]

In the right thigh, pain like growing pains. [*Htn.*]

Single itching pricks, like flea-bites, in the skin of the thighs, but especially on the sides of the hough, which was removed by scratching. [*Trn.*]

100. Drawing tearing from the middle of the left thigh to the knee. [*Htn.*]

Twitching tearing in the right thigh from its middle to the knee (aft. 1½ h.). [*Htn.*]

Obtuse stitches above the right knee. [*Htn.*]

Single stitches above the left knee from both sides, meeting in the middle (aft. 3 h.). [*Htn.*]

A drawing pain in the knee, which ends in a stitch. [*Htn.*]

105. Tingling in the skin of the whole leg, with hot feeling in it.

After walking the legs are as if bruised, as if brittle.

Tearing obtuse stitches from the middle of the left tibia to the toes. [*Htn.*]

Drawing tearing stitches from the middle of the right tibia to the knee (aft. 14 h.). [*Htn.*]

Dull drawing stitches from the right ankle-joint to the middle of the tibia (aft. 3½ h.). [*Htn.*]

110. Violent twitching stitches on the outer side of the calf.

A contractive, almost painless feeling in the right calf (aft. ¾ h.). [*Htn.*]

Betwixt the tibia and fibula shooting tearings to the patella, so violent as to jerk the leg upwards.

Long drawing, tearing stitches from the right tarsus into the knee. [*Htn.*]

A pain ending in a sharp stitch, on a small spot in the middle of the left instep, that goes off on moving. [*Htn.*]

115. Single sharp stitches in the right ankle-joint, when sitting (aft. ¼ h.). [*Htn.*]

Weariness of the lower extremities, especially of the thighs, as if he had walked far the previous day, and a similar weariness of the upper arms, as if he had done some hard work. [*Trn.*]

(Persons of a dry habit of body may get from it hectic fever or marasmus.) [P. A. MATTHIOLI,[1] *de Morbo Gallico*, 1537.]

General discomfort of the whole body (aft. 7 h.). [*Htn.*]

(Burning itching, increased by scratching.)

120. The symptoms almost all occur when sitting; most of them in the morning immediately after rising, then from 9 till 12 o'clock, and in the evening shortly before falling asleep. [*Htn.*]

Yawning and stretching of the limbs with comfortable feeling (aft. ½ h.). [*Htn.*]

Stretching of the upper extremities with yawning. [*Htn.*]

In the afternoon, great drowsiness (aft. 4½ h.). [*Lr.*]

He falls asleep later in the evening, and wakes earlier than usual; then all felt too narrow, and he tosses about in bed, but only when awake, not when asleep. [*Trn.*]

125. Dreams as if she would be stabbed with knives.

Dreams of fighting.

Vivid dream about scientific subjects (aft. 18 h.). [*Lr.*]

In the evening in bed he cannot fall asleep for two hours, tosses about in bed, dreams much in his sleep; and when he wakes up in the morning, he feels as if he had not slept at all. [*Trn.*]

In the evening in bed (when slumbering?) he felt as if some one threw a towel at his face, so that he started up in affright at it. [*Trn.*]

130. Frequent waking from sleep, as from a fright; he felt as if he were falling (aft. 21 h.). [*Lr.*]

Whilst he lay asleep on his back, he dreamt that some one was lying on him; from anxiety he could not fetch his breath nor cry

1 Observation.

out ; at last he emitted a cry and woke up quite beside himself (nightmare). [*Trn.*]

In the forenoon chilliness for two hours, and in the evening before going to sleep chilliness, which continued also in bed ; every morning some perspiration.

Shivering in the back, in the afternoon (aft. 6 h.). [*Lr.*]

Febrile chill in the back, in the afternoon (aft. 8 h.). [*Lr.*]

135. Internal chilliness in the whole body, followed immediately by heat, especially in the face, without thirst, towards evening. [*Trn.*]

Chilly, even close to the warm stove.

Heat in the whole face, without redness and perspiration, with thirst.

Much thirst.

When walking in the open air much perspiration, especially on the head ; on the forehead beads of sweat.

140. Profuse perspiration, at night, in the back.

Laziness for work. [*Htn.*]

Laziness and dislike to movement.

Morose disposition, he speaks little.

Great peevishness, contemptuous disposition.

145. Obstinacy.

HELLEBORUS NIGER.[1]

(*Christmas Rose.*)

(The juice of the fresh root mixed with equal parts of alcohol, and the alcoholic tincture of the dry root of the *Helleborus niger*.)

The symptoms which I and some of my disciples have observed from this root are but few in number ; still they constitute a commencement of the investigation of its properties. They serve to show that hellebore must prove useful in a peculiar kind of fever, some dropsical affections and mental derangements. When the morbid symptoms it can produce shall have been more completely ascertained, we shall then be able to see what the diseases were for the cure of which at their sanatory resorts the Greeks obtained such renown, for the plant they employed for this purpose was a species with pale red flowers closely allied to our hellebore. In large doses it acts for several weeks.

Camphor seems most frequently effectual in controlling its too energetic primary actions, but the untoward secondary effects yield most readily to cinchona bark.

I myself gathered the root which I used for my trials, and hence am convinced of its genuineness.

[HAHNEMANN was assisted in this proving by HARTMANN, HORNBURG, KUMMER, LANGHAMMER, MOSSDORF, E. F. RUCKERT, STAPF, WISLICENUS.

Symptoms were obtained from the following old-school sources :

ALBERTI, *Jurisp. Med.*, tom. vi.
BUCHNER, in *Samml. f. pr. Aerzte*, vol. i.
BISSET, *On the Med. Const. of Great Britain.*
COOK, JOHN, *Oxford Magazine* for March, 1769.
GESNER, *Entdeckungen*, i.
GREW, *Anatomy of Plants.*
HILDEN, VAN, *Opera Med. Chir.*, Cent. 4, Obs. 12.
MORGAGNI, *de Sedibus et. Caus. Morb.*, lix.
SCOPOLI, *Flora Carniolica.*
SCHULZE, *Materia Medica.*
STEGMANN, *Diss. de salut. et nox. Elleb. nigri usu.* Halæ, 1757.
TOURNEFORT, *Voyage dans le Levant*, t. ii.

In the 1st edit. Hellebore has 198 symptoms, in this 2nd edit. there are 288.]

HELLEBORUS NIGER.

Giddy in the head. [ALBERTI, *Jurisp. Med.*, tom. vi, p. 719.[2]]
Stupefaction of the head (immediately). [*Mss.*]
Giddy stupefaction of the head, in every position. [*Mss.*]

---

1 From vol. iii, 2nd edit., 1825.
2 The sixth volume of this work is not accessible.

On bending down and again raising the head vertigo, that passed off immediately after raising the head (aft. 10½ h.). [*Mss.*]

5. Stupefying headache, as from intoxication, all the afternoon (aft. 7 h.). [*Lr.*]

Stupefaction of the whole head during the fluent coryza (aft. 5½ h.). [*Lr.*]

Inability to think (aft. 10 h.). [*Mss.*]

Heaviness and heat internally in the head, with cold fingers and chilly feeling in the whole body, which is diminished when the hands are covered up and kept warm (aft. 1 h.).

Very painful heaviness in the head, with tension and pressure as from without inwards in the temples, but especially in the forehead; at the same time with every pulse a pressing drawing, as if the blood was forcibly propelled through the head (all day, especially in the fever), diminished in the open air.

10. Heaviness of the brain and sensation as if it was compressed by a tight membrane, with inability to think and to retain anything in the memory. [*Mss.*]

Weakness of memory: it was only by an effort that he could after some time remember what he wanted to say and what he had been questioned about (aft. ½ h.). [*Mss.*]

Weakness of memory: he could not retain what he had read one instant. [*Kr.*]

Confusion which makes the head stupid, a dull pain every afternoon from 4 to 8 o'clock.

Stupidity of the head, as if clouded, chiefly in the forehead (aft. ¾ h.). [*Lr.*]

15. Stupidity and heat in the head; burning in it.

Stupid* and heavy in the head.

Bruised pain as if combined with stupidity, now in one, now in another part of the brain, worst when stooping. [*Hbg.*]

Dazedness of the head, like a bruised sensation, during the fluent coryza (aft. 5 h.). [*Lr.*]

The head is painful as if bruised. [*Hbg.*]

20. Troublesome headache. [SCHULZE, *Materia Medica*, p. 152.[1]]

Headache, pressing from within outwards on the right side of the forehead. [*Ws.*]

Pain in the head, as if the whole brain were pressed inwards, at every step in the open air (aft. 1 h.). [*Htn.*]

Penetrating headache, which on sitting erect becomes a burning in the head.

* From various observations, I infer that stupor, obtuseness of the inner sensibility (*sensorium commune*), in which, though the sight is good, one sees only imperfectly, and does not observe what one sees; though the auditory apparatus is good, one hears or comprehends nothing distinctly; though the gustatory organs are all right, one relishes nothing; is always or often without thought, remembers little or not at all what has quite recently occurred, has no pleasure in anything, slumbers but lightly, and does not sleep soundly or refreshingly, attempts to work but without giving attention or energy to it—are primary effects of hellebore.

1 From continued use.

He knows not how to hold the head on account of the violent pain in it ; he lays it every instant on a different place ; it is most tolerable when he forces himself to lie still, and with closed eyes and in a half-slumber he forgets his pain.

25. Pressure as with a pointed instrument on the crown of the head. [*Hbg.*]

Violent aching pain in the head, with great heaviness, especially in the occiput, on awaking (aft. 41 h.).) [Mss.]

Uninterrupted aching pain in the occiput towards the nape. [*Rkt.*]

Aching pain in the right frontal eminence, increased when walking in the open air. [*Kr.*]

After enforced attention aching pain in the right temple, aggravated when walking (aft. 8 h.). [*Kr.*]

30. In both temples a compressive pain. [*Stf.*]

Pressure in the brain, just as if it were compressed from both sides towards the centre and upwards (aft. 9 h.). [*Mss.*]

An aching pain in the forehead, as if dazed (aft. 11 h.). [*Lr.*]

Semilateral headache, a tearing, with chilliness.

An aching, stupefying, giddy drawing, at one time in one half at another in the other half of the brain, and sometimes in the whole brain. [*Stf.*]

35. Drawing aching in the left half of the brain from behind to the forehead, as if the mass of the brain were heaped up there (immediately). [*Mss.*]

Drawing pain in the upper part of the head, in the morning in bed (aft. 24 h.). [*Ws.*]

Headache from the nape to the crown of the head.

Obtuse drawing in the forehead, causing the skin of the forehead to wrinkle. [*Hbg.*]

Pulsating throbbing in the left temple, each pulsation ending in a stitch (aft. ¾ h.). [*Kr.*]

40. Stitches as if rising up out of the brain, in the region of the coronal suture, right side. [*Kr.*]

Boring stitches going across the forehead (aft. 14 h.). [*Lr.*]

In the morning, several sharp stitches externally on the right, afterwards on the left side of the forehead (aft. 3, 4 h.). [*Lr.*]

Headache, as if bruised, in the occiput, especially when stooping (aft. 48 h.).

Bruised pain externally on the vertex and occiput, especially during the febrile chill ; at every movement, especially when stooping and going upstairs, the pain changes into a violent twitching in the integuments of the head, which is relieved by external pressure (aft. 48 h.). [*Ws.*]

45. Sensations, as if the integuments of the occiput were drawn down tightly (aft. 41 h.). [*Mss.*]

The frontal muscles contract into folds. [*Hbg.*]

Pulse-beats on the forehead and temples, with heat of face (aft. 6 h.). [*Mss.*]

Small swellings in the skin of the forehead, which pain as if bruised or as if from a blow.

A pimple on the left side of the forehead, which on being roughly touched pains as if bruised. [*Mss.*]

50. A prickly tension on the left palpebral arch when touched, as if a pimple would come there (aft. 46 h.). [*Mss.*]

Quivering in the muscles of the eye-brows and cheeks, with heat of face. [*Mss.*]

Pain drawing hither and thither in the palpebral arch, with spasmodic contraction of the muscle of the eye-brow (aft. 10 h.). [*Mss.*]

Aching in the orbits, as if the eyes would fall out. [*Rkt.*]

Painful aching in the right inner canthus, that is aggravated by closing the eyes (aft. 9 h.). [*Lr.*]

55. Itching in the canthi. (aft. $\frac{3}{4}$ h.). [*Lr.*]

Burning smarting in the eyes, especially the inner canthi. [*Ws.*]

Prickling in the eyes at if they would weep (immediately). [*Mss.*]

In the eyes sensation as if they were closed by something heavy pressing on them from above; he must make an effort to keep them wide open (in the open air) (aft. 7, 8 h.).

In the morning after waking, on shutting the eyes, violent prickling on the eye-ball and its coverings, as with sharp points (aft. 9 h.). [*Mss.*]

60. Prickling on the eye-ball from above. [*Mss.*]

In the morning, after waking, soreness of the canthi of the left eye, with some moisture in them. [*Stf.*]

In the morning the inner canthi are full of dry eye-gum (aft. 9 h.). [*Mss.*]

Quivering of the eyelids.

(Swollen, red eyelids.)

65. Daylight is painful to him; he does not like to look at surrounding objects, and lies with closed eyes (in the fever).

Dilated pupils.

Dilated pupils (the 1st hour). [*Stf.*]

Drawing pain from the temple to the ear (immediately). [*Mss.*]

In both ears a drawing as if the inner ear would burst, a kind of earache. [*Stf.*]

70. Along with the shooting tearing pains in the teeth, in the right ear a digging boring shooting all night long; in the morning and all day only the pain in the ear remained. [*Kr.*]

Near the ear, behind the ascending ramus of the lower jaw, a succession of needle-pricks (aft. 30 h.). [*Kr.*]

Aching in the depression behind the lobe of the ear.

Aching pain in the root of the nose.

Constriction of the nose as if he should be suffocated.[1] [SCHULZE, l.c.]

75. In the left ala nasi an itching burning. [*Hbg.*]

1 With S. 20.

Smarting itching underneath and about the nose and upper lip, as if coryza were coming on. [*Mss.*]

Yellowish complexion.

Paleness of the face during the heat of the head.

In the morning, after waking, a vesicular pimple on the middle of the red part of the upper lip. [*Hbg.*]

80. (Ulceration of the commissure of the lip, with itching.)

In the evening after lying down in bed, shooting tearing pain in the right lower and upper molars, which can bear neither warmth nor cold ; the pain torments him all night, so that he could sleep but little ; thereafter the lower molars are longer ; but little felt by day. [*Kr.*]

On biting the teeth together a tearing in both opposed third molars towards their roots (immediately). [*Mss.*]

Insensible stiffness of the tongue. [GREW, *Anatomy of plants*, p.280.[1]]

Quite dry, white tongue, in the morning on rising from bed (aft. 24 h.). [*Kr.*]

85. Vesicles on the tongue.

On the tip of the tongue a pimple with shooting pain when touched. [*Kr.*]

Swelling of the tongue. [BUCHNER, in *Samml. f. pr. Aerzte*, vol. 1, p. 3.[2]]

A scraping feeling on the back of the palate. [*Stf.*]

Tiresome dryness on the palate and cutting and scraping pain on the palate on moving the parts of the mouth engaged in swallowing (lasting many days). [*Ws.*]

90. Sore throat ; on swallowing, an aching, and the throat feels excoriated.

Dry slimy taste, with great thirst, for two hours. [*Mss.*]

Flow of saliva.

Accumulation of watery saliva ; he must spit out frequently.

Much watery saliva in the mouth. [*Stf.*]

95. Constant flow of saliva into the mouth, which he must spit out (aft. $1\frac{3}{4}$ h.). [*Htn.*]

Great hunger ; he is always hungry and everything tastes well. [*Kr.*]

Bitterness in the throat, but still more bitter when he eats anything.

He has appetite, but when he eats he does not relish it, and he gets nausea for a short time, which ceases immediately after eating.

Loathing of green vegetables and sourcrout, with good appetite for bread and meat (for more than a week.)

100. Dislike to food.

Loathing of fat meat (for more than a week), whereas bread and lean meat taste well.

Adipsia all day long.

---

1 From chewing root.

2 Observation.—"Swelling" should be "trembling."

Frequent tasteless, dry eructation (the first hour), then completely suppressed eructation. [*Stf.*]

Empty eructation, without any taste (aft. ½ h.) [*Kr.*]

105. Hiccup. [BUCHNER,—STEGMANN, *Diss. de salut et nox. Elleb. nigri usu.* Halæ, 1751, p. 22.[1]]

Hiccup (aft 2 h.). [*Lr.*]

Soon after dinner, discharge of strong, fœtid flatus (aft. 1¼ h.) [*Kr.*]

Feeling of nausea in the stomach ; he often feels hungry, but food is repugnant to him, though he has no abnormal taste either in the mouth or of food (aft. 24 h.). [*Mss*]

Inclination to vomit.

110. Inclination to vomit, rising up from the scrobiculus cordis.

Empty eructation and inclination to vomit, but yet he cannot vomit.

Continued inclination to vomit.* [GESNER, *Entdeckungen*, i, p. 167.[2]]

Vomiting. [JOHN COOK, in *Oxford Magazine* for March, 1769.[3]]

Vomiting of a greenish black matter, with bellyache; symptoms which recurred after ceasing for three hours, and lasted an hour, followed by apparent rest for two hours, then a violent cry, followed by death (aft. 38 h.) ; the limbs were relaxed and flaccid, the blood in the veins fluid, on the left side of the œsophagus and stomach, as also in the small intestines, a moderate inflammation ; the brain very soft and flaccid. [MORGAGNI, *de Sed. et Caus. Morb.*, lix, 15, 16.[4]]

115. Great bruised pain near and under the scrobiculus cordis in the region of the portal vein, where he feels every step painfully when walking ; the pain is aggravated by speaking aloud and by touching the part.

Sensation as if the scrobiculus cordis were drawn in.

Distension of the scrobiculus cordis and of the epigastric region, which impedes respiration, and is painful as from an internal ulcer.

Every step causes a painful impression on the scrobiculus cordis.

Excessive pain in the scrobiculus cordis. [GESNER, l. c.]

120. Pressure in the precordial region. [COOK, l. c.]

Scrapy rough sensation in the stomach (as from rubbing with a woollen cloth). [*Hbg.*]

A painful burning in the stomach, which rises up through the œsophagus. [TOURNEFORT, *Voyage dans le Levant*, t. ii, p. 180.[5]]

In the stomach, pinching (aft. 2½ h.). [*Hbg.*]

Pain in abdomen. [BUCHNER,—STEGMANN,—GESNER, l. c.]

125. Heaviness in the abdomen (aft. 2 h.) [*Hbg.*]

* From *Hel. fœtidus.*

1 Not accessible.
2 Statement.
3 Poisoning.
4 Effects of extract in a melancholic.
5 Statement.

A pinching, commencing in the hepatic region and twisting itself always deeper downwards and forwards (aft. 2½ h.). [*Htn.*]

Bellyache.

In the abdomen a couple of stitches and a tearing pain across it (aft. ½ h.).

(After a meal) severe dysentery-like pinching across the abdomen. [*Hbg.*]

130. Pinching in the abdomen (on going upstairs) (aft. 32 h.). [*Lr.*]

Sharp pressure across the abdomen, below the navel, from without inwards, especially severe when sitting (aft. 24 h.). [*Ws.*]

Cold sensation in the abdomen.

Grumbling in the abdomen.

Excessive rumbling and noises in the abdomen (immediately).

135. Audible painless grumbling below the umbilical region. (aft. 1 h.). [*Kr.*]

Movement in the abdomen, as if bubbles of air rose up and burst, followed by discharge of fœtid flatus (aft. 8 h.). [*Kr.*]

Flatulence moving about in the abdomen. [*Hbg.—Stf.*]

Transient distension of the abdomen, in the evening (aft. 5 d.).

In the morning after the accustomed draught of milk, discharge of fœtid flatus (aft. ½ h.). [*Kr.*]

140. Purging with nausea and bellyache. [Tournefort, l. c.]

Diarrhœa, and before each stool pain in the abdomen, which went off after each stool. [*Rkt.*]

Diarrhœa.

Diarrhœa. [Morgagni, l. c.]

Every day three or four times instead of the stool, there passes white gelatinous matter, like frog's spawn, with much pressing.

145. Stools of pure, viscid, white mucus.

Retained stool the first day, the next day in the morning an ordinary stool, and in the afternoon a diarrhœic stool.

Hard, scanty stool, during and immediately after which violent, cutting shooting in the rectum from below upwards, just as if it contracted tightly and as if a body with cutting edges stuck there. (aft. 12 h.). [*Mss.*]

Hæmorrhoidal irritation. [Schulze, l. c]

After an evacuation a burning smarting pain in the anus for a minute. [*Stf.*]

150. In the right inguinal region single pressures terminating in a stitch, a sensation as if a hernia would ensue. [*Kr.*]

Severe hard pressure on the middle of the os pubis (aft. ¼ h.). [*Hbg.*]

Frequent micturition.

Urging to urinate (micturition).

Copious discharge of urine, without any particular urging (aft. 24, 26 h.). [*Lr.*]

155. **Frequent urging to pass urine, with scanty discharge of urine** (aft. ¾, 2½, 3, 5½ h.). [*Lr.*]

Copious discharge of watery urine. [*Stf.*]

Several itching, fine pricks on the point of the glans penis (aft. ½ h.). [*Lr.*]

Seems to suppress powerfully the sexual desire. [*Stf.*]

Production of the menstrual flux (aft. 8 h).

* * *

160. Sneezing. [VAN HILDEN, *Opera Med. Chir.*, Cent. 4, Obs. 12[1].]

In the morning, when fasting, sneezing. (aft. 26 h.). [*Lr.*]

Spasmodic tickling irritation in the nose, as if about to sneeze (which however did not occur), with yawning (aft. 1 h.). [*Kr.*]

Sneezing, immediately after rising from bed in the morning, causing the upper lip to crack in the middle. [*Kr.*]

Short cough.

165. A suddenly arising, continued short coughing (whilst smoking the customary tobacco, when sitting) (aft. 15 h.). [*Lr.*]

Rapid breathing.

Dyspnœa ; he must breathe slowly and sometimes deeply (aft. ¼ h.). [*Mss.*]

Constriction of the glottis. [BUCHNER, l. c.]

Chest quite contracted, so that he gasped for breath with open mouth, but could not breathe. [ALBERTI, l. c.]

170. Sharp cutting in the lowest true ribs over the chest, from within outwards, increased by inspiration. [*Ws.*]

Elevated temperature in the lower part of the thoracic cavity. [*Hbg.*]

Scraping, rough sensation in the upper part of the sternum. [*Hbg.*]

When moving the neck some of its muscles are stiff and painful. [*Stf.*]

Rheumatic stiffness of the nape.

175. Pain of the cervical glands.

Stiffness of the muscles of the nape up to the occiput, even when at rest, but mostly when moving the head (in the morning) (aft. 41 h.). [*Mss.*]

Contractive pain in the sacrum.

A dull pain in the left scapula, more acutely painful when moving. [*Stf.*]

Betwixt the scapulæ, on the spine, bruised pain. [*Hbg.*]

180. Visible twitching of the muscles in the left upper arm, with pain as if something hard knocked violently against that part. [*Hbg.*]

Itching erosion on both arms, and after scratching, smarting as from salt-water, after going to sleep, in the evening and morning.

Yellowish, round tetters on both arms from which water exuded when scratched.

In the right upper arm, sensation as after a blow, but not when touched. [*Hbg.*]

Fine tearing in the shafts of the arm-bones. [*Ws.*]

1 From inhaling the odour.

185. Severe drawing from the middle of the forearm to the bend of the elbow. [*Mss.*]

Drawing pain from the right wrist to the index finger (aft. 10 h.). [*Mss.*]

In the evening when walking in the open air, severe needle-pricks in the left wrist-joint (aft. 13 h.). [*Lr.*]

Across the flexor tendons of the left hand needle-pricks dart (when walking in the open air) (aft. 12¾ h.). [*Lr.*]

Sweat on the palms of the hands, with coldness on the back of the hands (aft. 2 h.). [*Kr.*]

190. Tearing in the backs of all the fingers of the left hand (in the morning in bed) (aft. 18 h.). [*Mss.*]

Tearing in the left middle finger, especially in its middle joint. [*Mss.*]

Boring pain in the middle joint of the middle and index fingers (aft 20 h.). [*Mss.*]

Loss of power in both hands, so that he could grasp nothing, nor double the fingers up into a fist strongly. [*Mss.*]

Paralytic tearing in the right little finger (aft. 27 h.). [*Mss.*]

195. Paralytic tearing and spasmodic stiffening in the fourth finger of the right hand, going off when at rest. [*Mss.*]

A tickling on the right index (aft. 10 h.). [*Lr.*]

A painful aching across the right thumb. [*Lr.*]

An inflamed spot at the nails of the left index and right thumb, with pain like an ulcer when touched (aft. 20 h.) ; the following day some whitish humour escaped, whereupon it healed. [*Mss.*]

Betwixst the proximal joint of the right fourth and fifth fingers several small vesicles, which are sore when touched, exude moisture for some time, and then remain for a long time covered by a scab. [*Mss.*]

200. On the middle joint of the fourth right finger small, exuding, painless vesicles ; on applying strong pressure the bone seems to have sore pain. [*Mss.*]

A slight drawing pain in the right hip. [*Stf.*]

Sudden paralytic stiffness in the left hip-joint, when walking in the open air (aft. 23 h.). [*Mss.*]

Single pricks in the left hip, as with a needle. [*Hbg.*]

In the left hip several violent, rather slow pricks, as with several pins. [*Hbg.*]

205. Repeated burning aching in the left hip (aft. 2 h.). [*Hbg.*]

Stiffness and tension of the muscles of the thigh. [*Rkt.*]

Weariness of the thighs.

Very great weakness of the thighs and legs (aft. 1½ h.). [*Htn.*]

Stiffness in the houghs.

210. Unsteadiness of the limbs, weakness of the feet, staggering of the knees ; he can walk only slowly.

Digging pain in the right patella (aft. ½ h.). [*Lr.*]

Several times recurring, boring, obtuse stitches through the left knee-joint, in the open air, when walking and standing (aft. 26 h.). [*Mss.*]

Stiffness of the tendons in the hough, especially of the outer ones when walking in the open air (aft. 25 h.). [*Mss.*]

On the right leg, near the outer ankle, stitches darting upwards (aft. 3 h.). [*Lr.*]

215. In the inner ankle of the left foot, pain as if after an external blow. [*Hbg.*]

Dislocated pain in the left ankle-joint; he fears the foot will turn over (aft. 30 h.). [*Kr.*]

Feet heavy and tired.

A painful aching feeling on the right os calcaneum, in every position (aft. 11 h.). [*Lr.*]

A fine painful pressure in the right sole, when sitting (aft. 5 h.). [*Lr.*]

220. Tearing in the ball of the left foot (aft. ¼ h.). [*Mss.*]

Shooting twitching in the left big toe. [*Mss.*]

The hairs all over the body came out, the nails fell off. [COOK, l. c.]

The epidermis of the body scalded off. [COOK, l. c.]

Sharp tearing stitches in several parts of the body at once, on the upper and fore arms, chest, back, &c. (aft. 8 h.). [*Lr.*]

225. Paralytic weakness of the limbs and unusual stiffness. [SCOPOLI, *Flora Carniolica*, p. 557.[1]]

All the limbs are so heavy and painfully sensitive in the muscles, that he is unwilling to move them. [*Ws.*]

Stretching and straining of the limbs (aft. 1 h.). [*Kr.*]

Sudden relaxation of all the muscles; cold on the body and with cold sweat on the forehead he suddenly falls down on the ground and stammers, but retains his consciousness; the pulse is very slow and the pupils quite contracted (aft. 1 h.).

In the forenoon, weariness and drowsiness with yawning (aft. 2 h.). [*Kmr.*]

230. In the open air he feels better, the inclination to vomit goes off, and the headache is considerably relieved.

In the open air he feels as if he had been ill a long time; objects appear to him altered and novel.

Sudden œdematous swelling of the skin.*

(Sensation in the swollen parts as if they were distended and too heavy.)

Shooting boring pains in the periosteum of the bones.

* This symptom, combined with symptoms 154, 155, 156, seems to promise much for some dropsical diseases. These will certainly be rapidly and permanently cured by hellebore, if their other symptoms correspond homœopathically, *i.e.* in similarity with those which this powerful herb can excite in a peculiar manner in the healthy human subject. This is the reason of the occasional curative effect of Bacher's pills, which seem to be an accidental discovery of domestic practice, for the practitioners of ordinary medicine could know nothing about the homœopathic suitability of hellebore in certain dropsical affections, seeing that the peculiar morbific effects of this plant were unknown to them, and they had no suspicion what curative action could ensue from its employment.

1 Observation.—In the original "paralytic weakness" is represented by "torpor."

235. Shooting boring pains in various parts of the body, which are aggravated by cool air, exercise, and after eating and drinking.

Syncopes. [BUCHNER,—STEGMANN,—COOK, l. c.]

Convulsions, spasms. [BUCHNER,—STEGMANN,—VAN HILDEN, l. c.]

Spasms and convulsive movements, at the same time a blow on the brain as with an arrow. [TOURNEFORT, l. c.]

He slumbers with half opened eyes, the pupils directed upwards (immediately).

240. As soon as he opens his eyes in the morning in bed he must stretch himself, whereupon he becomes weary and his eyes close again. [*Kr.*]

Towards morning restless sleep; he turns first on one side, then on the other; in this slumber dark dream-pictures hover before him. (*Kr.*)

Towards morning restless slumber beset with historical fancies, during which he turns from side to side. [*Kr.*]

After lying down in bed, vivid fantasies, hundreds of figures hovered before his eyes, which disappeared as quickly as they came. [*Kr.*]

At night incessant confused, often very anxious, but unremembered dreams. [*Ws.*]

245. At night confused, unremembered dreams. [*Lr.*]

Slow pulse (aft. 1 and 16 h.).

Very small pulse.

He feels the beat of the pulse distinctly through the whole body, chiefly at the heart. [*Kr.*]

Strong pulse (aft. ¼ h.). [*Hbg.*]

250. Palpitation of the heart. [*Hbg.*]

Thirst. [BUCHNER,—STEGMANN, l. c.]

Fever. [SCHULZE, l. c.]

Coldness of the body, especially in the morning.

On account of shivering he wishes to lie down in bed, and his complexion appears yellowish.

255. The shivering commences in the arms.

After a thirstless rigor for five days, thirst.

Every time he lies down in the evening, chilliness, and every morning perspiration (aft. 10 d.)

General rigor with goose-skin, painful sensibility of the external head when it is touched and when moving, drawing tearing in the limbs and frequent stitches in the joints, especially of the elbow and shoulders without thirst for some days from the morning onwards (aft. 25 h.). [*Ws.*]

(In the evening, cold feet, which do not get warm even in bed.) [*Kr.*]

260. Coldness of the hands, whilst the face and the rest of the body were warm (aft. ¼ h.). [*Lr.*]

Fever: with excessive internal heat of head, coldness of the hands and feet, then slight sweat all over the body, for an hour (aft. 4 h.).

Fever of several days' duration: when out of bed constant thirstless chill over the body (when sitting, standing and walking), with cold hands, internal burning heat and stupidity of the head with great drowsiness, heaviness and weariness of the feet and stiffness of the houghs; after lying down in bed, immediately heat and sweat all over also without thirst.

Fever: constant chill over the body, without thirst, heat in the head and headache, like bruised pain, in the occiput.

In the evening (about 5 or 6 o'clock), and especially after lying down, burning heat all over the body, especially severe in the head, with internal shivering and chilliness, without thirst; when he attempted to drink, it was repugnant to him, he could only drink little at a time. [*Ws.*]

265. Frequent alternating attacks of general dry heat, then shivering and coldness, whereupon slight bellyache ensued.

After the fever a feeling as if he had long lain ill.

External heat of the face, the cheeks glow in the room (aft. 6 h.). [*Mss.*]

Slight sweat on the feet towards morning (the 1st night).

Heat and perspiration (aft. 36 h.).

270. **General sweat towards morning, for several nights, with only ordinary warmth of body** (aft. 48 h.). [*Ws.*]

Cold sweats. [BUCHNER,—STEGMANN, l. c.]

Pale, fallen-in face, pulselessness, icy coldness and cold sweat all over, so that a drop hung on every hair. [ALBERTI, l. c.]

Anxiety. [BUCHNER,—STEGMANN, l. c.]

Extreme anxiety.

275. Dreadful anxiety, which, however, went off after vomiting.* [BISSET, *Essay on the Med. Const. of Great Britain*, p. 333.[1]]

Such anxiety, nausea and suffering, that he thinks he is going to die. [ALBERTI, l. c.]

He could neither sit, stand nor lie, and always pointed to his heart. [ALBERTI, l. c.]

Restless and anxious, as if anticipating misfortune (aft. 5 d.). [*Kr.*]

Distraction of the mind when studying; he could not fix his thoughts.

280. (Irresolution.)

He despairs of his life.

He groans and grunts.

Home-sickness.

On seeing a happy person he becomes melancholy and then only he feels very unhappy.

* From *Hel. fœtidus.*

1 Poisoning.

285. (He puts on his clothes awkwardly.)

Sad disposition respecting his present position, everything seems to him so insipid and nothing interests him. [*Ws.*]

Wrapt up in his own thoughts, silent humour, all the afternoon. [Alberti, l. c.]

Disposition always cheerful and active (curative action). [*Kr*.]

HEPAR SULPHURIS CALCAREUM.[1]

(A mixture of equal parts of finely powdered oyster shells and quite pure flowers of sulphur, kept for ten minutes at a white heat, and stored up in well-corked bottles. I have found a very small portion of a grain of the million-fold attenuation (by means of three triturations, each of an hour's duration, with three times 100 grains of fresh milk-sugar) quite sufficient, often too large, for a dose.)

[HAHNEMANN was assisted in this proving by FRIEDRICH HAHNEMANN and STAPF.

Two symptoms are taken from

HINZE, A. H., in *Hufel. Journ. d. pr. A.*, Sept., 1815.

In the 1st edit. the number of symptoms of hepar is 206 ; in this 2nd edit. 298 ; in the *Chr. Kr.* there are 661.]

When driving in a carriage such great vertigo that on getting out she could not stand alone.

Faint vertigo and a staring of the eyes, as if he sat wrapped in thoughts, but without seeing anything.

On shaking the head vertigo and headache.

In the morning on awaking aching pain in the head.

5. In the morning in bed dull headache, which diminished after rising. [*Stf.*]

Drawing and aching in the temples by day.

In the right half of the brain a sharp pressure, varying in intensity.

Tensive headache above the nose.

In one half of the brain a continued pain as from a peg or blunt nail driven into the brain.

10. On rising up again after stooping and on every movement stitches in the head, especially after walking in the open air.

A boring pain on a small spot in the side of the head.

Boring pain in the right temple extending into the upper part of the head.

The hair falls out very much (aft. 5 d.).

The hair on several parts of the head falls out, and bald spots are formed.

15. Eruption of pimples, like wheals, on the hairy scalp and nape, which feel sore when touched, but not when let alone.

Eruption of many pimples on the side of the forehead, worst in the room, but which soon get better in the open air.

Two painless, swollen elevations on the forehead.

At night violent headache, as if the forehead would be torn out, with general heat without thirst.

---

1 From vol. iv, 2nd edit., 1825.

In the morning as soon as he wakes until some time after rising, pain in the forehead, as if sore, almost as if bruised, increased by moving the eyes ; at the same time a similar, slight, but very disagreeable pain in the abdomen.

20. Internal pain in the forehead, like needle-pricks.

From midnight onwards (in bed) until noon, pain like a boil in the forehead, and when stooping and coughing like needle-pricks ; externally when touched the forehead was also painful like a boil and needle-pricks, several mornings.

On lying down in the afternoon, a spasmodic twitching in the frontal muscles, which only went off on getting up.

Boring pain in the bones of the upper part of the orbit.

(In the outer canthus of the eye a cutting pain.)

25. Eruption of pimples on the upper eyelids and below the eyes.

Inflammation, redness and swelling of the upper eyelid, with pain more aching than shooting.

On waking the eyelids are closed, so that he is unable to open them for a long time.

The eyes get sore, they become gummed up in the night ; in the evening he cannot see the candle-light well, the eyes become dim and matter is secreted in them.

One eye sore, inflamed and swollen ; redness of the white.

30. The eyes are red and have aching pain, especially on moving.

Aching pain in the eyeballs and bruised feeling when touched.

Yellowness of the face, with blue rings round the eyes.

Yellowish skin and complexion.

All day sensible and visible redness of the cheeks, without thirst or shivering, for several days.

35. In the evening (about 7 o'clock) heat in the face.

Heat in the face in the night and on waking in the morning.

In the morning erysipelatous swelling of the cheeks (aft. 48 h.).

Swelling of the left cheek, for two days. [*Fr. H—n.*]

Heat, redness and itching of the outer ears, for six days.

On blowing the nose violent stitches in the ear.

40. In the evening on going to sleep, until he falls asleep, roaring and beating before the ears.

Drawing pain in the nose, which then goes into the eyes and becomes a smarting (in the morning).

Pain on the back of the nose on touching it, as if sore.

Bruised pain on the tip of the nose.

45. Feeling of ulcerated nostrils.

He blows coagulated blood from the nose.

Every morning some drops of blood come out of the nose.

Epistaixs, repeated two days.

Loss of the smell.

50. Very acute smell.*

In the middle of the upper lip a tensive pain.

Great swelling of the upper lip, which is very painful when grasped, but at othet times is only tense, for three days. [*Fr. H—n.*]

* Seems to be curative action.

An ulcer on the commissure of the lips.*

Eruption on the commissure of the lips, with hot feeling there.

55. On the right side of the chin, towards the under lip, vesicles and ulcers with burning sensation.

Eruption of pimples on the chin, above and below the lips and on the neck, like wheals, which are painful as if excoriated only when touched, not when let alone.

Swelling of the gums at the back molars, with some out-pressing pain, as if a new tooth were about to come there ; the pain is worst when he touches or bites on the teeth.

Twitching in the gums.

In the evening drawing toothache in a hollow tooth, as if too much blood were forced upon the nerves.

60. Toothache (aft. 1 h.). [*Fr. H—n.*]

Toothache, especially when eating.

Toothache (aft. 6 p. m.) : the tooth commences to be loose and has drawing pain, a pain that is worse in the warm room and better in the open air, neither aggravated nor ameliorated by cold water, nor yet by applying the warm hand ; not aggravated by speaking, but only by biting the teeth together, and then there is twitching in it.

A hollow tooth becomes loose and painful when biting on it (aft. 3 h.).

In the throat when swallowing and yawning, shooting pain, as if a splinter were sticking in it ; on yawning the shooting goes to the ear.

65. On breathing deeply there is shooting in the throat.

On turning the head there is shooting in the throat extending to the ear.

Single fine pricks on the external parts of the neck and behind the ears, like flea-bites.

Many small papules in the nape and on both sides of the neck, but not painful. [*Fr. H—n.*]

Bruised pain of the external cervical muscles, with sore throat ; there is pain on swallowing as from a swelling in the throat (aft. 24 h.).

70. In the morning, sensation in the throat as from a plug of mucus, which will not come away—a kind of internal swelling at the commencement of the œsophagus.

Immediately after supper a pressure under the larynx, as if something were sticking in the throat.

On swallowing, a feeling as if there were a swelling in the throat, over which he must swallow.

Scraping in the throat, for three days. [*Fr. H—n.*].

Rough and scrapy in the throat, even *per se*, but it feels most sore on swallowing solid food.

75. A choking and scraping feeling in the throat, as from burnt lard, in the morning.

Scraping in the throat : it is always so full of water, that she must be constantly spitting.

* Which belladonna removes, as it does also many other of the sufferings caused by hepar, where the symptoms correspond together in similarity.

In the evening after a meal he must hawk up much mucus from the throat.

She always felt as if water rose up in the œsophagus, as when one has partaken of something acid.

Flow of watery saliva from the mouth, like water-brash, which recurs next day at the same hour.

80. Flow of saliva from the mouth, with inclination to vomit.

In the morning bitter slimy taste in the mouth.

A bitter taste in the mouth ; the food also tastes bitter.

Bitterness at the back of the throat, but food tastes all right.

She has an earthy taste in the throat, although food tastes tolerably natural.

85. (Loss of the sense of taste.)

(He loathes everything, especially fat.)

(He has sometimes an appetite for something, but when he gets it, he does not like it.)

He has appetite only for sour and strong tasting (piquant) things.

More thirst than hunger.

90. Intolerable thirst for wine (which she usually disliked) ; this thirst was only allayed for a short time by wine and water (aft. 1 h.). [*Stf.*]

Uncommonly great thirst from morning till evening. [*Fr. H—n.*]

Eructation.

Burning in the throat during eructation.

Nausea, frequently during the day.

95. Qualmish, inclined to vomit. [*Stf.*]

In the morning **nausea** and inclination to vomit, when sitting and standing, which ceases on lying down.

Vomiting in the morning.

Sour vomiting in the afternoon.

Aching in the stomach, after eating but little.

100. Tension in the scrobiculus cordis ; he must unbutton his clothes and cannot bear to sit.

A hard pressure rising up out of the abdomen, which remains fixed in the scrobiculus cordis, and is only relieved by the discharge of flatus.

His abdomen is as hard as a stone, and there is pressure under the scrobiculus cordis.

Abdomen distended by flatulence, tightness of abdomen.

Distended, swollen abdomen, without flatulence.

105. Drawing pain in the epigastrium and at the same time over the sacrum (immediately).

Bellyache, like drawing pain.

Contractive pain in the abdomen.

Clawing in the umbilical region from both sides of the abdomen towards the middle, which sometimes rises up to the scrobiculus cordis, and causes nausea and anxious heat in the cheeks, in fits—almost as if from a chill or from the approach of the menstrual period (aft. 3 h.).

Twisting sensation above the navel.

110. Spasms in the abdomen (aft. 3 d.).

Pinching in the abdomen, as from a chill.

Violent stitches in the left side of the abdomen, just under the ribs.

A very disagreeable though slight pain in the abdomen, almost as from a bruise, from the early waking until some time after getting up, accompanied by a similar pain in the forehead.

(He feels much emptiness in the bowels.)

115. For several days, towards evening, cutting in the abdomen, without diarrhœa.

Cutting in the abdomen.

Every morning a wandering about of flatulence in the abdomen, accompanied by disagreeable feeling, especially in the sides of the abdomen ; a kind of colic.

Rumbling in the abdomen.

Discharge of flatus at night.

120. The glands in the groin become painful *per se*, and still more when touched ; they are painful as if they were swollen.

Buboes, abscesses of the inguinal glands.

With much urging very difficult evacuation of scanty, not hard fæces.

Frequent stools, also at night ; very little is evacuated, and yet it is with pressing and tenesmus and exhaustion.

Diarrhœa of bloody mucus, with rumbling as if behind in the back (without pain in the abdomen).

125. Three diarrhœic stools, and at the same time a qualmish feeling of nausea in the abdomen, with rumbling in it.

Every day a couple of slightly loose stools, preceded by some pinching ; there then comes some flatus before the loose stool and some more flatus afterwards.

For several days clay-coloured stool.

Greenish stool.

A pimple above the anus, and feeling of swelling there.

130. (Burning at the anus.)

Even when first passed the urine is cloudy like whey, and deposits a white sediment (aft. 12 h.).

Urine when first passed quite pale and clear, on standing cloudy, thick, and depositing a white sediment.

Dark yellow urine ; it scalds when passing.

When urinating the last drops of urine are bloody.

135. Great discharge of urine (aft. 4 d.).

He dare not urinate any more at night, at least he wakes up for it.*[1]

Impeded micturition : he must wait some time before the urine comes, and then it flows out slowly, for many days.

The urine scalds on the external parts of the genitals, and erodes the inner surface of the prepuce and makes it ulcerated.

The orifice of the urethra looks red and inflamed.

140. Itching externally on the penis and on the frenulum of the glans.

* Curative reaction of the organism.

---

1 The meaning of this symptom is obscure ; it is omitted in the *Chr. Kr.*

A stitch in the region of the frenulum glandis.

Shooting pain in the prepuce.

Externally on the prepuce ulcers appear resembling chancres.

* * *

Frequent sneezing (immediately).

145. Without having a cold the child blows much from its nose, of an evil odour.

Coryza and spitting of much saliva.

Coryza and scraping in the throat.

Like catarrhal fever ; internally chilly and cross.

Tickle in the throat and suffocation making him cough.

150. Scrapy, scratchy-cough.

When the smallest member becomes cool, there immediately occurs a cough, as from a chill and oversensitiveness of the nervous system.

(The cough is particularly troublesome when walking.)

Cough day and night.

Cough ending in sneezing.

155. Cough evening and morning.

Dry, deep cough, from tightness of the breath (suffocation) when breathing ; with this deep cough there is pain in the upper part of the chest as if sore.

Suffocative cough ; cough not excited by a tickling but by tightness of breath.

Cough, and on breathing deeply the most severe cough, which makes him vomit.

Dry cough on going to bed, in the evening (aft. 4 d.).

160. In the evening impulses of dry cough.

In the evening the cough teases her much.

Dry, almost uninterrupted cough from an irritation in the upper part of the left side of the throat, which is worst when talking and stooping ; late in the evening it always increases and then suddenly ceases (aft. 2 h.).

After going to bed at night from 11 till 12 o'clock, violent cough (with expectoration of mucus).

Cough with expectoration of mucus, all day ; a scraping irritation in the wind-pipe, but especially in the throat, excites it. [*Fr. H—n.*]

165. Cough frequently wakes her early from sleep.

From time to time violent fits of coughing, almost causing suffocation or vomiting.

Cough which excites vomiting.

Violent, deep cough of several impulses, which strikes painfully on the larynx and causes retching.

First in the scrobiculus cordis a feeling as of a hard body, then coughing of blood, then fœtid perspiration—then weakness in the head (aft. 48 h.).

170. Bloody expectoration, with cross humour and exhaustion.

Every three or four hours a severe fit of coughing with much expectoration ; but the cough does not wake him out of sleep at night.

Cough with expectoration.

Viscid mucus in the chest (aft. 5 d.).

Shortness of breath.

175. Frequent deep breathing.

In the sternum shooting when breathing and walking.

In the side of the chest, towards the back, shooting pain.

Eruption of two pimples on the sternum, which are acutely painful, like wounds, and have pus in their apices.

A boil on the last right rib, which has stitches in it *per se*, and is very painful when touched.

180. **Abscess of the axillary glands.**

Frequently recurring pain in the sacrum.

In the sacrum a pain drawing hither and hither, worst when walking. [*Fr. H—n.*]

Severe pain in the sacrum, like a cutting through; she could neither stand, lie, nor walk, during movement and when at rest (aft. 14 d.).

In the morning in bed drawing in the sacrum and in the whole back; after rising the whole of the back was painful on moving, she could hardly move; at the same time weakness in the limbs, disinclination for eating and work, with shivering, chilliness, and adipsia.

185. A pain compounded of bruised sensation and sharp pressure in the sacrum and lumbar vertebræ, but especially in the junction of the sacrum with the pelvic bones, which causes a sort of limping when walking; there is also pain when standing, sitting, and lying, which extends down into the lower extremities.

In the loins and ossa ischii pain as if dislocated, when sitting and turning the body when walking.

At night tensive pain in the back, worst when turning the body.

Some violent stitches in the back.

Pain between the scapulæ.

190. Fine tearing in the left shoulder.

Some twitching here and there in the left arm.

(At night the arm on which he has lain goes to sleep.)

Bruised pain in the shafts of the humeri.

In the point of the elbow pain as if contused or aching, only on moving after a long walk; it went off in the open air.

195. Drawing pain in the flexor tendons of the forearm (not in the joints).

Drawing tearing pain in the extensor tendons of the fingers and in the muscles belonging to them in the forearm.

After midnight pain in the inner side of the forearm, and over the back of the hand, aching, boring, and as if excoriated, more painful when touched, less by day.

Pain in the wrist.

On the hand and wrist a small gritty eruption with itching.

200. Swelling of the right hand.

Hot swelling and redness of one hand, which causes an intolerable sprained pain when moved, that extends into the arm.

On pressing the spread-out fingers against something they knuckle up; a sort of tendency to dislocate readily.

The finger-joints are swollen and the seat of gouty pains.

Needle-pricks in one finger.

205. Two boils on one of the nates.

A red itching lump on the upper part of the left natis.

Excoriation in the fold between the scrotum and thigh.

A formicating pain in the inferior extremity which drew it quite crooked ; most pain when walking and standing.

Bruised pain in the anterior muscles of the thigh.

210. All night long painful tension in the thighs and legs that prevents sleep.

Sudden pain of exhaustion in the thigh whilst walking, so that he is unable to walk further.

In the right thigh tearing pain (immediately).

On the outer side of the knee-joint and in the thigh and legs tearing pain, even when at rest, as from excessive fatigue and over exertion.

Swelling of the knee.

215. Aching pain in the hough on moving.

Great weariness in the feet, especially on ascending.

Stiff feeling in the ankle-joint, with a sensation of numbness and stiffness there.

In the evening, after having slept rather restlessly and tossed about in bed, there came on the outer side of the foot, on which he had lain without feeling pain, a pain for half an hour that made him cry out as from a violent knock or blow ; the pain was allayed only by grasping the foot and stroking it with the fingers, but not by moving (aft. 36 h.).

Pain in the foot, especially in the ankle-joint, as if gathering.

220. A tearing pain in the foot at night.

Drawing burning pain in the feet to the ankles, in the evening in bed.

Burning pain in the feet, especially on their dorsum, in the morning in bed.

Swelling of the feet about the ankles, with dyspnœa.

When walking, stitch in the tendo Achillis, and when lying in bed tearing in it.

225. Some stitches on the **instep.**

Formication in the sole of the foot.

Tearing in the big toe, worse when walking than when standing.

A severe stitch through the big toe.

A corn that had hitherto been free from pain commences to have burning pain when pressed slightly, mingled with a stitch-like sensation.

230. The nail of the right big toe pains violently (simple or ulcerative pains) on slight pressure.

On the toes a burning itching.

Formication in the toes and, tips of the fingers (aft. 24 h.).

Stitches in the joints when at rest and when moving.

Drawing and paralytic **pain in the limbs**, namely, in the fleshy parts of the arms, but especially of the thighs and legs.

235. **Cracked lines and chaps in the hands and feet.**

Even small wounds and slight injuries on the body suppurate, will not heal, and become ulcers (unwholesome, festering skin).

The ulcer bleeds on being merely gently wiped.

The affected part becomes inflamed (aft. 3 h.).

Burning and throbbing in the ulcer at night.

240. The wart inflames : stitches in it as if it would ulcerate.

Single severe stitches in the ulcer (on laughing) (aft. 4 h.).

(Fine prickly itching)

Burning itching on the body, especially in the morning on rising ; after scratching white blisters appear which exude white drops and soon afterwards disappear.

Eruption of pimples the size of a pea here and there on the body.

245. Nettle rash, *e.g.* on the wrist.

Eroding pain in the ulcer.

An itching erosion in the ulcer.

While walking in the open air a trembling in the knees, anxiety and heat in the whole body ; the soles of the feet burned.

After dinner he was weak when walking in the open air ; all the limbs were fatigued and there was a stretching in them, as if he were about to have ague ; on continuing to walk a cold sweat came over him ; thereafter in the evening in bed he could not go to sleep on account of hot feeling ; he did not fall asleep until 2 a. m.

250. Excessive excitability and sensitiveness of the nerves, *e. g.* on the septum of the nose.

Towards evening, from a slight pain, suddenly severe syncope.

Towards evening great drowsy weariness, with frequent, violent, almost convulsive yawning ; he can hardly keep from lying down.

In the evening so weary that he fell asleep while sitting.

In the morning very tired on rising from bed, after good sleep ; everything feels very heavy to her.

255. Restless sleep ; he cannot go to sleep.

Sleeplessness after midnight.

An excess of thoughts will not allow him to sleep after midnight (from 1 to 3 a. m.).

After a meal when slumbering, violent starting up in affright.

Before midnight he sprang up out of sleep, full of anxiety, called for help, and he felt as if he could not get his breath.

260. **At night the pains are worst.**

In the nocturnal fever, especially during the chill, the pains are worst.

The side of the body on which he lies at night becomes gradually insufferably painful ; he must turn round.

Dreams full of quarrels.

Dreams of fire ; he feels tumbling, &c.

265. He dreamt immediately on going to sleep, and dreamt much and anxiously, without waking.

Chilliness ; she sought the heat of the stove. [*Stf.*]

Rigor.

Frequent shivering, up to the hairy scalp, where the hairs felt painful.

Rigor for an hour (aft. 10 m.).

270. In the open air she is quite depressed by a painful sensation, like a shiver ; on account of chilliness she must walk all bent together. [*Stf.*]

Every evening (about 6 or 7 o'clock) severe chill not followed by heat.

In the evening (8 o'clock) severe chill with chattering of the teeth, for a quarter of an hour, with coldness of the hands and feet, then heat with sweat, especially on the chest and forehead, with slight thirst.

In the morning very bitter taste in the mouth, then after some hours fever first of chill with thirst, and after an hour much heat with disturbed **sleep** ; this fever recurred twice during the day.

Nocturnal **dry** warmth (heat) of the body, with perspiration only in the hands, which do not bear to be uncovered.

275. Fever : burning heat with almost unquenchable thirst, tiresome headache and slight wandering, from 4 p. m, onwards through the night, for three successive evening. [A. H. HINZE,[1] in *Hufel. Journ. d. pr. A.*, 1815, Sept., pp. 77, 79.]

Fever with severe oft-repeated vomiting of a green, excessively acrid water and viscid mucus, with constant nausea.[1] [HINZE, l. c.]

Perspiration in bed from midnight onwards, then she was chilly in bed, and also after rising every morning.

Perspiration about midnight, especially on the back.

Night sweat.

280. Perspiration, from the evening onwards in bed, especially on the head, so that beads of sweat stood on the face.

Profuse, sour smelling perspiration at night.

Before midnight in bed perspiration.

Profuse clammy night-sweat.

Night-sweat all over the body when awake.

285. In the morning profuse sweat all over the body.

In the morning profuse, continued sweat only on the head.

He perspires very readily during every, even slight, movement.

Profuse sweat day and night. [*Fr. H—n.*]

The slightest thing put him into a violent passion, he could have murdered any one without hesitation.

290. He was cross, and had such weakness of memory that he required three or four minutes to remember anything, and when at his work the thoughts often left him all at once.

Very cross ; every trifle annoyed him (aft. some h.).

Cross about trifles.

Extremely fretful and wayward.

Disposition sad, for many hours ; she must weep violently.

295. Sad, dejected, anxious.

---

1 Effects of large doses of hepar given for whooping-cough.—These two symptoms occurred together.

In the evening a frightful anxiety for two hours; he thought he must be ruined, and was sad to that degree that he could have killed himself.

Very hypochondriacal.

In the morning in bed after waking, when conscious, he had the visionary appearance of a deceased person, which frightened him, and he also imagined he saw a neighbouring house in flames, which terrified him.

SULPHURETTED HYDROGEN GAS IN MINERAL WATERS.

Violent ophthalmia.[1] [WAITZ, *Hufel. Journ*, xvi, ii, p. 63.*]

Black, pitch-like stools.[2] [WAITZ, l. c., p. 80.*]

Flying tearing pains in the feet.[3] [WAITZ, l. c., p. 37.*]

Pulse at first slower.[4] [KORTUM, l. c., iv, p. 24.†]

5. Pulse at first about eight or ten beats slower.[4] [WAITZ, l. c., xviii. i, p. 88.*]

Acute fever[5] (aft. 1 h.). [KORTUM, l. c., p. 25.†]

Fever with ophthalmia.[6] [WAITZ, l. c., xvi, p. 62.]

Fever with erysipelatous skin eruption all over the body.[7] [WAITZ, l. c., xvi, p. 34.]

* From Nenndorf water.
† From Aix la Chapelle water.

---

1 A lad of 15, subject to scrofulous ophthalmia, got a very severe attack of ophthalmia whilst taking the bath.

2 In a rheumatic patient while taking the baths and the water internally, the stools said also to be mixed with green mucus.

3 In a man disposed to rheumatism taking the baths for vertigo and noises in the ears; "flying" should be "wandering."

4 Statement of effects observed from baths.

5 General statement of effects of staying in bath longer than an hour; "fever" simply, not "acute fever."

6 A child of eight, subject to scrofulous ophthalmia, had an attack after the first baths.

7 Sixth day after commencing baths in a syphilitic subject who had been previously treated with mercurials.

HYOSCYAMUS NIGER.[1]

(Henbane.)

(The expressed juice of the fresh plant, *Hyoscyamus niger*, mixed with equal parts of alcohol.)

When dried the plant loses a great portion of its medicinal powers.

The following symptoms, which were produced by this drug on healthy persons, show the mental and emotional disorders and the derangements of the senses in which it is of use.

A dose containing a quadrillionth of a drop of the juice, or better, a small portion of such a drop, is more than sufficient for all homœopathic curative purpose when all other foreign irritants and drugs are kept away from the patient.

Frequent smellings at a saturated solution of camphor removes the troublesome effects of hyoscyamus when it has been given in too large a dose or in an unhomœopathic case.

Although the symptoms of this plant recorded below are very numerous, they require to be added to in order to make them complete.

[HAHNEMANN was assisted in this proving by FLAMING, FRANZ, FR. HAHNEMANN, LANGHAMMER, STAPF, WISLICENUS.

Symptoms are taken from the following old-school authorities :

BARRERE, *Observat. d Anatomie*, 1753.

BARTON (same as SMITH).

BERNIGAU, in *Hufel. Journ*, v.

BLOM. C. M., in *Kon. Vetensk. Acad. Handl.*, 1774, and in *Bergius' Mat. Med.*

BORELLI, PET., *Cent.* iv.

CAGNION, in *Desault's Journal de Chirurgie*, tom. i.

CAMERARIUS, in *Acta Nat. Cur.*, vol. i.

CLAUDER, G., in *Misc. Nat Cur.*, Dec. i, Ann. 3.

COSTA, in *Journ. de Medec*, tom. xxv, Febr.

EEMS, VAN, in *Prælect. Boerhavii de Morb. Nerv.*, ad tom. i.

FABER, J., in *Schenck*, lib. vii.

GARDANE, *Gazette de Sante*, 1773, 1774.

GESNER, J. A. PH., *Samml. von Beobacht.*, i,

GMELIN, J. F., *Reise durch Sibirien*, Gott., 1752, vol. iii.

GREDING, in *Ludwigii Advers. Med. pr.*, i.

GRUNEWALD, M., in *Miscel Nat Cur.*, Dec. iii, Ann. 9, 10, App.

HALLER, A. v., in *Vicat's Mat. Med.*, i.

HAMBERGER, *Diss. de Opio.*

HAMILTON, ARCH., in *Neue Edinb. Versuche.*, ii.

HEILBRONN, DAV., in *Neues Journal der Ausland. Med. Chir. Lit. v. Hufel. u. Harles*, i, 1804.

HELMONT, J. B. VAN, *Fus. duumv.*

HUNERWOLF, J. A., in *Misc. Nat. Cur.*, Dec. iii, Ann. 2.

---

1 From vol. iv, 2nd edit., 1825.

JASKIEWITZ, J., *Diss. Pharmaca regni veget.*, Vindob., 1775. JOERDENS, in *Hufel. Journal*, iv.
KIERNANDER, *Utkast til Medicinal Lagfar*, 1776.
MATTHIOLUS, *Comment in Diosc.*, lib. vi.
NAVIER, in *Recueil period. d'Obs de Med.*, tom. iv.
PLANCHON, in *Journal de Medecine*, tom. xix. *Pyl's Neues Magazine*, ii, B. iii, St.
RUEF, DE, in *Nova Acta Natur. Cur.*, t. iv.
SAUVAGES, *Nosol.*, ii. SCHULZE, S., in *Misc. Nat. Cur.*, Dec. i, Ann. 4, 5. SELIGER, CHPH., in *Misc. Nat. Cur.*, Dec. ii, Ann. 1. SERRE, J. LA, in *Misc. Nat. Cur.*, Dec. ii, Ann. 5. SLOANE, H., in *Philos. Transact.*, No. 457. SMITH, in *Med. Comment.*, vol. ii. Dec, ii. STEDMAN, J., in *Philos. Transact.*, vol. xl, vii. STOERCK, *Lib. de Stram., Hyos., Acon.*, Vien., 1762.
TOZZETTI, TARG., *Relaz. di alcuni viaggi*, vol. vi.
VICAT, *Mat. Med.*, i.
WEDEL, G. W., in *Misc. Nat. Cur.*, Dec. i, Ann. 3. WENDT, in *Hufel. Journ.*, v. WEPFER, *Hist. Cicut. aquat.*, Bas. 1716.

In the *Frag. de Vir.* hyoscyamus has 335 symptoms ; in the 1st edit. 539, and in this 2nd edit. 582.]

HYOSCYAMUS.

Vertigo.

Vertigo. [J. A. HUNERWOLF,[1] in *Miscel. Nat. Cur.*, Dec. iii, Ann. 2, Obs. 92.—M. GRUNEWALD[2] (1), in *Miscel. Nat. Cur.*, Dec. iii, Ann. 9, 10, app., p. 179*—C. M. BLOM,[3] in *Kon. Vetensk. Acad. Handl.*, 1774, p. 52.—NAVIER,[4] in *Recueil period d'Obs. de Med.*, tom. iv —PLANCHON,[5] in *Journal de Medecine*, tom. xix, p. 42.—H. SLOANE,[6] in *Philos. Transact.*, No. 429.—GREDING,[7] in *Ludwigii Advers. Med.*, pr., i, pp. 86, 91.—WEPFER,[1] *Hist. Cicutæ aquat.*, Bas., 1716, p. 230.—VICAT,[8] *Mat. Med.*, i, p. 185.—BERNIGAU,[9] in *Hufel. Journ.*, v, p. 905.]

Violent vertigo. [J. STEDMAN,[10] in *Philos. Transact.*, vol. xl, vii, p. 194.]

* A vertigo lasting 14 days from the exhalation of the seeds.

1 From cooked roots, eaten by several persons.

2 Three observations :—1. Effects of exhalations from seeds. 2. Do. of a clyster containing H., with turpentine and carminatives. 3. Do. of fomentations of it in the girls who had applied them.

3 From root eaten by an adult man.

4 From herb eaten as salad by an adult.

5 From repeated doses given to an adult.

6 From seeds eaten by children.

7 From gr. iij—xij daily given to patients. Those referred to pp. 73—78 were melancholico-maniacs, those of pp. 79—87 maniacs, of 89—99 epileptics, 103—107 epilepto-maniacs.

8 General statement

9 From a clyster of H. in an adult man.

10 From leaves boiled in broth, in several persons.

Vertigo, with obscuration of vision.* [SMITH,[1] in *Med. Comment.*, vol. ii, Dec. ii.]

5. Vertigo, as from intoxication (immediately). [*Stf.*]

Swaying about from one side to the other. [*Stf.*]

Staggering. [J. LA SERRE,[2] in *Misc. Nat. Cur.*, Dec. ii, Ann. 5, Obs. 78.—GRUNEWALD, l. c.]

They staggered as if intoxicated.† [CAGNION,[3] in *Desault's Journal de Chirurgie*, tom. i, p. 370.]

Intoxication. [SLOANE, l. c.—J. F. GMELIN,[4] *Reise durch Sibirien*, Gott., 1752, vol. iii, pp. 84, 85.‡]

10. Unconsciousness : he is insensible to pinching and nipping,§ [ARCH. HAMILTON,[5] in *Neue Edinb. Versuche*, ii, p. 275.]

Stupefaction.[6] [STEDMAN, l. c.]

Staring at objects devoid of thought, tendency to self-forgetfulness (aft. ½ h.). [*Fz.*]

He involuntarily remembers persons and events, which he had no wish to think about (aft. ½ h.). [*Fz.*]

Remembrance of long forgotten things.‖

15. Weak memory.

Complete loss of memory.

Loss of memory. [J. JASKIEWITZ,[7] *Diss. Pharmaca Regni Veget.*, Vindob., 1775, p. 53.]

Things he did not wish to remember come back into his thoughts, and he can with difficulty recall things he wishes to remember (aft. 3 h.). [*Fz.*]

Want of recollection : he remembers what he had thought and done the last few days only as if in a dream (aft. 24 h.). [*Ws.*]

20. Forgetfulness of all he had previously heard. [WENDT,[8] in *Hufel. Journal*, v, p. 390.]

Forgetfulness : he knows not whether he really said what he wished to say (aft. ¼ h.). [*Fz.*]

He complains of heaviness of the head and violent headache.[9] [HAMILTON, l. c.]

Continued violent headache. [PLANCHON, l. c.]

Heavy, dazed head. [COSTA,[7] in *Journ. de Medec.*, tom. xxx, Febr.]

* From four grains of the resinous extract in a healthy man 24 years old.

† Several children who had eaten the roots for carrots.

‡ From *Hyoscyamus physaloides*.

§ From *Hyoscyamus albus*.

‖ Curative action (?)

---

1 As in Hahnemann's note.

2 From clyster of H. given for dysentery.

3 From root in children.

4 General statement.

5 ii, 243, of original English edition, from which corrections have been made.—From gr. xxv of seeds of H. *albus* in a young man.

6 In original, "stupor, as if drunk."

7 From seeds in an adult man.

8 From a clyster of H. in an adult man.—This symptom not found.

9 This occurred 24 hours after the poisoning, with S. 467.

25. Heaviness in the head, [GREDING, l. c., p. 91.—VICAT, l. c.—MATTHIOLUS,[1] *Comment in Dios.*, lib. vi, p. 1064.]

Heaviness of the head with swollen eyelids. [GREDIND, l. c., p. 89.]

Dulness of the head, costiveness and pains in the loins. [GREDING, l. c., p. 95.]

The thoughts sometimes refuse to come (the 2nd d.) [*Stf.*]

His head is very much affected, like an absence of thoughts ; he is troubled about everything, and hence goes to sleep for some hours in the afternoon (without dreams), and though he often half awakes, he continues to sleep on (aft. 9 h.). [*Ws.*]

30. Confusion and dazed state of the head, such as occurs from excessive bodily weakness, especially in the morning.

Headache of several hours' duration.* [GARDANE,[2] *Gazette de Santé*, 1773, 1774, p. 294.]

Headache. [STEDMAN, l. c.—GREDING, l. c., pp. 73, 76, 86.—SAUVAGES,[3] *Nosol.*, ii, p. 242.]

(Fine shooting pain in the head.]

(Shooting tearing headache) (aft. 2 h.).

35. Obtuse headache in the base of the brain.

In the room he gets headache, after having felt nothing of it in the open air (aft. 2 h.). [*Fz.*]

Obtuse pain in the forehead, especially in the membranes of the brain.

Aching stupefying pain in the brain, especially in the forehead, with needle-pricks, especially on the left side, recurring alternately (aft. 4 h.). [*Lr.*]

Aching stupefying pain, especially in the whole forehead, that at length changed into an intermittent tearing (aft. 10½ h.). [*Lr.*]

40. Shooting in the head over the right eye, on coughing.

By fits, sometimes constrictive, dazing headache on the top of the forehead and general discomfort, sometimes freedom from all sufferings and comfort with exalted imagination, the latter continuing much longer (aft. 1 h.). [*Fz.*]

(Tearing headache in the occiput.)

Headache as if the brain shook and splashed when walking (aft. 5 h.).

An undulation in the brain as from violent beating of the arteries, with aching in the forehead ; worst after stooping (aft. ½ h.). [*Ws.*]

45. Headache with unnatural heat. [GREDING, l. c., p. 82.]

Heat and formication in the head (aft. 24 h.).

Formication on the crown of the head (aft. 1 h.).

Gnawing aching in the integuments of the head, increased by moving them and touching them (aft. 15 h.). [*Ws.*]

A dull stiff pain in the nape. [*Stf.*]

* From the odour and exhalations of the plant.

---

1 General statements.
2 From exhalations of H., in several persons
3 From root, in several persons.

50. Headache alternating with pain in the nape. [GREDING, l. c., p. 77.]

On turning the head an aching in the crown and drawing in the nape (aft. 3 h.). [*Fz.*]

Dazed state, dulness of senses. [GARDANE, l. c.]

Dimness of vision. [HUNERWOLF, l. c.]

Dimness of vision ; objects appear indistinct ; he is more short-sighted and must hold the book nearer when reading (aft. 1 h.). [*Ws.*]

55. Contracted pupils.

Very dilated pupils (aft. ½ h.). [*Fz.*]

Sensation before the right eye as if a veil were drawn before it (aft. 3 h.).

Dim vision, as if a veil were before the eyes. [BERNIGAU, l. c.]

Glittering before the eyes ; dark points played rapidly hither and thither (aft. 1 h.). [*Ws.*]

60. Diminution of the vision. [BLOM, l. c.]

When consciousness returned the eyes were dim and without lustre, and the brain was dazed.[1] [HAMILTON, l. c.]

Darkening of the vision. [GRUNEWALD,—JASKIEWITZ,—SLOANE,—WEPFER, l. c.]

Weakness of vision. [STOERCK,[2] ***Lib. de Stram.***, ***Hyosc.***, ***Acon.***, Vien., 1762, pp. 36, 39, 47, 55.]

Transient amaurosis. [SAUVAGES, l. c.]

65. Blind and senseless he wanders about the town. [HUNERWOLF, l. c.]

Myopia : he could scarcely recognise objects at three paces distance. [BERNIGAU, l. c.]

Longsightedness combined with great clearness of vision, with dilated pupils ; the longsightedness lasted several days and then declined gradually* (aft. 3 h.). [*Lr.*]

Myopia lasting four days. [COSTA, l. c.]

Chronic presbyopia.[3] [WEPFER, l. c.]

70. Deception of sight : nine persons after partaking of the root of henbane saw all objects of a scarlet colour. [DAV. HEILBRONN,[4] in *Neues Journ. d. Ausland. Med. Chir. Lit. v. Hufel. u. Harles*, i. 1804, p. 199.]

Deception of sight : objects appear fiery red. [WENDT, l. c.]

Deception of sight : everything appears made of gold. [S. SCHULZE,[5] in *Misc. Nat. Cur.*, Dec. i, Ann. 4, 5, Obs. 124.]

Deception of sight : small things appear very large to him. [GRUNEWALD,†—GMELIN,‡—WENDT,§ l. c.]

* In a very myopic person, as curative reaction of the body.
† He takes a lark for a goose.
‡ He takes a straw for a beam, and a drop of water for a pond.
§ The letters appear to him unusually large.

---

1 On the following morning.
2 Observations on patients.
3 In the original, "sight for a long time not so acute."
4 Not accessible.
5 From cooked roots, in several persons.

False sight: the flame of one candle appears smaller, of the other large, although both flames are the same size (aft. 10 h.).

75. False sight: when reading the letters appear to move, and look like ants running about. [WEPFER, l. c.]

False sight: when sewing he stuck the needle into a wrong place. [WEPFER, l. c.]

Staring, distorted eyes. [EL CAMERARIUS,[1] in *Acta Nat. Cur.*, vol. i, Obs. 12.]

Staring look. [LA SERRE, l. c.]

With a fixed look he stares at those about him. [HUNERWOLF, l. c.]

80. Intoxicated appearance, for a long time. [CAGNION, l. c.]

Twitching in the eye (aft. 8 h.).

Distorted eyes. [HUNERWOLF. l. c.]

Open eyes turned towards different sides. [HAMILTON, l. c.]

Convulsively moved, projecting eyes. [PLANCHON, l. c.]

85. Sparkling eyes.[2] [STEDMAN, l. c.—BLOM,[3] in *Bergius' Mat. Med*, p. 128.]

Red, sparkling eyes. [COSTA, l. c.]

Inflammation of the eyes.[4] [NAVIER, l. c.]

Itching tearing in both canthi, worst in the outer canthus, going off by rubbing (aft. 8 h.). [*Ws.*]

Gnawing aching in the superior orbital border, which goes off on touching the spot (aft. ½ h.). [*Fz.*]

90. Aching in the eyes, as if sand had got into them (aft. 12 h.). [*Lr.*]

The eyelids are as if swollen, the whites of the eyes here and there reddish; the eyes look as if he had been crying. [*Stf.*]

Inability to open the eyelids. [WEPFER, l. c.]

Heat in the face, particularly in the lobes of the ears, with somewhat increased redness of the face and very dilated pupils. [*Stf.*]

In the warm room burning heat in the face. [*Stf.*]

95. Distorted features, bluish, earthy complexion, with open mouth. [CAMERARIUS, l. c.]

Bluish[6] complexion (aft. 2 h.). [COSTA, l. c.]

Cold pale face* [HAMBERGER,[7] *Diss. de Opio*, § 18.]

Paleness of face. [SMITH, l. c.]

Frequent change of complexion. [STEDMAN, l. c.]

100. Heat and redness in the face.

Red, swollen face. [BLOM, in *Bergius*, l. c.]

Brownish red, swollen face. [BERNIGAU, l. c.]

* Before death.

---

1 From root, in children.
2 Stedman says "fiery-looking," Blom "glittering."
3 Same case as Blom's in S. 2.
4 In the original, "the eyes appeared inflamed."
5 In the original, "his distorted face becomes blue with a lurid and livid pallor."
6 In the original, "livid."
7 From root, in a boy of three.

Twitching in the cheeks.

Small pox-like pustules, chiefly on the right side of the chin. [*Fr. H—n*]

105. Painful heat-papules on the lip.

Thick eruption of pustules full of yellow pus breaks out on the cheeks and skin, whereupon the nose becomes ulcerated, [GREDING, l. c., p. 82.]

Sharp stitches into the ears ; aching in the temples ; confusion of the head (aft. 1 h.). [*Ws.*]

Towards evening a quick (indescribable) pain in the right ear. [*Stf.*]

Tearing in the whole of the ear cartilage, increased by pressing on it (aft. 15 h.). [*Ws.*]

110. (Noises in the ears, like bells) (aft. 1 h.).

When hawking he feels as if something fell before the ears. [*Fz.*]

Sudden twitching inside the root of the nose downwards (aft. 1 h.). [*Ws.*]

Heat, also perceptible externally, in the lower part of the nose, internally and externally (aft. 1 h.). [*Ws.*]

Dryness in the nose.

115. **Pressive squeezing on the root of the nose** and the zygomatic processes (aft. 1 h). [*Ws.*]

Epistaxis.

Epistaxis. [GARDANE, l. c.]

Distorted neck.[1] [PLANCHON, l. c.]

Closure of the jaws with perfect consciousness (aft. 24 h.). [*Fg.*]

120. On the left side of the neck a swelling that goes on to suppuration.[2] [GREDING, l. c.]

Stiffness of the muscles of the nape ; on bending the head forwards they feel stretched, as if too short, for some hours (aft. 1 h.). [*Ws.*]

Clean, parched tongue. [COSTA, l. c.]

Burning and dryness of the tongue and lips, which look like burnt leather. [WEPFER, l. c.]

On the middle of the tongue, a feeling of numbness as if it had been burnt with hot food, very much increased when speaking and drawing in the breath. [*Stf.*]

125. Dumbness. [TARG. TOZZETTI,[3] *Relaz. di alcuni viaggi*, vol. vi, p. 279.—JASKIEWITZ,—SAUVAGES, l. c.]

He does not answer. [GREDING, l. c., p. 77.]

Impeded speech. [BERNIGAU, l. c.]

Unconscious ; she lost the power of speech. [HUNERWOLF, l. c.]

Toothache ; the gums on the left side seem to be swollen, and the teeth of the upper jaw are affected with dull pain. [*Stf.*]

---

1 In recurring attacks.

2 The abscess was in the parotid gland. It never closed, and the patient died with pulmonary disease.

3 From root, in an adult.

130. Behind the rows of teeth, betwixt the cheek and gums, pain of the soft parts, as if they were gathering (in the evening during the febrile heat). [*Fz.*]

A painful drawing in a single tooth, now here, now there, just as if a tooth were about to become decayed. [*Stf.*]

Impediment to chewing. [HAMBERGER, l. c.]

Toothache. [GREDING, l. c., pp. 80, 106.]

Toothache during the perspiration,[1] [GREDING, l. c, p. 109.]

135. Toothache, especially when chewing, as if the teeth would fall out.

Toothache : tearing in the gums, especially on the access of cold air.

Tearing toothache, in the morning, with a rush of blood to the head, as if an attack of hæmoptysis were coming on.

Aching jerking pain in a hollow tooth which extends over the temple ; on biting on the tooth it seems to be too long and loose (not increased by drawing in air) (aft. 4 h.). [*Ws.*]

Shaking of the teeth with vibration and tingling in them.

140. Impediment[2] to deglutition. [HAMBERGER, l. c.]

He feels something wrong in the throat; he points with his finger into it, just as if something were sticking in it. [HAMBERGER, l. c.]

Frequent expectoration of mucus from the throat by hawking (aft. $\frac{1}{4}$ h.). [*Lr.*]

Burning heat in the larynx. [VICAT, l. c.]

Dryness causing fine shooting in the larynx (aft. 1 h.). [*Fz.*]

145. Parched throat (fauces horridæ). [WEPFER, l. c.]

Great dryness in the throat and thirst. [*Fz.*]

Rough and scrapy in the throat and on the tongue, with very moist mouth. [*Stf.*]

A scraping, tiresome feeling in the throat and palate, as from speaking too much. [*Stf.*]

Dryness in the throat. [BERNIGAU, l. c.]

150. Thirst and dryness in the throat. [CAGNION, l. c.]

Thirst from the shooting dryness in the throat (aft. $2\frac{1}{2}$ h.). [*Fz.*]

A smarting sensation in the back of the throat.

The throat is so contracted[3] and dry, that a mouthful of tea almost chokes him.* [HAMILTON, l. c.]

* When we take together symptoms 140 to 146, 149 to 151 and 153, 155, to 162, 164, 165, 166, with the mental and emotional symptoms 513, 515, 520, 547 to 551, 559, 565 to 573, 575, 580, the convulsions 441, 475, 480, and some others 101, 102, 427 to 429, we have a tolerably accurate picture of the ordinary hydrophobia caused by the bite of a mad dog, which therefore will and *must* be not unfrequently curable by henbane. The true histories of this frightful disease show us several varieties of this malady in human beings, for each of which there will be a perfectly suitable remedy, among which henbane is one of the best. For the other cases either stramonium or belladonna is the suitable homoeopathic remedy, according to the character of the totality of the symptoms.

1 Nine days after leaving off the medicine.
2 In the original, "impossibility."
3 "Uneasy," in the original.

In the throat a pressure as from a tumour when swallowing and at other times. [*Stf.*]

155. The throat feels constricted, with impeded deglutition. [BERNIGAU, l. c.]

Constriction of the throat. [SAUVAGES,—HUNERWOLF, l. c.]

Inability to swallow. [TOZZETTI, l. c.]

Inability to swallow, the fluids introduced into the mouth were twice spat out. [HAMILTON, l. c.]

Hydrophobia. [BARRERE,[1] *Observat d'Anatomie*, 1753.]

160. Intolerable thirst. [BLOM, l. c.]

Unquenchable thirst.[2] [SLOANE, l. c.]

Horror of drinks. [COSTA, l. c.]

After great thirst, profuse sweat. [GREDING, l. c., p. 78.]

After drinking tea he soon fell into convulsions, he did not know those about him. [HAMILTON, l. c.]

165. He wishes to drink, but cannot swallow. [HAMBERGER, l. c.]

Frequent spitting of saliva. [GREDING, l. c., p. 87.]

Great collection of saliva. [*Stf.*]

Ptyalism.

Ptyalism.[3] [STEDMAN, l. c.]

170. The saliva tastes salt.

Collection of saliva of a salt taste. [*Stf.*]

Bloody saliva in the mouth, with bloody, sweetish taste (after some h.). [*Stf.*]

Loss of appetite with proper taste.

Loss of appetite. [PLANCHON, l. c.]

175. Appetite and strength diminish from day to day. [GREDING, l. c., p. 102.]

Loss of smell and taste.

Belladonna has already effected some perfect cures, and would have done this more frequently, had not either other interposing remedies been administered at the same time, or, and especially, had it not been given in such enormous doses that the patients were sometimes killed by the remedy. Large doses of drugs, homœopathically suitable, are much more certainly injurious than such as are given without any similar (homœopathic) relation to the disease, or such as have an opposite (antipathic) relation to the case, that is to say, are quite unsuitable (allopathic). In the homoeopathic employment of medicines, where the totality of the morbid symptoms has a great similarity to the action of a drug, it is really criminal not to give quite small doses, indeed as small as possible. In such cases doses of the size prescribed in the routine practice become real poisons and murderous agents. Convinced by a thousand-fold experience, I assert this of the homoeopathic employment of medicines universally and invariably, particularly when the disease is acute; and this is especially true of the employment of belladonna, stramonium, and hyoscyamus in hydrophobia. So let it not be said, "One of these three medicines was given in the strongest doses, and not too seldom, but every two or three hours, and yet the patient died." "*That was precisely the reason.*" I reply with firm conviction, "*that was precisely the reason why the patient died, and you killed him.* Had you let him take the smallest portion of a drop of the quintillion-fold or decillion-fold attenuation of the juice of one of these plants for a dose (in rare cases repeating the dose after three or four days) then the patient would have been easily and *certainly saved.*"

---

1 Not accessible.

2 Original has simply "great thirst."

3 In original, "slavering."

Bitterness in the mouth, in the morning; but food did not taste bitter (aft. 24 h.). [*Fg.*]

Bitterness in the mouth and bitter eructation. [GREDING, l. c., p. 95.]

A kind of scurvy in the mouth.

180. Frequent tasteless eructation. [*Stf.*]

Frequent empty eructation (aft. 1½ h.). [*Lr.*]

Baulked inclination to eructate; half-suppressed, imperfect eructation, for 10 hours. [*Fz.*]

From external pressure on the scrobiculus cordis he has nausea, which then continue *per se*, but goes off on stooping (aft. ½ h.). [*Fz.*]

Nausea.

185. Nausea. [HUNERWOLF, l. c.—GREDING, l. c., p. 78.]

Nausea and vertigo. [GREDING, l. c., p. 80.]

Nausea, vomiting. [BARTON, l. c.]

Nausea, inclination to vomit. [*Stf.*]

Inclination to vomit.

190. Vomiting. [HUNERWOLF,—GRUNEWALD,—GARDANE, l. c.—GREDING, l. c., pp. 75, 76.]

Frequent vomiting. [GRUNEWALD, l. c. (I).]

Frequent vomiting of white but very viscid mucus. [GREDING, l. c., p. 87.]

Watery vomiting with vertigo. [GREDING, l. c., p. 94.]

For some days he could only with difficulty keep down the food without vomiting. [BARTON, l. c.]

195. After vomiting green bile and profuse perspiration, his mind became tranquil.[1] [GREDING, l. c., p. 80.]

Frequent hiccup (aft. 1¼ h. and later). [*Lr.*]

Hiccup with spasms and rumbling in the abdomen. [GREDING, l. c., p. 94.]

Severe hiccup on two successive midnights, with involuntary micturition and foam before the mouth. [GREDING, l. c., p. 104.]

The most violent hiccup with costiveness. [GREDING, l. c., p. 95.]

200. At night extremely violent hiccup with diarrhœa. [GREDING, l. c., p. 94.]

After dinner, extremely violent, long-continued hiccup. [GREDING, l. c., p. 89.]

After a meal, headache, aching in the temples and painfulness of the whole external head (aft. 4½ .). [*Fz.*]

Immediately after a meal, as if drunk. [*Fg.*]

Most of the sufferings and the most severe of them occur after eating. [*Fz.*]

205. Soon after dinner there occurs great anxiety, as if some sad event was about to take place (aft. 6 h.). [*Fz.*]

After a meal, frequent and continued erections of the penis (aft. 5 h.). [*Fz.*]

---

1 After rage.

The region of the scrobiculus cordis is sensitive and painful when touched.

Frequent attacks of pressure in the scrobiculus cordis which cause dyspnœa.

Tightness about the scrobiculus cordis. [CAMERARIUS, l. c.]

210. Weakness of the stomach.[1] [STEDMAN, l. c.]

Pain in the stomach. [GREDING, l. c., p. 87.]

After eating, quick pressure on the scrobiculus cordis in the sternum (aft. ¼ h.). [*Fz.*]

Stomach-ache.[2] [STEDMAN, l. c.]

Burning in the stomach. [BLOM, l. c.]

215. Inflammation of the stomach. [BARRERE, l. c.]

Fulness in the gastric region, with a tiresome feeling of tension of the abdomen, in the evening. [*Stf.*]

Cutting pains in the abdomen.

Bellyache.[3] [STEDMAN,—WEPFER,—HAMILTON, l. c.—GREDING, l. c., p. 105.]

Single stitches in the hepatic region (aft. ½ h.).

220. An aching in the umbilical region.

A shooting in the umbilical region when drawing a breath (aft. 5 h.).

Colicky pains. [STOERCK, l. c.]

Shooting pain below the navel when walking. [*Fr. H—n.*]

Drawing pain in the bowels (aft. 9 h.). [*Fg.*]

225. Pinching drawing in the abdomen, with discharge of much flatus (aft. 3 h.). [*Fz.*]

Pinching in the abdomen (aft. 26 h.). [*Fg.*]

He cries out about pains in the abdomen, which seem like to burst the abdomen open, and he digs his fists into his sides. [WEPFER, l. c.]

In the morning, on rising from bed, horrible flatulent colic, a pinching down-pressing, like a weight, in the hypogastrium, with inclination to vomit, and pain in the back as if it were bruised, without any flatus passing, when moving and when at rest (aft. 24 h.).

Aching flatulent colic in the epigastrium, his abdomen is distended, in the evening after lying down. [*Fg.*]

230. **Cutting, deep in the abdomen.**

Short attacks of cutting on a small spot deep in the hopogastrium, under the os pubis (aft. 6 h.).

Painful sensitiveness of the abdominal integuments.

Spasmodic contraction in the abdominal muscles, as if something alive were inside* (aft. 3 h.).

Pain of the abdomen (abdominal muscles), as if he had over-exerted and strained himself, in the morning immediately after waking.

* From the emanations of the plant.

1 The day after.
2 The day after. Literally, "weight at the stomach."
3 "Gripes," in Hamilton.

235. Pains of the abdominal muscles as though he had fallen on them (when sitting) (aft. 2 h.). [*Fr. H—n.*]

Uncommonly great development of flatulence after a very moderate supper ; and frequent, but difficult, discharge of flatus (aft. 14 h.).

Flatulent distension of the abdomen, which is painful to the touch. [COSTA, l. c.]

Feeling of hardness of the abdomen.

Rumbling in the abdomen,[1] also during the diarrhœa. [GREDING, l. c., p. 81.]

240. Rumbling in the abdomen, with violent diarrhœa. [GREDING, l. c., p. 98.]

Frequent urging to stool.*

Urging to stool (aft. 1 h.). [*Fz.*]

Urging to stool with feeling in the rectum as if diarrhœa would ensue (aft. $\frac{3}{4}$ h.). [*Fz.*]

Urging in the rectum as if he must go to stool (aft. $\frac{1}{4}$ h.). [*Fz.*]

245. Stool the first day three hours later than usual, the second day four hours earlier. [*Fg.*]

He must often go to stool ; but the stools are natural.

Frequent stools. [GRUNEWALD, l. c. (I).—GREDING, l. c., p. 74.]

The stool passes unconsciously in bed (aft. 2 h.).

Diarrhœa. [HUNERWOLF,—BLOM, l. c.—GREDING, l. c., p. 80.]

250. A single pappy stool, five hours before the usual time (aft. $1\frac{1}{4}$ h.). [*Fz.*]

Evacuation of a large pappy stool, with scanty flow of urine (aft. $\frac{3}{4}$ h.). [*Lr.*]

Soft stool in small thin pieces. [*Stf.*]

Diarrhœa, day and night. [*Fr. H—n.*]

Moderate diarrhœa. [BARTON, l. c.—GREDING, l. c., p. 76.]

255. Slimy diarrhœa. [GREDING, l. c., p. 84.]

Slimy debilitating diarrhœa.[2] [STOERCK, l. c.]

Watery diarrhœa. [GREDING, l. c., p. 94.]

Frequent discharge of thread-worms. [GREDING, l. c., p. 97.]

Costiveness, hard stool covered with mucus, and during its evacuation pain in the anus, for five successive days. [*Fr. H—n.*]

260. One very firm stool, some hours after the usual time (aft. 6 h.). [*Fz.*]

Constipation for four days, and frequent pressure in the umbilical

* The calls to stool and the frequent evacuations of henbane are alternating actions with the delayed stool and the absence of call thereto ; but the former appear to be the principal primary action. There seems, indeed, to be a twofold alternating action : much urging with rare evacuation, S. 242—244, 261, and more frequent evacuation with rarer calls, with little or no evacuation, S. 263, 264, also with more frequent evacuation, S. 248 ; but the frequent urging with the scanty and rare evacuations is the principal alternating action.

---

1 In original, "hypogastrium."

2 During resolution of pulmonary consumption : stools compared to sputa, which they possibly were.

region, as from fulness of the abdomen, during which he has often call to stool, without tenesmus in the rectum and anus.

The bowels are confined and the discharge of urine stopped, with pressing to urinate.

Constipation.[1] [HAMILTON, l. c.]

Sluggish action of the bowels. [STOERCK, l. c.]

265. Hæmorrhoidal discharge for eight days. [J. A. PH. GESNER,[2] *Samml. von Beobacht.*, i, p. 165.]

Yellow urine, clouded at the time of discharge, afterwards with whitish-grey sediment. [*Fg.*]

(The first two days, frequent urging with scanty discharge of urine; the third and following days, copious flow of urine.) [*Lr.*]

Copious flow of urine. [GREDING, l. c., pp. 74, 76, 80.]

Very frequent urination, with rumbling in the abdomen. [GREDING, l. c., p. 83.]

270. Frequent discharge of urine as clear as water; he must pass urine several times at night, contrary to custom. [*Stf.*]

Copious discharge of urine, sleep, transpiration, diarrhœa, followed by cheerfulness of mind.[3] [GREDING, l. c., p. 81.]

Diuresis. [STEDMAN, l. c.]

Dysuria. [SAUVAGES, l. c.]

Difficult micturition, performed not without pressing. [GREDING, l. c., p. 79.]

275. Suppressed discharge of urine with vesical tenesmus.

Retention of urine. [COSTA, l. c.]

Paralysis of the bladder.

Feeling of excoriation and burning at the entrance of the vagina (aft. 1 h.).

Profuse discharge of menses.† [GREDING, l. c., p. 81.]

280. Profuse discharge of menses, with delirious chattering. [GREDING, l. c., p. 81.]

Catamenia delayed some days.

Suppressed catamenia.

Retardation of the menstrual period. [GREDING, in several places.]

Before the occurrence of the menses, labour-like pains, as in childbirth, in the womb, with drawing in the loins and sacrum.

285. The catamenia appear on the fourteenth day.

Hands and feet tremble violently, almost convulsively, and she is

* The excitation of the bladder to urinate and its loss of irritability—the scanty flow of urine and the copious diuresis are in henbane alternating actions, so that much urging to urinate with scanty and copious flow of urine—as also inactivity of the bladder with scanty and very copious secretion of urine may be present at the same time; but much urging to urinate with scanty flow of urine seems to be the principal, more frequent primary action.

† The hæmorrhages of henbane seem all to be primary actions, hence its utility in metrorrhagia when the other symptoms of the disease correspond in similarity to those of henbane.

1 Merely a statement that no stool had passed from the ingestion of the poison at 4.30 p.m. till night.

2 Observation made after removal of a colic by H.

3 Curative effect.

as if maniacal during the catamenial period. [GREDING, l.c., p. 83.]

Diuresis during the catamenia. [GREDING, l. c., p. 83.]

Diuresis and perspiration during the catamenia. [GREDING, l. c., p. 84.]

Perspiration during the catamenia [GREDING, l. c., p. 86.]

290. Before the appearance of the catamenia hysterical pains. [GREDING, l. c., p. 106.]

Almost incessant loud laughter before the appearance of the catamenia. [GREDING, l. c., p. 106.]

The catamenia came on with profuse perspiration, headache and nausea. [GREDING, l. c., p. 98.]

Excitation of the sexual organs and erection of the penis, without excitement of the imagination (aft. ½ h.). [*Fz.*]

Sexual desire.*

295. Impotence in the male.† [DE RUEF,[1] in *Nova Acta Natur. Cur.*, t. iv, Obs. 59.]

* * *

Fœtid breath and exhalation from the mouth, which he himself perceives, on rising in the morning (aft. 24 h.). [*Fg.*]

Frequent sneezing, without coryza (aft. 1½ h.). [*Lr.*]

Sensation as if something were sticking in the wind-pipe and could not be dislodged by coughing.

Much mucus in the trachea and larynx, which makes the voice and speech not clear (aft. ½ h.). [*Fz.*]

300. Tightness of the chest. [HUNERWOLF, l. c.]

A squeezing in the upper part of the chest, tiresome and yet not painful, not increased either by walking or by speaking (aft. 6 h.). [*Stf.*]

Dyspnœa. [HUNERWOLF, l. c.—GREDING, l. c., p. 90.]

Difficult breathing, with occasional rattling. [CAMERARIUS, l. c.]

A tight feeling across the chest as from too great exertion by speaking or running. [*Stf.*[

305. Oppression of the chest, like shortness of breath, and at the same time strong cardiac impulse (aft. 3 h.). [*Ws.*]

During an oppressive aching in the chest, at the same time internal shooting, worst during inspiration (aft. ¾ h.). [*Fz.*]

Aching inferiorly in the right side of the chest, which when going upstairs is accompanied by great anxiety and dyspnœa (aft. 6 h.). [*Fz.*]

Pressure on the right side of the chest, near the ensiform cartilage and the last true rib, with great anxiety and oppression of the breath (aft. 6½ h.). [*Fz.*]

Hard pressure with stitches on the chest (aft. 3 h.). [*Fz.*]

310. (A burning pain in the left side, in the evening.)

Shooting in the side of the chest. [STEDMAN, l. c.]

Shooting in the right side. [*Fr. H—n.*]

* See 293. † For two months.

1 Effect of inhaling vapour for toothache.

A dry tickling short cough, which seems to come from the trachea. [*Stf.*]

Short dry cough.

315. Dry, spasmodic, continued cough. [GREDING, l. c., p. 96.]

At night, dry cough.

Nocturnal cough.

He coughs often at night, and wakes up every time and then goes to sleep again (aft. 30 h.).

Whilst lying almost incessant cough, which goes off on sitting up.

320. Greenish expectoration with the cough.

Cough, which is worst at night.[1] [GREDING, l. c., p. 109.]

Shooting in the scapulæ.

(A warm feeling in the back, immediately.) [*Stf.*]

(Tearing pain in the back.)

325. Tension of the pectoral and dorsal muscles at the shoulder-joint, especially when raising up the arm, as if they were too short (aft. 6 h.). [*Ws.*]

Backache. [GREDING, l. c., p. 99.]

Fixed pains in the loins.

Repeated pains in the loins. [GREDING, l. c., p. 106.]

Pain in the loins and swelling about the ankles. [GREDING, l. c., p. 108.]

330. Shooting pain in the loins and side. [GREDING, l. c., p. 108.]

(In the evening after bodily exercise, trembling of the arm.)

Externally on the elbow a couple of pimples with some pain when touched (aft. 9 h.). [*Ws.*]

Aching in the bend of the elbow when he holds the arm still in a bent position (aft. $\frac{3}{4}$ h.). [*Fz.*]

A dull pain in the wrist- and elbow-joints, which extended farther, and was alleviated by movement. [*Stf.*]

335. Itching pricks on the flexor side of the forearm (aft. 1 h.). [*Ws.*]

Continued prick as with a needle on the flexor side of the forearm (aft. 5 h.). [*Ws.*]

Painful numbness (stupor) of the hands. [G. CLAUDER,[2] in *Misc. Nat. Cur.*, Dec. v, Ann. 6, Obs. 178.]

Numbness of the hands.[3] [STEDMAN, l. c.]

A formication in the left hand, as if gone to sleep. [*Stf.*]

340. Drawing aching pain about the wrist-joint and knuckles of the hand (aft. $\frac{1}{4}$ h.). [*Fz.*]

Swelling of hands.[4] [STEDMAN, l. c.]

An aching drawing on the inner borders of the fingers on movement (aft $1\frac{1}{2}$ h.). [*Fz.*]

---

1 After a cold.

2 From preparing a fomentation of H., therefore local effect.

3 This and S. 341 occurred in one woman only. Qy. did she prepare the leaves for the broth ?

4 See note to S. 338.

In the left gluteus muscle, sharp stitches with cramp-pain (aft. 5 h.). [*Ws.*]

Redness of the nates and feet. [HAMBERGER, l. c.]

345. A boil on the left thigh. [GREDING, l. c., p. 106.[

A tensive pain across the middle of the thighs, as if they were too short, on going up-stairs.

Shooting drawing in the thighs; worse when at rest (aft. 1 h.).) [*Ws.*]

A paralytic drawing in the thighs, especially when walking.

Gangrenous spots and blisters break out, chiefly on the lower limbs (aft. 24 h.). [BLOM, l. c.]

350. While walking in the open air, stiffness and weariness in the knee-joints (aft. 3 h.). [*Fz.*]

Weariness and weakness of the feet.[1] [GREDING, l. c., p. 76.—STEDMAN, l. c.]

Swelling of the foot. [GREDING, l. c., p. 82.]

On moving pain in the calves, like cramp, in the afternoon.

Pinching in the calves (aft. 1 h.). [*Ws.*]

355. (When walking, pain in the left tibia, as if bruised, especially in the evening, whilst the side of the calf is hot, swollen, and covered with red, miliary rash, but without pain and without itching (aft. 72 h.).

Shooting pinching on the tibia (aft. 5 h.). [*Ws.*]

In the ankle-joint a cutting pain when walking.

The ankle-joint is painful as if bruised, in the afternoon.

When walking and advancing the feet and when ascending the toes are spasmodically flexed, as if from cramp.

360. He cries out from (pinching) twitching pains in the feet. [GREDING, l. c., p. 106.]

The limbs go to sleep.

The limbs go to sleep. [NAVIER, l. c.]

Drawing tearing in the soles of the feet, mostly when at rest; it went off by walking and returned when sitting (aft. 36 h.). [*Ws.*]

Pain in the feet.

365. Cold feet.

Rheumatic pains. [GREDING, l. c., p. 87.]

Pains in the limbs and loins. [GREDING, l. c., pp. 89, 107.]

Sharp continued stitches in the joints of the arms and legs (aft. 1 h.). [*Ws.*]

In the joints, but more in the muscles near the joints, a dull drawing pain. [*Stf.*]

370. Cutting tearing in almost all the joints, especially when moving (aft. 3 h.). [*Ws.*]

Pains in the limbs. [WEPFER, l. c.]

The symptoms seem to occur most severely in the evening. [*Sft.*]

Itching, compelling him to scratch the skin till it bleeds. [COSTA, l. c.]

---

1 "Feet and legs" in original.

Fine pricks out at the finger tips and out of all parts of the body (aft. a few m.). [WENDT, l. c.]

375. When he laid the warm hand on any part of the body, *e.g.* the back, arm, &c., for an instant, there occurred a long-continued, very considerable feeling of warmth, like burning, on that part (aft. some h.). [*Stf.*]

Numerous, large boils.

Cutaneous eruption of large pustules, accumulated on several spots, from the region above the hips to the knees, in appearance like confluent small-pox; they do not contain any fluid and scab off after 4 days (aft. 3 d.).[1] [COSTA, l. c.]

Alternate appearance and disappearance of brown spots all over the body. [GREDING, l. c., p. 81.]

Tettery spots on the nape. [GREDING, l. c., p. 96.]

380. Bruised pain in the ulcer, on moving the part (aft. 24 h.).

The ulcer becomes bloody and excessively painful (aft. 24 h.).

Obstinate dropsy. [BARRERE, l. c.]

Swelling.[2] [CLAUDER, l. c.]

Weakness. [SAUVAGES,—NAVIER,—PLANCHON, l. c.—GREDING, l. c., pp. 87, 90.]

385. Disinclination for and dislike to movement and work. [*Fg.*]

Weariness, exhaustion of the whole body.[3] [HAMILTON, l. c.]

When walking in the open air he very soon becomes hot and exhausted (aft. 12 h.). [*Ws.*]

Staggering. [STEDMAN, l. c.]

Uncommon sinking of the strength (aft. 4 h.). [WEPFER, l. c.]

390. Weakness: he can hardly stand on his feet and seems always inclined to fall. [BERNIGAU, l. c.]

Long-continued weakness of the legs.[4] [CAGNION, l. c.]

General debility with trembling of all the body, and extraordinary coldness of the surface of the limbs, until syncope became threatened. [SMITH, l. c.]

Syncope. [HUNERWOLF, l. c.]

Attacks of faintness. [STOERCK, l. c.]

395. Repeated fainting. [NAVIER, l. c.]

Death-like syncope. [J. FAVER,[5] in *Schenck*, lib. vii, obs. 152.]

Quite lying down.[6] [HAMBERGER, l. c.]

Drowsiness (aft. 2 h.). [HAMBERGER, l. c.]

In the morning, very over-busy, like a weak wakefulness; in the afternoon, drowsiness, exhaustion, and irresolution.* [*Fz.*]

400. Sleep.[7] [HAMILTON, l. c.]

* The over-wakefulness, see also 416 to 420, 422, 423, 426, 515 to 518, is in henbane an alternating action with drowsiness and sleep, but the over-wakefulness seems to be the chief primary action.

---

1 On seat of dartres thought to have been cured by mercury.
2 Of hands only as local effect. See S. 337 and note.
3 In half an hour. "General lassitude and inactivity."
4 In original, "lower extremities"
5 From gr. xxv of seeds in an adult.
6 Eight hours after.
7 After relief of condition shown in S. 22 and 467 by venesection.

Sleep for two days. [HUNERWOLF, l. c.]
Sleep for three days. [HUNERWOLF, l. c.]
Profound sleep. [HUNERWOLF, l. c.—GREDING, l. c., pp. 76, 78.]
Long, deep sleep. [SLOANE, l. c.—BLOM, in *Bergius*, l. c.]

405. Immediate sleep. [HUNERWOLE, l. c.]
Gentle sleep.[1] [GREDING, l. c., p. 76.]
Quiet sleep, with profuse sweat and frequent urination. [GREDING, l. c., p. 79.]
During sleep, perspiration.* [GREDING, l. c., p. 109.]
Irresistible inclination to sleep.[2] [HAMILTON, l. c.]

410. Drowsy inability to open the eyelids. [HAMILTON, l. c.]
Very profound slumber. (aft. 5 h.). [*Fg.*]
Long-continued slumber. [KIERNANDER,[3] *Utkast til Medicinal Lagfar*, 1776, p. 267.]
Coma vigil.
Coma vigil. [G. W. WEDEL,[4] in *Misc. Nat. Cur.*, Dec. i, Ann. 3, Obs. 21.]

415. In his sleep he has a comical look.
More sleepless nights. [GREDING, l. c., p. 74.]
He is late of falling asleep. [*Fr. H—n.*]
Sleeplessness. [BLOM, l. c.]
Sleeplessness on account of quiet exhilaration of mind. [*Stf.*]

420. Long-continued sleeplessness. [PLANCHON, l. c.]
Anxious sleeplessness.
Though he only fell asleep long after midnight, he woke unusually early, and felt very cheerful and disposed to engage in works of the fancy, wide awake and strong. [*Stf.*]
Frequent waking from sleep at night as if he had been disturbed, or had already slept enough, for two successive nights. [*Lr.*]
In bed he sometimes raised up the knees, sometimes stretched them out, sometimes he turned about, turned the head sometimes here sometimes there, sometimes he lifted up his hand and struck the bed with it, sometimes he plucked straw out of his bed, crept about on it, and did not talk while doing so; at the same time he was neither cross nor timorous (aft. 3½ h.).

425. In unconscious sleep (at 9 p. m.) he began to whine, then raised up the healthy arm, which soon fell down again, immediately afterwards the shoulder was violently jerked upwards; then the head was tossed about; then the affected leg rose up, then there was rapid jerking in the healthy leg; in the healthy hand, the fingers were often quickly extended and then again firmly closed; during this he sometimes emitted complaining sounds.
All night long he could not sleep; whatever side he lay on he

* Scarcely any perspiration occurred except when asleep.

1 Curative effect.
2 In half an hour. "Much inclined to sleep."
3 Not accessible.
4 From seeds, in a boy.

could get no rest; it was only when the day began to dawn that he occasionally slept, but in the short sleep he always sweated all over, most profusely in the neck (aft. 5 h.). [*Lr.*]

Nocturnal sleeplessness, mingled with convulsions and startings as from fright.[1] [HAMILTON, l. c.]

Frightful dreams. [PLANCHON, l. c.]

In the evening soon after going to sleep he has anxious dreams of mad cats jumping upon him (aft. 46 h.). [*Ws.*]

430. He wakes up spontaneously out of sleep with a cry. [HAMBERGER, l. c.]

Sleep interrupted by grinding of the teeth. [GREDING, l. c., p. 91.]

In sleep, suffocating snoring on inspiration (aft. 14 h.). [*Fg.*]

Starting up out of sleep. [*Fg.*]

He chatters in his sleep about war. [*Fg.*]

435. Lascivious dreams, the first two nights, without seminal emission, though the genitals are excited. [*Lr.*]

Apoplexy with snoring.[2] [COSTA, l. c.]

Hemiplegia. [A. V. HALLER,[3] in *Vicat's Mat. Med.*, i, p. 184.]

He suddenly falls to the ground. [CAMERARIUS,—HUNERWOLF, l. c.]

He suddenly falls to the ground with a cry and convulsions.* [*Pyl's Neues Magazine*,[4] B. ii, St. iii, p. 100.]

440. He is stiff all over, as in tetanus. [HUNERWOLF, l. c.]

Slight convulsive movements, sometimes of the upper, sometimes of the lower extremities. [PLANCHON, l. c.]

Convulsive movements. [HUNERWOLF, l. c.]

In the convulsions he stamps upon the ground first with one foot and then with the other. [CAMERARIUS, l. c.]

Convulsions. [COSTA,—JASKIEWITZ, l c.]

445. Convulsions for five days. [JASKIEWITZ, l. c.]

Frequent twitchings. [CAGNION, l. c.]

The spasms flex the limbs, and the bent body is thrown up high. [CAMERARIUS, l. c.]

The body is thrown about terribly with convulsions. [CAMERARIUS, l. c.]

Convulsions with foam before the mouth. [CAMERARIUS, l. c.]

450. In the convulsions the thumbs are turned in (upon the fist). [HUNERWOLF, l c.]

Epilepsy.† [CHPH. SELIGER, in *Misc. Nat. Cur.*, Dec. ii, Ann. i, Obs. 138.]

* From bathing the head with a decoction of henbane.

† From eating the seeds, in two boys, one of whom died after a few hours.

---

1 Literally, "he passed the night after without sleeping, and was alternately seized with convulsions, startings, and catched with his hands at everything.

2 Literally, "stertorous breathing as in apoplexy."

3 From seeds, in a male adult.

4 From seeds, in a boy.

5 No such observation occurs here; but the author relates how a fomentation of the seeds applied for menstrual headache caused epileptic symptoms to come on.

Little attacks of epilepsy, alternating with paroxysms of apoplexy.[1] [PLANCHON, l. c.]

Subsultus tendinum. [HAMILTON, l. c.]

Spasms with watery diarrhœa and diuresis. [GREDING, l. c., p. 94.]

455. Spasms, diarrhœa, and coldness of the whole body. [GREDING, l. c., p. 94.]

(He cannot get warm in bed at night.]

Chilliness and shivering all over the body for half an hour. [STOERCK, l. c.]

Rigor all over the body, with hot face and cold hands, without thirst (aft. 1 h.), recurring the following day (aft. 24 h.). [*Lr.*]

In the afternoon fever abounding in coldness and pain, *e. g.* of the back.

460. In the evening, violent and long-continued chilliness with restless sleep, followed by profuse sweat. [GREDING, l. c., p. 79.]

After twelve minutes the number of beats of the pulse diminished, and continued to do so, so that in an hour it fell from 85 to 59 beats, and was very small.* [BARTON, l. c.]

Very small, low pulse. [HAMILTON, l. c.]

Weak, irregular pulse. [STEDMAN, l. c.]

Hard pulse. [BLOM, in *Bergius*, l. c.]

465. Small, quick, intermittent pulse. [COSTA, l. c.]

Stronger pulse. [HAMILTON, l. c.]

Quick, full, strong pulse[2] [HAMILTON, l.c.]

Heightened circulation, for twelve hours. [COSTA, l. c.]

Distended blood-vessels all over the body. [COSTA,—MATTHIOLUS, l. c.]

470. (The blood burns in its vessels.)

Burning heat internally in the whole body. [COSTA, l. c.]

External burning heat of the whole body, without redness. [HAMBERGER, l. c.]

In the evening great heat all over the body with much thirst, putrid taste, and much mucus in the mouth ; the lips stuck together. [*Fz.*]

The skin of the whole body is inflamed[3] and of a cinnabar red colour (soon after the heat). [HAMBERGER, l. c.]

475. Transpiration. [GREDING, l. c.]

Profuse perspiration.[4] [HAMILTON,—STEDMAN, l. c.,—GREDING, l. c., p. 76, 78.]

Profuse sweats. [PLANCHON, l. c.]

Perspiration growing always more and more profuse. [GREDING, l. c., p. 74.]

Extremely profuse perspiration. [GREDING, l. c., p. 86.]

480. General perspiration, especially on the thighs and legs, for two days (aft. 24 h.). [COSTA, l. c.]

* From four grains of the resinous extract in a healthy man of 24 years.

---

1 In original "each fit followed by sopor."

2 Twenty-four hours after, with S. 22.

3 "As if inflamed."

4 In Stedman's case, curative reaction ; in Hamilton's, after bleeding.

Sour perspiration. [GREDING, l. c., p. 103.]

Perspiration with exhaustion and obtuseness of the senses. [GREDING, l. c., p 78.]

Cool perspiration. [STOERCK, l. c.]

Obtuseness, insensible laziness.[1] [HAMILTON, l. c.]

485. He is in danger of becoming senseless.* [VAN EEMS, in *Praelect. Bœrhavii de morb. nerv.*, ad. tom. i, p. 236.]

He lies bereft of reason and lazy. [GREDING, l. c., p. 78.]

Complete stupefaction. [WENDT, l. c.]

He does not know those belonging to him. [FAVER,—WEDEL,—STEDMAN, l. c.]

Bereft of all his senses, he sits in bed immovable, like a statue. [LA SERRE, l. c.]

490. Complete loss of reason. [J. B. VAN HELMONT,[2] *Jus Duumv.*, § 22.]

Complete loss of consciousness. [CAGNION, l. c.]

Stupidity. [WEDEL, l. c.]

Stupid[3] and sunk in constant sleep. [GREDING, l. c., p. 96.]

Imbecility, senselessness. [KIERNANDER, l. c.]

495. Senselessness (amentia). [WEPFER,—STEDMAN,—HALLER,—TOZZETTI, l. c.]

Insanity (insania). [BLOM, l. c.—GREDING, l. c., p. 78.]

Insanity with diarrhœa. [GREDING, l. c., p. 80.]

Extreme disorder of the intellect. [FAVER, l. c.]

He spoke many incoherent things. [HAMILTON, l. c.]

500. They babble out almost everything a sensible person would have kept silence about all his life, [GRUNEWALD, l. c. (II).]

Exhausted he rambles on about things to himself. [GREDING, l. c., p. 82.]

He speaks more than ordinarily, with greater liveliness and in a more hurried manner. [*Stf.*]

Loquacity. [GREDING, l. c., p. 75.]

Foolish laughter. [SAUVAGES, l. c.]

505. When reading he mixes up improper words and modes of speech. [WEPFER, l. c.]

He chatters incoherent things. [STEDMAN, l. c.]

He murmurs nonsensical things to himself. [WEPFER, l. c.]

He murmurs and chatters to himself. [KIERNANDER, l. c.]

Confusion of the mind with talk about various things.[4] [MATTHIOLUS, l. c.]

510. Unconnected words. [WEDEL, l. c.]

Floccillation and murmuring at the same time. [COSTA, l. c.]

Talking nonsense. [BERNIGAU,—WEDEL,[5]—HUNERWOLF, l. c.]

* Happened to Boerhave himself from the exhalations from henbane.

1 "Insensibility so that he did not know those about him," in original.
2 From ℨij of seeds, in an adult.
3 Increase of previous (morbid) dulness.
4 The last phrase in the original is "altercatio."
5 In Wedel's case, with red face.

When awake he talks nonsense ; says a man has been there—which was not the case.

He is delirious as in acute fever. [STEDMAN, l. c.]

515. Exalted state of mind (for 12 hours) with almost incessant delirium.* [JOERDENS, in *Hufel. Journal*, iv, p. 539.]

Extreme liveliness, restlessness, hurry. [*Stf.*]

Over-busy : he thought he was more active and stronger than he actually was (aft. 2, 4, 8 h.). [*Fz.*]

Thousands of fanciful ideas play about his mind. [PLANCHON, l. c.]

In the confusion of his fancy he thinks men are swine. [SCHULZE, l. c.]

520. He is silently wrapt up in his own thoughts.

Imbecility (stupor), shown in words and acts. [HUNERWOLF, l. c.]

Bereft of reason he knew not what he did. [GREDING, l. c., p. 90.]

Foolish acts. [GRUNEWALD, l. c.]

He sings love-songs and street ballads. [GRUNEWALD, l. c. (1).]

525. Chattering he prepares for a journey. [GREDING, l. c., p. 76.]

Chattering he makes preparations for a wedding. [GREDING, l. c., p. 76.]

A very peculiar feeling of lightness and mobility. [*Stf.*]

He dances. [COSTA, l. c.]

Comical confusion of mind† : they perform all sorts of ridiculous antics, like monkeys. [PET. BORELLI, *Cent.*, iv, Obs. 45.]

530. He makes ridiculous grimaces, like a dancing fool. [GRUNEWALD, l. c.]

Ridicuolus grimaces, like those of a drunken person. [GRUNEWALD, l. c.]

Gesticulations. [GRUNEWALD, l. c. (I).]

He gesticulates like a harlequin.[1] [SCHULZE, l. c.]

In his delirium he acts as if he were cracking nuts. [WEPFER, l. c.]

535. In his mania, he acts as if he must drive away peacocks with his hands. [WEPFER, l. c.]

He clutches about him, without knowing at what. [HAMILTON, l. c.]

He fumbles about his head, his face, his nose, and grapples the bed-clothes, as in floccillation.[2] [HAMILTON, l. c.]

He puts his arms round the stove and tries to climb up it as if it were a tree. [WEPFER, l. c.]

They cried out that near objects were going to fall and seized hold of them. [STEDMAN, l. c.]

* From a henbane clyster.

† From eating the root, in a whole family.

---

1 In original, "like an actor."

2 "As patients frequently do in nervous fevers."

540. They ran against all objects that stood in their way, with open, wild eyes. [CAGNION, l. c.]

Mania, as if possessed by the devil. [MATTHIOLUS, l. c.]

He strips himself naked. [GREDING, l. c., p. 81.]

He lies naked in bed and chatters. [GREDING, l. c., p. 76.]

Naked and enveloped in a fur cloak, he senselessly wanders about to a great distance in the summer heat. [GRUNEWALD, l. c. (I).]

545. Ridiculously solemn acts in improper clothing,* mixed with fury. [GRUNEWALD, l. c. (II).]

Along with constant burning heat and crying out he breathes with difficulty and makes violent movements with the hands. [HAMBERGER, l. c.]

The first day extremely lively and very crotchety, the second cross and much disposed to scold. [*Lr.*]

Alternations of calmness and fury. [GREDING, l. c., p. 85.]

Mania, he can scarcely be restrained.[1] [STEDMAN, l. c.]

550. He displays incontrollable strength in his fury. [GREDING, l. c., p. 76.]

Extremely furious and naked he passes the day and night without sleep and crying out. [GREDING, l. c.]

Jealousy.

Abusive talk, scolding, noise. [GRUNEWALD, l. c. (III).]

Quarreling.

555. Quarreling. [GRUNEWALD, l. c.]

Quarreling and abusive talk. [SCHULZE, l. c.]

He is violent and strikes at people. [GRUNEWALD, l. c.]

He lays violent hands on others. [GRUNEWALD, l. c. (III).]

Fury ; he tries to inflict injury on and hurt others.

560. Fury.[2] [SLOANE, l. c.—GREDING, pp. 75, 79, 81.]

Incontrollable frenzy. [COSTA, l. c.]

Extreme fury : he rushes at people with knives. [KIERNANDER, l. c.]

He strikes and tries to murder those he meets. [SCHULZE, l. c.]

Cross, sad (the 2nd day). [*Stf.*]

565. Dejection, sadness.[3] [HAMILTON, l. c.]

Restlessness. [HAMBERGER, l. c.— GREDING, l. c., p. 78.]

Extreme restlessness.[4] [STEDMAN, l. c.]

They always moved from one place to another (for two days). [SAUVAGES, l. c.]

Anxiety. [HUNERWOLF, l. c.]

570. Anxieties. [STOERCK, l. c.]

Horrible[5] anxiety. [WEDEL, l. c.]

* In a priest's cassock, put on over nothing but a shirt, and in fur boots, he wishes to go to church, in order to preach and perform clerical offices there, and furiously attacks those who try to prevent him.

---

1 Not found.
2 "Ravings" in Sloane's cases.
3 "Spirits dejected," in original.
4 The author adds, "cannot be restrained."
5 In original, "the utmost."

Shocks of fright, alternating with trembling and convulsions.[1] [HAMILTON, l. c.]

He complains that he has been poisoned.[2] [HAMILTON, l. c.]

(He considers himself a criminal.)

575. Peculiar fear of being bitten[3] by beates. [CAGNION, l. c.]

Irritable, morose, despairing. [GREDING, l. c., p. 104.]

(He reproaches himself and has scapules of conscience.)

He reproaches others, and complains of injustice that he imagines has been done him.

In despair he wishes to take his life, and throw himself into the water. [GREDING, l. c., p. 104.]

580. Extreme fearfulness.

Long-continued fearfulness. [CAGNION, l. c.]

Impatient ; he thought he should die when he had to wait for something of quiet a trivial nature. [*Stf.*]

---

1 Literally, "tremors, startings, and convulsions."
2 Merely a statement of the fact.
3 In original "devoured."

IGNATIA.[1]

(The seed of the Ignatia amara.)

(One grain of the pulverised* seed is first brought to the million-fold (third) trituration in the way taught in the introduction to arsenic, and of this one grain, after being dissolved, is brought by means of 27 diluting phials to the thirtieth potency ($\overline{X}$).

The characteristic peculiarities of this very powerful vegetable substance, as far as they are known to me, are pointed out in the foot notes.

On account of the alternating actions, that follow one another very rapidly, which it excites, it is particularly suitable for acute diseases, and for a considerable number of these, as may be seen from the symptoms corresponding in similarity to symptoms of disease frequently met with in daily life. It is therefore very properly regarded as a medicine created for great usefulness (polychrest).

Its action is usually exhausted in a few days; yet there are constitutions and states of the body where it cannot effect any evacuation, and in such cases I have sometimes observed its action last nine days. It is suitable for but few cases of chronic disease, and then only with the intermediate employment of some other suitable medicine of more persistent action.

In its employment it sometimes happens, which is seldom the case with other medicines, that where the first dose has not done what was intended, because (for some unknown cause) it first acted on the disease with its opposite symptoms and consequently soon caused an aggravation of the disease in its secondary action, like a palliative remedy, then (without any intermediate medicine having been given in alternation) *a second dose* of the same dilution can be given with the best curative effect, so that the cure is only obtained by the second dose. This is no doubt owing to the directly opposite symptoms (alternating actions) of this remarkable drug, of which I shall speak further on. But such cases do not often occur, for, as a rule, in an acute disease, the first dose effects all that this medicine can do in a homœopathic way, if it has been accurately selected according to similarity of symptoms.

Where in the case of an over-excitable system, perhaps also given in too large a dose, it produces too great sensitiveness, or an anxious, exalted states of the sensibility, hastiness, &c., coffee is serviceable as

* If the mortar is kept constantly standing in very hot water, and thus maintained at a moderately high temperature, then this seed (as is the case with nux vomica) may be easily reduced to a fine powder without diminution of its medicinal power.

1 From vol. ii, 3rd edit., 1833.

a homœopathic antidote. When it has been unsuitably chosen so that its symptoms do not correspond in sufficient similarity to those of the disease, the sufferings it causes may, according to their character, be relieved by the antidotal power of pulsatilla or chamomilla, and in rarer cases by cocculus, arnica, camphor or vinegar.

Although its positive effects have a great resemblance to those of nux vomica (which indeed might be inferred from the botanical relationship of these two plants) yet there is a great difference in their therapeutic employment. The emotional disposition of patients for whom ignatia is serviceable, differs widely from that of those for whom nux vomica is of use. Ignatia is not suitable for persons or patients in whom anger, eagerness, or violence is predominant, but for those who are subject to rapid alternations of gaiety and disposition to weep, or in whom we notice the other emotional states indicated at the end of the following list of ignatia symptoms, provided always that the other corporeal morbid symptoms resemble those that this drug can produce.

Even in a high potency, ignatia is a main remedy in cases of vexation in subjects who have no tendency to break out violently or to revenge themselves, but who keep their annoyance to themselves; in whom, in a word, the resemblance of the vexatious occurrence is wont to dwell in the mind, and so also especially in morbid states which are produced by occurrences that cause grief. So also attacks of even chronic epilepsy, which only occur after mortification or some similar vexation (and not from any other cause), may always be prevented by the timely administration of ignatia. Epileptic attacks that come on in young persons after some great fright, before they become very numerous, may also be cured by a few doses of ignatia. But it is very improbable that chronic epileptic fits of other kinds can be cured, or have ever been cured, by this medicine. At all events, the cases recorded in medical writings as having been cured by ignatia are not to be relied on, for other powerful drugs were almost always administered at the same time or as intermediate remedies, or there is no evidence that the cure was permanent.

When a person has, for the first time in his life, in consquence of some external disturbing circumstance, been seized with epilepsy which assumes a serious character by its duration or rapid recurrence, a single small dose of ignatia-tincture may be relied upon for relief and generally for permanent cure (as I have seen). But it is otherwise with chronic epilepsies. In these cases it cannot be of permanent benefit for the same reason that it is of no use in other chronic diseases. For its peculiar opposite primary actions (alternating actions) follow one another in this opposite way when it is given in diseases, so that, if the first dose has removed the morbid state, a second must not be given soon afterwards, for this would cause a recurrence of the morbid state, because its opposite alternating action comes into play, which produces the injurious effects of the secondary action of a palliative.* Hence it is proved that it is only applicable and curative in sudden attacks and in acute diseases.

* Thus, also, as above stated, a second dose of ignatia-tincture only acts curatively (in opposition) in those cases in which a first dose of the same remedy, though

It is best to administer the (small) dose *in the morning,* if there is no occasion for hurry. When given shortly before bed-time it causes too much restlessness at night. For all therapeutic purposes the administration of one small globule moistened by the thirtieth attenuation is sufficient, and still better, the olfaction of a globule the size of a mustard seed imbibed with the same potency, repeated once or twice daily.

[HAHNEMANN was aided in this proving by GROSS and FR. HAHNEMANN. The symptoms referred to HARTLAUB and TRINKS are those of JORG'S proving, which HAHNEMANN took from their *Arzneimittellehre.*

The old-school authorities whence symptoms were obtained are :

BERGIUS, *Mat. Med.*

CAMILLI, *Philos. Transact.*, vol. xxi, No. 250.

DURIUS, *Misc. Nat. Cur.*, Dec. iii, Ann. 9, 10, Obs. 126.

GRIMM, J. C., *Eph. Nat. Cur.*, Obs. 72.

VALENTINUS, *Hist. Simpl. reform.*

In the *Frag. de Viribus* Ignatia has 176 symptoms, in the 1st edit. of the 'R. A. M. L.' 624, in the 2nd edit. 674, and in this 3rd edit. 794.]

IGNATIA.

Heat in the head.

Feeling of hollowness and emptiness in the head.

Weak, fallacious memory (before the 8th and 10th h.).

Thinking and speaking are difficult for him, towards evening [*Hb. Ts.*[1]]

5. He is unable to concetrate the thoughts for an instant. [*Hb. Ts.*]

Vertigo. [BERGIUS,[2] *Mat. Med.*, p. 150.]

Slight vertigo which changed into aching pain in the right half of the occiput (all the 1st d.). [*Hb. Ts.*]

Vertigo with some stitches in the head. [*Hb. Ts.*]

A kind of vertigo : feeling of swaying hither and thither.

10. Vertigo : he staggerd when walking and could only with difficulty keep himself upright. [*Hb. Ts.*]

Dazedness of the head, in the morning after rising (2nd d.). [*Hb. Ts.*]

Dulness and confusion of the head. [*Hb. Ts.*]

Intoxication* (aft. 1 h.). [J. C. GRIMM, *Eph. Nat. Cur.*, Cent. x, Obs. 72.]

homoeopathically selected (for some unknown reason) only acted on the disease with its palliative alternating symptoms, whereby it must have caused an aggravation in the secondary action.

* From a drachm.[3]

---

1 Proving of the drug by Jorg and twelve associates, taking from 10 to 200 drops of the tincture, and from 1 to 4 grains of the powdered bean.

2 General accounts of the drug. All his symptoms, save 431, are evidently taken from Camelli.

3 Taken by a man. The symptoms appeared in an hour.

A strong feeling in the head, a kind of intoxication, as from brandy, with burning in the eyes (immediately). [*Fr. H—n.*]

15. **Head is heavy** (aft. 4, 6 h.).

He hangs the head forwards.*

He lays the head forwards on the table.

He feels as if the head were too full of blood; and the interior of the nose is very sensitive to the air, as if epistaxis were coming on.

Heaviness of the head as if it were too full of blood (as after stooping too low), with tearing pain in the occiput, which is alleviated by lying on the back,† is aggravated by sitting up, but is most relieved by stooping the head low when sitting.

20. **Headache which is increased by stooping forwards** (aft. 1 h.).

Headache coming on immediately after stooping low, which soon goes off on raising it up again (aft. 18 h.).

In the morning, in bed, on awaking and opening the eyes, severe headache, which goes off on rising (aft. 40 h.).

Confusion of the head with pains in its right side, especially in the occiput, rendering thinking and speaking difficult. [*Hb. Ts.*]

Confusion of the head, which changed into aching pain in the vertex; this afterwards extended to the forehead and down to the left eye. [*Hb. Ts.*]

25. Heaviness and confusion of the head. [*Hb. Ts.*]

Confusion of the head like intoxication, lasting all day, and frequently passing into actual aching pains in the forehead and especially the right half thereof, rendering thinking very difficult. [*Hb. Ts.*]

Confusion of the head, in the morning on awaking, changing into actual aching headache, that fixed itself particularly in the forehead, and affected the eyes so much, that the movement of the eyelids, and eyeballs caused pain in them (3rd d.), aggravated by going upstairs and every other bodily movement. [*Hb. Ts.*]

Pain in the frontal region, that extended sometimes into the right, sometimes into the left eyeball, and was aggravated by bodily movement. [*Hb. Ts.*]

Pain in the occiput on the side above the mastoid process, which sometimes was communicated to the auditory organs, and then seemed to blunt the sense of hearing. [*Hb. Ts.*]

30. Dull headache, which was chiefly confined to the right half of the forehead and thence extended at the same time to the right eye, rendering this organ very sensitive to the light. [*Hb. Ts.*]

Sensation in the head, as if suddenly attacked by coryza; a dull aching in the sinciput extended markedly down into the nasal cavity, and produced there for ten minutes the feeling that a violent coryza usually causes there; this aching went after ten minutes into other parts of the head and went on changing about in this way, came again and disappeared. [*Hb. Ts.*]

* 16, 17, 19, 47, contrasted with 20, 21, 22, are alternating actions of the primary sort, both of almost equal importance.

† See note to 599.

Slight aching pains in the frontal region, aggravated by the light of the sun. [*Hb. Ts.*]

Violent aching pains in the head, especially in the frontal region, and round about the orbits, becoming always more violent and lasting till the evening. [*Hb. Ts.*]

Aching pain behind and above the upper eyelids of both eyes, for two hours. [*Hb. Ts.*]

35. Aching pain in the right half of the forehead, going thence into the left side, latterly involving the whole head. [*Hb. Ts.*]

Aching in the frontal region, that extended at one time to this, at another to that part of the head, but was nowhere persistent; this pain extended even to beneath the orbits and into the cheeks. [*Hb. Ts.*]

Aching pain, especially in the right half of the forehead, which extended down to the right eye, and there particularly assumed such a character, that it seemed as if it would press out the right eyeball, in the afternoon. [*Hb. Ts.*]

Aching contractive pain in the vertex spreading to the forehead. [*Hb. Ts.*]

Violent pain of an aching character in the temples. [*Hb. Ts.*]

40. Aching pains in the right side of the head and in the occiput. [*Hb. Ts.*]

Aching pain that extended from the forehead to one side, either the right or the left. [*Hb. Ts.*]

Aching and pressing pain in the right half of the occiput, until he went to sleep. [*Hb. Ts.*]

Aching pains in the right side of the occiput. [*Hb. Ts.*]

Dull aching pain that spread all over the head. [*Hb. Ts.*]

45. Aching pain in the head increased by taking food. [*Hb. Ts.*]

Immediately after the midday sleep headache: a general pressure through the whole brain, as if there were too much brain or blood in the head, gradually increased by reading and writing (aft. 20 h.).

Tearing headache in the forehead and behind the left ear, which is tolerable when lying on the back, increased by raising up the head, with heat and redness of the cheeks and hot hands (aft. 5 h.).

Lacerating headache after midnight when lying on the side, which goes off by lying on the back.*

Twitching pain in the head on ascending.

50. Twitching headache, which is increased on opening the eyes (aft. 1 h.).

Aching pain in the forehead above the root of the nose which compels him to bend forward the head,† followed by inclination to vomit (aft. 5 h.).

Extreme aching in both temples especially the right one. [*Gss.*]

* See note to 599.

† The relief caused here and in 19 by stooping forwards stands with the other symptoms, 20, 21, 58, where stooping forward aggravates, in the position of alternating action; but the latter seems to be the best adapted for homoeopathic curative purposes, and is more frequent and more strongly marked.

An aching pain deep under the right side of the frontal bone. [*Gss.*]

Under the left frontal protuberance a stupefying intermitting aching. [*Gss.*]

55. Under the left palpebral arch a violent aching. [*Gss.*]

Pain as if the occipital bone were pressed in.

Cramp-like headache above the root of the nose in the region of the inner canthus (aft. 3 h.).

Above the right orbit, at the root of the nose, aching and somewhat drawing pain in the head, renewed by stooping low (aft. 10 h.).

Headache, like* a pressure with something hard on the surface of the brain, recurring in fits (aft. 6 h.).

60. An aching in the temples, sometimes accompanied by profound sleep.

Headache as if the temples were pressed outwards.†

In the morning (in bed), when lying on one side or the other, a furious headache as if it would force out at the temples, relieved by lying on the back‡ (aft. 48 h.).

Furious headache; a constant digging under the right frontal protuberance and on the right side of the frontal bone. [*Gss.*]

When walking in the open air aching pain in one half of the brain, increased by talking and reflection (aft. 2 h.).

65. When talking and speaking much there comes on a headache, as if the head would burst, which goes off entirely when reading and writing quietly (aft. 48 h.).

Headache increased by talking.

When reading and listening very attentively to a speech the headache is aggravated, but not by mere spontaneous reflection (aft. 6 h.).

Deep stitches in the right temple (aft. $\frac{3}{4}$ h.). [*Gss.*]

Throbbing headache.§

70. Throbbing in the head, above the right supraorbital arch.

Headache at every beat of the arteries.

Shooting pains in the forehead and above the eye-brows. [*Hb. Ts.*]

Shooting pains in the whole forehead and right side of the occiput, [*Hb. Ts.*]

Single stitches dart through his head. [*Hb. Ts.*]

75. External headache; the head is painful when touched.

External headache; drawing from the temples above the orbits; when touched there is pain as if bruised,

* Comp. note to 297. This and almost all the other kinds of headache from ignatia are soon removed by coffee.

† 61, 62, 65. The out-forcing and out-pressing headache in the temples, as also the pain as if the head would burst, is related to the bursting feeling in the bowels 283, and even to the sore throat 164, and also to 172 and 297; for the internal feeling of compression and constriction and the pressing asunder easily become alternating sensations. At all events the pressing asunder is opposed to the marked constriction in hollow organs 366, 368, 431, 465, 468, 472, as alternating action.

‡ See note to 599.

§ This kind of headache is not unfrequently felt on the side of the occiput a few hours after taking the drug.

Pain in the head as if bruised (aft. 8 h.).

In the morning on awaking headache as if the brain were smashed and crushed ; on getting up it goes off and there comes on instead a toothache as if the dental nerve were smashed and crushed ; a similar pain then goes into the sacrum ; this headache is renewed on thinking.

(The hair of the head falls out) (aft. 36 h.).

80. In the evening the inner surface of the upper eyelid is painful, as if it were too dry.

In the evening when reading dimness before one eye, as if a tear were in it, which he should wipe away, and yet there is no moisture in it.

On closing the eyelids pain like excoriation in the outer canthus.

In the morning the eyelids are closed by purulent mucus, and when he opens them, the light dazzles.

In the outer canthus of the left eye, sensation as if some dust had got into it, which pressed on the membranes at intervals.* [*Gss.*]

85. In the outer canthus shooting tearing ; the eyes are sealed up in the morning and water in the forenoon.

In the morning the eyelids are sealed up ; there is aching in the inside of the eye, as if a grain of sand were in it ; on opening the eyelids there is shooting in it (aft. 36 h.).

Gnawing smarting on the edges of the eye-lids (when reading in the morning) (aft. 18 h.).

Smarting in the outer canthi (aft. 24 h.).

Pimples round the inflamed eye (aft. 2 h.).

90. Itching in the interior of the eye (aft. 2 h.).

Itching of the eyeball in the inner canthus (aft. 4 h.).

(Stitches in the right eye.)

Pressure outwards in the right eye, as if the eye-ball would come out of the orbit. [*Hb. Ts.*]

Painful aching over the eyes and in the eyeballs themselves, especially when looking into the light. [*Hb. Ts.*]

95. Burning and weeping of the eyes, especially the left. [*Hb. Ts.*]

Inflammation of the left eye (the 2nd d.). [*Hb. Ts.*]

Swelling of the eyelids ; the Meibomian glands excrete much mucus. [*Hb. Ts.*]

Increased secretion of mucus in both eyes (the 2nd d.). [*Hb. Ts.*]

Increased secretion of tears. [*Hb. Ts.*]

100. The objects apparently moved before the eyes. [*Hb. Ts.*]

Cannot bear the light of the candle† (aft. 8 h.).

The light of the candle is intolerable to him (aft. 10 h.).

After the midday sleep dimness of vision of the right eye, as if a veil were drawn over it (aft. 6 h.).

A circle of brilliant white, glittering zig-zags beyond the visual point when looking at anything, whereby the letters on which the

* Comp. 86. † Comp. 83.

sight is directed become invisible, but those at the side are more distinct* (aft. 16 h.).

105. A zig-zag-like and serpentine white glittering at the side of the visual point, soon after dinner (aft. 30 h.).

At first contracts the pupils.†

The pupils are more capable of dilatation than of contraction (later).

Pupils more easily dilatable and dilated (aft. 4 h.).

The pupils are easily dilated and equally easily contracted.

110. Fine stitches in the cheeks.

Before going to sleep pressure in both zygomatic processes. [*Gss.*]

Shooting pressure on the zygomatic process, in front of the left ear. [*Gss.*]

In the zygomatic process of the left upper maxilla an intermittent, paralytic pressure. [*Gss.*]

(Feels a throbbing in the interior of the ear.)

115. Ringing in the ears.

Roaring in the ears. [*Hb. Ts.*]

Pain in the inner ear.

Stitches in the interior of the ear (aft. 3 h.).

Itching in the meatus auditorius (aft. 3 h.).

120. Music causes an uncommon and agreeable sensation‡ (aft. 2 h.).

Insensibility to music (aft. 30 h.).

Shooting in the lips, especially when they are moved (aft. ¼ h.).

Shooting in the lower lip, also when it is not moved (aft. 8 h.)

A very penetrating fine shooting on the lower lip on touching a hair of the beard there, as if a splinter had stuck in there§ (aft. 3 h.).

125. **The inner surface of the lower lip is painful, as if it were raw and excoriated** (aft. 8, 10 h.).

The internal surface of the lower lip is ulcerated (without pain).

On the inner surface of the lower lip an elevated cutaneous gland become ulcerated, with sore pain (aft. 4 h.).

On the inner surface of the lower lip an elevated little gland, which pains as if excoriated.

The lips are cracked and bleed.

130. One of the commissures of the lips becomes ulcerated (aft. 2 h.).

Pimple-like lumps, only painful when touched, just under the lower lip (aft. 36 h.).

Pressure under both rami of the lower jaw as if the flesh under

* 104, 105, two alternating actions, very much resembling HERZ's so-called false vertigo.

† 106—109, alternating actions ; the contraction seems to be first in point of time, and thus has the chief rank.

‡ 120 and 121, alternating actions.

§ Comp. 533.

the lower jaw were pressed down, when at rest and when moving. [*Gss.*]

The lower jaw is involuntarily drawn up and the jaws closed, which impedes him in speaking, for half an hour (aft. ½ h.). [*Fr. H—n.*]

The inner side of the gums is painful as if numb, as though it was burnt.*

135. (In the morning) pain of the teeth, as from looseness.

One front tooth is painful as if numb and loose, more painful whenever it is touched by the tongue.

The teeth are loose and painful.

Immovable sore pain in the foremost molars, especially when reading (aft. 3 h.).

Toothache in the molars as if they and their nerves were smashed and crushed.

140. The toothache commences towards the end of a meal and grows worse after the meal.

Routing, digging pains in the incisors, in the evening (aft. ½ h.).

Pain in the maxillary joint, in the morning when lying.

The anterior half of the tongue when talking, as if numb—when eating as if burnt or sore.

(In the morning in bed after awaking) the tip of the tongue is extremely painful (sore, tearing) as if it were burnt or wounded.

145. An acrid feeling on the tip of the tongue, as if it were excoriated.

Fine shooting on the extreme tip of the tongue (aft. 2 h.).

Needle-pricks at the frenum of the tongue. [*Fr. H—n.*]

He is apt to bite on one side of the tongue posteriorly when speaking or chewing (aft. 5, 8, 30 h.).

Painful swelling of the orifice of the salivary duct.

150. When chewing he is apt to bite on the inside of the cheek near the orifice of the salivary duct.

Sensation in the palate as if it were excoriated (as from frequent swallowing of the saliva).†

Sensation as if the palate were swollen or covered with viscid mucus (aft. 4 h.).

Stitches in the palate extending into the internal ear (aft. 1½ h.).

Sensation as if the whole surface of the inside of the mouth were about to become excoriated. [*Hb. Ts.*]

155. Aching and drawing in the sublingual glands. [*Hb. Ts.*]

Difficulty of swallowing food and drink. [*Hb. Ts.*]

Stitches in the throat, when not swallowing; when swallowing feeling as if swallowing over a bone, during which it jerks‡ (aft. 3 h.).

* 134, 135, 136, 137 seem to be secondary action.

† Comp. 164, 166, 167.

‡ If there is an alternating action of ignatia, where it produces a sore throat with shooting when swallowing (though I have never observed such a symptom), it must be of very rare occurrence, and hence of very little use from a curative point of view.

Needle-pricks in quick succession, deep in the throat, when not swallowing.

Shooting when swallowing deep down in the œsophagus, which goes off on continuing to swallow and returns when not swallowing.

160. Sore throat : stitches in the throat when not swallowing, and to a certain degree when swallowing ; the more he swallows, the more it goes off ; when he has swallowed something solid, such as bread, it seemed as if the shooting went off entirely.

Sore throat : stitches that are not present whilst swallowing.

Sensation as if a plug were sticking in the œsophagus, observed when not swallowing.

(In the evening) choking (contractive) sensation in the middle of the œsophagus, as if a large morsel or a plug* were sticking there, felt more when not swallowing than when doing so (aft. 4 h.).

Sore throat, like a lump or knob in the throat, which pains as if excoriated when swallowing† (aft. 16 h.).

165. Aching in the throat.

Sore throat : the throat is painful as if it were raw and excoriated (aft. 1½ h.).

Pain in the throat, as from excoriation, only observed when swallowing.

Sore throat : tearing pain at the larynx, which is increased by swallowing, breathing, and coughing (aft. 1½ h.).

Formication in the œsophagus (aft. 1, 2 h.).

170. Shooting in the throat on one side, in the parotid gland, when not swallowing (aft. 20 h.).

Pain in the neck when touched, as if glands were swollen there.

Aching pain in the cervical glands (submaxillary glands).

In the anterior submaxillary gland pain as if it were compressed from without.‡

Painful submaxillary gland, after walking in the open air.

175. Pain in the gland beneath the angle of the lower jaw on moving the neck (aft. 18 h.).

First aching then drawing pain in the submaxillary glands (aft. 4 h.).

Drawing pain in the submaxillary glands, which extends into the jaws, whereupon these glands swell (aft. 5 h.).

Taste in the mouth as if the stomach were deranged.

Symptoms of impeded or weak digestion.

Consequently I have never been able to cure a sore throat with ignatia, even when the other symptoms resembled those of this drug, in which there was shooting only when swallowing ; but, on the other hand, when stitches in the throat were only felt when not swallowing, ignatia cured, and that the more certainly, more quickly and more permanently when the other morbid symptoms could be covered by similar ignatia symptoms.

* See note to 61.

† Comp. 166. The ignatia sore throat, in which there is felt, when not swallowing, internal swelling of the throat, like a lump, is generally attended by only sore pain in this lump when swallowing ; and the sore throat must be of this description which ignatia (when the other symptoms correspond) will remove, and under such circumstances it will be rapidly and certainly cured by ignatia.

‡ On moving the neck and at other times. See also note to 61,

180. **The mouth is always full of mucus.**

The inside of the mouth is covered with ill-smelling mucus in the morning on awaking.

The salivary glands excreted a perfectly white frothy saliva in great quantity. [*Hb. Ts.*]

Increased secretion of saliva. [*Hb. Ts.*]

Chalky taste. [*Hb. Ts.*]

185. Flat, insipid taste, as if chalk had been eaten (aft. ½ h.). [*Hb. Ts.*]

After eating (morning and noon) watery, flat taste in the mouth as from deranged or overloaded stomach (aft. 16 h.).

The taste of what has been taken especially of beer, is bitter and putrid.

Beer tastes bitter (aft. 8 h.).

Beer tastes flat, stale and flavourless (aft. 2, 5 h.).

190. Beer easily goes into the head and causes intoxication (aft. 3 h.).

At first the taste is bitter, afterwards (aft. 10 h.) sour, with sour eructation.

Sour taste of the saliva (a sour taste in the mouth) (aft. 1, 6 h.).

Dislike to acids (aft. 1st h.).

Appetite for sour things* (aft. 10 h.).

195. Dislike to wine.

Dislike to fruit, and it does not agree (aft. 3 h.).

Appetite for fruit, and it agrees very well (aft. 3, 10, 20 h.).

Extreme dislike to tobacco-smoking (aft. 6 h.).

Tobacco-smoke tastes bitter to him (aft. 5 h.).

200. Tobacco-smoke causes smarting on the fore part of the tongue and produces (obtuse ?) pain in the incisors.

Dislike to tobacco-smoking, though it does not taste disagreeably to him (aft. 2, 5 h.).

Repugnance to tobacco-smoking just as if he were satiated with it and had smoked enough.

Hiccup from tobacco-smoking in one accustomed to smoke tobacco.

Nausea from tobacco-smoking, in an accustomed tobacco smoker.

205. Complete want of relish for tobacco, food and drink, with copious flow of saliva into the mouth, but without disgust at these things or feeling that they taste badly (aft. 8 h.).

When he smokes tobacco in the afternoon, he feels so completely satiated that he can eat nothing in the evening.

Want of appetite for food, drink, and tobacco-smoking (immediately).

Dislike to milk (formerly his favourite drink); it is repugnant to him when drinking, although it tastes quite naturally, and not at all disgusting.

When he has drunk some boiled milk (his favourite drink) with relish, and his extreme necessity is assuaged, the remainder is suddenly repulsive to him, although it did not taste disgustingly and he felt no actual nausea.

* 194, 197 are alternating actions with 193, 196, 328.

210. He could not swallow bread, as though it were too dry for him.

He loathes warm food and meat ; will only take butter, cheese and bread (aft. 96 h.).

Dislike to meat and longing* for sour fruit (cranberries) (aft. 24 h.).

Want of appetite (from 1 to 7 h.).

Before taking the medicine considerable hunger, a short time after taking it he felt quite satiated, without having eaten anything. [*Hb. Ts.*]

215. Good appetite ; but on attempting to eat, he felt already satiated. [*Hb. Ts.*]

Want of inclination to eat. [*Hb. Ts.*]

Increased appetite. [*Hb. Ts.*]

Gnawing ravenous hunger, whereby he often became qualmish and sick ; he lay down after the lapse of half an hour, without having taken anything to satisfy himself. [*Hb. Ts.*]

Good appetite ; food and drink are relished.†

220. Great appetite.‡

When eating, drinking and smoking, as soon as his needs are satisfied, the good taste of all these things goes off suddenly, or changes into a disagreeable taste, and he is no longer capable of tasting the smallest quantity of them, although there still remains a sort of hunger and thirst.

He belches up a bitter fluid § (there is eructation, and a bitter fluid comes up into the mouth).

What he has ingested is belched up again into the mouth,|| comes up into the mouth by a kind of eructation (ruminatio).

When she has eaten something (at noon) she feels as if the food stuck above the upper orifice of the stomach and could not get down into the stomach.

225. In the evening before going to sleep, and in the morning, the food seems to be sticking up high (aft 2, 15 h.).

He wakes up at night about 3 a.m. ; he is hot all over, and he vomits the food he had taken for supper.

Unusual and violent thirst, even in the night. [*Hb Ts.*]

Loathing. [*Hb. Ts.*]

Nausea ; the saliva collected in his mouth. [*Hb. Ts.*]

230. Nausea and inclination to vomit. [*Hb. Ts.*]

Empty ineffectual attempts to vomit.

The inclination to vomit goes off after a meal (aft. 2 h.).

After breakfast a kind of anxiety rises up from the abdomen (aft. 20 h.).)

* Comp. 194, 197.

† Secondary or curative action after previous opposite state (anorexia).

‡ This kind of bulimia seems to stand in the relation of alternating action with 205, 207, 208, 209, 210, 213, but to be of rarer occurrence.

§ 222, 223, alternating action with 225.

|| Allied to this is a symptom not inserted in the text : "The taste of the milk taken in the morning can not be got out of the mouth for a long time" (aft. 21 h.).

During supper his feet grew cold, his abdomen distended (and he became perfectly hoarse).

235. After a meal the abdomen is as if distended.

After a meal the abdomen becomes tense, the mouth dry and bitter, without thirst; one cheek is red (in the evening).

Anxious painful fulness in the abdomen after supper (aft. 36 h.)

A scraping at the top of the larynx, as from heart-burn (in the evening) (aft. 8 h.).

Empty eructation, only of wind (aft. 2 h.).

240. Repeated eructation (soon after taking the drug). [*Hb. Ts.*]

Bitter eructation (the 2nd d.). [*Hb. Ts.*]

Eructation with the taste of the ingesta (immediately).

Sour eructation.

Musty, mouldy eructation (in the evening).

245. (Suppressed, ineffectual eructation (in the morning in bed), which causes aching pain at the mouth of the stomach, in the œsophagus up into the fauces) (aft. 48 h.).

Frequent ejection of saliva.*

Flow of saliva out of the mouth during sleep (aft. 1 h.).

Spitting of frothy saliva all day.

After eating and drinking, hiccup† (aft. 3 and 8 h.).

250. In the evening, after drinking, hiccup (aft. 6 h.).

Burning on the tongue (immediately).

Coldness in the stomach.

Burning in the stomach (aft. 1 h.).

Painful sensations arising in the stomach and spreading to the spleen and spinal column. [*Hb. Ts.*]

255. Aching in the region of the floor of the stomach, sometimes intermitting. [*Hb. Ts.*]

Fixed and aching pain in the region of the stomach, for ten minutes. [*Hb. Ts.*]

Aching in the stomach and in the region of the solar plexus. [*Hb. Ts*]

The stomach seemed alternately to be sometimes as if overloaded, sometimes as if empty, with which latter feeling ravenous hunger was always conjoined. [*Hb. Ts*]

Drawing as if the walls of the stomach were distended, sometimes also aching in the stomach.

260. Pains like spasm of the stomach.

Burning, aching, and drawing pains in the stomach, in the hepatic and splenic regions. [*Hb. T's*]

Increased warmth in the stomach. [*Hb Ts.*]

Sensation in the stomach as if he had fasted long, as from emptiness, with flat taste in the mouth and exhaustion in all the limbs.‡

With appetite and relish for food and drink, qualmish fasting taste in the mouth.

265. Sensation of fasting about the stomach and debility of the body.

* 246, 247, 248, comp with 283, 368.

† 249, 250, comp. with 203.

‡ Alternating action with 235, 236, 237.

Flabbiness in the stomach; the stomach and bowels seem to him to hang down in a relaxed state (aft. 24 h.).

A peculiar feeling of weakness in the epigastric region and scrobiculus cordis* (aft. 2 h.).

Aching in the scrobiculus cordis.

Violent shooting in the scrobiculus cordis. [*Gss.*]

270. Fine shooting in the stomach.

Slow succession of shooting twitching pain in the epigastric region and scrobiculus cordis (aft. ½ h.).

First strong then fine shooting in the scrobiculus cordis (aft. ½ h.).

A pain in the scrobiculus cordis as if it were sore internally, only felt when pressing on it.

Painful aching in the region of the spleen and the floor of the stomach, alternately disappering and recurring. [*Hb. Ts.*]

275. Shooting and burning in the region of the spleen, recurring several times. [*Hb. Ts.*]

Aching in the umbilical region. [*Hb. Ts.*]

Painful sensation as if something passed from the epigastrium up towards the thoracic cavity. [*Hb. Ts.*]

Stretching pains in the epigastrium (aft. 1 h.). [*Hb. Ts.*]

Sensation as if the abdominal walls were stretched outwards and the diaphragm upwards; this pain was felt most strongly in the splenic region and posteriorly towards the spinal column, alternately more in one place and then again in another; it also several times extended to the thoracic cavity, changed there into a painful burning; but was chiefly and most violently directed towards the spinal column in the neighbourhood of the solar plexus; eructation of wind diminished this pain. [*Hb. Ts.*]

280. Pain in the epigastrium as from over-lifting.

An aching in both sides of the epigastrium or the hypochondria.

A sharp pinching pressure in the scrobiculus cordis and the right sub-costal region (aft. ½ h.).

A colicky pain as if the bowels would burst in the epigastrium, almost like a gastralgia, which extends into the throat, in the morning in bed, when lying on the side; which goes off by lying on the back† (aft. 40 h.).

General pressing in the abdomen towards the anus. [*Hb. Ts.*]

285. Distension in the umbilical region and cutting there, for a quarter of an hour. [*Hb. Ts.*]

Distension of the abdomen. [*Hb. Ts.*]

Drawing pains in the left lumbar region, lasting a few minutes. [*Hb. Ts.*]

Cutting in the umbilical region. [*Hb. Ts.*]

Cutting pain in the right side of the abdomen. [*Hb. Ts.*]

290. Cutting and contractive pains in the hypogastrium. [*Hb. Ts.*]

* Comp. 335 and 630. This feeling of weakness in the region of the scrobiculus cordis is a characteristic symptom of ignatia.

† Comp. 48, 62, and note to 599.

Considerable cutting in the abdomen, urging him to go to stool, when soft fluid fæces are evacuated. [*Hb. Ts.*]

Cutting spreading all over the abdomen ending in a diarrhœic stool. [*Hb. Ts.*]

Shooting that extended from the epigastrium as it were upwards to the thoracic cavity, but not involving the abdominal organs. [*Hb. Ts.*]

Rumbling and rattling in the abdomen. [*Hb. Ts.*]

295. Sensation in the abdomen as if a purgative had begun to act. [*Hb. Ts.*]

A kind of bellyache; a contractive pain from both sides, just beneath the ribs (aft. ¼ h.).

Constrictive sensation in the hypochondria, as in constipation, with a semilateral headache, as from a nail pressed into the brain,* in the morning (aft. 20 h.).

Spasmodic flatulent colic in the epigastrium in the evening on going to sleep and in the morning on awaking (aft. 8 h.).

Bellyache; continued bruised pain of the bowels, in the morning in bed.

300. Sensation in the abdomen, in the region of the navel, as if something alive were in there (aft. 8 h.).

Easy discharge of flatus (aft. ½ h.). (The opposite is generally secondary action.)

Nocturnal flatulent colic.

Flatulent colic with stitches towards the chest.

In the morning flatulent bellyache in the hypogastrium, which gives off stitches towards the chest and towards the side.†

305. Flatulent colic above the navel alternating with copious flow of saliva‡ in the mouth (aft. 1 h.).

Discharge of much flatus at night, even during sleep, and always production of more, so that everything in the abdomen seems to turn to flatus.

Much troubled with flatus, which then presses on the urine (aft. 96 h.).

Unsatisfactory discharge of short interrupted flatus of fœtid odour. passed not without an effort of the abdominal muscles (aft. 24, 30 h.).

Flatulent distension immediately after a meal.§

310. Frequent discharge of flatus immediately after a meal (aft. 26 h.).

After a meal loud rumbling in the abdomen.

(Rumbling in the abdomen.)‖ [VALENTINUS,[1] *Hist. Simpl. Reform*, p. 198.]

* The ancients called this kind of headache *clavus*. This kind of pain is characteristic of ignatia: a pressure as from a sharp-pointed body, as shown in other symptoms also, as 365, 462, 485, to which also "pressure as with a hard body" seems to belong, as 59, 599.

† Comp. 332.

‡ Comp. 246, 247, 248, 368.

§ Alternating action with 310.

‖ Comp. 311, 314, 315.

1 Not accessible.

Grumbling in the abdomen as in a hungry person (aft. 1 h.).
Rumbling and rattling in the bowels.

315. **Throbbing in the abdomen.**
Itching exactly in the navel (aft. 2½ h.).
On the left near the navel a painful pressure. [*Gss.*]
On the left above the navel a sharp shooting. [*Gss.*]
Oppression in the abdomen and cutting.

320. Cutting in the abdomen (aft. 2 h.).
Immediately after a meal, cutting shooting pain in the abdomen, which changed into flatulent distension (aft. 4 h.).
A continual pinching on a small spot in the right hypogastrium, in the region of the cæcum, especially when walking (in the open air) (aft. 4 h.).
Aching in the hypogastrium (aft. ¼ h.). [*Gss.*]
Painful aching in the left side of the hypogastrium. [*Gss.*]

325. Violent aching in the left side of the abdomen. [*Gss.*]
A pinching distension in the whole abdomen, immediately after a meal, only when he is standing, and worse when he is walking, increased to an intolerable degree on continuing to walk, though flatulence does not seem to be the cause of it; on sitting still it soon goes off, without discharge of flatus (aft. 4 h.).
Shooting in the left side of the hypogastrium* [*Gss.*]
An aching pinching in the abdomen after eating the smallest quantity of fruit, especially when standing and walking, which goes off when sitting.
Pinching colic in all the bowels, even long after a meal, when walking in the open air.

330. Fine shooting pain below the navel (aft. 1 to 2 h.).
Pain, first pinching, then shooting, in one side of the abdomen (aft. 2, 10 h.).
Pinching pain in the abdomen, just in the umbilical region, the pain afterwards goes into the left side of the chest, where it is a mixture of pinching and shooting.
Pinching in the abdomen (aft. 1 h.).
Pinching pain in the abdomen in the open air, as if diarrhœa would come on.

335. Drawing and pinching in the abdomen: it came into the rectum like pressing, with qualmishness and weakness in the scrobiculus cordis† and paleness of the face (aft. 48 h., two days before the catamenia).
(Tearing pain in the abdomen.)
Shooting twitching pain in the left groin, in the evening when lying in bed.
Sensation in the left groin as if a hernia would protrude.
Above the left hip an intermitting, deep internal aching. [*Gss.*]

340. Stool first of hard and then of thin fæces.‡

* Comp. 330.

† Comp. 267, 630.

‡ Easy and satisfactory evacuation of fæces is generally only primary action, which comes on in half an hour or one hour.

Thin fæces pass involuntarily with flatulence (in 50 h.).

Soft stool immediately after a meal.

Three evacuations of soft fæces in the afternoon. [*Hb. Ts.*]

Three moderate evacuations of the bowels. [*Hb. Ts.*]

345. Two evacuations of the bowels of thin consistence (2nd d.). [*Hb. Ts.*]

Three diarrhœic stools (the 1st d.). [*Hb. Ts.*]

After cutting, diarrhœic stool. [*Hb. Ts.*]

Whitish yellow stools (aft. 3 h.).

Slimy stools.

350. Acrid stools.

Prolapsus of the rectum during moderate straining at stool.

Straining at stool without result. [*Hb. Ts.*]

Frequent almost ineffectual urging to stool, with bellyache, tenesmus, and tendency to prolapsus of the rectum (aft. 48 h.).

In the evening great desire and urging to go to stool, more in the middle of the abdomen ; but no stool came, only the rectum was forced out.

355. Yellowish-white stool of a very large size and passing through the rectum and anus with great difficulty.

Very large stool passing with great difficulty (aft. 12 h.).

Ineffectual urging to stool in the rectum, not in the anus (aft. 1½ h.).

Ineffectual call and straining to stool and urging in the intestines of the upper part of the abdomen,[1] chiefly soon after a meal.

Anxious urging to stool, with inactivity of the rectum ; he cannot press out the fæces without danger of prolapsus of the rectum.

360. **Violent urging to stool, more in the upper bowels and upper part of the abdomen ; he has great desire, and yet the stool although soft does not pass in sufficient quantity ;** the urging lasts long after the stool is passed (aft. 20 h.).

Ineffectual call and urging to stool.

After sudden urgent call an insufficient quantity of tenacious, clay-coloured, but not hard fæces is passed with difficulty and not without great straining of the abdominal muscles (almost as if there was a deficiency of the vermicular movement of the bowels) (aft. 3 d.).

Spasmodic tension in the rectum all day.

Sharp pressing pain deep in the rectum after the stool, as from incarcerated flatus (such as usually occurs after a too hasty evacuation—a kind of proctalgia)* (aft. 2 h.).

365. In the evening after lying down, for two hours, sharp pressing pain in the rectum (proctalgia), without relief in any position, which is allayed spontaneously without discharge of flatus.

Painless contraction of the anus,† a kind of stricture for several days (aft. 12 h.).

---

* Comp. note to 297.

† 366, 368. See note to 61.

1 Hahnemann's "Oberbauch," usually rendered "epigastrium," sometimes means, as here, the abdomen above the navel.

Creeping and burning in the anus. [*Hb. Ts.*]

Contraction of the anus (in the evening), which returns next day at the same hour, painful when walking, but most so when standing, but painless when sitting, with flow of insipid saliva* into the mouth (aft. 4, 12, 36 h.).

Several times cutting, rather deep in the rectum (aft. 20 h.).

370. **A coarse stitch from the anus deep into the rectum.**

Coarse stitches in the anus (aft. 2 h.).

Violent itching in the rectum in the evening in bed.

Creeping in the rectum, as from thread-worms.

In the lower part of the rectum, towards the anus, disagreeable creeping as from thread-worms (aft. 24 h.).

375. An itching lump at the anus, which is not painful during stool, but which causes an aching when sitting.

Hæmorrhoidal sufferings along with soft stool (aft. 5 h.).

Soon or immediately after a stool, pain in the anus, as from blind piles, and like **sore pain.**

Sore pain in the anus when not at stool (aft. 1 h.).

Pain in the rectum, as from hæmorrhoids, constrictive and sore as when a wound is touched (aft. 3 h.).

380. **From one to two hours after stool, pain in the rectum, as from blind piles, compounded of contraction and sore pain** (aft. 2 and 36 h.).

After straining the mind with thinking, soon after a stool, pain as from blind piles, aching and as if excoriated (aft. 36 h.).

Swelling of the border of the anus round about, as from distended blood-vessels.

Blind hæmorrhoids with pain compounded of aching and soreness (at the anus and in the rectum), more painful when sitting and standing, slighter when walking,† but recurring most severely after enjoying the open air.

(Flow of blood from the anus, with itching of the perinæum and anus.)

385. Thread-worms crawl out at the anus (aft. 16 h.).

Itching at the anus.

Itching in the perinæum, especially when walking.

(Exhaustion after the stool.)

A sharp pressure on the bladder, as from misplaced flatulence, after supper.

390. A scraping, aching pain on the region of the neck of the bladder, especially when walking and after a meal, when not urinating; the urine passes without pain.

Frequent micturition. [*Hb. Ts.*]

Frequent discharge of much watery urine (aft. 2, 6, 20 h.).

Lemon-coloured urine with white sediment (aft. 16 h.).

Cloudy urine.

395. Stiffness of the penis for some minutes (aft. ¼ h.).

* Comp. 246, 247, 248, 305.

† Alternating action with 368.

Stiffness of the penis every time he goes to stool.

During the urging to stool much mucus (prostatic fluid) escaped from the urethra (aft. 5 d.).

(Dark urine passes with burning sensation.)

Coarse stitches along the urethra when walking* (aft. 5 h.).

400. **Soon after dinner a stitch in the anterior part of the urethra, that ends in a tearing.**

In the middle of the urethra (when sitting in the evening) a scraping tearing pain (aft. 1 h.).

In the middle of the urethra a scratching scraping and scraping tearing pain (in the evening when lying in bed) (aft. 5 h.).

Creeping and burning in the urethra, especially when urinating, also combined with stitches. [*Hb. Ts.*]

An itching in the anterior part of the urethra (aft. 2 h.).

405. In the morning scalding of the urine (aft. 12 h.).

Violent, intermitting, racking, tearing aching pain in the root of the penis, especially when walking, which goes off when he stands leaning against the sacrum.

Along with flatulent distension of the abdomen, burning itching in the neck of the bladder, which excites the sexual desire.

In the very next night a great pollution (in a young man who scarcely ever had anything of the sort).

Itching all around the genitals and on the penis, in the evening after lying down, which goes off by scratching (aft. 3 h.).

410. Smarting burning in the anterior part of the urethra when urinating.

Smarting itching on the glans penis (aft. 4 and 20 h.).

Smarting itching pain on the inner surface of the prepuce (aft. 12 h.).

Sore pain as if excoriated on the seam of the prepuce (aft. 1 h.).

Excoriation and ulcerative pain combined with itching on the border of the prepuce (aft. 24 h.) (aft. 3 and 27 h.).[1]

415. (Spasmodic pain on the glans penis.)

Itching shooting on the scrotum as from innumerable fleas, especially when at rest.

Perspiration of the scrotum.

In the evening swelling of the scrotum (aft. 5 h.).

A rigid, strangling sensation in the testicles, in the evening after lying down in bed.

420. Aching in the testicles.

Lascivious, amorous fancies and rapid excitation of the sexual desire, with weakness of the genitals and impotence, and external disagreeable bodily heat.

Irresistible tendency to seminal emission, with soft penis (aft. 24 h.).

* Comp. 370, 371.

[1] There is an error in the numeration here. This symptom ought to be 414, and not 415 as numbered in the original.

Lasciviousness with impotence (aft. 10, 20 h.).

Lasciviousness with uncommon prominence of the clitoris, with weakness and relaxation of the other sexual parts, and cool temperature of the body (aft. 40 h.).

425. Impotence in the male, with feeling of weakness in the hips.

The penis is contracted so that it becomes quite small (after urinating).

The prepuce is retracted and the glans penis remains uncovered, as in impotence (aft. 24 h.).

Complete absence of sexual desire.*

Chronic leucorrhœa.

430. Promotion of the menstrual period.†[1] [BERGIUS, l. c.]

Violent spasmodic pressing together in the uterus, like labour-pains, followed by a purulent, eroding leucorrhœa.‡

Menstrual discharge in coagulated masses.

During the catamenia scanty but black blood of a putrid, nasty smell is discharged.

Catamenia retarded several days.§

* * *

435. In both nostrils a crawling itching.

Sensation of ulceration and soreness on the inner angle of one or both nostrils (aft. 12 h.).

The nostrils are ulcerated.

Tickling in the nose.

(Immediately epistaxis.)

440. First dropping from the nose, then coryza (aft. ½ h.).

Fluent coryza. [*Gss.*]

Stoppage of one nostrils as if a leaf obstructed it internally; not as from stuffed coryza.

Catarrh, stuffed coryza.

A feeling of catarrh on the chest; his air-tubes are full of mucus (aft. ¼ h.).

445. Hollow, dry cough, in the morning on waking from sleep.

In the evening after lying down, on going to sleep, irritation to cough (aft. 6 h).

In the evening after lying down, a (not tickling) constant irritation to short cough in the larynx, which does not go off by coughing, but rather by suppressing the cough (aft. 5 h.).

Very short, often quite dry cough, the irritation to which is in

* I have observed this alternating state with the lascivious symptoms 421—424 remain for a long time just like a secondary action; cocculus removed it.

† From the large dose of scruple. See note to 434.

‡ See note to 61.

§ Appears to be rare alternating action, if not secondary action. At all events, ignatia has in many cases often seemed to me to produce the opposite, namely, too early occurrence of the catamenia in its primary action, and hence has homoeopathically cured the too early (and too profuse) catamenia when the other symptoms corresponded.

1 Bergius merely says that the drug is emmenagogue. From Hahnemann's note it would seem that the latter thought him to refer to Camelli's observations, in which scruple doses were used; but this is doubtful.

the pit of the throat, as from feather dust being inhaled, that does not go off by coughing but which is renewed all the oftener the more he abandons himself to the cough, especially aggravated towards evening.

A sudden (not tickling) interruption of the breathing in the upper part of the trachea above the pit of the throat, which irresistibly excites to short violent cough, in the evening (aft. 1 h.).

450. A constricting sensation in the pit of the throat, which excites coughing as from sulphur vapour.*

(Every impulse of the cough causes a painful sensation in the penis, like a sudden penetration of blood into it.)

Difficult expectoration from the chest.

Yellow expectoration, smelling and tasting like old catarrh (aft. 12 h.).

Palpitation of the heart.[1] [*Hb. Ts.*]

455. Shooting in the cardiac region during expectoration (aft. ¼ h.).

Shooting in the left side (aft. ¼ and 3 h.).

Frequent stitches in the side of the chest, in the region of the last rib, when not breathing, synchronous with the pulse.

Single coarse stitches on the right side of the chest when not breathing, also on the tibia (aft. 1 h).

First aching in the left side of the chest, followed by fine shooting in the right side of the chest (aft. 1 h.).

460. Aching first in the left, then in the right side of the chest, then in the ankle-joint (aft. 1 h.).

Aching in the thoracic cavity, just behind the sternum. [*Hb. Ts.*]

A pressure in the region of the middle of the sternum, as with a sharp body† (aft. 20 h.).

An aching in the middle of the sternum soon after a meal (aft. 24 h.).

Along with oppression of the chest aching in the scrobiculus cordis, which is increased by inspiration and soon changes into stitches in the scrobiculus cordis (aft. 2 h.).

465. Oppression of the chest and respiration‡ (aft. 5 h.).

Tightness of the chest. [*Hb. Ts.*]

Feeling of anxiety and oppression of the chest wakes him at 12 o'clock at night from sleep ; he had to breathe often and deeply, and could only get to sleep after an hour. [*Hb. Ts.*]

Oppression of the chest after midnight, as if the chest were too narrow, whereby the respiration was impeded (aft. 12 h.).

On stooping forward a pain on the front of the chest, from both sides of the sternum, as if the ribs pushed together pressed painfully against one another (in the morning) (aft. 15 h.).

470. A tensive pain on the front of the chest when he raises himself straight up (when sitting) (aft. 16 h.).

* See note to 61.
† See note to 297.
‡ 465, 468, 472. See note to 61.

1 Other symptoms of the heart and circulation will be found from 741 to 748.

A tensive pain over the chest on standing upright (aft. 24 h.).

Aching and pressing on the chest (aft. 7 and 9 d.).

When walking his breath fails him, and when he stands still he gets a cough.

(When he shut his mouth he could get no air through the nose.).

475. Very exhausted in the whole body; when he walks he feels as if his breath would fail him, he becomes qualmish in the scrobiculus cordis and then he coughs.

Fulness in the chest.

Inspiration is impeded as by a weight lying upon him, expiration is all the easier.

Slow inspiration, quick expiration* (aft. 3 h.).

(Must often breathe deeply, and deep breathing momentarily diminished the pressure on the chest.)

480. Slow inspiration, for which he must heave up from the depths of the abdomen; (he must fetch his breath from low down in the body) (aft. 1 h.).

Short breathing alternates with longer, gentle with violent breathing† (aft. 2 h.).

Pain on the sternum, as if bruised, also excitable by touch (aft. 14 h.).

A throbbing on the right side of the chest (aft. 1½ h.).

On breathing deeply a stitch in the nipple, with flatulent movements in the abdomen (aft. 5 h.).

485. In the morning in bed, sharp pressive pain in the cervical vertebræ, when at rest.‡

Shooting in the nape.

Shooting tearing pain in the nape (aft. 2½ h.).

Tearing pain in the nape on moving the neck, as from a twist of the neck (aft. 12 h.).

Stiffness of the nape.

490. Heat and burning in the nape, or on one side of the neck, externally.

On the neck just above the left shoulder a painful pressure.§ [*Gss.*]

On the left, not far from the spinal column, where the true ribs are separated from the false, an obtuse shooting.‖

In the middle of the spinal column, rather towards the left side, a deep, tearing pain. [*Gss.*]

Aching shooting pain in the spinal column when walking in the open air.

495. Simple pain in the scapula increased by moving the arm and by letting it hang down (aft. 20 h.).

(In the morning some stitches at the apex of the scapula.)

A throbbing in the sacrum (aft. 7 h.).

* Alternating action with 656.
† Comp. 657.
‡ See note to 297.
§ Comp. 485.
‖ Comp. 494.

(In the sacrum (and on the chest) a tensive pain on standing upright) (aft 24 h.).

Stitches in the sacrum (aft. 48 h.).

500. **Pain in the sacrum, also when lying on the back, in the morning in bed.***

Aching bruised pain in the sacrum when lying on the back, in the morning in bed.

In the shoulder-joint pain as if dislocated when moving the arms.

In the joint of the humerus, when bending the arm back, a pain as from prolonged hard work, or as if bruised.

In the joint of the humerus a griping, clutching, beating and partly drawing pain when at rest (which becomes shooting on moving).†

505. In the joint of the humerus a rheumatic pain, or as if bruised, when walking in the open air (aft. 10 h.).

Pain in the humeral joint as if it were dislocated (aft. 10 h.).

In the deltoid muscle of the upper arm a quivering twitching. (aft. 24 h.).

On turning the arm inwards simple pain in the biceps muscle (aft. 2 h.).

In the muscles of the arm pain, as if bruised, when the arm hangs or is raised up.

510. The arm on the side he lies on goes to sleep (aft. 8 h.).

When lying on the right side, in the evening in bed, the head of the shoulder of the left side is painful as if bruised, and the pain goes away when he lies on the painful arm (aft. 12 h.).

Intolerable (indescribable) pain in the shafts of the bones and in the joints of the arm, on which he is not lying, in the evening in bed, which only goes off when he lies on the painful arm (aft. 12 h.).

Intolerable (indescrilable) pain in the shafts of the bones and in the joints of the arm on which he is lying, in the morning in bed, which only goes off when he lies on the other painless side‡ (aft. 20 h.).

In the morning in bed, pain as if bruised in the head of the shoulder of the side on which he lies, which goes off when he lies on the opposite side or on the back. (aft 24 h.).

515. In the evening after lying down, in one part of the muscles of the forearm, a twitching as if a mouse were crawling under the skin (aft. 36 h.).

Drawing pain in the arms.

* 500, 501. An alternating action with the disappearance of an ignatia symptom by lying on the back (see 19, 47, 48, 62, 5: 9, 600).

† Comp. 452.

‡ 513, 514 (and probably also 515) stand towards the symptoms 511, 512 as alternating states, and are both primary actions. Their difference seems to depend on the different periods of the day in which each chiefly manifests itself, evening and morning. Even the kind of pain appears to be different in each of these alternating states. See also 599, 601.

From the upper arm to the wrist and as far as the fingers a pulsating drawing.

From cold air (a chill ?) tearing in the right arm and on the right side of the head (aft. 12 h.).

Just above the right elbow painful drawing* (aft. 36 h.). [*Gss.*]

520. On the wrist tearing pain in the morning after waking.

On the wrist and in the fingers tearing pain.

In the thumb-joint tearing pain as if it were dislocated, in the morning while slumbering in bed.

A stiffness in the right wrist and sensation as if it were asleep.

In the carpal bones of the right hand a drawing† (aft. 36 h.). [*Gss.*]

525. On the left wrist a paralytic pain as if the hand were sprained or dislocated.

Some stitches in the last joint of the thumb (aft. 10 h.).

Itching pricks on the thumb-joint, which make him scratch.

In the proximal phalanx of the index finger pain as if it were dislocated, on moving.

Warm sweat on the inner surface of the hand fingers (aft. 16 h.).

530. Copious warm sweat of the hands, in the evening (aft. 8 h.).

Warm sweat of the palms (aft. 36 h.).

Transient yellowness of the hands, as from jaundice.

On touching a hair on the hand a penetrating, fine prick, as if a splinter were sticking there.‡

In the evening after lying down spasmodic movement hither and thither of the index finger.

535. On exerting the fingers, out-stretching cramp of the middle finger (which is relieved by stroking).

Shooting in the hip-joint (aft. 24 h.).

In the morning (from 4 to 8 o'clock), in the hip-joint and knee, shooting pain when walking and moving the legs (aft. 8 h.).

Almost paralytic immobility of the inferior extremities, with single twitchings in them.

In the morning on rising from bed, stiffness of the knees and ankle-joints, of the thigh and sacrum (aft. 38 h.).

540. When sitting, pain in the posterior muscles of the thigh, as if they were bruised (aft. 5 h).

On the centre of the thigh a deep violent pressure. [*Gss.*]

Violent shooting on the inner side below the left knee.§ [*Gss.*]

He could not walk and is forced to sit down, because when walking the knees are involuntarily drawn up (aft, ½ h.). [*Fr. H—n.*]

After going upstairs a stiffness in the knee-joint, which impedes her movement.

545. Stiffness of the knees and loins, which causes pain on movement.

As if stiff in the feet, in the morning (aft. 24 and 96 h.).

Boil on the inner side of the thigh (aft. 12 h.).

* Comp. 516, 518.

† Comp. 520, 521.

‡ Comp. 124.

§ Comp. 537.

After a meal, when sitting, the (thigh and) leg goes to sleep (aft. 5 h.).

Formication in the feet.*

550. Formication as if on the bones of the feet, not as if asleep (aft. 10 h.).

Fine pricking formication on the legs (the skin of the calves), after midnight, which does not permit him to rest or to remain in bed.

The legs to above the knee go to sleep in the evening when sitting.

In the whole of the left leg a paralytic pain, excited by walking, and continuing afterwards when sitting. [*Gss.*]

In the whole of the left leg painful drawing, in bed before going to sleep; it sometimes ceases, but returns all the more violently. [*Gss.*]

555. The leg goes to sleep when sitting at dinner (aft. 6 h.).

A tension in the legs to above the knee, with **heaviness of the limbs.**

A stretching† in the calves on extending the legs or walking.

Cramp of the calf when walking, which goes off when standing and when at rest‡ (aft. 4 h.).

Attacks of cramp in the muscles of the foot and toes, when sitting.

560. Attacks of cramp in the calf when sitting at dinner.

Cramp in the calf quite early in bed, on flexing the limb, which goes off on extending the limb or pressing against something (aft. 8 h.).

Intermittent shooting on the inner border of the foot (aft. 5 h.). [*Gss.*]

Above the right outer ankle intermittent pressure. [*Gss.*]

In the right foot violent drawing. [*Gss.*]

565. In the ball of the heel a numbness (as if asleep) when walking.

In the ball of the heel or rather in the periosteum of the astragalus, a pain as if contused, or as from a jump from a great height (aft. 3 h.).

In the ball of the heel or rather in the periosteum of the os calcis pain when walking as from internal soreness (aft. 4 h.).

Aching pain in the tibia when walking (aft. 2 h.).

In the anterior tibial muscles an undulating, as it were griping and beating, tearing aching pain, especially on moving.

570. Aching in the left ankle-joint (with an internal tickle) which forced him to make a trembling movement of the left foot in order to get relief.

In the ankle-joint, in the morning, when walking, pain as from dislocation§ (but not shooting).

* 549 551 (and again 548), and 552, 555 constitute three different alternating states.

† A kind of cramp, or, at least, the commencement thereof.

‡ 558 is alternating action with 559—561; both apparently of the same rank.

§ Comp. 506.

On the dorsum of the foot a tearing pain (aft. 20 h.).

Internally in the ball of the heel, are itching twitching pain, especially in the morning in bed.

Tearing burning pain in the heel bone, in the morning on waking (aft. 8 h.).

575. On the dorsum of the foot a spot the seat of burning itching pain when at rest.

Burning pain in the corn when sitting.

Burning pain on pressure in a hitherto painless corn on the foot.

The shoes press painfully on the upper part of the toes; corns commence to have burning pain.

An itching burning (as from chilblains) in the heel and other parts of the foot (aft. 8 h.).

580. On the side of the foot burning shooting, or burning cutting pain.

Shooting pain under the ankle on moving.

Early in the morning several stitches in the heel (aft. 20 h.).

In the dusk of the evening weariness of the feet as from a long walk, with quiet disposition.

Could not drag the feet along, as if he had walked a long way.

585. Heaviness of the feet.*

Heaviness of one foot.

Weakness of the feet.

Creaking and cracking in the knees (aft. 2 h.).

Coldness of the feet and legs to above the knee.

590. Chill about the knee, that is not cold externally.

Hot knees (with tickling itching of one knee) **with cold nose** (aft. 3 h.).

(Stiffness of the ankle-joint.)

Painful sensitiveness of the soles when walking (aft. 4 h.).

Feet are burning hot.

595. A creeping as if internally in the bones of the whole body.

Creeping, gone-to-sleep feeling in the limbs† (aft 4 h. several times).

Weariness of the legs and arms.

Sensation of weakness and exhaustion in the arms and legs.

Here and there in the periosteum in the middle of the shafts of the bones (not in the joints) a transient pressure, as with a hard body, like contused pain, by day, but especially when lying on one side or the other, in the evening in bed, that goes off by lying on the back‡ (aft. 20, 36 h.).

600. At night on one or the other side, on which he is lying, pain as if bruised, in the joints of the neck, back, and shoulders, which only goes off when lying on the back (aft. 12 h.).

In the joints of the shoulders, hip and knees, a pain as from a sprain or dislocation (aft. 8 h.).

* Comp. 556.

† Comp. 548, 550, 555.

‡ 599, 600, and comp. 19, 47, 48, 62, in which the pain only goes off when lying on the k, constitute a third alternating action with 513, 514, and with 511 and 512.

About the joints or somewhat above them, a continued shooting pain.

A deep shooting burning pain on various parts,* without itching.

In the external elevated parts of the joints, a burning shooting pain accompanied by itching (aft. 1 h.).

605. In the evening on going to sleep, jerks and twitches through the whole body† (aft. 96 h.).

Jerks and single twitchings of the limbs (aft. 10, 12 h.).

Single twitchings of the limbs when going to sleep (aft. 3 h.).

After lying down twitching and quivering in single muscular parts, here and there on the body (aft. 2 h.).[1]

Innumerable fine stitches here and there, like flea-bites (especially in bed).‡

610. Itching here and there on the body, after getting somewhat heated by walking in the open air.

In the evening, after lying down in bed, itching here and there, which readily goes off by scratching.§

Itching here and there in the body, under the shoulder, &c., at night, which goes off by scratching.

Itching on the wrist-joint, on the elbow-joint, and on the neck.

The outer skin and the periosteum are painful (aft. 8 h.).

615. Sensitiveness of the skin to a draught of air ; he feels in the abdomen as if he should get a chill (aft. 4 h.).

Simple violent pain, only felt when touched, here and there, on a small spot, e.g. on the ribs, &c.

The symptoms of ignatia are aggravated by drinking coffee and smoking tobacco.

Burning in the ulcer.

Renewal of the pains immediately after dinner, immediately after lying down in the evening, and immediately after waking in the morning.

620. Leaves a tendency to swelling of the cervical glands, toothache, and looseness of the teeth, as also to stomachache.

Great general weariness from slight movement.

Is unwilling to move, shirks work.

Exhaustion, weariness, in the evening.

When walking in the open air a heaviness in the legs, with anxiety, which went off in the room, but depression of spirits came on instead.

625. The knees gave way under him from weakness.

Exhaustion and lassitude after dinner ; he felt unfit for his usual work, and contrary to custom fell asleep over it. [*Hb. Ts.*]

* *e. g.* on the corner of the mouth, under the first joint of the thumb, &c.

† 605, 607, comp. with 608, 665, 667.

‡ Comp. 604 and the alternating action 603.

§ 611, 612. Characteristic of ignatia is the itching *which is readily removed from the part by slight scratching.*

---

1 Another error in the enumeration of the symptoms occurs here in the original.

Discomfort in the morning after getting up (the 2nd d.). [*Hb. Ts.*]

Exhaustion in the limbs. [*Hb. Ts.*]

Great exhaustion and weariness, he felt as if he had had a very long walk. [*Hb. Ts.*]

630. Exhaustion, as from a weakness about the scrobiculus cordis ; he became qualmish ; he must lie down.*

So tired that he has no wish to dress himself and go out ; he has no pleasure in anything, prefers to lie down (aft. 4 h.).

Staggers when walking, readily falls and stumbles over the least thing that lies in his way.†

Weariness as if his eyelids would close.

He becomes very sleepy on hearing sad news.

635. He falls asleep when sitting reading (aft. 4 h.).

Drowsiness, which invites him to sleep when sitting ; but on lying down there ensues a half-waking, dreamful sleep (aft. $\frac{1}{4}$ h.).

Very profound and yet not refreshing sleep.‡

Profound sleep§ (aft. 3 h.).

Sleeplessness.

640. Frequent yawning. [*Hb. Ts.*]

Inclination to sleep. [*Hb. Ts.*]

Early sleepiness in the evening. [*Hb. Ts.*]

Drowsiness after dinner, and deep, sound, unrefreshing afternoon sleep for two hours ; after waking feeling of exhaustion. [*Hb. Ts.*]

Sound and continued sleep, from which he wakes still tired. [*Hb. Ts.*]

645. Uncommonly sound but not refreshing midday sleep. [*Hb. Ts.*]

Restless sleep. [*Hb. Ts.*]

Sleeplessness ; cannot go to sleep, and awakes (at night) from no perceptible cause (aft. 14 h.).

Sleep so light that he hears everything in it, *e.g.* the striking of a clock at a great distance.

In the evening in bed flatulent colic : a kind of pressure in the abdomen here and there, recurring every time he wakes at night.

650. In the night in bed he often changes his position, lies sometimes in one place sometimes in another.

Moaning talking in sleep ; he tosses about in bed ‖ (aft. 2, 5, h.).

Stamps with his feet in sleep¶ (aft. 4 h.).

He moves the mouth in sleep, as if he were eating (aft. 3 h.).

In sleep she moves the muscles of the open mouth in all directions, almost convulsively, and at the same time the hands are twitched inward (aft. 2 h.).

655. In sleep, groaning, grunting, sighing (aft. 4 h.).

* Comp. 267, 335.

† Comp. 754.

‡ He thinks he has not slept at all when he awakes.

§ 637, 638 constitute alternating actions with 639, 647, 648.

‖ Comp. 652.

¶ Comp. 662.

During sleep short inspiration* and slow expiration.

During sleep all kinds of breathing, alternately short and slow, violent and gentle, suspended, snoring.†

In the evening in bed, feeling as of an ebullition in the blood, on account of which he could not get to sleep.

During sleep snoring inspiration.

660. Lies in sleep on the back and lays the open hand under the occiput.

In the morning he lies on the back and puts one arm above the head so that the outspread hand comes to lie under the occiput or in the nape.

Starts up suddenly in sleep, moans with piteous expression of countenance, kicks and stamps with the feet, the hands and face being at the same time pale and cold.

Dreams full of sadness ; he wakes up weeping.

Talks in a lachrymose and complaining manner in sleep ; inspiration is snoring with quite open mouth, and sometimes one eye sometimes the other is slightly opened (aft. 10 h.).

665. Startings in affright, when about to go to sleep, on account of monstrous visions which present themselves to him, and hover before him after waking.‡

In the morning at the instant of waking he feels a heaviness, an accumulation, stagnation and ebullition of blood in the body, with sadness.

Starting in affright, in the morning, on waking out of a sleep so light that he hears every stroke of the clock.

Dreams full of frightful things.

Awakes with sulky expression.

670. Awakes with cheerful countenance (aft. 20 h.).

Awakes in the morning on account of horrible dreams (aft. 18 h.).

On awaking she rises up suddenly and talks nonsense before she comes to herself (aft. 4 h.).

(She dreams she is standing, but not standing firmly ; when awake she examines her bed to see if she is lying firmly, and curls herself up, in order to be sure not to fall ; at the same time she is always in some perspiration all over.)

Awakes on account of horrible dreams (*e. g.* of drowning) from the afternoon sleep (aft. 24 h.).

675. Dreams at night, that he has fallen into the water and weeps.

At night dreams full of disappointed and miscarried expectations and endeavours.

Fixed idea in dream : dreams all night of one and the same subject.

Dreams of the same subject for several hours.

Dreams with reflection and consideration (aft. 4 h.).

680. Slumbering dreams before midnight, with general heat, without perspiration.

* 656 in alternation with 479, 480.

† Comp. 481,

‡ 665, 667, comp. with 605, 607 (608).

At night general anxious heat with slight sweat round about the nose, the greatest heat on the hands and feet, which however he dislikes being uncovered but will always have covered, with cold thighs, palpitation of the heart, short breath and lascivious dreams; chiefly when he lies on either side, less when he lies on the back.

From 2 to 5 a.m. (while wide awake) heat all over, especially on the hands and feet, without sweat and without thirst, and without feeling of dryness.

He perspires every morning, when after previous waking he goes to sleep again, and when he gets up he is so tired and unrefreshed that he feels disposed to lie down again.[1]

At night dreams full of learned mental exercitations and scientific discussions.

685. Dreams which are a strain on the thinking power, towards morning (aft. 10 h.).

Nocturnal phantasies which strain the thinking power.

In dreams the thoughts are engaged on one subject all night through; a fixed idea, which does not leave him even after waking.

Tonic spasm of all the limbs, like stiffness.

Very frequent yawning (aft. $\frac{1}{4}$ h.).

690. Great yawning, even during a meal.

Frequent yawning after sleep.

Excessive yawning, in the morning (and chiefly after the midday sleep), as if the jaw would be dislocated.

Extreme convulsive yawning, so that the eyes run over with water, in the evening before going to sleep, and in the morning after rising from bed (aft. 28, 38 h.).

Frequent yawning interrupted by a kind of immobility and unyielding condition of the chest (between 8 and 10 o'clock).

695. In the afternoon and evening thirst.

During the febrile chill thirst.

Dreads the open air (aft. 6 h.).

In moderately cold though not open air he gets immoderate chilliness, and becomes cold all over, with semilateral headache (aft 4 h.).

Coldness and chilliness; the pupils dilate but little.

700. Chilliness and cold, especially on the posterior part of the body; but both can be dispelled immediately by a warm room or a warm stove* (aft. 6 h.).

Chill in the back and over the arms (aft. $\frac{1}{4}$ h.).

Rigor in the face and on the arms, with chattering of the teeth and goose-skin.

Becomes chilly at sunset (heat goes out of him).

Shivering with goose-skin over the thighs and forearms; afterwards also on the cheeks (immediately).

705. Chilliness, especially on the feet.

In the period of apyrexia, constant shivering.

* The febrile coldness removable by external warmth of ignatia is characteristic.

---

1 Another error of enumeration in the original occurs here.

Heat of the face with coldness of feet and hands.*

Chilliness over the upper arms with hot ears.

Heat of the hands, with shivering over the body and an anxiety terminating in weeping.

710. Along with redness of the face in the evening shaking shivering.

(After a meal chilliness and shaking shivering; at night anxiety and sweat.)

Fever, first chilliness over the arms, especially the upper arms, then heat and redness of the cheeks and heat of hands and feet, without thirst, whilst lying on the back.

In the afternoon, fever: shivering with bellyache; thereafter weakness and sleep with burning heat of the body.

One ear and one cheek are red and burning.

715. **Sudden attack of flying heat all over the body.**

The external temperature is increased.

External heat and redness, without internal heat.†

Feeling of general heat, in the morning in bed, without thirst, during which he does not like to throw off the clothes.

Nocturnal heat, during which he wishes the bed-clothes taken off, and allows himself to be uncovered.

720. Heat of the body, especially during sleep.

In the afternoon thirstless heat in the whole body, with a feeling of dryness of the skin, but with some sweat on the face (aft. 8 h.).

Heat mounts to the head, without thirst.

From internal restlessness, increased internal heat and thirst, disturbed sleep. [*Hb. Ts.*]

At 2 a.m. groaning from external heat, desires fewer bed-clothes (aft. 15 h.).

725. **External warmth is intolerable to him**; then quick breathing.

Feeling as if sweat would break out (anxious feeling of flying heat) (aft. 1½ h.).

Feeling as if sweat would all at once break out over the whole body, which did occur partially, in the forenoon.

General sweat.

Profuse perspiration.[1] [GRIMM, l. c.]

730. Cold sweats. [BERGIUS, l. c.]

Violent anxiety about the scrobiculus cordis, with vertigo, fainting, and very cold sweats.‡ [CAMELLI,[2] *Philos. Transact.*, vol. xxi, No. 250.]

* 707—710 single alternating states of the chief symptoms, namely, the heat of particular parts, with coldness, chilliness or shivering of other parts.

† 717, 718. The heat of ignatia is hardly ever anything but external; moreover, there is hardly ever any thirst accompanying it, not even when it occurs in the form of an intermittent fever. Hence ignatia in the smallest dose can only homœopathically and permanently cure those agues which have thirst during the chill but none during the heat.

‡ From a whole bean.

1 After bleeding and antidotes.

2 Observations of effects of scruple doses.

Trembling for several hours.

Trembling all over the body.* [BERGIUS, l. c.]

Trembling of the whole body for three hours, with itching and frightful convulsive twitchings (vellicationibus), so that he could hardly keep up on his legs; they were strongest in the jaws, so that the mouth is distorted as though he were laughing (immediately). [CAMELLI, l. c.]†

735. Constant moving of the body (agitatio continua).‡ [GRIMM, l. c.]

Convulsive movements. [BERGIUS, l. c.]

Convulsions. [DURIUS,[1] *Miss. Nat. Cur.*, Dec. iii, ann. 9, 10, Obs. 126.]

Insensibility of the whole body. [GRIMM, l. c.]

Syncope.[2] [GRIMM, l. c.]

740. The variety of pressure on and in several parts of the head at the same time makes him sullen and cross. [*Gss.*]

Palpitation of the heart.

Very moderate acceleration of the pulse. [*Hb. Ts.*]

Acceleration of the circulation, during which, however, the pulse had a small beat. [*Hb. Ts.*]

Pulse slower and smaller than usual in the first hours of the afternoon. [*Hb. Ts.*]

745. On thinking deeply, palpitation of the heart.

During dinner, palpitation of the heart (aft. 48 h).

After the (midday) sleep, palpitation of the heart (aft. 5 h.).

In the morning in bed he gets hot and has palpitation of the heart

Anxiety as if he had done something bad.

750. Anxiety of short duration (aft. ¼ h.).

Anxiety.§ [GRIMM, l. c.]

Goes about quite perplexed, dazed, stupefied.‖ [GRIMM, l. c.]

Extreme anxiety, which prevents speaking.

After exertion of the head, especially in the morning, a hurry of the will; he cannot express himself in talking, write, or do anything as quickly as he wishes; whereby there occurs an anxious behaviour, he makes mistakes in speaking and writing, and does everything awkwardly¶ and needs to be corrected (aft. 20 h.).

755. Excessively busy: he restlessly sets about doing first one thing then another.

Obtuseness of senses, with tendency to hurry; when he makes haste the blood mounts into his face (aft. 6 h.).

* Comp. 732.
† From a scruple.
‡ From a drachm.
§ Comp. 749, 750, 753.
‖ Comp. 782, 783, 786, 787, 788.
¶ Comp. 757.

---

1 No mention of any pathogenetic effects of I. here; it is simply reported as antiepileptic.

2 This symptom properly belongs to Bergius, and is not found in Grimm's narrative.

He imagines he cannot get on, cannot walk.
She fears she will get an ulceration of the stomach.
Fearfulness, cowardice, cannot trust himself to do anything, considers all is lost.

760. On awaking, after midnight, has fear of thieves (aft. 10 h.).
Uncommon tendency to be frightened.
Fears every trifle, is especially afraid of objects coming near him* (aft. 1 h.).
Audacity (aft. 3, 5 h.).
Slight blame or contradiction excites him to quarrel, and he is vexed at himelf for doing so (aft. 36 h.).

765. From slight contradiction he is irritated and angry (aft. 8 h.).
From slight contradiction his face gets red.
Quickly passing crossness and anger.
Towards evening he is discontented, sulky, stubborn, no one can do anything right, anything to please him (aft. 8 h.).
Is extremely sulky ; finds fault and makes reproaches

770. **Fickle, impatient, irresolute, quarrelsome** (recurring every 3, 4 h.).
Incredible changeableness of disposition, at one time he jokes and jests, at another he is lachrymose (alternately every 3, 4 h.).
Some hours after the angry humour jocularity comes on (aft. 6 h.).
Jesting, childish tricks (aft. 8 h.).
Desires improper things, and weeps aloud when they are denied him.

775. When one hesitates in the least to do what she wishes, or remonstrates much with her, though in a mild and friendly manner, or endeavours to persuade her, or wishes differently from what she wishes, she weeps aloud (aft. 1 h.).
Howling and crying, and beside herself about trifles (aft. 1 h.).
Unreasonable complaints about too much noise (aft. 2 h.).
Noise is intolerable to him, and then the pupils dilate more readily (aft. 6 h.).
Whispering low voice ; he cannot speak loudly.

780. Loss of the usual cheerfulness (2nd d.). [*Hb. Ts.*]
Loss of the usual liveliness, in the afternoon. [*Hb. Ts.*]
Avoids opening the mouth and speaking ; laconic (aft. 1 to 4 h.).
Is as if in slumber ; he dislikes opening the eyes to look, and the mouth to speak, with low, slow respiration.
A kind of apathy in the whole body (2nd d.). [*Hb. Ts.*]

785. Indifference to everything (2nd d.), [*Hb. Ts.*]
Quiet, serious melancholy ; cannot be induced to converse or be cheerful, with flat, watery taste of all food and small appetite (aft. 24 h.).
Quiet reserve, internally disposed to anger and irritable (aft. ½ h.).

* 762, 763 alternating states.

Sits to all appearance in deep thought, and looks staringly in front of him, but is all the time quite destitute of thought* (aft. 2 h.).

Fixed ideas, *e. g*, about music and melodies, in the evening, before and after lying down.

790. A fixed idea, which he follows out in thought, or pursues all too zealously and completely in conversation (aft. 2 h.).

Thinks against his will of annoying, vexatious things, and dwells on them (aft. ½ h.).

Delicate disposition, with very clear consciousness.

Sensitive disposition, delicate conscientiousness (aft. 20 h.).

Sad (towards evening).[1]

* 788 forms, as a rare condition, alternating action with the following symptoms.

---

1 The number of the symptoms given above does not correspond with those in the original (which are 795 in number). The reason of this is that in the original there are several errors in the enumeration from S. 415 onwards. There are also a few clerical errors, which have been corrected in the translation. The second edition has been of use in enabling these corrections to be made.

IPECACUANHA.[1]

(The alcoholic tincture of the root of *Cephaelis Ipecacuanha*, WILLD., from Brazil.).

It will be seen from the following symptoms, though they are not complete, that this powerful plant was not created merely for the purpose of causing a forcible evacuation of the stomach by vomiting (which *in most casss* is to be reckoned as one of the useless cruelties of ordinary practice), but that far higher and more important curative objects are attainable by its means. It was originally brought to Europe as a remedy for autumnal dysenteries, and hence it received the name of the dysentery-root. One hundred and twenty years have elapsed since it was, on Leibnitz's recommendation, misused for this purpose, on the false indication that because it relieves some kinds of diarrhœa it must therefore cure dysenteries, for these maladies are the exact opposite of diarrhœa, *i.e.* of too frequent loose motion. It is only quite lately that this practice has been abandoned, because on extensive employment of it for many years in dysenteries has shown that it is of no use in these affections. All these unfortunate trials, whereby many lives have been sacrificed, might have been spared if the pure peculiar action of this root had first been ascertained, and it had been learnt what morbid states it was capable of originating in the healthy subject, and consequently what similar states in the naturally sick it could remove and cure. It would have been seen, as is now seen from the following symptoms of ipecacuanha, that it, by similarity of action, can only diminish the excess of blood in the dysenteric stools and allay some kinds of abdominal pains in dysentery, but that it cannot remove the other far more important phenomena of this disease, because it cannot produce anything similar.

On the other hand, we may learn from its symptoms that, as it can relieve some cases of tendency to vomit similar to its own, so it must, as experience has shown, exert a specific curative action more particularly in hæmorrhages, in paroxysmal, spasmodic dyspnœa and suffocative spasms, and also in some kinds of tetanus (provided that in all these affections the other symptoms of the patient are met with of a similar character among those of ipecacuanha).

Certain kinds of agues are so constituted that this root is their appropriate remedy, as is to be inferred from its own symptoms, in so far as they present a greater homœopathic similarity to those of the case of ague than do those of other medicines. If the selection has not been quite

---

1 From vol. iii, 2nd edit., 1825.

suitable for this purpose it generally leaves the fever in a state in which arnica (in other cases china, ignatia, or cocculus) is the remedy.

Some after-sufferings from the unsuitable employment of arsenic and from the long-continued abuse of cinchona-bark may be removed by a few doses of ipecacuanha.

In all these cases of the homœopathic therapeutic employment of this root only very small doses are indicated. Hitherto I have employed the diluted tincture in the dose of a drop containing the millionth part of a grain of ipecacuanha, but I have seen, from the often unnecessarily strong action of this dose in many cases, that for homœopathic employment the dose should be still further diminished, care being, of course, taken that all other foreign and medicinal influences are avoided.

It is only when we have to treat serious poisoning by a large dose of opium that we must administer a large dose of ipecacuanha (30, 40, 60 drops of the strong tincture)—when the circumstances do not rather demand the administration of strong coffee (or camphor).

Ipecacuanha acts for but a short time ; in large doses hardly a couple of days, in quite small doses about a couple of hours.

[HAHNEMANN was assisted in this proving by LANGHAMMER, J. G. LEHMANN, STAPF.

The following old-school authorities are cited :

CLARKE, in *Murray's Apparat. Med.*, i.

CLEGHORN, *Diseases of Minorca.*

FOTHERGILL, *Medic. Obs. and Inqu.*, vi.

GEOFFROY, *Traite de la Mat. Med.*, ii.

GMELIN, EBERH., *Untersuch. ub. d. Thier. Magnetismus*, Heilbr., 1793.

HALLER, in *Hufel. Journ.*, xxvii, I.

HILLARY, *Air and diseases of Barbadoes.*

LEMERY, *Traite univ. des drog. simpl.*

MURRAY, *Medic. pr. Biblioth.*, iii.

PYE, S., in *Medic. Bemerk. und Unters.*, i.

SCOTT, W., in *Edinb. Med. Comment.*, iv.

In the *Frag. de Vir.*, Ipecacuanha has 83 symptoms, in the 1st edit. 231 ; only two more symptoms are added to this 2nd edit.]

IPECACUANHA.

Vertigo when walking.

Vertigo as if he would stagger hither and thither, with vanishing of thoughts for instants, only when walking, and especially when turning round (aft. 2 h.). [*Stf.*]

(In the evening) when walking in the open air a swaying of the body to and fro towards both sides, as from intoxication, with stupefaction of the head (aft. 10 h.). [*Lr.*]

Severe shooting pain in the crown of the head.

5. In short fits a fine and severe shooting headache, which in an hour changes to an aching (aft. 8 h.).

Fine shooting pain in the forehead, which is excited and increased by touching.

A violent tearing pain in the forehead, increased by stooping (aft. 31 h.). [*Ln.*]

External pain on the parietal bone of the head as from a blow with a blunt point (aft. $\frac{1}{2}$ h.).

Painful heaviness in the head (aft. 2 h.). [*Stf.*]

10. Heaviness in the head with drowsiness. [*Ln.*]

Headache : shooting and heaviness.

Tearing pain in the forehead which is excited and aggravated by touching the part.

In the morning after rising from bed tearing headache till noon, less in the afternoon (aft. 31 h.). [*Ln.*]

Headache as if the brain and skull were bruised, which penetrates through all the bones of the head down to the root of the tongue, with nausea.

15. Aching pain in the head.

Tensive headache.

A dull drawing here and there in the head (immediately). [*Ln.*]

(Constrictive pain in the left temple and above the orbit) (aft. 1 h.).

An outpressing and almost boring pain, sometimes in the temples, sometimes over the orbit on a small spot, which goes off by external pressure, and is alleviated by shutting the eyes (aft. 1 h.).

20. Tensive aching pain in the occiput and nape, which extends to the shoulders (aft. 3 h.). [*Stf.*]

Painfulness of the occiput and nape, excited by moving the head (aft. $2\frac{1}{2}$ h.). [*Stf.*]

On stooping severe stitches above the eye, with a feeling as if it were swollen (aft. 20 h.).

Pale face with blue rings round the eyes and great weakness, as after recovery from a severe illness.

(Miliary rash on the forehead up in among the hair and on the cheeks.)

25. **Pupils more readily dilatable** (aft. 8 h.).

Dilatation of the pupils (aft. $2\frac{1}{2}$ h.). [*Lr.*]

Dryness of the eyelids with drowsiness (aft. 8 h.).

Eye-gum in the outer canthi of the eyes (aft. $7\frac{1}{2}$ and 12 h.). [*Lr.*]

Red, inflamed eyes. [W. Scott,[1] in *Edinb. Med. Comment*, iv, p. 74.]

30. Inflammation of the eyes. [Geoffroy,[2] *Traite de la Mat. Med.*, ii, p. 157.]

Aching pain from the concha of the ear to the membrana tympani, which extends to the protuberance of the occiput (aft. 28 h.). [*Ln.*]

Dulness of hearing of the right ear, with aching in it. [*Ln.*]

---

1 Effects of emanations in a sensitive woman. The original is "eyes a little inflamed."

2 Accidents liable to happen to those who powder the drug.

Epistaxis. [MURRAY,[1] *Medic. pr. Biblioth.*, iii, p. 237—GEOFFROY, l. c.—LEMERY,[*2] *Traite univ. des drog. simpl.*, p. 438.]

Sensation of heat in the cheeks, also perceptible externally, but without redness (aft. 3 h.). [*Stf.*]

35. Lips externally covered with eruption. [HELLER,[3] in *Hufel. Journal*, xxvii, i, p. 51.]

Lips covered with aphthæ and eruption. [HELLER, l. c.]

Smarting on the borders of the lips, the tip of the tongue, and the sides of the tongue, with flow of watery saliva into the mouth and some pain in the abdomen (aft. ½ h.). [*Stf.*]

A smarting sensation on the lips.

In the corners of the lips sensation as if they were excoriated, on touching and moving the lips.

40. Very violent pain in the hollow tooth when biting, immediately, as if it were pulled out, causing loud howling and crying out, and thereafter constant tearing in it (aft. 1 h.).

A pain in the teeth as if they were pulled out, in fits (aft. 8 h.).

Excessive and almost painful sensitiveness of all parts in the mouth.

A smarting sensation on the border of the tongue.

On the back part of the tongue and on the palate a sensation as from chewing hepatica or tarragon, which excites great secretion of saliva.

45. He must constantly swallow the saliva (aft. 1 h.).

Great flow of saliva for some hours.

When lying the saliva pours from the mouth.

Flow of saliva. [S. PYE,[4] in *Med. Bemerk. und Unters.*, i, p. 244—HELLER, l. c.]

Great collection of saliva in the mouth (aft. 2½ h.). [*Ln.*]

50. Obtuse stitches across the throat into the inner ear.

Spasmodic contractive sensation in the throat and on the chest. [SCOTT, l. c.]

Sore throat. [GEOFFROY, l. c.]

A fine pricking in the œsophagus (aft. ½, 1 h.).

Pain on swallowing as if there were a swelling at the top of the gullet (aft. 1 h.).

55. Dryness and roughness in the mouth, especially in the top of the gullet (aft ½ h.).

* From the powder snuffed up into the nose.

---

1 Not accessible.

2 From taking I. in large doses of powder, obviated by moistening it, *i. e.* local irritation.

3 Effects when given in chronic agues. The subject of nearly all the symptoms extracted by Hahnemann had had six paroxysms already ; his face was yellow, and the præcordia tender.

4 After ineffectual attempts at vomiting. The work Hahnemann quotes from is a German translation of the *Medical Observations and Enquiries*. The symptoms have been compared with the English original.

Difficulty of swallowing, as from paralysis of the tongue and gullet (aft. 8 h.).

Pain in the gullet, as if it were too dry and rough and sore, which is allayed for a short time only by swallowing the saliva or ordinary liquids (aft. 1 h.).

Adipsia.

Flat taste in the mouth.

60. Whilst swallowing a taste in the throat as from rancid oil (aft. $\frac{1}{4}$ h.).

Beer tastes flat (aft. 2 h.).

The (accustomed) tobacco tastes nauseous when smoked and excites vomiting. [*Ln.*]

Immediately after the (accustomed) tobacco-smoking a nausea arising from the stomach, with hiccup, which only went off after several stools, the last of which were pappy (aft. 14 h.). [*Lr.*]

After eating yawning and stretching.

65. He is sick, qualmish, squeamish. [*Stf.*]

Loathing, nausea and heaving as if he would vomit (aft. $1\frac{1}{4}$ h.). [*Ln.*]

Troublesome nausea. [CLARKE,[1] in ***Murray's Appar. Med.***, i, p. 814.]

Sickness and vomiting.

(Nausea and heaviness in the abdomen.)

70. **Nausea as from the stomach, with empty eructation and great flow of saliva** (aft. $\frac{1}{2}$ h.). (*Lr.*]

Eructation every eight or ten minutes, also the following day, with grumbling in the abdomen. [*Ln.*]

On stooping vomiting and sensation as if he must fall down. [*Ln.*]

On stooping vomiting of the food he had eaten, without previous eructation (aft. $1\frac{1}{2}$ h.). [*Ln.*]

Vomiting of a yellow slimy mass. [HALLER, l. c., p. 54.]

75. Vomiting of large masses of mucus. [HELLER, l. c., p. 57.]

Vomiting of large fœtid lumps of mucus. [HELLER, l. c., p. 54.]

Vomiting of green gelatinous mucus. [HELLER, l. c., p. 51.]

Vomiting of grass-green mucus. [HELLER, l. c., p. 52.]

Sensation as if the stomach hung down loosely, with want of appetite (aft. 1 h.).

80. Sensation of emptiness and relaxation of the stomach.

Most violent pain in the stomach. [HELLER, l. c., p. 53.]

Horrible pains in the stomach. [HELLER, l. c., p. 57.]

Indescribable pain about the heart (scrobiculus cordis ?) [HELLER, l. c., 54.]

An obtuse shooting pain in the scrobiculus cordis, as with a pointed piece of wood. [*Ln.*]

85. Qualmishness in the abdomen, with commencing bellyache. [*Ln.*]

---

1 Effects of I. when given in dysentery without relief.

Uneasiness in the abdomen (aft. $\frac{1}{2}$ h.).
Contractive sensation under the short ribs.
Severe stitches in the left hypochondrium (aft. $\frac{1}{2}$ h.).
Feeling of extreme distension and swelling of the abdomen.

90. Flatulent colic.

A clutching pinching in the abdomen, as if grasped by the hand, so that each extended finger made a sharp impression on the bowels, alleviated by bodily rest, but aggravated to the highest degree by the slightest movement.

Pinching pain in both hypochondria and in the region of the scrobiculus cordis (aft. 3 h.).

Cutting pain about the navel, with shivering.

Cutting pain at the side in the umbilical region, which is aggravated by the touch and by external pressure, with white, frothy saliva in the mouth and dilated pupils (aft. $\frac{1}{8}$ h.).

95. Cutting pain about the navel, as if the menses were about to come on, with chilliness and coldness of the body, whilst internal heat rises to the head (aft. 2 h.).

Tearing pains above the navel.

Violent shooting in the right flank of the abdomen for some minutes. [*Ln.*]

(Shooting pains in the abdomen, and burning and shooting in the rectum, with urging to stool.)

(Leek-green stools.)

100. Grass-green stools. [HELLER, l. c., p. 53.]

(Lemon-coloured stools.)

(Thin stool, with burning shooting pain in the rectum and anus.)

Frequent fluid stools, with qualmish feeling in the abdomen. [*Ln.*]

Purging. [MURRAY, l. c.]

105. **Diarrhœic and, as it were, fermented stools** (aft. 1 h.).

Putrid smelling stools.

Fæces covered with red, bloody mucus.

Bloody stool. [SCOTT, l. c.]

Crawling in the anus, as if thread-worms would come out. [*Ln.*]

110. Shooting, cutting, burning pain on the border of the anus, as in obstinate hæmorrhoids (aft. $\frac{3}{4}$ h.).

Severe stitches in the anus.

Frequent call to urinate with scanty discharge of urine (aft. 2, $2\frac{1}{2}$ h.). [*Lr.*]

(Frequent micturition of straw-coloured urine, which, before the discharge, is preceded by great urging and burning, not followed by urinary tenesmus) (aft. 2 h.). [*Stf.*]

Scanty red urine.*

115. Bloody urine. [SCOTT, l. c.]

Urine cloudy, with sediment-like brick-dust. [HELLER, l. c., pp. 51, 65.]

* See 149.

(From the child's urethra there flows for several days a purulent fluid, with smarting pain.)

When standing a voluptuous itching on the glans penis, compelling scratching (aft. 3½ h.). [*Lr.*]

A twisting, drawing pain in the testicles (aft. 8, 10 h.).

120. On crossing the thighs a shooting in the testicles (aft. 2 h.). [*Lr.*]

An urging and pressing towards the womb and anus.

Metrorrhagia—recurrence of the catamenia that had ceased fourteen days previously.[1] [SCOTT, l. c.]

The blood coming away at the end of the catamenia was suppressed.*

* * *

Violent, repeated sneezing. [*Ln.*]

125. Like dry coryza in the nose, as if the nasal cavity were too dry. (aft. 3 h.).

Sensation of dryness in the nose and frontal sinuses (aft. 3 h.).

Coryza, with drawing pains in all the limbs.

Rattling noise in the bronchial tubes on drawing breath.

In the forenoon an oppression on the chest and short breath, as if he were in much dust, on account of which he could not breathe.

130. Tightness of the chest. [MURRAY, l. c.]

Tightness of the chest.

Tightness of the chest for several hours.

Tightness of the chest in the evening.

Spasmodic asthma with great contraction in the throat and chest, during which a peculiar kind of wheezing noise was heard.† [SCOTT, l. c.]

135. Sudden attacks of troublesome dyspnœa, with a wheezing noise in the air-tubes. [SCOTT, l. c.]

Contraction in the chest, with dyspnœa and wheezing respiration; she must go to the open window and gasp for air, with paleness of face, scarcely perceptible pulse, and danger[2] of suffocation, from the evening until 9 a. m. [SCOTT, l. c.]

Recurrence of the tightness of chest after twenty-four hours, from 10 p. m. until 10 a.m. for eight days. [SCOTT, l. c.]

Attack of suffocation for two or three days. [SCOTT, l. c.]

Oppression of the chest after eating.

140. The chest is painful internally, as if sore.

A cough, that impedes the breathing to suffocation.

* By the secondary action or antagonistic reaction of the organism; for the primary action of ipecacuanha causes hæmorrhage from all the outlets of the body, and it particularly produces metrorrhagia, and cures the former as well as the latter homœopathically, when the other symptoms of the patient resemble those of ipecac ʼa (see 95, 121, &c.).

† In two women from the exhalation from the powder in a distant room; the illness lasted fourteen days.

1 Literally, "a show of the menses fourteen days before their time.'

2 "Apparent danger," Scott says.

Suffocative cough, during which the child becomes quite stiff and blue in the face (aft. 10 h.).

Towards evening a suffocative, fatiguing, very debilitating cough, lasting an hour. [EBERH. GMELIN,[1] *Untersuch. ub. d. Thier. Magnetismus*, Heilbr., 1793.]

In the evening, between 6 and 7 o'clock, extremely violent, convulsive cough. [GMELIN. l. c.]

145. About 7 p.m. a suffocative, extremely debilitating cough for half an hour, with coldness of the extremities. [GMELIN, l. c.]

Dry cough, from a tickle in the upper part of the larynx (aft. 2, 3, 5 h.).

Cough which arises from a contractive tickling sensation, extending from the upper part of the larynx to the lowest extremities of the bronchial tubes. (aft. 4, 6, 7 h.).

A cough which, after walking in cold air and on lying down, in the morning and evening, continues incessantly, excited by deep inspiration ; at the same time with a pain in the abdomen, as if the navel would be torn out, and heat in the (head) face, and sweat on the forehead.

On coughing pain in the abdomen, as if he had an urging to urinate and the urine could not pass, as in retention of urine.

150. Inclination to vomit without nausea is caused by coughing (aft. 1 h.).

After coughing throbbing pain in the head and scrobiculus cordis.

Cough with expectoration of a thick, disagreeably metallic tasting mucus[2] [SCOTT, l. c.]

Hæmoptysis. [GEOFFROY,—MURRAY,—SCOTT, l. c.]

(Pinching [twitching tearing ?] pains of short duration in the right side of the chest, under the shoulder.)

155. (Cramp-pain between the scapulæ on moving.)

Pinching pains in the right arm (aft. 3 h.).

One hand is cold.

(Tettery eruption on the wrist and anus, which itches most in the evening after lying down ; after scratching red lumps appear on the skin, but the itching does not cease.)

Pain in the knee, as if the tendons and ligaments were fatigued by over-exertion.

160. In the left knee a pain as if from a sprain, especially when walking, seldomer and less noticed when sitting (aft. 1 h.). [*Stf.*]

Weariness of the thighs and lower extremities (aft. 8, 9 h.).

In the muscles of the calf a quivering and formication, as if the limb had gone to sleep.

Pinching pain in the right foot (aft. 4 h.).

A drawing pain in the bone of the upper arm and thigh, in the evening after lying down (aft. 5 h.).

---

1 This edition not accessible. That of 1787 has no observations regarding ipecacuanha.

2 As the asthmatic paroxysm of S. 136 passed off.

165. Cracking and creaking in the joints.

(Here and there on the body shooting pain excited by movement, which end is burning.)

Pain in all the bones, as if bruised (aft. 3 h.)

Pain in the joints, such as usually occurs when the limbs go to sleep (aft. 3 h.).

Drowsiness and lassitude in all the limbs (aft. 2 h.). [*Ln.*]

170. Debility. [SCOTT, l. c.]

Drowsiness.

Drowsiness, weariness (aft. 2 h.). [*Stf.*]

Sleep (immediately).

Sleep with half-open eyes (aft. 6 h.).

175. Restless sleep. [SCOTT, l. c.]

Sleep full of restlessness and moaning.

When about to go to sleep she has shocks in all the limbs.

He starts up in his sleep.

Sleep broken by frequent waking, and frightful dreams (aft. 10 h.).

180. Vivid, unremembered dreams, with frequent waking, as from watchfulness, at night. [*Lr.*]

In the morning on awaking anxiety in the blood, as if he had great heat or had perspired profusely, or were wakened up out of anxious dreams, though he is neither hot nor perspiring to the touch; at the same time a heaviness in the head, as if the brain were pressed.

Moaning fearfulness in sleep.

Symptoms of emprosthotonos and opisthotonos* (aft. 10 h.).

The body of the child is stretched out stiffly.

185. Stiff extension of the whole body, followed by a spasmodic clapping together of the arms (aft. $\frac{1}{4}$ h.).

Sudden spasmodic jerking together of the arms.

Palpitation of the heart.

Palpitation, almost without anxiety.

Shivering with yawning (aft. $\frac{1}{2}$ h.).

190. Shivering with eructation.

He has no warmth in the body.

Chilliness; he cannot bear the slightest cold.

Always chilliness under the skin, and all the more when she sits near the warmth.

Over-sensitiveness to cold and heat.

195. He was cold all night in bed, and could not sleep for chilliness.

He becomes cold on the body.

(About 4 p.m.) first shivering, then chilliness with coldness without thirst (aft. 5 h.).

Shuddering coldness in the limbs just as when one is terrified at something. [*Ln.*]

Hands and feet are icy cold and dripping with cold perspiration, at the same time one cheek is red, the other pale, and he feels

* See 142, 184, 185.

miserable in disposition and exhausted in body, with dilated pupils (aft. 10 h.).

200. External cold and internal heat.

(External, not internal heat) (aft. several h.).

(Heat and redness in the face, without thirst.)

In the evening heat of the whole body.

Great increasing, almost burning heat (feeling of heat) in the head and the whole body, but with cold hands and feet ; when the heat increased to the highest degree, there occurred on the trunk and head some perspiration with a smarting itching, especially on the neck (aft. 1 h.). [*Ln.*]

205. In the afternoon and evening feeling of heat, almost burning in the head, forehead and cheeks, without thirst (aft. 6 h.). [*Stf.*]

In the afternoon (about 4 o'clock) sudden general heat, with sweat on the arms and back (aft. 16 h.).

Sweat. [FOTHERGILL,[1] *Medic. Obs. and Inqu.*, vi, art. 18.]

Sweat about midnight (aft. 12 h.).

Night sweat.[2] [CLEGHORN, *Diseases of Minorca*, p. 230.]

210. Sweat for some hours. [HILLARY,[3] *Air and Diseases of Barbadoes.*]

Sour-smelling sweat. [HELLER, l. c., pp., 51, 54.]

Profuse, sour sweat, with cloudy urine. [HELLER, l. c., p. 74.]

He will not speak a word.

The flow of his ideas is very slow.

215. He has pleasure in nothing, nothing is agreeable to him.

Everything is repugnant to him.

Dislike to work. [*Ln.*]

Repugnance to literary work ; thoughts fail him (aft. 29 h.). [*Ln.*]

Sullen unsociable moroseness, that makes him disdain everything.

220. All day long ill-humour ; he had no inclination to talk and was disposed to weep. [*Lr.*]

Sulky humour, that despises everything, and he desires that others also should not esteem or care for anything.

Moroseness : he considers himself unfortunate.

He is scrupulous, apprehensive, and thinks trifles of importance (aft. 6 h.).

He is morose and vexed that his business is not performed quick enough.

225. He is clumsy and awkward and knocks against everything.

Extreme impatience.

He lets his courage sink, and is greatly given to be vexed and to get angry.

His disposition is full of wishes and longing he knows not for what.

---

1 When given in chronic diarrhoea.

2 Merely, "sweat on the night after it was given."

3 Effects when given in dysentery.

He very often gets angry about the merest **trifle, and can just as** easily and quickly become calm (aft. 5 h.).

230. He is irritated by the slightest noise.

He is much inclined to become cross and angry.

The child cries and howls violently and **uninterrupted**ly, **and shoves** its fists into its mouth ; the face is pale and the **body rather cool** (aft 1 h.).

Cheerful humour : he likes to talk and even to joke.* [*Lr.*]

***Curative secondary action after a previous opposite state of the disposition.**

END OF VOL. I.